Manual of Office Medicine

edited by

Kenneth R. Epstein, MD, FACP

ASSOCIATE DIRECTOR
Division of Internal Medicine

CLINICAL ASSISTANT PROFESSOR
Department of Medicine

*Jefferson Medical College of
Thomas Jefferson University
Philadelphia, Pennsylvania*

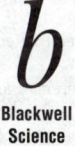

Blackwell
Science

BLACKWELL SCIENCE

Editorial offices:
238 Main Street, Cambridge, Massachusetts 02142, USA
Osney Mead, Oxford OX2 0EL, England
25 John Street, London WC1N 2BL, England
23 Ainslie Place, Edinburgh EH3 6AJ, Scotland
54 University Street, Carlton, Victoria 3053, Australia
Arnette Blackwell SA, 1 rue de Lille, 75007 Paris, France
Blackwell Wissenschafts-Verlag GmbH, Kurfürstendamm 57, 10707 Berlin, Germany
Blackwell MZV, Feldgasse 13, A-1238 Vienna, Austria

Distributors:
North America
Blackwell Science, Inc.
238 Main Street
Cambridge, Massachusetts 02142
(Telephone orders: 800-215-1000 or 617-876-7000)

Australia
Blackwell Science Pty, Ltd.
54 University Street
Carlton, Victoria 3053
(Telephone orders: 03-347-5552)

Outside North America and Australia
Blackwell Science, Ltd.
c/o Marston Book Services, Ltd.
P.O. Box 87
Oxford OX2 0DT
England
(Telephone orders: 44-865-791155)

Acquisitions: Victoria Reeders
Development: Coleen Traynor
Production: Michelle Choate
Manufacturing: Kathleen Grimes
Typeset by Octal Publishing, Salem, NH
Printed and bound by Edwards Brothers, Inc. Ann Arbor, MI

© 1995 by Blackwell Science, Inc.
Printed in the United States of America
95 96 97 98 5 4 3 2 1

All rights reserved. No part of this book may be reproduced in any form or by any electronic or mechanical means, including information storage and retrieval systems, without permission in writing from the publisher, except by a reviewer who may quote brief passages in a review.

Library of Congress Cataloging-in-Publication Data

Manual of office medicine / edited by Kenneth R. Epstein.
    p.   cm.
  Includes bibliographical references and index.
  ISBN 0-86542-340-7
  1. Family medicine—Handbooks, manuals, etc. 2. Ambulatory medical care—Handbooks, manuals, etc.   I. Epstein, Kenneth R.
  [DNLM: 1. Family practice—methods. 2. Primary Health Care. WB 110 M294 1995]
RC55.M27   1995
616—dc20
DNLM/DLC
for Library of Congress   94-20423
                                                                    CIP

To Suzanne and Meghan, whose enthusiasm, support, and patience were essential to the completion of this book.

NOTICE

The indications and dosages of all drugs in this book have been recommended in the medical literature and conform to the practices of the general medical community. The medications described do not necessarily have specific approval by the Food and Drug Administration for use in the diseases and dosages for which they are recommended. The package insert for each drug should be consulted for use and dosage as approved by the FDA. Because standards of usage change, it is advisable to keep abreast of revised recommendations, particularly those concerning new drugs.

Contents

Contributors • *xiii*

Preface • *xv*

Part I. Medical Emergencies

1. **Anaphylaxis,** *Karen S. Scoles* • *3*
2. **Status Asthmaticus,** *Ellen M. O'Connor* • *7*
3. **Cardiac Emergencies,** *Daniel Holleran* • *11*
4. **Diabetic Ketoacidosis,** *Barry Ziring* • *16*
5. **Ophthalmologic Emergencies,** *Marvin E. Gozum* • *20*
   A. Corneal Abrasions • *20*
   B. Foreign Bodies • *23*
   C. Red and Painful Eye • *26*
6. **Status Epilepticus,** *Robert D. Aiken* • *29*

Part II. Screening/General Care

7. **Screening for Breast Cancer,** *Kenneth R. Epstein* • *35*
8. **Screening for Colorectal Cancer,** *Kenneth R. Epstein* • *40*
9. **Screening for Prostate Cancer,** *Kenneth R. Epstein and Daniel Holleran* • *45*
10. **Screening for Cervical Cancer,** *Kenneth R. Epstein* • *49*
11. **The Yearly Physical Examination,** *Barry Ziring* • *55*
12. **Travel Medicine,** *Carol M. Reife* • *59*
13. **Involuntary Weight Loss,** *Kenneth R. Epstein* • *65*

14. Evaluation of the Chronically Fatigued Patient, *Kenneth R. Epstein* • *69*

15. Smoking Cessation/Nicotine Dependence, *Susan E. West* • *76*

Part III. Allergy

16. Allergic Rhinitis, *Karen S. Scoles* • *85*

17. Insect Allergies, *Karen S. Scoles* • *92*
    A. Insect Sting Allergy • *92*
    B. Insect Bites • *95*

18. Plant Dermatitis, *Karen S. Scoles* • *100*

19. Urticaria, *Karen S. Scoles* • *103*

Part IV. Cardiology/Hypertension

20. Hypertension: Individualizing Therapy, *James Witek* • *109*

21. Angina Pectoris, *Rosemarie A. Leuzzi* • *122*

22. Valvular Heart Disease, *Gregg Fromell* • *138*
    A. Aortic Stenosis • *138*
    B. Aortic Insufficiency • *146*
    C. Atrial Septal Defect • *154*
    D. Mitral Valve Prolapse • *158*

23. Prescribing Safe Exercise, *Karen G. Kelly* • *168*

24. Office Management of Arrhythmias, *Arnold J. Greenspon* • *172*
    A. Palpitations • *172*
    B. Paroxysmal Supraventricular Tachycardia (PSVT) • *175*
    C. Atrial Fibrillation • *179*
    D. Ventricular Arrhythmias Including Premature Ventricular Contractions (PVCs) and Ventricular Tachycardia • *183*

25. Congestive Heart Failure, *Karen G. Kelly* • *186*

Part V. Consultative Medicine

26. Outpatient Preoperative Evaluation, *Barry Ziring* • *195*

Part VI. Dermatology

27. **Acne,** *Guy F. Webster* • *207*
28. **Alopecia,** *Guy F. Webster* • *209*
29. **Pruritis,** *Guy F. Webster* • *212*
30. **Dermatitis,** *Guy F. Webster* • *214*
    A. Atopic Dermatitis (Eczema) • *214*
    B. Contact Dermatitis • *216*
    C. Seborrheic Dermatitis • *217*
31. **Xerosis (Dry Skin),** *Guy F. Webster* • *218*
32. **Fungal Infections,** *Guy F. Webster* • *220*
33. **Psoriasis,** *Guy F. Webster* • *222*
34. **Benign and Malignant Growths,** *Guy F. Webster* • *225*

Part VII: Endocrinology/Metabolism

35. **Adrenocortical Hyperfunction,** *Rosemarie A. Leuzzi* • *231*
    A. Cushing's syndrome • *231*
    B. Hyperaldosteronism • *238*
    C. Pheochromocytoma • *243*
36. **Adrenocortical Insufficiency (Addison's Disease),** *Rosemarie A. Leuzzi* • *251*
37. **Management of the Patient on Glucocorticosteroids,** *Karen G. Kelly* • *258*
38. **Diabetes Mellitus,** *Richard G. Paluzzi* • *262*
    A. Clinical Presentation and Diagnostic Approach • *262*
    B. Potential Complications of Diabetes Mellitus • *265*
    C. Treatment of Diabetes Mellitus • *269*
    D. Monitoring of Therapy and Management of Complications • *273*
39. **Hypercholesterolemia,** *Barry Ziring* • *276*
40. **Hypercalcemia,** *Karen G. Kelly* • *284*

41. **Osteoporosis,** *Kenneth R. Epstein* • 289
42. **Thyroid Diseases,** *Richard G. Paluzzi* • 295

Part VIII. Foot Problems

43. **Hyperkeratotic Lesions (Corns and Calluses),** *Arthur E. Helfand* • 309
44. **Foot Pain,** *Arthur E. Helfand* • 313
    A. Digital Deformities • 313
    B. Anterior Foot Pain • 317
    C. Posterior Foot Pain • 320
    D. Heel Pain • 323
    E. Assorted other Foot Pain Disorders • 325
45. **Foot Care in the Diabetic Patient,** *Arthur E. Helfand* • 326

Part IX. Gastroenterology

46. **Acute Nausea and Vomiting,** *David S. Weinberg and Christine Laine* • 335
47. **Bowel Symptoms,** *Christine Laine and David S. Weinberg* • 341
    A. Constipation • 341
    B. Diarrhea • 347
    C. Colonic Diverticulosis and Diverticulitis • 354
    D. Irritable Bowel Syndrome • 359
    E. Lactose Intolerance • 365
48. **Epigastric Pain,** *David S. Weinberg and Christine Laine* • 369
    A. Peptic Ulcer Disease • 369
    B. Nonulcerative Dyspepsia • 376
49. **Evaluation of Heme-Positive Stool,** *David S. Weinberg and Christine Laine* • 380
50. **Gastroesophageal Reflux Disease,** *David S. Weinberg and Christine Laine* • 386
51. **Hepatic and Biliary Disease** • 392
    A. Abnormal Liver Function Tests, *Karen S. Scoles* • 392

B. Cholelithiasis, *Christine Laine and David S. Weinberg* • 397

C. Viral Hepatitis: A, B, and C, *Carol M. Reife* • 402

Part X. Geriatrics

52. **Dementia,** *Karen G. Kelly* • 413

53. **Functional Assessment of the Elderly,** *Karen G. Kelly* • 421

54. **Prevention in the Elderly,** *Karen G. Kelly* • 426

Part XI. Gynecology

55. **Estrogen Replacement Therapy,** *Kenneth R. Epstein* • 433

56. **Menstrual Abnormalities,** *Rosemarie A. Leuzzi* • 440

57. **Genital Infections,** *Rosemarie A. Leuzzi* • 450
    A. Vaginitis • 450
    B. Cervicitis • 457
    C. Pelvic Inflammatory Disease • 462
    D. Human Papillomavirus Infection • 467

Part XII. Hematology

58. **Abnormal Coagulation Tests,** *Barry Ziring* • 471

59. **Anemia,** *Barry Ziring* • 479

60. **Lymphadenopathy,** *Barry Ziring* • 486

Part XIII. HIV Disease

61. **Pretest and Posttest HIV Counseling,** *Carol M. Reife* • 493

62. **Management of the Symptomatic Patient,** *James Witek* • 498

63. **Management of Early HIV Infection,** *James Witek* • 506

Part XIV. Infectious Diseases

64. **Aphthous Stomatitis,** *Richard G. Paluzzi* • 517

65. **Ear Infections,** *Richard G. Paluzzi* • 520
    A. Otitis Externa • 520
    B. Otitis Media • 524

66. **Lyme Disease,** *Richard G. Paluzzi* • 527
67. **Genitourinary Tract Infections** • 533
    A. Cystitis/Pyelonephritis, *Richard G. Paluzzi* • 533
    B. Urethritis, *Kenneth R. Epstein* • 540
    C. Epididymitis, *Richard G. Paluzzi* • 545
    D. Prostatitis, *Richard G. Paluzzi* • 549
    E. Genital Ulcers, *Rosemarie A. Leuzzi* • 552
68. **Management of Positive PPD,** *Richard G. Paluzzi* • 558
69. **Respiratory Tract Infections,** *Richard G. Paluzzi* • 562
    A. Pharyngitis • 562
    B. Acute Sinusitis, *Kenneth R. Epstein* • 568
    C. Chronic Sinusitis • 573
    D. Acute Bronchitis • 576
    E. Pneumonia • 579
    F. Influenza • 594
70. **Selected Skin Infections,** *Richard G. Paluzzi* • 598
    A. Animal Bites • 598
    B. Cellulitis and Erysipelas • 601
    C. Herpes Simplex • 607
    D. Herpes Zoster • 611
    E. Pediculosis and Scabies • 614
71. **Syphilis,** *Rosemarie A. Leuzzi* • 618

Part XV. Neurology/ENT

72. **Carpal Tunnel Syndrome,** *Carol M. Reife* • 629
73. **Cerebrovascular Disease,** *Robert D. Aiken* • 633
74. **Headache,** *Barry Ziring* • 640
75. **Hoarseness,** *David Zwillenberg* • 650
76. **Peripheral Neuropathy,** *Kenneth R. Epstein* • 656
77. **Seizures,** *Robert D. Aiken* • 663
78. **Tinnitus,** *David Zwillenberg* • 669

79. Tremor, *Karen G. Kelly* • 675

80. Vertigo, *David Zwillenberg* • 679

Part XVI. Psychiatry/Behavioral Medicine

81. Anxiety, *Susan E. West* • 687

82. Bipolar Affective Disorder, *Susan E. West* • 693

83. Depression, *Susan E. West* • 697

Part XVII. Pulmonary

84. Asthma, *Marvin E. Gozum* • 705

85. Chronic Cough, *Sandra B. Weibel* • 709

86. Chronic Obstructive Pulmonary Disease, *Sandra B. Weibel* • 714

87. Hemoptysis, *Sandra B. Weibel* • 720

88. Pulmonary Function Tests, *Daniel Holleran* • 726

89. Pulmonary Nodule, *Sandra B. Weibel* • 731

Part XVIII. Renal/Urologic Diseases

90. Evaluation of Renal Dysfunction, *Herman J. Michael, Jr.* • 739

91. Hematuria, *Herman J. Michael, Jr.* • 746

92. Urinary Incontinence, *Karen G. Kelly* • 752

93. Impotence, *Daniel Holleran* • 759

94. Prostatic Hyperplasia, *Daniel Holleran* • 762

95. Proteinuria, *Herman J. Michael, Jr.* • 766

96. Kidney Stones, *Karen G. Kelly* • 772

Part XIX. Rheumatology/Orthopedics

97. Serologic Testing in the Evaluation of the Rheumatologic Patient, *John M. Spandorfer* • 779

98. Degenerative Joint Disease, *John M. Spandorfer* • 785

99. Evaluation of the Hot, Tender Joint, *John M. Spandorfer* • 791

100. Joint Pain, *Barry Ziring* • 796
   A. Ankle Pain • 799
   B. Shoulder Pain • 802
   C. Knee Pain • 808
   D. Wrist Pain • 815

101. Neck and Back Pain, *Ellen M. O'Connor* • 818
   A. Cervical Pain Syndromes • 818
   B. Low Back Pain • 825

102. Myalgias, *John M. Spandorfer* • 830
   A. Fibrositis • 830
   B. Polymyalgia Rheumatica • 833

103. Common Sports Injuries, *Ellen M. O'Connor* • 836

Part XX. Vascular Disease

104. Peripheral Vascular Disease, *Geno J. Merli* • 849

105. Peripheral Venous Disease, *Geno J. Merli* • 855
   A. Deep Venous Thrombosis • 855
   B. Chronic Venous Insufficiency • 862

Appendices

Appendix A: Adult Immunizations, *Kenneth R. Epstein* • 869

Appendix B: Subacute Bacterial Endocarditis Prophylaxis, *Kenneth R. Epstein* • 877

Appendix C. Topical Corticosteroid Potencies, *Guy F. Webster* • 883

Index • 885

Contributors

Robert D. Aiken, MD
Assistant Professor of Neurology, Jefferson Medical College, Thomas Jefferson University, Philadelphia, Pennsylvania

Kenneth R. Epstein, MD, FACP
Associate Director, Division of Internal Medicine, Clinical Assistant Professor, Department of Medicine, Jefferson Medical College, Thomas Jefferson University, Philadelphia, Pennsylvania

Gregg Fromell, MD
Clinical Professor of Medicine, Hospital of the University of Pennsylvania, Havertown, Pennsylvania

Marvin E. Gozum, MD
Clinical Assistant Professor of Medicine, Chief, Section of Medical Informatics, Chief, Section of Medical Consultation, Wills Eye Hospital, Division of Internal Medicine, Department of Medicine, Jefferson Medical College, Thomas Jefferson University, Philadelphia, Pennsylvania

Arnold J. Greenspon, MD
Division of Cardiology, Jefferson Medical College, Thomas Jefferson University, Philadelphia, Pennsylvania

Arthur E. Helfand, DPM
Professor and Chairman, Department of Community Health and Aging, Pennsylvania College of Podiatric Medicine; Adjunct Professor, Department of Orthopedic Surgery, Jefferson Medical College, Thomas Jefferson University Hospital; Consultant, Wills Eye Hospital, Department of Verterans Affairs Medical Center, Philadelphia, Pennsylvania

Daniel Holleran, MD
Clinical Instructor in Medicine, Division of Internal Medicine, Jefferson Medical College, Thomas Jefferson University, Philadelphia, Pennsylvania

Karen G. Kelly, MD
Clinical Assistant Professor of Medicine, Department of Medicine, Jefferson Medical College, Thomas Jefferson University, Philadelphia, Pennsylvania

Christine Laine, MD, MPH
Clinical Instructor in Medicine, Division of Internal Medicine, Center for Research in Medical Education and Health Care, Jefferson Medical College, Thomas Jefferson University, Philadelphia, Pennsylvania

Rosemarie A. Leuzzi, MD
Clinical Instructor in Medicine, Division of Internal Medicine, Jefferson Medical College, Thomas Jefferson University, Philadelphia, Pennsylvania

Geno J. Merli, MD
Clinical Associate Professor of Medicine, Division of Internal Medicine, Jefferson Medical College, Thomas Jefferson University, Philadelphia, Pennsylvania

Herman J. Michael, Jr., MD
Assistant Clinical Professor of Medicine, Thomas Jefferson University, Philadelphia, Pennsylvania

Ellen M. O'Connor MD
Clinical Instructor, Department of Medicine, Thomas Jefferson University Hospital, Philadelphia, Pennsylvania

Richard G. Paluzzi, MD
Clinical Assistant Professor of Medicine, Division of Internal Medicine, Jefferson Medical College, Thomas Jefferson University, Philadelphia, Pennsylvania

Carol M. Reife, MD
Clinical Assistant Professor of Medicine, Jefferson Medical College, Thomas Jefferson University, Philadelphia, Pennsylvania

Karen S. Scoles, MD
Clinical Assistant Professor of Medicine, Division of Internal Medicine, Jefferson Medical College, Thomas Jefferson University, Philadelphia, Pennsylvania

John M. Spandorfer, MD
Clinical Instructor, Division of Medicine, Jefferson Medical College, Thomas Jefferson University, Philadelphia, Pennsylvania

Guy F. Webster, MD, PhD
Assistant Professor of Dermatology, Department of Dermatology, Jefferson Medical College, Thomas Jefferson University, Philadelphia, Pennsylvania

Sandra B. Weibel, MD
Instructor, Department of Medicine, Division of Pulmonary and Critical Care Medical Director, Pulmonary Function Laboratory, Jefferson Medical College, Thomas Jefferson University, Philadelphia, Pennsylvania

David S. Weinberg, MD
Fellow in Gastroenterology, Division of Gastroenterology, Hospital of the University of Pennsylvania, Philadelphia, Pennsylvania

Susan E. West, MD
Clinical Assistant Professor of Medicine, Division of Internal Medicine, Jefferson Medical College, Thomas Jefferson University, Philadelphia, Pennsylvania

James Witek, MD
Clinical Instructor of Medicine, Division of Internal Medicine, Department of Medicine, Jefferson Medical College, Thomas Jefferson University, Philadelphia, Pennsylvania

Barry S. Ziring, MD
Clinical Assistant Professor of Medicine, Division of Internal Medicine, Jefferson Medical College, Thomas Jefferson University, Philadelphia, Pennsylvania

David A. Zwillenberg, MD
Clinical Associate Professor, Department of Pediatrics, Assistant Professor, Department of Otolaryngology, Jefferson Medical College, Thomas Jefferson University, Philadelphia, Pennsylvania

Preface

Over the past decade, there has been an increasing emphasis on the outpatient setting as the focus of medical care. The vast majority of diagnostic evaluations and therapeutic administrations can be done in the office setting, and the hospital is becoming increasingly the setting for those who are critically ill or require procedures. The health care needs of patients in the office setting are quite different from those in the hospital. This book was envisioned with the practitioner in this setting in mind. The goal of this book is to be practical and useful to the busy clinician, who may not have time to read a chapter in a textbook to clarify management of the patient waiting in his or her examining room. Although the main audience for this book is primary care clinicians, our hope is that those in other fields will find the book equally useful as they care for the diverse needs of their patients.

The practitioner in a busy office setting needs readily accessible information that highlights the diagnostic approach and therapeutic options for the patient. This book was therefore organized around a practical, easy-to-access format. The chapters highlight the key aspects of the clinical presentation and diagnostic approach to common medical conditions. Many of the chapters are oriented towards presenting symptoms rather than diagnoses. Treatment is divided into acute treatment of the patient, as well as the principles of long-term management. A major aspect of clinical practice in the office setting is deciding when to refer a patient to a specialist, and when to admit the patient. This manual therefore lays out for each condition the indications for referral or admission to the hospital. Pertinent annotated bibliographies are offered for each clinical condition if the reader desires more detailed reading.

This manual could never have come to be without the help and support of many people. I first want to thank all the contributors for their time and effort. I also want to acknowledge the patient and tireless efforts of the secretarial staff of the Division of Internal Medicine at

Jefferson Medical College, namely Frances Gamble, Cynthia Little, Kimberly Quigley, and Lisa Xavier, in the manuscript preparation for the book. I especially want to recognize the assistance provided by Marion Warchol and Joan Taylor, without whom this book never could have been done. Lastly, I want to thank Coleen Traynor and Dr. Victoria Reeders of Blackwell Science for their belief in this book and their patient help in moving it towards reality.

Kenneth R. Epstein

Part 1:
Medical Emergencies

Chapter 1: Anaphylaxis

Karen S. Scoles

I. Clinical Presentation

A. General Information

1. Anaphylaxis is an immune response to an agent to which an individual has become hypersensitive by previous exposure. It is generally an acute IgE reaction. However, a syndrome indistinguishable from IgE-mediated *anaphylaxis* may occur without IgE, called *anaphylactoid* reactions.

2. Common causes of anaphylaxis/anaphylactoid reactions
    a. Foods—shellfish, nuts, eggs, milk, celery
    b. Food additives—aspartame, monosodium glutamate, sulfites
    c. Biologic products—insulin, seminal fluid, allergen extracts, blood products, γ globulin
    d. Drugs—especially antibiotics, opiates, iodinated radiographic contrast materials, nonsteroidal anti-inflammatory drugs (NSAIDs)
    e. Physical stimuli—cold, exercise
    f. Other—latex, insect stings, idiopathic

B. Symptoms

1. Symptoms generally begin within minutes of exposure to the inciting agent, peak within 15–30 min and the episode is generally completed within hours. Some patients may have a recurrence of the episode as long as 8–24 h later.

2. Cutaneous—flushing, pruritis

3. Cardiovascular—faintness, palpitations, weakness

4. Respiratory—nasal congestion, hoarseness, dyspnea, wheezing

5. Gastrointestinal—nausea, vomiting, cramps, abdominal pain, bloating

C. Physical Examination

1. Cutaneous—erythema, urticaria, angioedema

2. Cardiovascular—tachycardia, arrythmias, hypotension, shock, syncope

3. Respiratory—respiratory distress, tachypnea, laryngeal edema, wheezing, asphyxiation

4. Gastrointestinal—abdominal distension, vomiting, diarrhea

II. Diagnostic Approach

The diagnosis is not difficult if a patient presents with the typical array of acute symptoms and physical findings after exposure to an offending agent.

III. Differential Diagnosis

A. Can be confused with a vasovagal reaction

B. Diagnosis more difficult if the patient is sedated

C. Can also be difficult in the syncopal patient. However, anaphylaxis should be considered if the patient presents with urticaria, angioedema, or wheezing in addition to syncope.

D. Other conditions that may be included in the differential diagnosis include:

1. Serum sickness
2. Hereditary angioedema
3. Systemic mastocystosis
4. Pheochromocytoma
5. Carcinoid syndrome

IV. Treatment

A. Goals

1. Prompt treatment of the acute potentially life-threatening episode
2. Prevention and prophylaxis of recurrent episodes

B. Treatment of Acute Anaphylaxis

1. When applicable, place tourniquet above the site of injection or the sting to obstruct venous return or stop the administration of the causative agent. Remove the tourniquet temporarily every 10–15 min.
2. Place patient in recumbent position and elevate lower extremities.
3. Epinephrine is the drug of choice for initial treatment:
    a. For life-threatening reactions 5mL of 1:10,000 solution should be given IV and repeated q 5–10 min as needed.
    b. For less severe reactions administer aqueous epinephrine 1:1000, 0.3–0.5 mL SQ or IM q 20–30 min for three doses.
4. When applicable, inject aqueous epinephrine 1:000, 0.1–0.3 mL at the site of the injection or sting.

5. Establish and maintain airway; if necessary, use endotracheal tube.
6. Give oxygen as needed.
7. Monitor vital signs frequently.
8. If patient is not responding, give diphenhyramine hydrochloride (Benadryl), 25–50 mg IV over 3 min (maximum, 5 mg/kg in 24 h). May be given IM as well.
9. In addition, cimetidine, 300 mg IV or ranitidine 50 mg IV should be given over 3–5 min.
10. If blood pressure cannot be obtained, give normal saline IV and maintain blood pressure with levarternol bitartrate (Levophed), 1 or 2 ampules (8–16 mg) in 500 mL of 5% glucose in water. Titrate to maintain blood pressure.
11. If severe asthma without shock give aminophylline, 500 mg IV over 10–20 min.
12. Although corticosteroids will not be helpful for the acute anaphylaxis, they may prevent protracted anaphylaxis; hydrocortisone sodium succinate, 500 mg IV q 6 h or equivalent.
13. In patients chronically treated with β blockers, the treatment of acute anaphylaxis may complicated. The use of glucagon (5–15 µg/min IV) has been useful in these patients.

V. Prevention of Recurrent Episodes

A. Patients should be counseled to avoid the offending agents.

B. Those patients who may be accidentally reexposed to the offending agent should obtain and be instructed in the use of an emergency kit that contains self-administered epinephrine and antihistamine.

C. Chronic β-blocker therapy should be avoided in patients with a history of recurrent anaphylaxis.

D. Patients at risk for reaction to iodinated contrast material should be pretreated with prednisone 50 mg q 6 h for three doses before exposure. Dephenhydramine 50 mg and ephedrine, 25 mg, 1 h before exposure may be helpful as well.

VI. Prophylaxis

A. Patients with a history of hymenoptera reactions should be referred for immunotherapy.

B. Skin testing and desensitization may be appropriate for patients with a history of penicillin or other antiobiotic reactions if the use of these drugs is urgent.

C. Immunotherapy and skin testing are contraindicated in patients being treated with β blockers.

VII. Indications for Referral to an Allergist

Any patient with a significant anaphylatic/anaphylactoid reaction may need referral to an allergist to help identify the offending agent, administer appropriate immunotherapy, and instruct the patient in the use of emergency treatment kits.

VIII. Indications for Hospitalization

Because symptoms may recur over a number of hours, patients should be closely observed or admitted to the hospital during the 12–24 h after anaphylaxis.

IX. Annotated Bibliography

Atkinson T, Kaliner M. Anaphylaxis. Med Clin North Am 1992;76:841–855. A practical discussion of the classification, presentation, and management of anaphylaxis.

Valentine M. Allergy and related conditions. In: Principles of Ambulatory Medicine, 3rd ed. Baltimore:Williams & Wilkins;1991:253–269.

Chapter 2: Status Asthmaticus

Ellen M. O'Connor

I. Clinical Presentation

A. General Information

1. See Chapter 84 chronic management.
2. 5–8% of general population is affected by asthma.
3. Physician awareness of high-risk patient profile is needed:
    a. History of respiratory failure and mechanical ventilation
    b. History of corticosteroid use
    c. History of ICU care secondary to asthma
4. Expeditious referral to ER is mandatory in any case unresponsive to initial therapy.
5. Mortality from asthma, though rare, is a real threat.

B. Precipitating Events

1. Allergic reactions
2. Respiratory infections
3. Exercise
4. Occupational exposure

C. History

1. Breathless speech
2. Extreme chest tightness
3. Wheezing
4. Exercise intolerance
5. Near syncope or syncope
6. Intense breathlessness

D. Physical Examination

1. General—restless, diaphoretic patient
2. Cardiac
   a. Tachycardia
   b. Paroxidal pulse
3. Respiratory
   a. Respiratory rate > 30/m
   b. Accessory respiratory muscle use
   c. Diffuse wheezes, expiratory or both inspiratory and expiratory
   d. Decreased air movement
   e. Absent breath sounds unilaterally consistent with pneumothorax

II. Diagnostic Approach

A. Suspect of history and physical. Treatment should not be delayed for diagnostic testing. Immediate referral to the ER may be indicated before any tests are performed.

B. Pulmonary Function Testing.

1. Peak expiratory flow rate (PEFR) < 200 L/min
2. Forced expiratory volume (FEV1) < 1 L/min
3. Oxygen saturation < 90%
4. Arterial blood gas with PO_2 < 60 mm Hg or PCO_2 > 40 mm Hg

C. Radiographic Testing

1. Chest x-ray to rule out pneumothorax, pneumonia, atelectasis secondary to mucous plugging

III. Differential Diagnosis

A. Cardiac asthma secondary to left-sided ventricular failure

1. History of coronary artery or valvular heart disease
2. Associated symptoms of pedal edema, S_3

B. Pulmonary embolism

1. Acute onset of symptoms
2. Unilateral wheezes
3. Evidence of deep venous thrombosis

C. Upper airway obstruction, ie, foreign body, tumor, excretions, inflammation, thyromegaly

1. Inspiratory wheezes

IV. Treatment

A. Goals

1. Rapid reversal of airway obstruction
2. Relief of respiratory distress

B. Acute Management

1. Subcutaneous β_2-agonist
   a. Use with caution in patients with cardiac disease or hyperthyroidism, elderly patients, pregnant patients, or patients taking tricyclic antidepressants or monoamine oxidase inhibitors
   b. Epinephrine 0.3 mL SQ every 20–30 min
   c. Terbutaline 0.25 mg sq 30–60 min
2. Albuterol 2.5 mg by nebulizer q 20 min
3. Oxygen therapy—2–3 L via nasal canula
4. Corticosteroids may be considered if unresponsive to bronchodilation; however, their therapeutic effect does not begin for 6–12 h.
5. Peak expository flow rate—check q 20 min

V. Patient Education

A. Follow-up visit after resolution of acute symptoms should be made within 24–48 h.

B. Stress importance of regular outpatient appointments to decrease acute exacerbations.

C. Recommend regular or increased use of medications at first sign of viral infection to decrease severity of exacerbation.

D. Ensure correct usage of inhaler device by thorough instruction.

E. Discourage smoking in any asthmatic.

VI. Long-Term Management (see Chapter 84)

A. Emphasis on anti-inflammatory inhaled therapy for control.

B. Compliance with medication and outpatient follow-up decreases acute exacerbations.

VII. Indications for Referral/Hospitalization via ER

A. Syncope or near syncope

B. PEFR < 300L/min after above therapy

C. No change in patient's subjective feelings after one h

D. Presence of pneumonia or pneumothorax

VIII. Annotated Bibliography

Lane D, Storr A. Asthma, The Facts, 2nd ed. Oxford: Oxford University Press; 1987. A good personal accounting of asthma with practical guidelines.

Sheth K, Busse W. Asthma in the adolescent and adult. In: Rokel RE, ed. Conn's Current Therapy, 28th ed. Philadelphia: WB Saunders; 1992:684–691. An excellent, concise explanation of the disease and treatment.

Chapter 3: Cardiac Emergencies

Daniel Holleran

I. General Information

A. This chapter deals with two common and potentially life-threatening cardiac emergencies.

1. *Chest pain* due to myocardial infarction, unstable angina, or aortic dissection (see Chapter 21 for more general description of evaluation of chest pain)

2. *Dyspnea* due to pulmonary edema

B. Unfortunately, physicians are at a potential disadvantage when an emergency occurs in the office.

1. They may not have immediate access to ECG, x-ray, or laboratory facilities.

2. Time is critical.

3. Calling an ambulance to transport the patient to the nearest ER may be the most prudent action.

II. Acute Chest Pain

A. Clinical Presentation
1. History
   a. Quality of pain
      1) Myocardial ischemia classically described as "crushing."
      2) Other types of pain, such as sharp or burning, are less likely but still possibly ischemic.
   b. Duration
      1) Few seconds or days—virtually excludes ischemia
      2) Minutes—nonspecific
   c. Radiation
      1) Classical ischemia radiates down left arm or up to jaw.
      2) Radiation from the xyphoid process up to sternum implies reflux dyspepsia.
   d. Epiphenomena—diaphoresis and shortness of breath

e. Association with activity—exertional chest symptoms suggest ischemia.
   f. Atherosclerosis risk factors—helpful in excluding coronary ischemia in an unlikely patient (eg, 24-year-old woman).
2. Physical Examination
   a. Vital signs
      1) Hypotension (systolic BP < 90) mandates immediate transfer to the ER.
      2) Decrease in BP of > 20 mm of left arm or leg compared to right arm suggests aortic dissection.
      3) Bradyarrhythmia and tachyarrhythmia-treatment according to ACLS protocols.
   b. Chest
      1) Bibasilar rales may be due to severe coronary ischemia (congestive heart failure [CHF]).
      2) Other findings depend on the exact etiology of the chest pain.
         a) Decreased breath sounds and increased tympany suggest pneumothorax.
         b) Examination may be normal if pulmonary embolism.
   c. Cardiac
      1) Tachycardia—nonspecific
      2) S_4 may be due to ischemic left ventricular stiffness in diastole.
      3) Murmur
         a) New aortic insufficiency may be due to aortic dissection.
         b) Acute mitral regurgitation can be caused by ischemic papillary muscle dysfunction.
   d. Extremities
      1) Edema suggests possible cardiac etiology.
      2) Unilateral leg edema with palpable venous cord suggests pulmonary embolism—insensitive.

B. Diagnostic Approach

1. ECG
   a. Necessary if there is even a remote possibility of coronary ischemia.
   b. Pulmonary embolism may show right ventricle (RV) strain or an SIQIII pattern.

2. Chest x-ray
   a. Diagnostic for pneumothorax
   b. May be normal for pulmonary embolism or cardiac ischemia

3. Other tests: arterial blood gas, upper GI, ultrasound, and CT
   a. Available in the ER and radiology department
   b. Should not delay the management of ischemic pain

C. Differential Diagnosis
See Chapter 21 for nonemergent diagnostic evaluation.

Part I: Medical Emergencies • 13

D. Treatment of Acute Chest Pain

1. *Empirical*—sublingual nitroglycerin 1/150 q 5 min PRN and oxygen 2 L/min via nasal cannula
   a. May relieve pain if anginal, but also relieves esophageal spasm
   b. Risk of hypotension even if true angina
2. *Specific:* based on etiology of pain
3. Once stabilized, the patient should be transferred to the ER.

E. Indications for Referral

All patients with suspected ischemia should be referred to the ER. Possible exception is the patient with chronic stable exertional angina who develops typical episode, eg; walking up steps to office, who promptly responds to rest or sublingual nitroglycerin.

F. Indications for Hospitalization

1. Safest approach is "guilty (of ischemia) until proven otherwise" especially in patients > age 40.
2. Noncardiac etiologies may require hospitalization.
   a. Pulmonary embolism (PE)
   b. Aortic dissection
   c. Pneumothorax (PTX)
   d. Biliary colic

III. Acute Dyspnea

A. Clinical Presentation

1. History
   a. Exertional dyspnea implies CHF or angina.
   b. Acuteness of onset
      1) Abrupt suggests PTX or PE.
      2) Onset over seconds to minutes implies ischemia.
   c. Associated chest pain occurs with angina, PTX, and PE.
   d. Recent bed rest or travel and use of oral contraceptives increase risk of PE.
2. Physical Examination
   a. Neck
      1) Use of accessory muscles is nonspecific.
      2) Deviated trachea suggests tension PTX.
      3) Jugular venous distension suggests cardiac etiology.
   b. Cardiac
      1) S_3 suggests CHF.
      2) Systolic murmurs of aortic stenosis or mitral regurgitation or diastolic rumble of mitral stenosis suggest CHF due to an abnormal valve.

c. Chest—variable findings depending on etiology
   1) Clear—suggests pulmonary embolism
   2) Rales—suggests pulmonary edema
   3) Wheezing—bronchospasm
   4) Decreased breath sounds with increased tympany: suggests PTX.
   5) "Clear" with decreased aeration—suggests severe bronchospasm with impending respiratoty failure
d. Extremities—dependent edema suggests CHF

B. Diagnostic Approach

1. Physical examination may reveal problem but not underlying etiology.

    a. Wheezing may be due to asthma or CHF.
    b. Clear lungs may represent PE or severe bronchospasm.

2. ECG helpful to exclude ischemia.

3. Chest x-ray, arterial blood gas, and ventilation/perfusion scans usually only available at hospital.

C. Differential Diagnosis

1. Cardiac

    a. CHF (see also Chapter 24)
    b. Ischemia

2. Pulmonary

    a. Bronchospasm
    b. PE
    c. PTX

D. Treatment of Acute Dyspnea

1. CHF

    a. Loop diuretic, eg; furosemide 40–120 mg IV depending on renal function
    b. Nitrates—topical or IV drip
    c. Angiotensin-converting enzyme inhibitor; eg; enalapril 0.625–1.25 mg IV
       1) Can cause hypotension due to profound arterial vasodilation, so should have IV fluids available.
       2) Probably reserved for use in hospital setting (ER, CCU).
    d. O_2 at 6 L/min via nasal cannula
    e. See Chapter 24

2. Angina—see Section II-D of this chapter.

3. Bronchospasm (asthma)—see Chapter 84.

4. PTX

    a. Chest tube placed by surgeon or ER physician.

b. NB: clinical suspicion of tension PTX with associated circulatory collapse requires immediate placement of 20-gauge needle into third intercostal space on affected side before chest x-ray available.
5. PE: hospitalization for parenteral heparin

E. **Indications for Referral**
   Most patients should be sent to the ER with a few possible exceptions:

1. Asthmatic who can cooperate with the use of a metered-dose inhaler and can take oral corticosteroids within 1 h

2. Chronic stable exertional angina: see II-E of this chapter

F. **Indications for Hospitalization**

1. Congestive heart failure
   a. Suspicion of underlying coronary ischemia or worsening pattern in patient with known coronary disease

2. PTX

3. Evidence of or clinical suspicion of PE

4. Asthmatic bronchospasm unresponsive to inhaled β-agonist and IV steroid therapy given in the ER—see Chapter 84

IV. Annotated Bibliography

Emergency Cardiac Care Committee and Subcommittee, American Heart Association. Guidelines for cardiopulmonary rescue and emergency/cardiac care. JAMA 1992;268:2171–2295. Excellent source for management of cardiac arrhythmias.

Goldman L, Braunwald E. Chest discomfort and palpitation In: Wilson JD, Braunwald E, Isselbacher KJ, eds. Harrison's Principles of Internal Medicine, 12th ed. New York:McGraw-Hill;1991. Well within approach to the evaluation of chest pain and palpitations. This article describes the differential diagnosis and the importance of the history in evaluating cardiac symptoms.

Gottlieb SH. Heart failure. In: Barker JR, Zieve PD, eds. Principles of Ambulatory Medicine, 2nd ed. Baltimore: Williams & Wilkins; 1986. Clear concise discussion of heart failure, very readable.

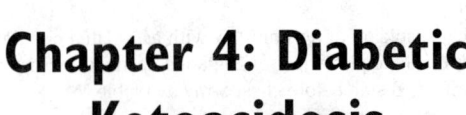

Chapter 4: Diabetic Ketoacidosis

Barry Ziring

I. Clinical Presentation

A. General Information

1. Diabetic ketoacidosis (DKA) is initiated either by cessation of insulin therapy, new presentation of diabetes, or stress (myocardial infarction, infection, steroids) that renders the normal dose of insulin inadequate.
2. Gluconeogenesis is heightened while glucose consumption outside the brain is decreased.
3. Hyperglycemia results in osmotic diuresis, with resultant electrolyte loss, volume depletion, and cellular dehydration.
4. Acidosis and ketosis result from increased production of acetoacetic acid and β-hydroxy butyric acid.

B. Symptoms

1. Common

    a. Vomiting
    b. Thirst
    c. Polyuria
    d. Weakness
    e. Altered sensorium (drowsiness)—occurs in approximately 40% of cases of DKA
    f. Air hunger

2. Less common

    a. Stupor (approximately 14%)
    b. Coma (approximately 5%)
    c. Abdominal pain

C. Physical Examination

1. Tachycardia
2. Blood pressure—hypotension is poor prognostic indicator.

3. Body temperature may range from below normal to severe hyperthermia.
4. Respiratory rate
   a. Rapid (Kussmaul's respiration)
   b. Suppressed with severe acidosis
5. Altered sensorium
6. Muscle weakness
7. Acetone smell on breath

II. Diagnostic Approach

A. Features of the History and Physical

1. Rapid determination blood sugar has become so readily available that diagnosis can be confirmed easily in most cases. However, if a patient presents in coma (and blood sugar determination is unavailable) initial treatment should be for presumed hypoglycemia.
2. Initial evaluation should be directed at assessment of airway patency and adequacy of hydration, as well as cardiovascular, renal, and mental status.
3. Patient should be screened for precipitating events including infections, myocardial infarction, stroke, and steroid use.

B. Laboratory Tests

1. Serum glucose generally > 250 mg/dL
2. Electrolytes
   a. Hyperglycemia—results in factitious (pseudo-) hyponatremia: for each 100 mg/dL elevation in serum glucose above 100 mg/dL, the measured serum sodium must be corrected upward by 1.6 mEq/L.
   b. Typically serum potassium is initially high due to acidosis.
   c. Serum bicarbonate level is low.
3. Complete blood count
   a. Leukocyte counts are usually elevated due to stress and acidosis but may be a sign of infection.
4. Arterial blood gas
   a. pH < 7.3
   b. Bicarbonate < 15 mEq/L
5. Serum ketones—usually present at a dilution > 1:2.
6. Other useful tests may include urinalysis, chest x-ray, ECG, drug screen, amylase, and thyroid function.

III. Differential Diagnosis

A. Hyperglycemia (glucose > 250 mg/dL)—nonketotic hyperosmolar coma, stress, hyperglycemia

B. Ketosis—alcoholic ketosis, hypoglycemic ketosis, starvation

C. Metabolic Acidosis—lactic acidosis, uremia, drug/toxin-induced acidosis

IV. Treatment

A. Goals of Therapy

1. Rehydration
2. Reduction of hyperglycemia
3. Treatment of acidosis
4. Replacement of potassium
5. Management of precipitating cause

B. Acute Management

1. Fluids—usually up to 1 L fluid may be given over the first hour followed by 200–1000 mL/h of normal or half normal saline. D5 should be added to the solution when blood glucose level reaches 200 mg/dL.

2. Insulin—A 10–15 unit bolus of regular insulin is given followed by an IV infusion of 5–7 units/h.

3. Bicarbonate—The use of bicarbonate remains somewhat controversial but may be helpful if the arterial pH is below 7.0.

4. Potassium—patients with ketoacidosis are potassium depleted due to loss of potassium in urine. Initially the serum potassium may be high due to cellular displacement in response to acidosis. As acidosis corrects, potassium will fall and must be replaced to keep serum K+ at 4–5 mEq/L.

5. Precipitating causes—Infection or myocardial infarction must be aggressively treated.

V. Patient Education

A. All of the usual diabetic teaching should be reinforced including dietary instruction, home glucose monitoring, foot and eye care, etc.

B. Patients should be instructed to never miss an insulin dose without discussing this with a physician. Sick patients who are not eating should take half of their usual dose of NPH insulin and no regular insulin.

C. Families should be instructed to recognize the early signs of DKA. Patients and families should always assume that mental status changes are caused by hypoglycemia and treat initially with sugar or glucagon.

VI. Referral to an Endocrinologist

A. Patients with frequent episodes of DKA

B. Patients with extremely labile blood sugars

C. Patients requiring extensive teaching if this is unavailable in general practice

VII. Annotated Bibliography

Kitabchi AE, Murphy MB. Diabetic ketoacidosis and hyperosmolar hyperglycemic nonketotic coma. Med Clin North Am 1988;72:1545–1563.

Kitabchi AE, Rumbak M. The management of diabetic emergencies. Hosp Pract 1989;24:129–160. A recent review of diabetic emergencies focusing on treatment.

Chapter 5: Ophthalmologic Emergencies

Marvin E. Gozum

5A Corneal Abrasions

I. Clinical Presentation

A. General Information

1. Follows nonpenetrating trauma to the cornea. As trauma varies, so can the extent of a corneal abrasion.
2. The cornea can easily be devastated, scarred, or infected.
3. Infections may extend to the entire eye if an early corneal ulcer is unrecognized.

B. Symptoms

1. Eye pain
2. Photophobia
3. Foreign body sensation

C. Physical Signs

1. Abrasion is visible grossly with fluorescein dye.
2. Abrasions are better visualized under blue filtered light but *not* strictly necessary.
3. Redness or injection of the eye around the area of injury on the cornea may occur with an abrasion.

II. Diagnostic Approach

A. Obtain history of injury
B. Determine contact lens use

C. Examine with fluorescein dye

1. Method

    a. Apply topical anesthetic.
    b. Apply flourescein. Touch flourescein paper moistened with 1 drop sterile saline onto the affected eye's everted lower eyelid, then close eye for 5 sec.
    c. View eye preferably under blue filtered light.
    d. Evert the eyelids. Examine the entire eye ball for foreign bodies.

2. Interpretation

    a. Note size and location of the abrasion.
    b. Small abrasions are < 2 mm in diameter.
    c. Central and large abrasions need an ophthalmology referral.

3. Problems

    a. Small penetrating foreign bodies may be missed.
    b. Nonresolution of pain 24 h after injury and worsening signs and symptoms suggest a persistent foreign body or a developing corneal ulcer.

III. Differential Diagnosis

A. Early corneal ulcers may be mistaken for a corneal abrasion. Corneal ulcers have infiltrates (their early appearance may be subtle), an abrasion does not.

B. The development of eyelid edema, hyphema, purulent discharge and a red eye (see Chapter 5B) clarifies the diagnosis of corneal ulcer.

IV. Treatment

A. Goal—control infection

B. Acute Therapy

1. Noncontact lens wearer

    a. Antibiotic ointment, eg, erythromycin tid for 4 days.
    b. Consider follow up with ophthalmologist if pain unresolved in 24 h.
    c. Using a firm patch, keep eye closed overnight.

2. Contact lens wearer, large abrasion, or central abrasion

    a. Consider cycloplegic such as cyclopentolate 2%.
    b. Tobramycin drops q.i.d for 4d. Tobramycin ointment qhs may be added.
    c. Using a firm patch, keep eye closed overnight.
    d. Refer to an ophthalmologist.

V. Patient Education

A. Persistent pain, swelling, or redness over 24 h requires an evaluation by ophthalmology.

B. Eye protection and goggles

VI. Indications for Immediate Referral to Ophthalmologist

A. Large or centrally located corneal abrasion

B. Suggestion of whitish infiltrate around the abrasion

C. Suggestion of intraocular foreign body

D. Contact lens wearer

VII. Bibliography

See end of chapter.

5B Foreign Bodies

I. Clinical Presentation

A. General Information

1. The location and size of foreign bodies in the eye determine its urgency or degree of ocular emergency.

2. Foreign bodies may be divided into:

   a. Superficial penetrating foreign bodies, usually visible on the sclera or cornea
   b. Deep penetrating foreign bodies
   c. Foreign bodies on the conjunctiva or subconjunctiva
   d. Foreign bodies within the orbit

B. Symptoms

1. Foreign body sensation
2. Eye pain
3. Blurred vision

C. Physical Signs

1. Conjunctival injection
2. Eyelid edema
3. Small infiltrate may surround the foreign body or its penetration site. Degree of inflammation will depend on time elapsed from the moment of injury.

II. Diagnostic Approach

A. History of Injury:

1. Was the patient sanding, grinding, or hammering at the time of injury?
2. Was patient wearing safety goggles?

B. Clinical Examination

1. Method

   a. Irrigate the eye with saline solution. Large foreign bodies in the conjunctiva or subconjunctiva may be removed with a blunt instrument, such as a cotton-tipped applicator.
   b. Examine both upper and lower eyelids.
   c. Determine extent of ocular motion.
   d. Determine visual acuity with corrective lenses.
   e. Apply flourescein dye to evaluate for corneal abrasions (see Chapter 5A).

2. Interpretation
   a. Inability to perform normal occular range of motion suggests foreign body within the orbit.
   b. Change in visual acuity suggests penetrating foreign body.
3. Problems
   a. Small foreign bodies (injuries sustained from grinding, hammering, or sanding material) may not be easily visible.
   b. Patients may complain of persistent pain or foreign body sensation despite no visible irritant.

III. Differential Diagnosis

A. Red Eye (see Chapter 5C)

IV. Treatment

A. Goal—control infection

B. Removal of superficial conjunctival or subconjunctival foreign bodies immediately without further injury to the eye

C. If corneal abrasions are present, see Chapter 5A.

D. Artificial tears, "Refresh" q.i.d $\times$ 2 d.

V. Patient Education

A. Need for goggles or eye protection

VI. Indication for Immediate Referral to an Ophthalmologist

A. Large or centrally located corneal abrasion

B. Suggestion of whitish infiltrate around the abrasion

C. Suggestion of intraocular foreign body

D. Contact lens wearer

E. Pain or foreign body sensation 24 h after examination (particularly if the injury occurred while grinding, sanding, or hammering material)

Part I: Medical Emergencies • 25

F. Change in visual acuity

G. Limitation of ocular motion

VII. Bibliography

See end of chapter.

5C Red and Painful Eye

I. Clinical Presentation

A. General Information

1. Presuming no injury to the eye, red or painful eyes can be diagnosed by the presence or absence of a discharge and degrees of pain.

B. Symptoms

1. Eye pain
2. Blurred vision

C. Physical signs

1. Conjunctival injection, bulbar injection or palpebral injection or circumcorneal (surrounding the cornea)
2. Blood in the conjunctiva
3. Discharge: purulent or clear

II. Diagnostic Approach

A. Obtain history of onset of red eyes and pain.

B. Obtain allergic history and history of associated symptoms.

C. Clinical Examination

1. Method
    a. Obtain Gram stain and culture of the discharge, if purulent, to identify potential organism and its susceptibility.
    b. Examine the eye with flourescein dye to identify corneal abrasions (see Chapter 5A).
    c. Perform visual acuity testing.
2. Interpretation
    a. Clear discharge suggests allergic etiology.
    b. Clear discharge with palpable cervical nodes suggests a viral etiology.
    c. Purulent discharge suggests infectious etiology.
    d. Visual acuity changes require an ophthalmology evaluation.

III. Differential Diagnosis

A. Conjunctivitis—red eye with discharge present and mild pain or discomfort

1. Allergic conjunctivitis—suspect if discharge is clear, the patient complains of marked itching or burning eye sensation, and the history supports additional allergic symptoms.
2. Viral conjunctivitis—(usually adenovirus) suspect if discharge is clear, cervical nodes are enlarged, the history suggests a prior upper respiratory infection and an initially monocular complaint becomes binocular.
3. Bacterial conjunctivitis—suspect if discharge is purulent.

B. Blepharitis—suspect if discharge is primarily on eyelids and patient complains of mild pain or discomfort.

C. Keratitis, acute angle closure glaucoma, scleritis or anterior uveitis—suspect if patient has a red eye with no discharge and patient complains of eye pain.

D. Subconjunctival hemorrhage or conjunctival tumor—suspect if patient has a red eye with no discharge and patient has *no* eye pain.

IV. Treatment

A. Allergic Conjunctivitis

1. Treat systemic allergy with oral histamines (see Chapter 16).
2. Eliminate allergen.
3. Use antihistamine/vasoconstrictor eye drops such as naphazoline/pheniramine q.i.d. until symptoms abate.

B. Viral Conjunctivitis

1. Treat with artificial tears q 4–8 h.
2. Use naphazoline/pheniramine q.i.d. for duration of symptoms.
3. Do not rub eyes.

C. Bacterial Conjunctivitis

1. Can be treated empirically with topical sulfacetamide 10% solution or erythromycin ointment for 5–7 d.
2. Choice of antibiotics can be altered depending on the culture results and sensitivities.

D. Subconjunctival hemorrhages require no treatment.

E. Blepharitis

1. Warm water compresses for 10 min
2. Erythromycin ointment q.i.d. for 7–10 d

F. Keratitis—refer to ophthalmologist immediately

G. Acute angle closure glaucoma—refer to ophthalmologist immediately

H. Scleritis—refer to ophthalmologist immediately

I. Anterior uveitis—refer to ophthalmologist immediately

V. Patient Education

A. Viral and allergic conjunctivitis is self-limiting but may be worsened by rubbing eyes.

B. Subconjunctival hemorrhages are self-limiting and have no clinical significance although may appear alarming.

VI. Indications for Immediate Referral to an Ophthalmologist

A. Purulent discharge

B. Change in visual acuity

C. Large or centrally located corneal abrasion

D. Suggestion of whitish infiltrate around the abrasion

E. Suggestion of intraocular foreign body

F. Contact lens wearer

G. Red eye with absence of discharge or trauma precipitating symptoms—suggestive of keratitis, acute angle closure glaucoma, scleritis or anterior uveitis

VII. Annotated Bibliography

Eva P, Vaughn D. Eye. In: Tierney LM, McPhee SJ, Papadokis MA, Schaeder SA, eds. Current Medical Diagnosis and Therapy. Norwalk, Connecticut: Appleton-Lange, 1993:125–148. A very concise, well written, up to date text (revised annually) and geared toward clinicians. For many topics, this book may be all you need to read. Highly recommended.

Friedberg M, Rapuano C. Wills Eye Hospital Office and Emergency Room Diagnosis and Treatment of Eye Disease. Philadelphia: JB Lippincott; 1990:20–24, 64–68, 103–118. An easy to digest comprehensive manual of eye disorders edited by chief residents at Wills Eye Hospital.

Chapter 6: Status Epilepticus

Robert D. Aiken

I. General Information

A. See Chapter 77 for discussion of seizure disorders

B. Definition
   Generalized Status Epilepticus (GSE)—Prolonged or recurrent generalized seizures lasting 30 min or more or recurrent generalized seizures that occur without an intervening period of consciousness

C. Incidence
   18–28/1000; 9–14,000 new cases/y in United Kingdom. 45–70,000 new cases/y in United States. More than 50% of cases of status epilepticus are GSE.

D. Classification of Status Epilepticus

1. Generalized status epilepticus
   a. Convulsion status
      1) Tonic-clonic (grandmal)
      2) Tonic
      3) Clonic
      4) Myoclonic
   b. Absence status

2. Partial status epilepticus
   a. Simple partial status
      1) Somatomotor
      2) Dysphasia or aphasia
      3) Adversive
      4) Somatosensory
      5) Elementary visual
      6) Autonomic
   b. Complex partial seizures

3. Neonatal status epilepticus

II. Clinical Presentation

A. Adults—repeated generalized seizures without recovery of consciousness between seizures or prolonged/unremitting seizures

B. Children—continuous or serial seizures; serial seizures usually last 2–3 min.

C. General Signs

1. Respiration may be halted during tonic-clonic seizures—patient often appears cyanotic.
2. Cardiovascular system stressed by repeated seizures—tachycardia, bradycardia, or cardiac arrhythmias
3. Hyperpyrexia
4. Paralysis of cerebral autoregulation may lead to hypoperfusion and result in cerebral ischemia
5. Pulmonary edema may occur due to altered lymph flow
6. Autonomic failure may cause hyperpyrexia, excessive tracheobronchial secretions, hypertension, or hypotension.

D. Laboratory findings

1. Blood sugar initially elevated 200–250 mg/dL, but hypoglycemia may develop after many seizures.
2. Rhabdomyolysis may lead to myoglobinuria and acute renal failure.
3. See treatment below and Chapter 77 for laboratory evaluation.

III. Diagnostic Approach

See Chapter 77 for diagnostic approach to seizure disorders.

IV. Differential Diagnosis

A. Metabolic/Toxic

1. Exacerbation of seizures in established epileptic patient often due to antiepileptic drug (AED) noncompliance
2. Alcohol or drug abuse
3. Drug or alcohol withdrawal
4. Miscellaneous or undetermined (eg, encephalitis, hyponatremia)

B. Structural Derangement

1. Anoxic/hypoxic
2. Acute cerebrovascular event (ischemic stroke, intracerebral hemorrhage, subarachnoid hemorrhage)
3. Brain/intracranial abscess or neoplasm
4. Penetrating or blunt head trauma
5. Metabolic (eg; hepatic encephalopathy, uremia)
6. Infection—meningitis, encephalitis

V. Treatment

A. General Measures

1. 0–10 min
   a. Assess and maintain cardiorespiratory function.
   b. Establish and maintain airway.
   c. Initiate supplemental 0_2.
   d. Secure IV access.

2. 0–60 min
   a. Monitor regularly.
   b. Administer AEDs in loading dose (see below).
   c. Emergency investigations—arterial blood gases, glucose, renal and hepatic function, Ca, mg, complete blood count, differential, platelets, coagulation studies, and anticonvulsant levels, if applicable
   d. Give thiamine 50 mg IV, then glucose 50 ml of a 50% solution.
   e. Treat acidosis, if severe.

3. 0–90 min
   a. Search for cause (see Chapter 77).
   b. Identify and treat medical complications.
   c. Monitor intracranial pressure, if appropriate to manage cerebral edema.
   d. Initiate long-term AED.

B. Anticonvulsant Drug Therapy Principles

1. Diazepam (5 mg/min) or lorazepam (2 mg/min) until seizures stop
2. Start phenytoin (20 mg/kg) at rate of 50 mg/min.
3. Use diazepam or lorazepam q 15 min PRN during phenytoin loading if seizures occur.
4. If seizures persist, intubate, then load with phenobarbital 20 mg/kg at 100 mg/min IV.
5. If seizures persist more than 30–60 min, give phenobarbital 5 mg/kg loading then 1–3 mg/kg 1 h and *adjust* dose to obtain burst-suppression pattern on continuous on-line EEG, but avoid hypotension.

6. AED levels should be drawn from opposing antecubital vein after anticonvulsant infusion, reaching phenytoin level of 25 µg/mL and phenobarbital level of 35–40 µg/mL.
7. Other forms of GSE—not usually life-threatening emergencies
   a. Tonic status epilepticus—most frequently occurs in children and adolescents; not usually life-threatening and may continue for days or weeks
   b. Clonic status epilepticus—most often occurs in infants and young children, often due to acute brain lesion or chronic encephalopathy and often exacerbated by fever
   c. Myoclonic status epilepticus
   d. Absence status epilepticus—responds to IV diazepam. Ethosuxamide or valproate should be given for chronic control.
   e. Simple and complex partial status epilepticus should be treated with IV benzodiazepine, phenytoin, then, if needed, phenobarbital.

VI. Indications for Referral to a Neurologist

A. All patients with no history of prior seizures

B. Patients in whom an obvious cause is not apparent

C. Patients who do not respond promptly to IV benzodiazepines and phenytoin

VII. Indications for Hospitalization

Patients with GSE usually require hospitalization to treat seizures and establish their cause.

VIII. Annotated Bibliography

Leppik I. Status epilepticus. In: Wyllie E. The Treatment of Epilepsy: Principles and Practice. Philadelphia: Lea & Febiger; 1993:678–685. Excellent up-to-date review of the approach to treatment of status epilepticus.

Ropper A. Neurological and Neurosurgical Intensive Care. New York: Raven Press; 1993. Comprehensive current review of critical care problems in clinical neurology.

Shorvon S. Tonic-clonic status epilepticus. J Neurol Neurosurg Psychiat 1993;56:125–134. British approach to management of this problem.

Part II:
Screening/General Care

Chapter 7: Screening for Breast Cancer

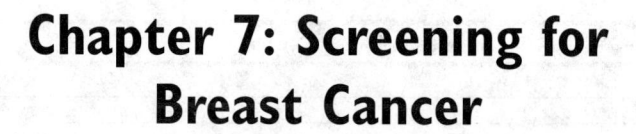

Kenneth R. Epstein

I. Epidemiology

A. General

1. Most common cancer in American women
2. Second leading cause of cancer death in women (after lung cancer, which passed breast cancer in mortality in early 1980s); leading cause of cancer death in women aged 40–55 y
3. 12% of all women in the United States will be given a diagnosis of breast cancer and 3.5% will die from the disease.
4. The mortality rate is increasing for African American women, while remaining unchanged for white women. Mortality rate for African American women now exceeds that of white women.
5. The failure to diagnose breast cancer is the second most frequent reason for claims brought against physicians and the most expensive.

B. Risk Factors

1. Incidence rate increases with increasing age.
2. Risk increases significantly if a primary relative (mother or sister) had breast cancer. This risk is even higher if primary relative had premenopausal cancer.
3. Benign breast disease
   a. Mild hyperplasia or fibroadenoma—no increased risk
   b. Proliferative or with atypia—increased risk
4. Nulliparity or first pregnancy after age 30 y
5. Risk increases with longer period of cyclic ovarian function. Therefore, risk higher for early menarche or menopause after age 55 y.
6. Oral contraceptive use > 8 y
7. Alcohol use > 3 drinks per day

C. Prognosis by Stage

1. See Table 7-1 for staging

Table 7–1. Staging Systems for Breast Cancer

Symbol	Meaning
TNM System	
TX	Primary tumor cannnot be assessed
T0	No evidence of primary tumor
Tis	Carcinoma in situ: intraductal carcinoma, lobular carcinoma in situ, or Paget's disease of the nipple with no tumor
T1	Tumor ≤ 2 cm
a	Tumor ≤ 0.5 cm
b	Tumor > 0.5, but not > 1 cm
c	Tumor > 1 cm, but not > 2 cm
T2	Tumor > 2 cm, but not > 5 cm
T3	Tumor > 5 cm
T4	Tumor or any size with direct extension to chest wall[†] or skin[‡]
a	Extension to chest wall
b	Edema (including peau d'orange), ulceration of the skin or the breast, or satellite skin nodules confined to the same breast
c	Both of the above
d	Inflammatory carcinoma
NX	Regional lymph nodes cannot be assessed (eg, previously removed)
N0	No regional lymph node metastases
N1	Metastasis to movable ipsilateral axillary nodes
N2	Metastases to ipsilateral axillary nodes fixed to one another or to other structures
N3	Metastases to ipsilateral internal mammary lymph nodes
M0	No evidence of distant metastasis
M1	Distant metastases (including metastases to ipsilateral supraclavicular lymph nodes)
Clinical Stage	
I	T1.N0.M0
IIA	T0.N1.M0
	T1.N1.M0
	T2.N0.M0
IIB	T2.N1.M0
	T3.N0.M0
IIIA	T0 or T1.N2.M0.
	T2.N2.M0
	T3.N1. or N2.M0
IIIB	T4, any N.M0
	Any T.N3.M0
IV	Any T, any N.M1

* According to the Union Internationale Centre le Cancer and the American Joint Commission on Cancer Staging and End-Results Reporting.

† The chest wall includes the ribs, intercostal muscles, and serratus anterior muscle, but not the pectoral muscle.

‡ Dimpling of the skin, nipple retraction, or any other skin changes except those listed for T-b may occur in T1, T2, or T3 without affecting the classification.

SOURCE: Reprinted by permission of the New England Journal of Medicine from Harris JR, Lippman ME, Veronesi U, Willett, W. Breast cancer. N Engl J Med 1992;327:390–398.

2. 5-year survival rates
   a. Stage I: 85%
   b. Stage II: 66%
   c. Stage III: 41%
   d. Stage IV: 10%

II. Screening

A. Screening Modalities

1. Definition of terms
   a. Sensitivity—true positives/(true positives + false negatives)—Of all those with cancer, in what percentage is the test positive.
   b. Specificity—true negatives/(true negatives + false positives)—Of all those without cancer, in what percentage is the test negative.
   c. Positive predictive value—true positives/(true positives + false positives)—Of all those with a positive test, in what percentage is cancer really present.
   d. Negative predictive value—true negatives/(true negatives + false negatives)—Of all those with a negative test, in what percentage is there really no cancer present.
2. Breast self-examination
   a. Technique—Perform visual examination with arms at sides, arms overhead, and then hands on hip. Look for differences in contour, retracted or elevated areas, nipple abnormalities, prominent venous patterns, and dimpling. After visual inspection, then perform palpation of breasts and axillae. See Clinical Breast Examination below for findings on palpation suggestive of malignancy.
   b. Sensitivity and specificity are both low. Detection of lesions is increased by breast self-examination, but there is limited evidence that mortality is decreased.
   c. Breast self-examination is an important means of increasing patient awareness of importance of breast cancer screening. However, it is not adequate as the sole screening recommendation, and it should not give patient a false sense of security that she does not require a clinical breast examination or mammography.
3. Clinical breast examination
   a. Physical findings that are suggestive of malignancy include
      1) Firm mass with indistinct borders
      2) Attachment to skin or deep fascia
      3) Dimpling of skin, retraction of nipples
      4) Bloody discharge from nipples
      5) Lack of tenderness
   b. It is important that examination includes careful palpation of the axillary tail, axillary nodes, and supraclavicular nodes.

c. Clinical breast examination has been shown to increase detection rate. The sensitivity is 50%, meaning that half of the breast cancers will be missed, especially lesions < 1 cm. The specificity is 95–99% using the above criteria for a positive test.
d. Clinical breast examination can detect masses that are malignant in the presence of a negative mammogram, so it remains an essential part of screening.

4. Mammography
   a. Mammography is a primary screening modality. It can pick up tumors even < 1 cm.
   b. Mammography has been definitely shown to decrease mortality for women over age 50 y.
   c. The sensitivity is > 90% at good centers, and the specificity is 88–99%.
   d. Findings suggestive of malignant lesion include
      1) Spiculated density
      2) Diffuse dense tissue
      3) Cluster microcalcification
   e. The benefits of mammography in women ages 40–50 y remains controversial. Breast cancer in these women grows and metastasizes early, making detection by mammography problematic. Additionally, the denser breasts of younger women increase the difficulty in reading mammograms.
   f. Newer mammographic techniques use much lower doses of radiation than older machines.

B. Screening Recommendations

1. Breast self-examination: monthly after age 20 y
2. Clinical breast examination: between 20 and 40 years, q 3 y; after 40 y, perform annually
3. Mammography
   a. For an average risk woman, annually after age 50. Consider annually between 40 and 50 y.
   b. For a woman at increased risk, perform annually after age 40 y. If the woman's mother or sister had premenopausal breast cancer, may consider starting at an even earlier age.
4. It is important to realize that mammography and careful clinical examination are complementary, and *both* are necessary.

III. Evaluation of a Palpable Mass

A. If a mass is palpated on examination, perform a mammogram. However, it is essential to pursue evaluation of the mass even if the mammogram is negative.

B. Fine-needle aspiration (FNA) is the first step in evaluation. The fluid should be sent for cytology.

1. If FNA reveals the presence of a *cyst* and the cytology is positive, the fluid is bloody, the lesion recurs, or the lesion is suspicious on mammogram, then proceed with an *outpatient biopsy*. If all of the above are negative, then follow lesion with observation.

2. If FNA reveals the presence of a *solid mass*, and the cytology is negative or only suspicious of malignancy, then regardless of mammographic appearance, proceed with outpatient biopsy. If the cytology is positive for cancer, then proceed with *intraoperative biopsy*.

IV. Evaluation of Nonpalpable Mass

A. If a suspicious lesion is noted on mammography, but is not palpable, then perform FNA for cytologic examination, using either ultrasound or mammography for localization.

B. Findings on cytology guide the next step.

1. If the cytology reveals malignant cells, then the woman will require an interoperative biopsy.

2. If the cytology reveals atypical, but not clearly malignant cells, then the woman will need an outpatient biopsy.

3. If the cytology is benign, then follow the woman with periodic mammography.

V. Annotated Bibliography

Council on Scientific Affairs. Mammographic screening of asymptomatic women aged 40 years and older. JAMA 1989;261:2535–2542. The American Medical Association's Council on Scientific Affairs official recommendations regarding mammographic breast cancer screening.

Donevan WL. Evaluation of a palpable breast mass. N Engl J Med 1992;327: 937–941. Good review, with recommendations, of literature on subject of the title.

Eddy DM. Screening for breast cancer. Ann Intern Med 1989;111:389–399. Good review of the literature regarding the benefits and costs of various strategies for breast cancer screening. Recommendations are then made based on mathematical modeling.

Harris JR, Lippman ME, Veronesi U, Willett W. Breast cancer. N Engl J Med 1992;327:319–328, 390–398, 473–479. Three-part review article on breast cancer, including screening. Part one discusses prevention, risk factors, and screening. Parts two and three review staging and treatment.

Jackson VP. The status of mammographically guided fine needle aspiration biopsy of nonpalpable breast lesions. Rad Clin North Am 1992;30:155–166. More detailed review of state of the art of fine-needle aspiration biopsies of breast lesions.

Chapter 8: Screening for Colorectal Cancer

Kenneth R. Epstein

I. Epidemiology

A. General

1. Most common noncutaneous cancer in the United States, with the second highest mortality rate; 157,500 new cases and 60,500 deaths were estimated to occur in 1992. The lifetime probability of any one person developing colorectal carcinoma is approximately 6%.
2. The incidence of colorectal carcinoma increases with age.
3. Colorectal carcinoma may arise anywhere within the colon.
   a. < 10% occur in the distal 7.5 cm of the colon.
   b. 40% occur in the distal 35 cm.
   c. 55% occur in the distal 60 cm.
   d. Remaining 45% occur more proximally.
4. The current theory on the temporal sequence of evolution of colorectal carcinoma:
   a. It takes approximately 5 years to advance from a totally negative colon to the presence of an adenoma.
   b. It takes approximately 10 years to advance from a totally negative colon to a grossly infiltrating carcinoma.
   c. These numbers are important in devising a screening strategy.
5. Although 93% of invasive cancers arise from adenomas, < 10% of adenomatous polyps will eventually become malignant.

B. Risk Factors

1. Incidence rate increases with increasing age.
2. High-fat, high-animal protein diets have been linked to increased incidence of colorectal carcinoma. Conversely, low-fat, high-fiber diets increase transit time and may decrease cancer incidence.
3. Risk of colorectal carcinoma is increased 2-3 times in persons with a first-degree relative with colorectal carcinoma. Risk is also higher in persons with a personal or family history of cancer of the breast or genitourinary tract.

4. Risk is further increased for persons with a family history of the cancer family syndrome and persons with a previous colorectal adenoma or carcinoma.
5. Tubulovillous, villous, or large (> 1 cm) adenomas found on screening sigmoidoscopy suggest increased risk of future colorectal carcinoma. Hyperplastic polyps and single, small tubular adenomas do not increase risk of subsequent cancer.
6. Risk is highest for those with familial polyposis or ulcerative colitis.
   a. Individuals with the familial polyposis syndrome have a 50% probability of developing cancer by age 40 y.
   b. Persons with a > 10-year history of ulcerative colitis have a 20-fold increase in the annual risk of colorectal carcinoma.

C. Prognosis by Stage

1. 5-year survival rate by stage at diagnosis

Dukes class A—lesion limited to mucosa	95%
Dukes class B—lesion extends to serosa	65%
Dukes class C—lesion extends to regional lymph nodes	30%
Dukes class D—lesion metastatic to distant sites	5%

II. Screening

A. Screening Modalities

1. Digital rectal examination (DRE)
   a. Assesses approximately the distal 7.5 cm of rectum. Less than 10% of lesions are in this distribution.
   b. Low sensitivity: Many individuals with colorectal carcinoma may have negative DREs.
   c. If done as part of the routine physical examination, there is little additional cost to DRE.
2. Fecal Occult Blood Testing (FOBT)
   a. Method—Patient obtains two stool samples per day on 3 different days, for a total of six samples. A positive test is defined as any 1 out of 6 samples being positive.
   b. Guaiac testing is based on the principle that guaiac undergoes phenolic oxidation, turning blue in the presence of hemoglobin and hydrogen peroxide. Prepared slides decrease in positivity the longer they are stored before being developed. Rehydration with a drop of water before processing increases both true positive and false positive rate.
   c. False positives may occur with injestion of red meat, aspirin or nonsteroidal anti-inflammatory drugs, iron, and vegetables with high peroxidase activity (broccoli, turnips, cantaloupes, radishes, horseradish, parsnips). False negatives may occur after ingestion of ascorbic acid, an antioxidant.

d. The sensitivity is approximately 26%. The specificity is approximately 95%. There seems to be no significant difference in terms of sensitivity between the Hemoccult and HemoQuant FOBTs. Both will miss the majority of cancers or polyps.
e. 1–5% of unselected persons tested with FOBTs will have a positive test. The positive predictive value is 10% for cancer, and 30% for adenomas, ie; of those with a positive test, 10% will have colorectal carcinoma, and 20–30% will have adenomatous polyps.
f. Therefore, FOBT will detect some cancers, but will miss many. A decreased mortality from colorectal cancer has been demonstrated with annual FOBT and colonoscopic follow-up of positive results.
g. Costs and charges vary over time and between institutions. The charge for FOBT is usually in the range of $15.

3. Flexible Sigmoidoscopy

a. 35-cm flexible sigmoidoscopy reaches 40% of adenomas. There is a 0.02% risk of perforation. 60-cm flexible sigmoidoscopy reaches 55% of adenomas. The risk of perforation is 0.045%.
b. Sensitivity is 85% for lesions within the reach of the sigmoidoscope. The sensitivity for adenomatous polyps anywhere in the colon is 44%.
c. Specificity is very high, ie, there are very few false positives, because one may biopsy any positive lesions.
d. Main drawbacks are patient anxiety and discomfort.
e. Several case-control studies have demonstrated a 60–80% reduction in colorectal carcinoma mortality for those receiving screening sigmoidoscopy versus those who did not. Several randomized trials are currently underway.
f. The charge for flexible sigmoidoscopy varies in different offices but is usually in the range of $200. The charge may be higher if done in a hospital.

4. Colonoscopy

a. Colonoscopy can visualize the entire colon. Therefore, sensitivity is much higher, approximately 95%. The risk of perforation is 0.2%.
b. There are very few false positives (specificity is high) because one can biopsy any suspicious lesions.
c. The main drawbacks to screening colonoscopy are the high cost and patient anxiety and discomfort. The charge is variable, but is often $1000–1500, and may be considerably higher if biopsies are performed.

5. Double-contrast barium enema

a. Can visualize the entire colon although is less sensitive for rectal lesions than is colonoscopy.
b. Sensitivity is 85%, slightly lower than colonoscopy. The risk of perforation is 0.02%.
c. The specificity is 96–97%, lower than that of colonscopy. False positives may occur secondary to retained stool or other factors affecting visualization.

d. There are several disadvantages of barium enemas versus colonoscopy. First, barium enemas visualize the rectum poorly, so sigmoidoscopy is often still necessary. Secondly, suspicious lesions cannot be biopsied, so that follow-up colonoscopy may be necessary if the barium enema is abnormal.
e. Additional drawbacks to screening barium enema are cost and patient anxiety and discomfort. In most institutions, however, a barium enema is significantly less expensive than colonoscopy. The charge for a barium enema is often in the range of $400–600.

B. Screening Recommendations

1. Colorectal carcinoma is prevalent in both men and women. There is therefore no rationale for taking a differing approach to men and women when screening.

2. Although there are no randomized trials demonstrating a decrease in mortality from screening for colorectal carcinoma, case-control studies have supported a mortality reduction. The assumption is that detecting adenomas will prevent future carcinomas, and therefore decrease mortality. Most authors have concluded that colorectal carcinoma screening is both effective and cost effective.

3. One ideal screening strategy does not exist. There is a wide range of tests in terms of cost and effectiveness. FOBT is the simplest, most convenient, and least expensive, but least effective. Strategies that visualize the entire colon, either colonoscopy or barium enema, are the most effective, but involve greater patient discomfort, less patient acceptance, and greater cost. Based on the charges listed above, in most institutions a flexible sigmoidoscopy plus barium enema is still much less expensive than a colonoscopy.

4. Although population recommendations can be made, an individual health care provider needs to discuss with the individual patient what is best, based on that patient's own risk factors, values, and desires. The strategies below are therefore more options than recommendations.

5. A reasonable screening strategy for a man or woman at average risk would be, at age 50 y to begin receiving an annual FOBT and a flexible sigmoidoscopy q 3–5 y.

6. Individuals at high risk of colorectal carcinoma should be encouraged to have an examination of their complete colon by either colonoscopy or barium enema. As discussed above, colonoscopy costs considerably more than barium enema, but allows direct visualization and biopsy of any suspicious lesions. Due to the slow growth of colorectal adenomas, and the slow conversion to carcinomas, a 5-y frequency of these tests is probably adequate.

7. If flexible sigmoidoscopy detects the presence of an adenoma, then full colonoscopy with biopsy and removal of all polyps is indicted.

8. For evaluation of a heme-positive stool detected on FOBT, see Chapter 49.

III. Annotated Bibliography

Ahlquist DA, Wieand HS, Moertel CG, et al. Accuracy of fecal occult blood screening for colorectal neoplasia. JAMA 1993;269:1262–1267. A comparison of the Hemoccult and HemoQuant FOBTs.

Atkin WS, Morson BC, Cuzick J. Long-term risk of colorectal cancer after excision of rectosigmoid adenomas. N Engl J Med 1992;326:658–662. Data assessing the long-term risk of colorectal carcinoma in over 1600 patients who had polyps on sigmoidoscopy who did not undergo follow-up surveillance. The risk of subsequent cancer developed on the type, size, and number of adenomas found.

Eddy DM. Screening for colorectal cancer. An Intern Med 1990;113:373–384. An excellent review of the various screening modalities, with calculations of expected costs and benefits of various screening strategies.

Mandel JS, Bond JH, Church TR, et al. Reducing mortality from colorectal cancer by screening for fecal occult blood. N Engl J Med 1993;328:1365–1371.

Ransohoff DF, Lang CA. Sigmoidoscopic screening in the 1990s. JAMA 1993;269:1278–1281. A good review of the state of the art regarding sigmoidoscopic screening, with discussion of the controversial questions that remain.

Selby JV, Friedman CD, Quesenberry CP, Weiss NS. A case-control study of screening sigmoidoscopy and mortality from colorectal cancer. N Engl J Med 1992;326:653–657. Data supporting a mortality reduction from colorectal carcinoma in those patients screened with sigmoidoscopy.

Chapter 9: Screening for Prostate Cancer

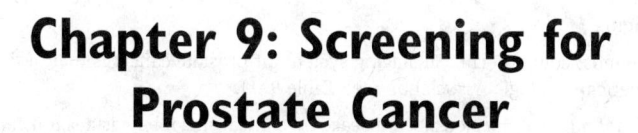

Kenneth R. Epstein and Daniel Holleran

I. Epidemiology

A. General

1. Adenocarcinoma of the prostate is the most common cancer in men and is the second leading cause of cancer deaths in men (equal to colorectal cancer).

2. 1 in 11 men will develop prostate cancer. For African Americans, this number is 1 in 9.

3. The peak age for prostate cancer is between 65 and 70 y. 70% of men aged 70 will have asymptomatic foci of prostate cancer. Therefore, it is said that many more men die with prostate cancer than of it.

B. Risk Factors

1. Age—Prostate cancer is rare in men < 40 y, but both the incidence and mortality rate increase exponentially with age, such that it is common by age 80 y.

2. Race—African American men have a higher incidence and mortality than do white men. Coversely, the incidence and mortality are much lower in Asian men.

3. Family history—A man with a brother or father with prostate cancer has a 2–8 fold increased likelihood of developing prostate cancer.

4. Occupation—Men who have worked with cadmium (eg; welding and electroplating) have an increased incidence of prostate cancer.

5. Diet—Current evidence supports a positive relationship between the incidence of prostate cancer and a diet high in animal fat. Conversely, a high-fiber, low-fat diet seems to be protective.

6. Vasectomy—Several studies have demonstrated a 1.6- to 1.9-fold increase in the risk of developing prostate cancer among men who have had vasectomies in the past.

7. Benign prostatic hyperplasia (BPH)—Data are still unclear. Some studies have demonstrated an increased risk in men with a history of BPH, whereas others have not demonstrated any change in risk.

C. Staging

1. The most common clinical staging system for prostate cancer is that of the American Urologic Association (see Table 9-1).
2. Even if a patient has localized disease by clinical stage, he has a significant likelihood of having spread of the cancer to regional lymph nodes found at the time of surgery. Although 65% of cancers are clinically localized (stage A, B, or C) at the time of diagnosis, only half of these prove to be confined to the prostate at surgery.
3. The degree of tumor differentiation may be even more important than clinical staging in determining prognosis. The Gleason grading system is used, with grade 1 being the most well differentiated and grade 5 the most poorly differentiated.

II. Screening

A. Screening Modalities

1. Definition of terms—see Chapter 7
2. Digital rectal examination (DRE)
   a. On digital rectal examination, prostate cancer usually presents as either a distinct nodule or diffuse area of induration. Only the lateral and posterior lobes of the prostate are palpable.
   b. The sensitivity of DRE for prostate cancer is reportedly to be 50-86%. However, the cancers that are not detected by DRE are usually small and localized. Therefore, DRE is not sensitive enough to detect prostate cancer at a stage when it is likely to be curable.
   c. The specificity of DRE is low, at 44%. It may be difficult to differentiate whether an indurated area represents cancer or benign hyperplasia.
   d. DREs are often performed to screen for colorectal carcinoma in addition to prostate cancer. If done as part of the routine physical examination, there is little additional cost to DRE.
   e. Due to DREs low sensitivity and poor performance at detecting early, curable cancers, it is not satisfactory as the sole screening test.
2. Transrectal ultrasound (TRUS)
   a. Prostate tissue normally has a finely stippled echo pattern. Prostatic cancer presents as hypoechoic lesions on ultrasound.
   b. The sensitivity of TRUS for detecting any prostate cancer is reported to be 60-92%. However, as with DRE, the lesions that often cannot be detected by TRUS are those that are small and localized.
   c. Specificity of TRUS is quite low, in the range of 25-30%.
   d. Advantage of TRUS is that suspicious lesions can be biopsied at the time of the procedure.
   e. TRUS is not adequate as a screening test for prostate cancer. Its utility is in the evaluation of patients suspected of having cancer based on abnormal DRE or prostate specific antigen (PSA) levels.
3. Prostate specific antigen
   a. PSA is a serine protease present exclusively in prostatic epithelial cells. It is measurable in all men with prostatic tissue.

Table 9–1.

Stage	Description	Frequency at Diagnosis
A_1	Not palpable, focal	10%
A_2	Not palpable, diffuse	
B_1	Palpable, one lobe, < 1.5 cm	10–15%
B_2	Palpable, two lobes or > 1.5 cm	
C	Local extension beyond prostate	40%
D_1	Regional lymph node involvement	35%
D_2	Distant metastases	

    b. PSA levels are increased in 30–50% of men with BPH, depending on the size of the gland.

    c. PSA is also elevated in men with prostatitis, following cystoscopy and other procedures involving the prostate, and in 25–92% of men with prostate cancer.

    d. Normal PSA levels are slightly different for different manufacturers of the assay, but are usually considered to be between 0 and 3.9 ng/mL. Levels between 4.0 and 9.9 ng/mL are common in both BPH and prostate cancer. Levels > 10.0 ng/mL are highly suggestive of the presence of cancer.

    e. The sensitivity of PSA is approximately 80%. As with other screening tests, the more advanced the cancer, the higher the likelihood of the PSA being elevated.

    f. The specificity of PSA is 60–70%.

    g. The advantage of PSA as a screening test is that it is objective, quantitative, and not dependent on the examiner's skill.

    h. In the range of 0–10.0 ng/mL, PSA levels are not significantly changed by recent digital rectal examination. Therefore, PSA levels can be drawn on patients following a physical examination that included DRE. For PSAs > 10 ng/mL, DRE can significantly elevate levels. However, in this range, all patients will require further evaluation and biopsy anyway.

    i. The level of PSA is proportional to tumor volume and the clinical stage of cancer in untreated patients. However, there is considerable overlap in the ranges of PSA for each stage, making it difficult to predict a patient's stage based solely on the PSA level. Most men with prostate cancer and a PSA between 4 and 10 ng/mL will have clinically localized disease, but many may have progression of disease beyond the prostate at the time of surgical staging. Most men with PSA levels > 10.0 will be found to have extracapsular spread of the disease.

    j. PSA levels are not satisfactory as the sole screening test for prostate cancer. It is possible to detect a clinically localized cancer on DRE in a man with a PSA < 4 ng/mL. Conversely, many men with PSA levels of between 4–10 ng/mL will have BPH as the cause of their PSA elevation. If a cutoff of 10 ng/mL were used as the cutoff for cancer detection, almost all men with early, potentially curable cancer would be missed.

B. Screening Recommendations

1. The value of screening for prostate cancer remains controversial. There is concern that screening will detect many occult cancers in men that never

would have become clinically significant. Therefore, the morbidity and mortality from the detection and treatment of these cancers may exceed that of the cancer itself.
2. There is increasing evidence that men with early, asymptomatic prostate cancer may live with their disease for more than 10 y if left untreated. Therefore, a criteria that is becoming increasingly accepted for prostate cancer screening is to limit screening for prostate cancer to men older than 50 y with an anticipated life span of > 10 y.
3. A prudent recommendation would be for all men over the age of 50 with an expected life span of > 10 years, as well as those between 40 and 50 y with a strong family history of prostate cancer, to undergo annual DRE and PSA determination.
4. Recommendations
   a. If DRE is negative, and the PSA is < 4 ng/mL, repeat both in 1 y.
   b. If DRE reveals a suspicious lesion, then regardless of the PSA level, obtain a TRUS with biopsy.
   c. If the PSA is > 10 ng/mL, then regardless of DRE findings, the patient requires TRUS with biopsy.
   d. For PSA levels of 4–10 ng/mL, there are two equally acceptable recommendations, depending on patient and physician preference.
      1) Obtain a TRUS on all patients, regardless of DRE findings.
      2) Obtain TRUS with biopsy only if the DRE reveals an abnormal lesion. If the DRE reveals only BPH, then repeat the PSA in 6–12 mo. If the PSA level increases by > 0.75 ng/mL over that time period, then TRUS with biopsy should be obtained.
   e.) If the TRUS reveals a suspicious lesion, then it is biopsied at the time of the ultrasound. If the TRUS does not reveal a lesion, then most authors recommend blind sextant biopsies to look for foci of tumor.

III. Annotated Bibliography

Catalona WJ, Smith DS, Ratliff TL, et al. Measurement of prostate-specific antigen in serum as a screening test for prostate cancer. N Engl J Med 1991;324:1156–1161. One of the best studies to date analyzing the value of DRE, PSA, and TRUS in the detection of prostate cancer.

Garnick MB. Prostate cancer: screening, diagnosis, and management. Ann Intern Med 1993;118:804–818. An excellent review of the current literature on prostate cancer.

Oesterling JE. Prostate specific antigen: a critical assessment of the most useful tumor marker for adenocarcinoma of the prostate. J Urol 1991;145:907–923. An excellent review of the literature on the biology of and clinical utility of PSA.

Pienta KJ, Esper PS. Risk factors for prostate cancer. Ann Intern Med 1993;118:793–803. A good review of the data on potential risk factors for prostatic carcinoma.

Roetzheim RG, Herold AH. Prostate cancer screening. Prim Care 1992:19:637–649. A good review of the issues related to screening for prostate cancer, with prudent recommendations.

Chapter 10: Screening for Cervical Cancer

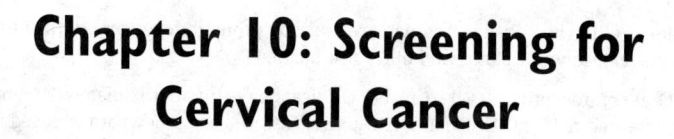

Kenneth R. Epstein

I. Epidemiology

A. General

1. There are 13,000 cases of invasive cervical carcinoma (ICC) per year in the United States, and 7000 women die of cervical carcinoma per year.

2. Both the incidence and mortality from ICC are inversely proportional to the rate of cytologic screening in a population.

3. 80-90% of ICC is squamous cell carcinoma, arising at the transformation zone between the squamous and columnar epithelium. The rest are adenocarcinoma, adenosquamous carcinoma, or undifferentiated cell type.

4. Definitions
    a. Carcinoma in situ (CIS)—carcinomatous changes confined to the epithelium of the cervix
    b. Cervical intraepithelial neoplasia (CIN)—includes all precancerous lesions, including CIS and dysplasia

B. Risk Factors

1. Age—The peak incidence of ICC in women is age 45-60 y. The peak incidence of CIN is approximately 10 y earlier, between 34-38 y. Although 14% of women in the United States are over age 65 y, 25% of cervical carcinoma cases and 41% of cervical carcinoma deaths are in this age group.

2. Sexual history—The incidence rises progressively with increasing total number of sexual partners and with an earlier age at first intercourse. It is unclear if age at first intercourse is a risk factor independent of the total number of sexual partners.

3. Male sexual history—Women whose male sexual partners have had multiple sexual partners are at increased risk. Likewise, the female partners of men who have had previous partners with cervical carcinoma are at increased risk.

4. Socioeconomic status—Incidence increases with decreasing socioeconomic status. This appears to be due to decreased access to screening as well as presence of other risk factors.

5. Race/ethnicity—Risk is not increased for any group independent of the effect of socioeconomic status and other risk factors.
6. Oral contraceptives (OC)—Current OC users have an approximately 1.5 times increased risk of CIN versus never users. Risk is also somewhat increased for past users. The increased relative risk seems to be independent of the number of sexual partners.
7. Cigarette smoking—Current smokers have a 2-3-fold increased risk versus nonsmokers. The risk increases progressively with the number of cigarettes smoked per day.
8. Human papillomavirus (HPV) infection—HPV may be a key etiologic agent in cervical carcinoma. At least 17 types of HPV have been associated with sexually transmitted infections of the female genital tract. HPV DNA has been found in both ICC and CIN lesions. 90-100% of cervical carcinomas have HPV DNA, especially HPV types 16 and 18. HPV infection may require the presence of cofactors to produce malignant transformation. The increased risk associated with the sexual history of the woman and her male partners mentioned above may be due to the increased risk of HPV infection.
9. Chronic immunosuppression—Immunosuppressed women have an increased risk of cervical carcinoma.

C. Staging

1. Staging of cervical cytology has changed several times. The most recently accepted nomenclature is the Bethesda system. Table 10-1 reviews the various nomenclature systems.
2. Clinical staging based on the CIN system:
    a. Stage 0—CIS
    b. Stage I—ICC confined to the cervix
    c. Stage Ia—early stromal invasion diagnosed microscopically
    d. Stage Ib—stromal invasion > 5 mm in depth or 7 mm in horizontal spread
    e. Stage II—ICC extending beyond cervix, but not to pelvic wall; may involve all but the lower third of vagina
    f. Stage III—ICC extending to pelvic wall, involvement of lower third of vagina, hydronephrosis, or nonfunctional kidney
    g. Stage IV—ICC extending beyond pelvis, clinical involvement of bladder or rectal mucosa
3. Cure Rates by stage:
    a. Stages 0, Ia   100%
    b. Stage Ib   90%
    c. Stage II   50-60%
    d. Stage III   30-40%
    e. Stage IV   5%

Table 10–1. Cervical Cytology Nomenclature Systems

Pap System	WHO System	CIN System	Bethesda System
Class I	Normal	Normal	Normal
Class II	Atypical		Other
			Infection
			Reparative
Class III	Dysplasia		Squamous intraepithelial lesion (SIN)
	Mild	CIN I	Low-grade SIN
	Moderate	CIN II	High-grade SIN
	Severe	CIN III	High-grade SIN
Class IV	Carcinoma in situ (CIS)	CIS	High-grade SIN
Class V	Invasive squamous carcinoma (ICC)	ICC	Squamous cell carcinoma
Class V	Adenocarcinoma	Adenocarcinoma	Glandular cell abnormality
			Adenocarcinoma
			Nonepithelial malignant neoplasm

SOURCE: Reprinted by permission from Dewar MA, Hall K, Perchalski J. Cervical cancer screening. Past success and future challenge. Prim Care 1992;19: 589–606.

II. Screening

A. Screening Modalities

1. Definition of terms—see Chapter 7

2. Papanicolaou (Pap) Smear—cytologic sampling of the surface of the uterine cervix for precancerous or cancerous cells.

   a. Method—Perform before the bimanual examination to maximize the number of cells available.
      1) Visualize the cervix using a vaginal speculum. Do not use lubricant to avoid obscuring cytologic examination.
      2) Obtain ectocervical sample using cervical spatula. Goal is to obtain cells from squamous epithelium and from transformation zone (squamocolumnar junction).
      3) Obtain an endocervical specimen, using either a cotton swab (moistened with saline to avoid dessication of cells), the extended tip of the cervical spatula, an endocervical brush, or an aspiration device. The endocervical brush is thought to be the most effective.

4) In perimenopausal and postmenopausal women, also obtain sample from vaginal pool to screen for endometrial and ovarian cancers.
5) Samples should be rapidly smeared on a clear glass slide. To prevent air drying of cells, smear should be fixed immediately, either by immersing in a fixative, such as 70% alcohol, for 15 min, or by spraying with a fixative, holding the nozzle of the spray can about 10–12 inches from the slide.
6) Quality of the samples is judged by the presence of endocervical cells. If patient is high risk, and no endocervical cells are seen, repeat the Pap smear.

b. Test characteristics: Sensitivity is 50–80%, meaning in 20–50% of cases of CIN will have false negative. The specificity is 98–99%, meaning there are relatively few false positives.

c. Interpretation of results: There have been several changes in the nomenclature for the reporting of Pap test results. The most recently adopted system is the Bethesda system, which incorporates a reporting of the adequacy of the specimen. Table 10-1 compares the various reporting systems.

3. Colposcopy—magnified binocular examination of the cervix.

   a. Used primarily to evaluate the cervix of women with abnormal Pap tests and to direct biopsy of tissue.
   b. Compared to Pap tests as a screening test, it is much more expensive and time consuming.
   c. Colposcopy is more sensitive than Pap test, meaning that there are fewer false negative examinations.
   d. However, specificity is much lower, meaning that there are many false positive examinations. This leads to many biopsies of normal tissue.
   e. Therefore, due to the time and expense involved, as well as the high false positive rate, colposcopy is much less cost effective as a screening test than is the Pap test.

4. Cervicography—magnified photography of the cervix. 5% acetic acid solution is applied to the cervix to maximize the appearance of any abnormal tissue.

   a. Has increased sensitivity over Pap test.
   b. Has decreased specificity, meaning that there will be many false positive cervicograms.
   c. Cervicography does not take significantly more time than Pap test. It is less expensive than colposcopy, although it does involve the purchase of specialized equipment.
   d. There is a high rate of unsatisfactory or technically defective cervicograms in many studies.
   e. Cervicography is more cost effective as a screening test than colposcopy, but due to the need for specialized equipment, Pap testing is still the preferred screening tool.

B. Screening Recommendations

1. Despite the lack of prospective randomized controlled trials demonstrating the Pap smear's effectiveness in reducing morbidity and mortality from cervical

carcinoma, data from historical surveys, cross-cultural correlational studies, and case-control studies document decreased morbidity and mortality. It is therefore no longer ethically possible to perform a prospective randomized controlled trial on Pap testing.

2. Regular Pap testing is recommended for all women who are or who have been sexually active. The controversy regarding Pap testing involves when to start, when to stop, and how often to perform it.

3. Pap testing should begin at the onset of sexual activity. Women who do not engage in sexual activity are at very low risk of cervical carcinoma and do not require screening. Many groups have recommended starting Pap testing at age 18 regardless of reported sexual activity, but this is controversial.

4. The frequency of performing Pap testing once it has been initiated is also controversial. Performing Pap testing q 5 y may decrease incidence of ICC by over 83%. Increasing the frequency to q 3 y decreases the incidence further to over 90%. Further increasing test frequency to yearly only provides an additional several percent reduction in incidence. Therefore, most groups recommend a frequency of q 1-3 y for Pap testing. A reasonable approach, given the long period from CIN to ICC might be to perform Pap testing annually for 3 y consecutively, then extend testing to q 3 y.

5. Whether to continue screening women over age 65 y has also been controversial. The incidence of new cervical carcinoma developing in elderly women is unknown, but is presumed to be quite low. For women who have had regular screening with negative results prior to age 65, there is little additional benefit to further screening. For women who have not had adequate screening previously, it is beneficial and cost effective to perform q 3 y Pap testing. There is little additional benefit of increasing the frequency to yearly.

III. Management of the Pap Test Results

A. Adequate specimen with normal results—repeat q 1-3 y as discussed above.

B. Inadequate specimen with no endocervical cells seen—repeat Pap test, particularly if woman is high risk.

C. Normal Pap test with visible cervical lesion—due to high false negative rate of Pap testing, all women with visible lesions should be referred to a gynecologist for colposcopy.

D. Abnormal smear suggestive of infection—test for infection, and treat empirically or based on findings. Repeat Pap test 1 mo after treatment. If normal, repeat according to regular schedule. If still abnormal, refer for colposcopy.

E. Abnormal smear suggestive of atrophy—if symptomatic, consider short-term treatment with estrogen, either intravaginally or orally.

F. Abnormal Pap smears with squamous intraepithelial lesions (SIN), abnormal glandular cells, or carcinoma (using Bethesda classification)—refer for colposcopy with biopsy. Recommendations the same for CIN, CIS, or ICC, using the older classifications.

IV. Annotated Bibliography

Dewar MA, Hall K, Perchalski J. Cervical cancer screening. Past success and future challenge. Prim Care 1992;19:589–606. A good review of the issues related to screening for cervical cancer.

Fahs MC, Mandelblatt J, Schechter C, Muller C. Cost effectiveness of cervical cancer screening for the elderly. Ann Intern Med 1992;117:520–527. An excellent analysis of the costs and the benefits of alternative screening recommendations for cervical carcinoma in the elderly.

Fink DJ. Change in American Cancer Society checkup guidelines for detection of cervical cancer. The most recent ACS recommendations. CA J Clin 1988;38:127–128.

National Cancer Institute Workshop. The 1988 Bethesda system for reporting cervical/vaginal cytological diagnoses. JAMA 1989;262:931–934. Describes in detail the Bethesda system.

United States Preventive Services Task Force. Screening for Cervical Cancer. Guide to clinical preventive services. Baltimore: Williams & Wilkins, 1989: 57–62. The recommendations of the U. S. Preventive Services Task Force.

Chapter II: The Yearly Physical Examination

Barry Ziring

Many patients and physicians believe that a comprehensive visit and good preventive health care include a thorough physical examination. Yet, when the various portions of the physical examination and routine yearly laboratory tests have been subjected to scientific scrutiny, remarkably few have been proven to have the ability to improve clinical outcomes.

Several commissions including the Canadian Task Force on the Periodic Health Examination, (CTF), the U. S. Preventive Services Task Force (USPSTF) and Obler and LaForce have made recommendations regarding various components of the yearly physical examination.

The recommendations of the various task forces are not identical. The following recommendations represent the ranges suggested by the CTF, USPSTF, and Obler/LaForce for the periodic examination in healthy patients. These recommendations take into account cost effectiveness. The patient's coincidental health problems, risk factors, and the preferences of patient and the physician should be considered.

I. Routine Periodic Examinations (Healthy 19–39 y, Performed q 1–3 y)

A. Leading Causes of Death

1. Motor vehicle accident
2. Homicide
3. Suicide
4. Injuries (non-motor vehicle)
5. Heart disease

B. History

1. Particular attention should be given to:
   a. Dietary intake
   b. Physical activity
   c. Tobacco/alcohol/drug use
   d. Sexual practices

C. Physical Examination

1. Features of demonstrated benefit:

    a. Height and weight
    b. Blood pressure on the initial visit and during visits scheduled for any reason

2. Examinations that are of benefit for particular risk groups

    a. Clinical breast examination—women with first-degree relative who have had premenopausal breast cancer
    b. Testicular examination—men with history of cryptorchidism, orchiopexy, or testicular atrophy
    c. Skin examination—personal history of skin cancer, dysplastic nevus, or unusual sun exposure
    d. Thyroid examination—upper body radiation
    e. Oral examination—heavy smoking or drinking

3. Additional examination is of no demonstrated benefit in large population trials but should be performed at the discretion of the physician and patient.

D. Testing

1. Tests that have demonstrated benefit

    a. Nonfasting total blood cholesterol
    b. Papinicolaou smears

2. Tests that are beneficial for particular risk groups

    a. Fasting glucose—obese or family or gestational history of diabetes
    b. Rubella titer—woman lacking evidence of rubella immunity
    c. High-risk sexual behavior—VDRL, chalymdial and gonorrhea testing, consider HIV testing
    d. Urinalysis for bacteriuria—diabetics
    e. Hearing testing—persons exposed to excessive noise
    f. Purified protein derivative—possible TB exposure
    g. ECG—men who would endanger public safety (such as airline pilots) should a sudden cardiac event occur
    h. Mammogram—women over 35 with first-degree relative with premenopausal breast cancer
    i. Colonoscopy—persons with a family history of familial polyposis or cancer family syndrome

E. Counseling

1. Diet and exercise
2. Substance use
3. Sexual practices
4. Injury prevention
5. Skin protection

F. Immunization (see Appendix A)

1. Tetanus-diptheria booster q 10 y
2. High-risk groups
   a. Homosexually active men, IV drug abusers, or persons with exposure to blood products should receive hepatitis B vaccine.
   b. Persons with chronic cardiac disease or pulmonary disease, sickle cell disease, nephrotic syndrome, Hodgkin's disease, asplenia, diabetes, alcoholism, cirrhosis, multiple myeloma, or leukemia should receive pneumococcal vaccine once and influenza vaccine yearly.
   c. Persons born after 1956 who lack evidence of immunity to measles (receipt of live vaccine on or after first birthday, laboratory evidence of immunity, or physician diagnosis of measles) should receive measles or measles-mumps-rubella vaccine.

II. Routine Periodic Examination (Patients 40 and Older)

A. Leading Causes of Death

1. Heart disease
2. Lung cancer
3. Cerebrovascular disease
4. Breast cancer
5. Colorectal cancer
6. Obstructive lung disease

B. History—similar to that for patients aged 19–39 y

C. Physical Examination

1. Features of demonstrated benefit
   a. Height and weight measurement q 1–4 y
   b. Blood pressure checked q 2–5 y and at the time of visits for other reasons
   c. Hearing screening after age 60 especially if history is positive for hearing loss
   d. Yearly vision screen after age 60
   e. Clinical breast examination—yearly after age 40
   f. Abdominal examination for aortic aneurysm—should be considered after age 60 yearly
2. Examinations that are of benefit for particular risk groups—similar to age 19–39
3. Additional tests—screening for colon cancer and prostate cancer discussed in Chapters 8 and 9.

D. Testing

1. Tests that have demonstrated benefit

a. Nonfasting total cholesterol levels should be checked q 5 y in patients with no history of elevated cholesterol.
b. Pap smear—q 1–5 y after age 18 (see Chapter 10)
c. Mammography—frequency is controversial (see Chapter 7)

2. Tests for particular risk groups are similar to age 19–40

E. Counseling

1. Diet and exercise
2. Substance use
3. Sexual practices
4. Injury prevention
5. Skin protection

F. Immunization (see Appendix B)

1. Tetanus-diptheria booster q 10 y
2. Consider giving pneumococcal vaccine once after age 55
3. Influenza vaccine yearly after age 65

III. See Chapter 54 for Preventive Issues in the Elderly

IV. Annotated Bibliography

Canadian Task Force on the Periodic Health Examination. The periodic health examination. Can Med Assoc J 1979;121:1193–1254. The landmark study of 78 elements of the periodic health examination.

Fink DJ. Guidelines for the cancer related check-up. Atlanta: American Cancer Society; 1991. Tend to recommend more aggressive screening guidelines than the national task forces.

Hayward RSA, Steinberg EP, Ford DE, et al. Preventative care guidelines: 1991. Ann Intern Med 1991;114:758–783. The most recent compilation of available guidelines from the ACP, CTF, USPSTF, and other well known authorities.

National Cancer Institute PDQ Cancer Information. Cancer screening guidelines. Bethesda, MD: National Cancer Institute; 1992.

Obler SR, LaForce FM. The periodic physical examination in asymptomatic adults. Ann Intern Med 1989;110:214–226. Also a compilation of available data but includes authors recommendations.

U.S. Preventive Services Task Force. Guide to clinical preventive services: an assessment of the effectiveness of 169 interventions. Baltimore: Williams & Wilkins; 1989. An exhaustive work evaluating 169 interventions by a panel of 20 experts from medicine and related fields.

Chapter 12: Travel Medicine

Carol M. Reife

Detailed information regarding recommendations for international travel is available from the Centers for Disease Control and Prevention (CDC) in the book *Health Information for International Travel*, which is published annually. It can be obtained by writing to:
Superintendent of Documents
U. S. Government Printing Office
Washington, DC 20402

Up-to-date automated information is also available by calling the CDC at 404-332-4559.

I. General Information

A. It is recommended that travelers carry information detailing any medical problems with them. The following may be useful as well:

1. Prescription medication—Extra amounts should be carried as well as a written prescription with the generic name of medications in case additional amounts are needed.

2. Pain relief—ASA, acetaminophen, ibuprofen

3. Cold symptoms—antihistamines, decongestants

4. Motion sickness—scopolamine, antihistamines

5. Sunscreen

6. Insect repellent

7. Eyeglasses/contact lenses—an additional pair as well as the lens prescription

II. AIDS

A. Travelers should be reminded of the risk of AIDS worldwide.

B. Risk is related *more to behavior than to area of travel* and may be transmitted through sexual contact, use of contaminated needles, or blood transfusion.

C. In some undeveloped areas, programs available for testing blood for HIV antibodies may be inadequate and transfusions should be avoided if possible.

III. Traveler's Diarrhea

A. Definition

1. Three or more loose bowel movements daily or loose stools associated with fever, vomiting or abdominal cramps.
2. Patients who develop acute diarrhea within a week of returning from abroad probably have traveler's diarrhea. Symptoms are usually self-limited.

B. Etiology

1. The most common cause of traveler's diarrhea is infection with enterotoxigenic *Escherichia coli, Campylobacter, Shigella, Salmonella,* viruses, and parasites are less common causes.
2. Risk of infection can be reduced by avoiding
    a. Uncooked vegetables
    b. Unpeeled fruit
    c. Foods cooked or stored at insufficient temperatures
    d. Ice or nonbottled water

C. Prophylaxis

1. Although antibiotics have been proven to be effective in preventing diarrhea, their routine use has been discouraged due to the risk of emergence of resistant strains, medication side effects, and cost.
2. Prophylactic regimens should be considered in travelers with concomitant illnesses for whom an episode of diarrhea could cause decompensation in their medical condition. Protection is limited to the time of administration.
3. Various prophylactic regimens include:
    a. Bismuth subsalicylate (Pepto-Bismol) 2 tablets q.i.d.
    b. Trimethoprim/sulfamethoxazole (TMP/SMX) (160/800 mg): 1 tablet daily
    c. Doxycycline 100 mg once daily
    d. Trimethoprim 200 mg once daily
    e. Ciprofloxacin 500 mg once daily
    f. Norfloxacin 400 mg once daily

D. Treatment

Adequate replacement of fluid and electrolytes with juices, soft drinks or electrolyte-containing solutions plays a key role in the treatment of diarrheal episodes. Recommended treatment regimens include:

1. Bismuth subsalicylate 2 tablets 4 times daily

2. Loperamide hydrochloride (Imodium): 4 mg to start, then 2 mg after each loose bowel movement to a maximum of 16 mg daily—to be taken in combination with one of the antibiotic regimens below.
3. TMP-SMX (160/800 mg) 1 tablet b.i.d.
4. Ciprofloxacin 500 mg b.i.d.
5. Norfloxacin 400 mg b.i.d.
6. Ofloxacin 300 mg b.i.d.
7. Antibiotic should be started when diarrhea begins and should be continued for 3–5 d or until symptoms resolve.

IV. Tuberculosis

A. Travelers taking short trips for business or pleasure are not at great risk for developing tuberculosis.

B. Travelers working in hospitals, schools, or other facilities abroad may be at increased risk of exposure to TB.

C. Travelers at risk should have purified protein derivative (PPD) placed prior to travel and again approximately 12 wk after return if the original PPD is negative.

D. Management of those who convert to a positive PPD should be in keeping with guidelines for any PPD conversion.

V. Malaria Chemoprophylaxis

A. Countries that carry a risk of malaria can be determined by called the CDC at 404-332-4559.

B. Risk of acquiring malaria varies depending on itinerary, length of stay, and underlying medical condition of the traveler.

C. No prophylactic regimen is completely effective in preventing malaria. Because mosquitoes feed from dusk to dawn, travelers should leave areas where malaria is transmitted before dusk. Risk of mosquito bites can be decreased by wearing clothing with long sleeves and long pants, and by using window screens, room sprays, mosquito nets for beds, and insect repellents containing 15–20% diethyltoluamide.

D. The following are recommended regimens for prevention
1. Chloroquine-sensitive areas (Mexico, Haiti, Dominican Republic, parts of Central America, and most of the Mideast): chloroquine 300 mg weekly beginning 1 wk prior to and continuing for 4 wk after exposure. (This is the drug of choice.)

2. Chloroquine-resistant areas (check with the CDC at the number on page 59)
   a. Mefloquine 250 mg weekly beginning 1 wk prior to and continuing for 4 wk after exposure. (This is the drug of choice.)
   b. Doxycycline 100 mg daily beginning 1 wk prior to and continuing for 4 wk after exposure.
   c. Chloroquine phosphate 300 mg weekly beginning 1 wk prior to and continuing for 4 wk after exposure **plus** either:
      1) Pyramethamine/sulfadoxine (25 mg/500 mg) 3 tablets to be taken together at the first sign of fever
         or
      2) Proguanil 200 mg daily beginning 1 wk prior to and continuing for 4 wk after exposure

VI. Immunizations

A. Cholera

1. The risk of cholera for travelers is generally so low that benefit of vaccination is questionable. Cholera vaccine provides only about 50% protective immunity and is not generally recommended for tourists.
2. Travelers to areas at increased risk (Peru, Ecuador, Colombia) should avoid drinking untreated water or eating raw fish, uncooked vegetables, or unpeeled fruit.
3. Some countries do require a validated cholera vaccination for travelers coming from cholera endemic areas.
4. Primary vaccination for cholera consists of 2 doses of the inactivated parenteral vaccine SQ or IM at least 1 wk apart. Booster doses are given every 6 mo if risk of exposure continues.

B. Hepatitis A

1. Risk of acquiring hepatitis A is increased in areas where hygiene is poor, especially areas outside of the usual tourist routes. Infection can be prevented by giving immune globulin.
2. A dose of .02 mL/kg IM (usually a total dose of 2 mL) is recommended for trips of < 3 mo and a dose of .06 mL/kg IM (usually a total dose of 5 mL) for longer stays, repeated q 5 mo. Immune globulin should be given close to the time of travel.
3. A vaccine against hepatitis A is currently available in Europe but is not currently licensed for use in the United States.

C. Hepatitis B

1. Hepatitis B vaccine is not recommended for routine travel.
2. It may be indicated for those at risk for exposure to blood or body fluids such as medical personnel and relief workers, those who expect to have sexual

contact abroad, or those who spend long periods of time in areas where hepatitis B is endemic, such as parts of Asia and Africa.

3. There is currently a plasma-derived inactivated viral vaccine as well as two recombinant vaccines produced from yeast.
4. Vaccination consists of 3 doses—1 cc given at 0, 1 and 6 mo.
5. Testing is advised after vaccination to confirm the presence of antibody.

D. Polio

1. Polio vaccine is indicated for travelers to certain developing countries where polio is endemic.
2. If a primary series has never been completed, enhanced potency inactivated polio vaccine (eIPV) should be given as a 3-dose series: Doses 1 and 2 are given SQ or IM 4–8 wk apart and dose 3 is given 6 wk after dose 2.
3. If there is insufficient time to complete the full primary series, a single dose of eIPV or OPV (trivalent live oral polio vaccine) should be given.
4. Travelers who completed a primary series in childhood should receive a booster dose of either eIPV or OPV.

E. **Tetanus and Diptheria**

1. Tetanus and diptheria still pose significant health problems in certain areas of the world, especially for those who are unimmunized or inadequately immunized.
2. Everyone (regardless of travel plans) should receive a primary series as well as a booster dose q 10 y.
3. The primary series consists of Td (tetanus and diphtheria toxoids absorbed) in 3 doses of 0.5 mL given SQ or IM. Doses 1 and 2 are given 4–8 wk apart and dose 3 is given 6 mo later.

F. **Typhoid**

1. The risk of typhoid fever to Americans traveling abroad is small but may be increased in some areas (Mexico, India, Peru, Pakistan, Chile).
2. The parenteral vaccine has been found not to be fully protective but is sometimes easier to obtain than the newer oral vaccine. Parenteral vaccine is given in 2 doses 4 wk apart as a primary series and a booster after 3 y or more. Side effects may be troublesome and include soreness at the injection site, headache, fever, and malaise.
3. The live oral vaccine is at least as effective and has fewer side effects. It is given as one enteric-coated capsule every other day for a total of 4 capsules beginning at least 2 wk before departure.

G. Yellow Fever

1. Risk of transmission of yellow fever to travelers is low but may be increased when epidemic conditions arise. Vaccination is recommended for travel to rural areas of yellow fever endemic countries (parts of South America and Africa). Some countries require a certificate of vaccination prior to entry especially if travel is from an infected or endemic area.

2. The vaccine is only available in centers specifically designated by local or state health departments. A single dose of vaccine is given SQ for primary vaccinations and becomes effective after 10 d. Boosters are given q 10 y.

VII. Annotated Bibliography

Advice for travelers. Med Lett 1992;34 (issue 869): May 1. Concise summary of major topics a physician should be familiar with when advising travelers.

Drugs for parasitic infections. Med Lett 1992;34 (issue 865): March. Concise summary of recommendations for treatment of parasitic infections including prophylaxis for maleria.

Health Information for International Travel. U.S. Department of Health and Human Services, Centers for Disease Control and Prevention. U.S. Government Printing Office, Washington, DC. Easy to use reference including recommendations for all countries as well as detailed information on different immunizations and treatment regimens.

Wolfe MS. Travel medicine. Med Clin North Am 1992;7:1261–1294, 1327–1374. Concise summary of major topics a physician should be familiar with when advising travelers.

Chapter 13: Involuntary Weight Loss

Kenneth R. Epstein

I. General Information

A. Obesity is a major health problem in this country, and many people present to their physicians asking for assistance with losing weight. This chapter, however, will only deal with those persons presenting with involuntary weight loss, defined as an involuntary loss of > 5% of an individual's usual body weight in a 6–12-mo period.

B. It is important to identify weight loss even in those individuals with known diagnoses. For instance, survival with cancer is shorter in those patients with weight loss. This worse prognosis is independent of tumor extent or performance status.

C. The mechanisms of weight loss include decreased food intake, increased metabolism, or a loss of calories in the urine or stool. Frequently, several of these mechanisms exist in an individual patient.

D. Although it is important to differentiate anorexia from weight loss, the differential diagnoses are similar. It is particularly important to consider anorexia in the evaluation of weight loss in the elderly.

II. Diagnostic Approach

A. In an individual with a history of weight loss, try to document the actual loss of weight. Approximately one half of patients who claim to have lost weight have not by objective recordings. Conversely, some elderly patients may not complain of weight loss, so it is important to document weights with each visit.

B. The key to diagnosing the etiology of involuntary weight loss is a thorough history and physical, searching for the presence of a systemic illness. This includes a good psychiatric history looking for depression (see Chapter 83). Section III below reviews some of the specific diseases to look for.

C. Several screening tests are indicated in almost all patients with unexplained weight loss.

1. Chest x-ray—the most useful test. In one study, 41% of patients with a physical cause of weight loss had abnormalities on radiography, such as an infiltrate, mass, pulmonary edema, or adenopathy.
2. Serum chemistries—look particularly for abnormalities on hepatic function tests and serum calcium.
3. Complete blood count—many patients will be anemic.
4. Urinalysis—particularly look for glycosuria or proteinuria.
5. In one study, 66% of patients with a physical cause of weight loss had an abnormality on one of the above four tests.
6. In patients with gastrointestinal symptoms, an upper GI series is useful.
7. Additional laboratory and radiologic tests should be based on the diagnoses suspected by history and physical examination. Physical causes will almost always declare themselves within 6 mo. Watchful waiting is therefore appropriate if the initial evaluation is negative.

D. In 65% of patients with weight loss, a physical cause can be found, and in another 10%, a psychiatric cause will be found. In approximately 25% of patients, no identifiable cause is found.

III. Differential Diagnosis

A. Medical Causes

1. Neoplasia

    a. Lung
    b. Gastrointestinal especially gastric and pancreatic
    c. Lymphomas
    d. Genitourinary—prostrate and ovarian
    e. Any cancer may present with weight loss.

2. Gastrointestinal

    a. Inflammatory bowel disease
    b. Malabsorption from a variety of diseases
    c. Esophageal dysmotility
    d. Peptic ulcer disease
    e. Diabetic enteropathy
    f. Cholelithiasis
    g. Atrophic gastritis
    h. Oral disease, including dental disease and poorly fitting dentures

3. Metabolic

    a. Hyperthyroidism
    b. Hypothyroidism—in the elderly, may cause anorexia and apathy resulting in weight loss
    c. Diabetes mellitus—may be associated with increased food intake

4. Cardiovascular

    a. Class III or IV congestive heart failure
    b. Mesenteric ischemia

5. Pulmonary

    a. Chronic obstructive pulmonary disease

6. Infectious

    a. Tuberculosis
    b. HIV infection
    c. Abscesses
    d. Subacute bacterial endocarditis
    e. Systemic fungal infections

7. Alcoholism—often related to the social/psychiatric causes listed below

8. Renal failure—One of the first manifestations of uremia is anorexia.

9. Connective tissue diseases

    a. Rheumatoid arthritis
    b. Scleroderma

10. Drug-induced—anorexia or gastrointestinal side effects of medications. This risk is increased by the prescription of multiple medications, particularly in the elderly.

11. Neurologic

    a. Advanced parkinsonism
    b. Stroke

B. Psychiatric Causes

1. Depression

2. Dementia

3. Paranoid psychosis

C. Social Causes

1. Economic hardship

2. Social isolation in those who live alone

3. Inability to shop for food

4. In an institutional setting, failure to consider ethnic tastes

IV. Treatment

A. The most important aspect of treatment is to treat the underlying medical or psychiatric cause of the weight loss.

B. If social causes are responsible for weight loss in the elderly, consider

1. Have patient eat in a congregate setting
2. Meals-on-Wheels programs
3. Economic assistance programs

C. If the patient is in nutritional deficit, then consider oral nutritional supplementation.

D. Megestrol Acetate

1. Has been studied in both cancer and AIDS patients
2. Is a synthetic, orally active progestational agent; it is extremely expensive
3. Has been documented in several studies to increase appetite, resulting in increased caloric intake and nonfluid weight gain
4. Dosage range is 400–1600 mg/d. Usually start with 160 mg, and titrate up as necessary. Increasing doses have been shown to increase appetite and weight gain.

E. Corticosteroids have also been shown to increase appetite in cancer patients.

V. Indications for Hospitalization

If patient requires enteral or parenteral nutritional support due to life-threatening malnutrition

VI. Annotated Bibliography

Loprinzi CL, Goldberg RM, Burnham NL. Cancer-associated anorexia and cachexia. Implications for drug therapy. Drugs 1992;43:499–506. A review of the literature on the use of various agents, including megestrol acetate, for the treatment of cancer-related weight loss.

Marton KI, Sox HC, Krupp JR. Involuntary weight loss: diagnostic and prognostic significance. Ann Intern Med 1981;95:568–574. A prospective study of patients presenting with involuntary weight loss, identifying the causes, and useful diagnostic tests.

Morley JE. Anorexia in older patients: its meaning and management. Geriatrics 1990;45:59–66. A good review of the evaluation and management of anorexia and involuntary weight loss in the elderly.

Chapter 14: Evaluation of the Chronically Fatigued Patient

Kenneth R. Epstein

I. Clinical Presentation

A. General Information

1. Fatigue is the seventh most common complaint in primary care, accounting for over 10 million office visits per year.

2. The prevalence of fatigue is in the range of 21–24% and is higher for women than for men.

3. Fatigue is classified as acute when it has been present < 6 mo. This chapter specifically deals with evaluation of the chronically fatigued patient and reviews the chronic fatigue syndrome (CFS).

B. Symptoms

1. By definition, the patient's primary complaint is > 6 mo of fatigue.

2. A complete and detailed history should be obtained to rule out the presence of an organic or psychiatric illness causing the chronic fatigue.

3. Table 14–1 presents the Centers for Disease Control and Prevention (CDC) definition of CFS.

4. The CDC definition was created to provide uniformity for research and epidemiologic purposes. Only 19–30% of patients with chronic fatigue meet the CDC criteria for CFS.

5. The frequency of symptoms in patients who meet the CDC definition of CFS is shown in Table 14–2.

6. As described in more detail under diagnosis, the symptoms of CFS can overlap the symptoms of psychiatric illness such as depression and fibrositis (fibromyalgia), as well as other psychophysiologic diseases such as irritable bowel syndrome, chronic headaches, and primary dysmennorrhea.

C. Physical Examination

1. A careful and detailed physical examination should be performed to rule out the presence of an organic illness causing the chronic fatigue.

2. There are usually no physical signs in the patient with CFS.

3. Physical findings consistent with the diagnosis of CFS are listed in Table 14–1.

Table 14-1. Center for Disease Control and Prevention Case Definition of Chronic Fatigue Syndrome

A case of CFS must fulfill major criteria 1 and 2, and 8 of the symptom criteria, or 6 of the symptom criteria with 2 of the physical criteria.

Major Criteria

1. New onset of persistent or relapsing, debilitating fatigue in a person with no previous history of similar symptoms, that does not resolve with bed rest, and that decreases daily activity by $> 50\%$ for > 6 mo.
2. Other clinical conditions that may produce chronic fatigue must be ruled out, based on history, physical examination, and selected laboratory tests.

Minor Criteria

Symptom Criteria:

1. Mild fever ($< 38.6°C$) or chills
2. Sore throat
3. Painful cervical or axillary lymph nodes
4. Unexplained generalized muscle weakness
5. Muscle discomfort or myalgia
6. > 24 h of generalized fatigue after levels of exercise easily tolerated previously
7. Generalized headaches
8. Migratory arthralgias without arthritis
9. Neuropsychologic complaints (photophobia, transient visual scotomata, forgetfulness, irritability, confusion, difficulty thinking, inability to concentrate, depression)
10. Hypersomnia or insomnia
11. Onset of the symptom complex over a few hours to days

Physical Criteria:

1. Low-grade fever ($< 38.6°C$ orally or $38.8°C$ rectally)
2. Nonexudative pharyngitis
3. Palpable or tender cervical or axillary lymphadenopathy, 2 cm.

SOURCE: Adapted from Holmes GP, Kaplan JE, Gantz NM, et al. Chronic fatigue syndrome: a working definition. Ann Intern Med 1988;108:387–389.

II. Diagnostic Approach and Differential Diagnosis

A. General Guidelines

1. A complete history and physical examination are essential to look for the presence of primary organic or psychiatric disease as the etiology of the chronic fatigue.

Table 14-2. Frequency of Symptoms in Patients with Chronic Fatigue Syndrome

Symptom	Frequency (%)
Fatigue	100
Impaired cognition	90
Arthralgias	85
Postexertional malaise	85
Depression	80
Fever	80
Myalgias	80
Headache	75
Muscle weakness	75
Pharyngitis	75
Sleep disorder	75
Enlarged or painful lymph nodes	50

SOURCE: Reprinted by permission from Klonoff DC. Chronic fatigue syndrome. Clin Infect Dis 1992;15:812-823.

2. Of patients presenting with chronic fatigue
   a. 20-45% will have an organic etiology
   b. 40-45% will have primary psychiatric diagnoses
   c. 19-30% will meet CDC criteria for CFS

B. Medical Disorders

1. Almost any chronic disease may result in fatigue. The differential diagnosis for chronic fatigue includes infections, malignancies, connective tissue disease, endocrinopathies, neurologic diseases, and primary sleep disorders. Almost all of these can be excluded by history and physical examination.

2. A few selected laboratory tests are usually indicated to screen for the presence of organic disease. Baseline laboratory tests that should be ordered include
   a. Complete blood count with differential
   b. Chemistry profile (including creatinine, glucose, calcium, and liver enzymes)
   c. Erythrocyte sedimentation rate
   d. Thyroid-stimulating hormone
   e. Urinalysis

3. Additional laboratory and radiologic tests should be based on clinical suspicion. For instance, if myalgias and arthralgias are prominent symptoms, then an antinuclear antibody (ANA) and rheumatoid factor might be ordered.

4. In the absence of clinical suspicion, a "fishing expedition" to find an organic disease to explain the patient's symptoms is not indicated and can be potentially detrimental to the patient.

C. Psychiatric Disorders

1. As with medical disorders, almost any psychiatric disease may present as chronic fatigue. The most common disorders include affective disorders (depression, bipolar disorder), anxiety disorders, and somatoform disorders. Most of these disorders can be excluded by history.
2. A psychiatric disorder as the etiology of chronic fatigue should be especially suspected in the presence of
    a. A gradual or insidious onset of symptoms
    b. No accompanying somatic symptoms
    c. A history of prior psychiatric disorders
    d. Presence of other symptoms suggestive of psychiatric disease

D. Chronic Fatigue Syndrome

1. The etiology of CFS is currently unknown. Much of the controversy centers around whether CFS represents a specific disorder or a common biologic response to disparate conditions. There are three main theories at present—postinfectious, psychiatric, and immunologic.
2. Postinfectious—No one infectious agent has been found to be causally related to CFS.
    a. Upper respiratory infection (URI)—Since viral URI's are so common, many patients with any illness will have recently recovered from one. There does not seem to be a causal relationship between prior viral URI's and CFS.
    b. Epstein-Barr virus (EBV)—95% of adults over age 30 will have serologic evidence of prior EBV infection. This is usually manifested as positive anti-Epstein-Barr nuclear antigen (anti-EBNA), IgG antibody to viral capsid antigen (IgG-VCA), and rarely antibody to the early antigen (anti-EA). Therefore, many patients with CFS will have serologic evidence of past EBV infection. It does not appear that CFS patients are any more likely to have positive titers than are non-CFS patients.
    c. Other viruses—Several other viruses have been studied as potential etiologic agents for CFS. These include enteroviruses, human herpesvirus 6, herpes simplex virus, cytomegalovirus, and retroviruses, specifically human T lymphotropic virus type 2 (HTLV-2). In no case has a causative relationship been found on subsequent investigation.
3. Psychiatric—The degree to which psychiatric illness plays a role in CFS is controversial.
    a. The initial CDC definition of CFS excluded patients with psychiatric illness from meeting the criteria for CFS.
    b. A recent National Institutes of Health workshop proposed a clarification. Patients with nonpsychotic depression, somatoform disorders, and

generalized anxiety or panic disorders may now be considered to have CFS. Exclusions remain for psychotic depression, bipolar disorder, and schizophrenia.

c. In some studies, up to two thirds of CFS patients have coexistent psychiatric illness. Half the patients have depression, and the remainder have anxiety or somatoform disorders.

d. To further confuse the picture, the direction of causality can be unclear. A patient with depression may develop the symptoms of CFS, but a patient with CFS for another reason may also develop a secondary, reactive depression due to the profound loss of function that may result from this disorder.

4. Immunologic

a. Immunologic defects that have been reported in CFS include partial hypogammaglobulinemia, elevated circulating immune complex levels, decreased interferon and interleukin synthesis, increased helper to suppressor lymphocyte ratios, and decreased natural killer cell activity.

b. Most of these immunologic findings are highly variable, and no one abnormality occurs in the majority of patients. Additionally, the degree of abnormality does not correlate with the severity of symptoms.

c. It has been hypothesized that some degree of immune dysfunction may result from many of the infections and psychiatric illnesses described above, and that it is the resultant immune dysfunction that causes CFS.

III. Management

A. Goals

1. Provide emotional support

2. Educate patient

3. Relieve symptoms

B. Patient Education and Support

1. Explain to the patient that fatigue is a common symptom and the symptoms are legitimate.

2. It is essential that the physician not underestimate the degree of functional disability that the patient is suffering from. Most patients with CFS have significant functional limitations.

3. Explain that CFS is a real illness. Although it is poorly understood, it is not life threatening and is rarely progressive. Many patients have significant symptomatic improvement over the course of months or years.

4. Initially, it may be useful to minimize stressful activities, both to improve energy and to avoid any potential immunosuppression.

5. It is important to acknowledge the patient's diagnostic and therapeutic beliefs, even if the physician disagrees.

C. Symptomatic Therapy

1. The choice of agents is based on the predominant symptoms that the patient is uncomfortable from.
2. For headaches, myalgias, and arthralgias, nonsteroidal anti-inflammatory agents may be helpful.
3. For depressive symptoms and sleep disturbances, antidepressants are indicated. Antidepressants are also useful for the chronic pain.
   a. The choice of agents is based on the desired effects and the side effect profile.
   b. If treating symptoms of insomnia and restlessness, then a sedating antidepressant is indicated. Start with a low dose of an agent such as amitriptyline 25 mg qhs or doxepin 10–20 mg qhs.
   c. If primary complaints are excess fatigue, hypersomnia, and psychomotor retardation, then use a selective serotonin reuptake inhibitor such as fluoxetine or sertraline or a less sedating tricyclic agent such as nortriptyline.
   d. Some patients are resistant to the concept that depression may be playing a role in their illness. It is therefore useful to explain that antidepressants are the indicated medication for their symptoms even if they are not depressed.

D. Other Medications

1. No data support the use of other agents for the treatment of CFS.
2. Medications that have been discussed in the literature for which there is no proven benefit include antivirals such as acyclovir, vitamins, γ globulin, liver extract-folic acid-cyanocobolamin, or trace minerals.
3. The potential for a strong placebo effect in CFS must be kept in mind in evaluating any reported therapy.

IV. Indications for Referral

A. If a primary psychiatric illness is suspected, then referral to a psychiatrist is appropriate. Some patients resist referral, but will allow the prescription of psychopharmacologic agents.

B. If an organic illness is determined to be the etiology of the chronic fatigue, then referral to the relevant specialist may be indicated.

V. Annotated Bibliography

Holmes GP, Kaplan GP, Gantz NM, et al. Chronic fatigue syndrome: a working case definition. Ann Intern Med 1988;108:387–389. The article that first officially defined the term "chronic fatigue syndrome," and presented the CDC definition of the syndrome.

Klonoff DC. Chronic fatigue syndrome. Clin Infect Dis 1992;15:812–823. An excellent review of the current state of knowledge as of 1992.

Kroenke K, Wood DR, Margelsdorff A, Meier NJ, Powell JB. Chronic fatigue in primary care. JAMA 1988;260:929–934. A good epidemiologic review of the prevalence, etiology, and outcome of chronically fatigued patients in a primary care setting.

Schluederberg A, Straus S, Peterson P, et al. Chronic fatigue syndrome research. Ann Intern Med 1992;117:325–331. A review of the outcome of a National Institutes of Health workshop held in 1991 to review the strengths and weaknesses of the CDC definition of CFS and to present recommendations for modifications of the definition.

Chapter 15: Smoking Cessation/Nicotine Dependence

Susan E. West

I. Clinical Presentation

A. Tobacco use is the single largest cause of preventable morbidity and mortality in this country; it is responsible for 1 in every 5 deaths.

B. Adult smoking prevalence has decreased to about 25%.

C. Teen smoking has not decreased; smoking among teenage girls has increased.

II. Health Consequences

A. Cancer
1. Lung
2. Larynx
3. Mouth
4. Esophagus
5. Bladder
6. Kidney
7. Pancreas
8. Smoking has also been associated with stomach, cervical, and hematopoietic cancers.

B. Cardiovascular
1. Myocardial infarction
2. Sudden death
3. Stroke
4. Peripheral vascular disease

C. Pulmonary

1. Chronic obstructive pulmonary disease
2. Airway hyperresponsiveness
3. Recurrent sinusitis
4. Recurrent upper respiratory illnesses

D. Environmental Tobacco Smoke

1. Lung cancer in nonsmokers
2. Children have higher incidence of respiratory infections and asthma.

E. Pregnant women who smoke have a higher incidence of babies with low birth weight, sudden infant death syndrome (SIDS), behavior problems, and learning disabilities.

F. Other

1. Accelerated osteoporosis
2. Peptic ulcer disease
3. Skin wrinkling
4. Diminished fertility

III. Health Benefits of Smoking Cessation

A. Substantially reduced morbidity and mortality following smoking cessation, even in smokers > 65 y old.

B. Lung cancer risk drops significantly after 10 y of abstinence but never reaches the low levels of those who never smoked.

C. After 10 y of abstinence, the risk of head and neck, esophagus, pancreas, and bladder cancers approaches that of nonsmokers.

D. Smoking cessation rapidly reduces the risk of myocardial infarction (50% decrease in risk of second infarction within first postinfarct year). Risk of stroke, abdominal aortic aneurysm, and peripheral vascular disease greatly diminish.

E. Ex-smokers have fewer respiratory infections, cough, wheezing and dyspnea; the improvement occurs immediately.

F. Health benefits of stopping smoking far exceed the risks from the average 5-lb weight gain.

IV. Why Should Physicians Intervene?

A. At least 70% of American smokers visit a doctor each year.

B. 70% of smokers say firm, supportive messages from their physician would be very important in stopping smoking.

C. However, up to 75% of smokers state their physicians never counseled them to quit.

D. The public does not understand the risk of smoking. Half of smokers surveyed did not know that smoking causes heart attacks, and even fewer knew smoking is the major cause of emphysema and chronic bronchitis.

V. Smoking Cessation Intervention—4 As

A. Ask all patients about smoking at every opportunity.

B. Advise all smokers to quit, citing consequences of smoking that are meaningful to them as individuals.

C. Assist patients in quitting.

D. Arrange follow-up.

VI. History

A. Ask patients about smoking.
1. Place smoking on problem list.
2. Ask whether the patient has ever thought about, tried or actually did quit. Assess whether patient is in
    a. Precontemplation—not seriously considering quitting
    b. Contemplation stage—seriously planning to stop
    c. Action—trying to stop
    d. Maintenance—trying to avoid relapse
3. If patient is in precontemplative stage, motivate patient to stop based on factors important to that individual.
    a. Fear of death or lung disease may not impress teenagers; discussing issues of decreased attractiveness (tobacco smell, stained teeth, wrinkles) or decreased athletic prowess may be better inducements.
    b. Fear of death or loss of limb may be a powerful motivation in a patient with atherosclerotic disease.
    c. Fear of harming children in the house may induce parents to quit.

4. If patient is in contemplative stage:
   a. Set a quit date
   b. Provide self-help material. Call 1-800-4-CANCER for material from National Cancer Institute
   c. Consider nicotine replacement therapy—assess the degree of nicotine addiction. Patients may benefit from nicotine replacement therapy if
      1) Patient smokes while bedbound from illness
      2) Patient smokes within 30 min of arising
      3) Ask which cigarette of the day is most important. If it is the first cigarette of the day, it is likely he or she experiences nicotine withdrawal in the morning.
      4) Patient craves a cigarette in situations in which smoking is not allowed (eg, domestic flights, smoke-free office)
      5) Patient smokes one pack per day or more

VII. Nicotine Replacement Therapy

A. Nicotine Gum

1. Requires detailed instruction in its use; slow methodical chewing and pauses are necessary.

2. Improperly trained and supervised patients may become ill from chewing too much or too rapidly, with nausea, abdominal pain, dizziness, and headaches.

3. Not as effective as nicotine patches.

B. Nicotine Transdermal Patches

1. Patient must stop smoking altogether; smoking in addition to nicotine patches or gum may produce a nicotine overdose.

2. Usual starting dose of Habitrol, Nicoderm, and Prostep is 21 mg/d patch, applied to skin of upper body or arm daily. Recommended dosing schedule is 6 wk at 21 mg/d, 2 wk at 14 mg/d, and 2 wk at 7 mg/d. Another brand, Nicotrol, recommends 15 mg/d patch for 12 wk, then 10 mg × 2 wk and 5 mg × 2 wk.

3. Start with smaller dose, eg, 14 mg/d patch if patient
   a) Has cardiovascular disease
   b) Weighs < 100 lb
   c) Smokes < 1/2 pack/d

4. Nicotine patches should not be removed at bedtime because patients may awaken with withdrawal symptoms

5. NOTE: At cessation of smoking, may require an increased dose of imipramine, oxazepim, pentazocine, propranolol, theophylline, insulin, and adrenergic antagonists. May require a decreased dose of adrenergic agonists.

VIII. Behavior Modification to Break the Habit

A. Advise ways to break familiar habit chains, and help patient find other ways to relax.

1. Stop automatic smoking. Keep cigarettes in a different place and use opposite hand to hold it.

2. Make smoking inconvenient
   a. Don't buy cartons.
   b. Don't carry cigarettes with you.
   c. Fill the car ashtray with potpourri.

3. Make smoking unpleasant. Do not watch TV, talk to others, or perform other activities while smoking. Only smoke standing up, outside if possible, and focus only on the cigarette and its consequences.

4. Consider occupying your hands or mouth with gum, low-calorie foods, fake cigarette.

5. Exercise

6. Initially, avoid situations strongly associated with smoking (eg, cocktails).

7. Relaxation training

8. Reward abstinence (eg, using money previously spent on cigarettes)

IX. Other

A. Standardized programs, such as multiweek Smoke-Enders and other programs are available for patients who can afford them. Studies have shown that a brief physician intervention in the office has the same success rate.

B. Hypnosis has helped some patients refractory to all other therapies.

X. Helping Patient Maintain Abstinence

A. Schedule follow-up visits or phone calls.

B. Ask about smoking at each visit.

C. Advise about weight gain. Average of 5 lb can be minimized by initiation or increase in exercise programs.

XI. Annotated Bibliography

Fiore MC, ed. Cigarette smoking: a clinical guide to assessment and treatment. Med Clin North Am 1992;76(2). Entire volume is devoted to cigarette smoking, including health risks, environmental smoke, the health benefits of quitting, and ways to combat nicotine dependence.

Fiore MC, Jorenby DE, Baker TB, Kenford SL. Tobacco dependence and the nicotine patch: clinical guidelines for effective use. JAMA 1992;268:2687–2694. Practical discussion of the pharmacology and use of nicotine patches, including recommendations for special populations such as those with cardiovascular disease.

How to help your patients stop smoking: Guideline for diagnosis and treatment of nicotine dependence, 1994 published by the American Medical Association.

Samet JM, Coultas D. Smoking cessation. Clin Chest Med 1991;12(4). Again, an entire volume of well-written articles on smoking, nicotine addiction, health effects, and ways to assist patients in smoking cessation. Unfortunately, its discussions precede the introduction of nicotine patches.

Part III:
Allergy

Chapter 16: Allergic Rhinitis

Karen S. Scoles

I. Clinical Presentation

A. General Information

1. 20% of U.S. population will experience allergic rhinitis at sometime in their lifetime.

2. Symptoms decrease after age 40 in most patients.

3. Allergic rhinitis can have several etiologies.

   a. Seasonal allergic rhinitis caused by pollens, pollen fragments, and mold spores
   b. Perennial allergic rhinitis: chronic nasal symptoms due to perennial allergens, such as household dust mites, resembles seasonal allergic rhinitis, but symptoms are present year round.
   c. Food-associated allergic rhinitis
   d. Occupational allergic rhinitis

B. Symptoms

1. Paroxysms of sneezing
2. Rhinorrhea
3. Nasal and palatal pruritus
4. Nasal stuffiness
5. Poor appetite and nausea due to swallowing excessive mucus
6. Fatigue and irritability
7. Itchy eyes, lacrimation, chemosis, conjunctival hyperemia
8. Earache

C. Symptom Patterns

1. Often start in childhood
2. Generally recur each year at the same time

3. Often worse in the morning
4. 60% of patients have a positive family history.

D. **Physical Examination**

1. Tearing, conjunctival injection, and edema
2. Periorbital cyanosis (allergic shiners)
3. Crease across lower nose secondary to repeated rubbing
4. Pale, bluish, edematous nasal turbinates
5. Thin, clear nasal secretions
6. Mouth breathing
7. Fluid in the middle ear

II. Diagnostic Approach

A. Diagnosis is generally based on history.

B. Tests may be useful to differentiate allergic rhinitis from other syndromes.

1. Nasal cytology
   a. Method—The mucosal surface of the inferior turbinates is scraped with a flexible, disposable, plastic probe.
   b. Interpretation
      1) Normal nasal mucosal cytology usually has no eosinophilic or basophilic cells and few neutrophils or bacteria.
      2) The main use of nasal cytology is to differentiate infectious rhinitis (increased neutrophils) from allergic rhinitis (eosinophilia).
   c. Problems
      1) Absence of eosinophilia does not rule out allergic rhinitis.
      2) Eosinophilia may be seen in nonallergic conditions.
2. Allergen skin testing: the most useful procedure to detect specific allergic triggers in allergic rhinitis
   a. Method
      1) The skin is pricked with appropriate antigens and control substances to detect specific triggers of allergic rhinitis symptoms.
      2) The testing should be done with extracts prevalent in the region where the patient lives.
   b. Interpretation—A positive skin test is a wheal and flare reaction.
   c. Problems—may not be useful in following situations
      1) Patients who are unable to stop antihistamine therapy
      2) Patients with severe dermatitis or dermatographism
      3) Patients with anaphylactic sensitivity

3. IgE determination
   a. Method—In vitro blood tests such as the RAST (radioallergosorbent test) for specific IgE or PRIST (paper disc radioimmunosorbent test)
   b. Interpretation
      1) These tests measure total serum IgE or specific IgE antibodies directed at specific antigens.
      2) May be of use for patients who cannot be evaluated by skin testing.
   c. Problems
      1) Less sensitive and more expensive than skin testing
      2) Wide variation in normal values and overlap in patients with clinical disease
4. Rhinoscopy
   a. Method
      1) The flexible fiberoptic rhinoscope is used to visualize the upper respiratory tract, nasopharynx, openings of the eustachian tubes, and vocal cords.
      2) The rigid endoscope is used to visualize the middle meatus and maxillary sinus ostia.
   b. Interpretation
      1) Useful for the determination of the presence of nasal obstruction or postnasal drip
      2) May discover polyps or tumors responsible for symptoms
5. Imaging studies
   a. Method: The coronal CT scan with bone windows is used to visualize sinuses and detect obstruction in the ostiomeatal complex to rule out chronic sinusitis.

III. Differential Diagnosis

A. Perennial nonallergic rhinitis

B. Nonallergic rhinitis with eosinophilia

C. Atrophic rhinitis

D. Rhinitis medicamentosa

E. Rhinitis induced by hormones

F. Nasal mastocytosis

G. Chronic sinusitis

H. Nasal neoplasms

Table 16–1. Antihistamines Used to Treat Allergic Rhinitis

Class	Generic Name	Trade Name	Sedation	Dose for Adults (mg)	Generic Available	OTC Drug
Ethanolamines	doxylamine	Decapryn	+ +	12.5–25 q.i.d.	no	no
	carbinoxamine	Clistin	+ +	4 q.i.d	no	no
	diphenhydramine	Benadryl	+ + +	25–50 q.i.d.	yes	yes
Ethenediamines	tripelennamine	Pyribenzamine	+ +	50 q.i.d.	yes	no
Alkylamines	chlorpheneramine	Chlor-trimeton	+	4 q.i.d.	yes	yes
	dexchlorophenirmaine	Polaramine	+	2 q.i.d.	yes	yes
	triprolidine	Actia	+	2.5 q.i.d.	yes	yes
Phenothiazines	promethazine	Phenergan	+ +	12.5–25 q.i.d.	yes	no
	trimeprazine	Temaril	+ +	2.5–7.5 q.i.d.	yes	no
Piperidines	azatidine	Optimine	+ +	1–2 q.i.d.	no	no
	cyproheptadine	Peri-actin	+ + +	4 q.i.d.	no	no
Butyrophenone	terfenadine	Seldane	− to +	60 q.i.d.	no	no
Piperazine	hydroxyzine	Atarax/Vistaril	+ +	10–25 b.i.d. or t.i.d.	yes	no
Miscellaneous	astemizole	Hismanal	− to +	10 daily on empty stomach	no	no
	loratidine	Claritin	− to +	10 daily	no	no

IV. Treatment

A. Goals

1. Avoid and control environmental factors
2. Symptom reduction with pharmacologic and nonpharmacologic methods, finding the appropriate balance between benefits of the medications and undesirable side effects
3. Appropriate use of allergy immunotherapy

B. Initial Treatment

1. Antihistamines (Table 16–1)

    a. Antihistamines are generally first-line therapy, most helpful in controlling sneezing, itching, and rhinorrhea.
    b. Antihistamines are less effective for nasal congestion.
    c. Patients will generally respond to a particular class of antihistamine; preference within a class may be determined by lack of side effects.
    d. Cost can be a significant factor and generic equivalents should be used when possible.
    e. Older agents, ie, diphenhydramine, chlorpheniramine, may cause some sedation and mucous membrane drying; this is less common with newer agents such as astemizole and terfenidine.
    f. Antihistamines are more effective if taken in anticipation of symptoms, ie, before exposure or before the start of the pollen season.

2. Decongestants (Table 16–2)—Can be added or combination products used for patients who experience nasal congestion

3. Topical nasal corticosteroids (Table 16–3)

    a. Useful for patients whose symptoms are not relieved by oral antihistamines or decongestants, or patients who do not tolerate systemic side effects of oral therapy

Table 16–2. Examples of Decongestant Preparations Used in Allergic Rhinitis

Trade Name	Generic	Mg/tablet	Dose	OTC
Sudafed	pseudoephedrine	30	1–2 q.i.d	yes
Trinalin	azatidine	1	1 b.i.d.	no
	pseudoephedrine	120		
Actifed	triprolidine	2.5	1 t.i.d.	yes
	pseudoephedrine	120		
Dimetapp	bromphenerimine	12	1 b.i.d.	yes
	phenylpropanolamine	75		

Table 16–3. Topical Nasal Steriod Preparations

Trade Name	Generic	Dose
Beconase Beconase AQ*	beclomethasone diproprionate	1 spray in each nostril b.i.d.–q.i.d.
Nasalide	flunisolide	1 spray b.i.d.–t.i.d.
Nasacort	trimcinolone	2 sprays qd
Decadron Turbinaire**	dexamethasone	2 sprays b.i.d.–q.i.d.
Vancenase Vancenase AQ*	beclomethasone diproprionate	1 spray in each nostril b.i.d.–q.i.d.

* aqueous prep
** increased risk of adrenal supression

    b. Very helpful for obstructive nasal symptoms
    c. May decrease late response to allergen challenge
    d. There are no systemic side effects associated with their use; however, local nasal irritation, nasal burning, drying and epistaxis may occur.
    e. Usually effective within 7–14 d
    f. Most effective for long-term prophylaxis rather than acute symptom relief
    g. Patients should be reminded that they should be used regularly, rather than PRN, for maximal effectiveness.
    h. The nasal mucosa should be examined approximately q 6 mo in patients receiving long-term treatment.

4. Systemic steroids

    a. Occasionally necessary for treating seasonal allergy
    b. May be especially helpful to gain control before topical therapy becomes effective
    c. The course is generally a 3–4-d regimen of the equivalent of 20 mg prednisone a day; only rarely should longer regimens, ie, 2–4 wk be administered.
    d. Depot steroid injections should be avoided because of the risk of adrenal suppression.

5. Nasal cromolyn (Nasalcrom)

    a. Inhibits mast cell mediator release in the nasal mucosa
    b. Must be administered q 4 h
    c. More effective in controlling sneezing, rhinorrhea, and nasal itching than nasal congestion
    d. Mild local side effects common
    e. Relatively high cost

V. Patient Education

A. Patients are counseled to avoid and remove environmental factors where possible.

1. Control dust
2. Limit exposure to offending animals
3. Seal mattresses and use polyester pillows
4. Use air conditioning and close windows

B. Use pharmacologic agents as directed.

1. Oral antihistamines and decongestants in appropriate doses and intervals
2. Counsel on risks of drug interactions and side effects
3. Use in anticipation of exposure to allergens
4. Appropriate use of nasal corticosteroids

VI. Indications for Referral to an Allergist

A. Patients who fail to respond to the treatment described above should be referred to an allergist for the following:

1. Confirm the diagnosis of allergic rhinitis
2. Rule out any other causes of nasal symptoms
3. Consider use of immunotherapy

VII. Bibliography

Badhwar A, Druce H. Allergic rhinitis. Med Clin North Am 1992;76:789–803.
Kaliner M, Lemanske R. Primer on allergic and immunologic diseases. JAMA 1992;268:2807–2829.
Valentine M. Allergy and related conditions. In: Barker LR, Burton JR, Zieve PD, eds. Principles of Ambulatory Medicine, 3rd ed. Baltimore: Williams & Wilkins; 1991:253–269.

Chapter 17: Insect Allergies

Karen S. Scoles

17A Insect Sting Allergy

I. Clinical presentation

A. General Information

1. In the United States, four major winged insects are responsible for stings—yellow jackets, hornets, wasps, and honeybees.

2. Most commonly stings are secondary to yellow jackets.

3. The fire ant, a nonwinged insect, is becoming an increasing source of sting reactions.

B. Four Types of Reactions Secondary to Stings

1. Normal reactions result in local pain, redness, and swelling. They usually subside in 1-2 h.

2. Large local reactions result in swelling extending from the sting site over a large area. If severe, they can be associated with systemic symptoms such as fatigue and nausea. They peak at 48 h and can last as long as a week.

3. Anaphylaxis, which is a serious systemic reaction associated with generalized urticaria, angioedema, upper airway obstruction and circulatory collapse. This kind of reaction usually occurs within 15 min of a sting but can also occur as long as 3 d after a sting. Anaphylaxis is responsible for 40 or more deaths each year in the United States. More commonly it occurs in patients with a history of atopy. Approximately 0.4% of the population experiences anaphylaxis secondary to insect stings. These reactions are mediated by IgE antibodies reacting with insect venom (see Chapter 1).

4. Unusual reactions—vasculitis, serum sickness, nephritis, neuritis and encephalitis

II. Diagnostic Approach

A. The diagnosis is made by history and physical. Insect stings are always painful as compared to insect bites.

B. Patients may not always be able to identify the particular winged insect responsible for the sting, but the setting may help determine the likely agent. Fire ant stings are notable for the development of a sterile pustule at the sting site within 24 h. These insects are also known for stinging at multiple sites in a circular pattern.

C. Allergic symptoms generally occur within 15–20 min. However, because delayed reactions can occur, the cause of the allergic or anaphylactic reaction may not be obvious.

D. Confirmation of stinging insect allergy should be carried out by skin testing in those patients who have acute allergic reactions.

III. Treatment

A. Acute

1. Normal reactions—Apply local cold compresses and use oral analgesics where necessary.

2. Large local reactions—Use aspirin and antihistamines. Prednisone 40 mg q d for 2–3 d is helpful for extensive large local reactions.

3. Anaphylaxis—Patients should receive prompt medical attention and treatment guidelines followed as described in Chapter 1.

4. Unusual reactions—Steroids are often used if these complications occur.

B. Preventive

1. Patients can avoid stings by minimizing exposure. Avoid going barefoot, wear dark-colored clothing, and avoid perfumes and hairspray.

2. Patients who have had a serious reaction should acquire and be instructed in the use of emergency kits containing epinephrine for injection. This should not substitute for prompt medical attention, but treatment should be initiated at the time of the sting.

IV. Indications for Referral to an Allergist

A. Any adult patient who has a past history of a serious allergic reaction, ie, systemic anaphylaxis or urticaria/angioedema, should have sensitivity confirmed.

B. Because there can be a > 50% chance of potentially life-threatening reaction recurring, these patients should be referred to an allergist for immunotherapy with the appropriate venoms. This can provide almost 100% protection against serious re-sting reactions.

V. Indications for Hospitalization

Patients with anaphylaxis may need hospitalization for treatment and observation.

VI. Annotated Bibliography

Atkinson T, Kaliner M. Anaphylaxis. Med Clin North Am 1992;76:841–855. A complete review of the pathogenesis, clinical presentation, and state of the art treatment of anaphylaxis.

Valentine M. Allergy and related conditions. In: Barker LR, Burton JR, Zieve PD, eds. Principles of Ambulatory Medicine, 3rd ed. Baltimore: Williams & Wilkins;1991:253–269.

17B Insect Bites

I. Spider Bites

A. Bites of many types are locally irritating.
B. Two types of spiders cause clinically significant problems in North America.
1. Widow spiders (*Lactrodectus* species)
    a. Clinical presentation
        1) Widow spiders are glossy black with characteristic red hourglass mark.
        2) The bite causes momentary sharp pain at the site. This is followed by cramping, which begins locally and spreads within 15–60 min.
        3) Excruciating waves of pain can be accompanied by labored respirations, nausea, vomiting, and headache.
        4) The venom causes increased autonomic activity, diffuse central and peripheral nervous system excitation, muscle spasm, vasoconstriction, and hypertension.
        5) Slight fever may be present.
        6) The pains subside over several hours. Mild recurrences may occur over several days. The symptoms may take a week to resolve.
        7) Deaths have occurred in young children and the elderly secondary to cardiorespiratory failure.
    b. Diagnosis
        1) Patients may appear to have a perforated ulcer, appendicitis, or acute pancreatitis. However, the abdomen is not tender after a spider bite and the above conditions are not usually associated with extremity pain.
        2) Other conditions with similar symptoms such as renal colic, myocardial infarction, tetanus, strychnine poisoning, and lead colic need to be ruled out by history and differential diagnosis.
    c. Treatment
        1) Relief of pain with analgesics
        2) Hot tub bath
        3) Calcium gluconate (10 mL) injected IV over 10–20 min may transiently relieve cramps.
        4) Patients at special risk, ie, small children or those with coexisting medical problems, should be treated with *Lactrodectus* antivenin. An IV solution of 2.5 mL antivenin is diluted in 50 mL saline and administered over 15 min.
2. Recluse spiders (*Loxosceles* species)
    a. Clinical presentation
        1) Initially bites cause minor stinging discomfort.
        2) In severe bites, intense local pain appears within 2–8 h, with bullae formation, erythema then ischemic necrosis, and a deep ulcer with a necrotic base.

3) In some patients a systemic reaction occurs, characterized by fever, myalgias, and a rash 24–28 h after the bite.
4) Intravascular hemolysis and in severe cases hemoglobinuria and acute renal failure may occur.
5) Deaths have been reported in children.
  b. Treatment
    1) Depends on the severity of the bite
    2) If bullae formation, pain and progressing ischemic necrosis do not occur within the first 6–8 h, then the bite is probably not severe and treatment is not necessary.
    3) With more serious local reactions, IV glucocorticoids are advocated to prevent progression.
    4) Dapsone and brown recluse antivenin have been used experimentally.
    5) Other treatment includes
       a) *Local wound care*
       b) *Cool compresses*
       c) *Elevation of extremity*
       d) *Treatment of secondary infection*
    6) Patients with systemic illness should be hospitalized and monitored for hemolysis, disseminated intravascular coagulation, and acute renal failure.

II. Tick Bites

A. Clinical Presentation

1. Can be associated with serious illnesses such as Lyme disease and Rocky Mountain spotted fever (see Chapter 66).
2. Local reaction is itching papule, which resolves in a few days.
3. If mouth parts are incompletely removed, a granuloma may occur, requiring surgical excision.
4. Ticks should be removed intact with tweezers or forceps. If fingers are used, they should be covered and washed afterwards. Mineral oil or other organic solvents may facilitate removal. Hot matchsticks or other heated objects should not be used to attempt removal.

B. Complications

1. Ticks may serve as vectors for other diseases.
2. Tick paralysis is primarily caused by wood ticks.
   a. Caused by neurotoxin secreted in saliva of the engorging tick
   b. Causes a progressing, ascending, flaccid paralysis and acute ataxia
   c. Differential diagnosis includes poliomyelitis, Guillain-Barre syndrome, myasthenia gravis, Eaton-Lambert syndrome, diptheric polyneuropathy, and botulism

d. The treatment is to remove the tick, including any retained mouth parts.
   e. Death can occur if respiratory or bulbar paralysis is present and the tick is not removed in time.
   f. Deaths occur primarily in children.

III. Flea Bites

A. Many types of fleas attack human beings.

B. In sensitive individuals, the salivary secretions cause large, pruritic papules.

C. Treatment is symptomatic using antipruritics and antihistamines.

D. The fleas should be eradicated.

IV. Caterpillar Rash

A. An erythematous, pruritic rash can occur secondary to contact with the early larval or caterpillar stage of several species of moths, not secondary to a bite.

B. Occasionally the reaction is complicated by urticaria and bullae.

C. Treatment is with local soaks and antihistamines.

V. Centipede Bites

A. The giant desert centipede can deliver an intensely painful bite associated with erythema, edema, and sometimes regional lymphangitis.

B. Rhabdomyolysis and acute renal failure have occurred secondary to these bites.

C. Treatment is with analgesics and aggressive wound cleansing.

VI. Bedbug Bites

A. Bedbugs can bite, causing reactions varying from simple puncture to large urticarial lesions.

B. The type of reaction depends on the sensitivity of the individual.

VII. Kissing Bug Bites

A. The members of the family Reduviidae are associated with severe bite reactions.

B. Bites occur nocturnally and in multiple groups.

C. Reactions to the bites are thought to be allergic in nature.

D. Reactions vary from pruritic and painful papules to vesicles, giant urticaria, hemorrhagic nodular to bullous lesions, or anaphylaxis.

E. Differential diagnosis includes necrotizing spider bites or erythema multiforme.

F. Treatment

1. Local reactions are treated symptomatically.

2. More severe allergic reactions should be treated appropriately.

3. Patients with significant reactions should obtain and be instructed in the use of allergy kits.

VIII. Chiggers

A. Chiggers are tiny mites.

B. In the United States, the larval form attacks the skin, secreting a substance that digests tissue creating a red, intensely pruritic papule.

C. Treatment is with antipruritics.

D. Preventive treatment consists of insect repellents, protective clothing, and bathing after exposure.

IX. Scorpion Stings

A. Glands in the scorpion produce venom, injected in the victim by a stinger in the tail.

B. They often get into clothing and shoes at night and the accidental contact results in a sting.

C. Most nonlethal species in United States cause only minor local reactions like a bee sting.

D. Some produce local edema and ecchymosis, with burning local pain.

E. Many of the species whose venom has potentially lethal systemic effects may have little or no visible cutaneous reaction at the site of the sting.

1. A burning sensation occurs followed by local parathesia, hyperesthesia, or numbness.

2. The whole extremity becomes involved, followed by malaise, restlessness, neurologic hyperreactivity, lacrimation, rhinorrhea, salivation, perspiration, nausea, and vomiting.
3. Convulsions and coma may follow and catecholamine release can lead to hypertension and arrhythmias.
4. Death usually occurs in 12 h but sometimes as late as 2 d after the sting.
5. Deaths generally do not occur in healthy adults, but more commonly occur in children and elderly persons.

F. Treatment

1. Most stings are not lethal and the treatment is at home with analgesics and cool compresses.
2. Specific antivenin is available in some areas and should be considered for patients who develop signs of cranial nerve dysfunction and increased involuntary activity in skeletal muscles.
3. Supportive therapy is used for shock, dehydration, and other complications.

G. Prevention

1. Examine objects and clothing carefully before use to avoid hidden scorpions.
2. Prevent them from entering the home by
   a. Closing or covering areas of entry
   b. Removing debris, woodpiles, and so forth away from the home
   c. Applying a hydrocarbon mixture between the ground and house foundation
3. Extermination may be necessary if an infestation is present.

X. Fly Bites

A. Horseflies and deerflies attack and feed on human beings and other warm-blooded animals.

B. Transmission of serious disease can occur, such as anthrax and tularemia.

C. In North America bites are painful, pruritic lesions, which can be followed by delayed, localized allergic reactions.

D. Treatment includes thorough cleaning of the bite site, topical steroids, and oral antihistamines.

XI. Annotated Bibliography

Wallace J. Disorders caused by venoms, bites and stings. In: Wilson JD, Braunwald E, Isselbacher RJ, et al, eds. Harrison's Principles of Internal Medicine, 12th ed. New York: McGraw-Hill;1991:2187–2194. A fairly detailed, practical description of the presentation and management of various bites and stings.

Chapter 18: Plant Dermatitis

Karen S. Scoles

I. Clinical Presentation

A. General Information

1. Poison ivy, poison oak, and sumac are the major plants responsible for allergic contact dermatitis caused by plants.
2. The dermatitis is secondary to exposure to the plant's resin, which persists on clothing, pets, tools, and the like, and may take as long as 3 wk to evaporate.
3. The history is key in making the diagnosis.

B. Symptoms

1. All cause an acute dermatitis characterized by an eczematous or blistering eruption, often with linear streaking, angular lesions, and oozing lesions.
2. Lesions are often delayed in appearance because of continuing exposure and not "spread" from weeping blisters or lesions.

C. Physical Examination

1. Pattern of involvement is helpful.
    a. Usually restricted to exposed areas
    b. Weeping or vesicular eruption with prominent linear streaking

II. Differential Diagnosis

A. Contact dermatitis secondary to other irritants or allergens

B. Atopic dermatitis

C. Stasis dermatitis

D. Psoriasis

E. Photosensitivity

F. Herpes zoster or herpes simplex

G. Primary bullous dermatoses

H. See Part 6: Dermatology

III. Treatment

A. When possible after recognized exposure, patients should wash the exposed skin and clean items that may have had contact with the resin. Pets should be bathed.

B. If dermatitis occurs, treatment includes

1. Application of cooling compresses with saline or Burow's solution, for 20 min q 2–3 h

2. Oral antihistamines such as diphenhydramine 50 mg or chlorpheniramine 4 mg, q 4–6 h or terfenadine 60 mg q 12 h

3. Corticosteroid creams, lotions, or sprays (depending on area of involvement, triamcinolone 0.1% or higher potency). High-potency topical steroid use should be avoided on the face or skin folds (see Appendix C Topical Corticosteroid Potencies).

4. Systemic corticosteroids may be necessary for

   a. Extensive involvement over a large area
   b. Facial lesions
   c. Significant edema and blisters
   d. Patients known to have had severe reactions to the same contactant in the past
   e. Generally high doses are needed, ie, prednisone 60 mg/d in divided doses, tapered over a 2–3 wk period

5. Antibiotics may be necessary for the rare secondary bacterial infection.

   a. Dicloxacillin 250 q.i.d.
   b. Erythromycin 250 q.i.d.
   c. Cephalexin 250 q.i.d.
   d. Amoxicillin-clavulanic acid 250 q.i.d.

IV. Indications for Referral to an Allergist or Dermatologist

A. Patients should be referred to a dermatologist if the diagnosis is in question or if the patient does not respond as expected to therapy.

B. There is a very limited role for hyposensitization therapy and these patients should be referred to an allergist or dermatologist.

V. Annotated Bibliography

Horan R, Schneider L, Sheffer A. In: Primer on Allergic and Immunologic Diseases, Chapter 8. JAMA 1992;268:2858-2868. A thorough review of the common and uncommon immunologically mediated diseases of the skin.

Lamberg S. Common problems of the skin. In: Barker LR, Burton JR, Zieve PD, eds. Principles of Ambulatory Medicine, 3rd ed. Baltimore: Williams & Wilkins;1991:1345-1379.

Chapter 19: Urticaria

Karen S. Scoles

I. Clinical Presentation

A. General Information

1. Approximately 20% of the population is affected.
2. Onset is generally rapid with resolution over hours.
3. Acute attacks are more common in children and young adults.
4. *Acute urticaria* refers to eruptions occurring over a period of < 6 wk.
5. *Chronic urticaria* refers to episodes that persist for > 6 wk.
6. Angioedema differs from urticaria pathologically only in that the deeper skin structures are affected, with swelling of the subcutaneous and submucosal tissues. Often the skin appears normal in angioedema. The patient may experience burning or tingling rather than pruritus.

B. Symptoms

1. Characterized by blanchable, erythematous, edematous papules and plaques, usually pruritic
2. Angioedema can result in airway obstruction.

C. Physical Examination

1. Size rages from 1 mm to several centimeters with serpiginous borders.
2. The eruption does not generally persist in the same area of skin for > 24 h.
3. In typical episodes eruptions may arise in different areas over a 1–3-d period.

II. Diagnosis

A. Diagnosis is predominately based on history and physical examination.

B. Etiology

1. Acute

    a. Allergy to foods, drugs, insect stings, food additives
    b. Infection
        1) Viral—mononucleosis, hepatitis
        2) Bacterial—β-hemolytic streptococcus
    c. Idiosyncratic—aspirin or nonsteroidal anti-inflammatory drugs, contrast materials
    d. Physical factors
        1) Dermatographism
        2) Heat
            a) Generalized "cholinergic"
            b) Localized
        3) Cold
        4) Solar
        5) Pressure
    e. Idiopathic

2. Chronic

    a. Hereditary angioneurotic edema
    b. Hepatitis
    c. Parasitic infestation
    d. Neoplasms, especially Hodgkin's disease
    e. Collagen vascular disease
    f. Polyarteritis
    g. Endocrine disorders, especially thyroid disease
    h. Idiopathic

3. Work-up of chronic urticaria

    a. May be necessary if etiology not determined by history
    b. Limited diagnostic testing:
        1) Complete blood count with differential
        2) Sedimentation rate
        3) Stool for ova and parasites
        4) Hepatitis serologies
        5) Monospot
        6) Complement levels
        7) Antinuclear antibody
    c. Yield often poor, with no etiology found in > 70% cases

III. Treatment

A. Patients should avoid aggravating factors and agents where possible.

B. If underlying disease is present, treatment of that condition will often resolve the urticaria.

C. Acute attacks respond well to epinephrine 0.2–0.5 mL of a 1:1000 solution SQ, repeated after 15 min.

D. Oral antihistamines can be given at the same time.

1. Diphenhydramine (Benadryl) 50 mg PO, half dose if used IM
2. Chlorpheniramine (Chlor-trimeton) 4 mg

E. Antihistamines should be continued for prolonged symptoms.

1. Hydroxyzine (Atarax) may be especially effective in controlling symptoms in chronic urticaria, starting with 10 mg q 8 h with titration to 25 mg q 8 h if necessary.
2. Cyproheptadine (Periactin) starting 2 mg q 12 h and titrating to 4 mg q.i.d.
3. Second-generation agents such as astemizole and terfenadine can be used; they are:
   a. Less sedating
   b. Equally efficacious
   c. Dosed q d or q 12 h
   d. More expensive

F. H_2 antagonists can be added if more control is needed.

G. For severe cases, corticosteroids may offer symptomatic relief and may resolve urticaria.

1. 0.5–0.1 mg prednisone equivalent/kg/d with taper over several weeks

IV. Indications for Referral to an Allergist or Dermatologist

A. Patients suspected to have hereditary angioneurotic edema should be referred to an allergist for diagnosis and management.

B. Patients with lesions not resolving over typical time course should be referred to a dermatologist to rule out other skin conditions.

V. Indications for Hospitalization

A. Patients should be counseled that urticaria/angioedema can progress to a life-threatening situation and they should seek prompt medical attention.

B. Patients with severe attacks of hereditary angioneurotic edema should be hospitalized.

VI. Annotated Bibliography

Bruce R, ed. Clinical allergy. Med Clin North Am 1992;76:4. A complete review of the pathogenesis, clinical presentation, and state of the art treatment of allergic diseases.

de Shazo R, ed. Primer on allergic and immunologic diseases. JAMA 1992;268:20. A review of applied immunology; although directed to medical students, it is a useful review for practicing physicians as well.

Part IV:
Cardiology/Hypertension

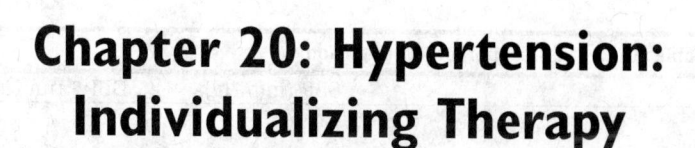

Chapter 20: Hypertension: Individualizing Therapy

James Witek

I. Clinical Presentation

A. General Information

1. Hypertension is defined as a diastolic blood pressure (DBP) > 90 and a systolic blood pressure (SBP) > 140.

2. Isolated elevations of SBP are frequently seen in the elderly and carry similar risks of morbidity and mortality; this is defined as isolated systolic hypertension (ISH).

3. Hypertension is one of the most common medical illnesses encountered.

4. More common in African Americans and Hispanics; prevalence increases with age.

5. Occurs more commonly in men than women until after menopause when the incidence in women is greater than in men.

6. Although generally easily treated, can cause significant mortality if untreated. Morbidity and mortality increase independently with increasing levels of DBP and SBP.

7. BP elevations should be documented on two, or preferably three, occasions and the readings averaged before diagnosis made; an exception to this is when there are marked elevations of DBP ≥ 120 or SBP ≥ 210 or evidence of target organ damage. In these later cases diagnosis is obvious and urgent treatment is required.

B. Classification—Developed by Joint National Committee on Detection, Evaluation, and Treatment of High Blood Pressure (Table 20-1).

C. Essential versus Secondary Hypertension

1. Essential hypertension
    a. > 90% of cases
    b. Due to a variety of abnormalities in the regulatory systems of arterial pressure although the specific etiology is currently unclear.
    c. Often recognized at ages 30-55
    d. Family history usually significant for hypertension

Table 20-1. Classification of Hypertension

	SBP (mm Hg)	DBP (mm Hg)
Normal	< 130	< 85
High normal	130–139	85–89
Hypertension		
Stage 1 (mild)	140–159	90–99
Stage 2 (moderate)	160–179	100–109
Stage 3 (severe)	180–209	110–119
Stage 4 (very severe)	≥ 210	≥ 120
Isolated systolic hypertension (ISH)*	> 160	< 90

*ISH should be classified into stages 2–4 based on level of SBP
SBP, systolic blood pressure; DBP, diastolic blood pressure

SOURCE: Adapted from the Fifth Joint National Committee on Detection, Evaluation and Treatment of High Blood Pressure (JNC V). Arch Intern Med 1993;153:154–183.

2. Secondary hypertension
    a. Accounts for 5–10% of cases
    b. Refers to those cases where abnormalities in a specific organ create an elevation in BP
    c. Should be suspected when hypertension first diagnosed in patients < 35 or > 55 y
    d. Treatment ultimately directed toward correcting the organ defect, if possible
    e. Organ defects causing secondary hypertension (Table 20-2)

D. Presentation

1. Often initially discovered at routine health screening or during visits for other medical problems
2. May present as medical emergency
3. Patients may present with evidence of target organ damage.
    a. Cerebrovascular—strokes or transient ischemic attacks
    b. Retina—retinopathy characterized by exudates or hemorrhages; papilledema
    c. Cardiac—left ventricular hypertrophy (LVH) or dysfunction; diastolic or systolic congestive heart failure (CHF)
    d. Renal—microalbuminuria, proteinuria, or elevated creatinine
    e. Peripheral vascular—intermittent claudication
4. Patients may present with hypertension with an obvious secondary cause.

E. Symptoms

1. Usually asymptomatic

Table 20-2. Organ Defects Causing Secondary Hypertension

Organ System	Disease	Suggestive Symptoms/Findings
Vascular	Renal artery stenosis	Abdominal bruit
	Coarctation of aorta	Disproportionate upper to lower extremity size
Endocrine	Acromegaly	Weakness, characteristic bone and soft tissue enlargement
	Cushing's syndrome	Weight gain, truncal obesity, polyuria, moon facies
	Hyperthyroidism	Palpitations, diarrhea, weight loss
	Hypercalcemia (hyperparathyroidism)	Weakness, anorexia, depression
	Pheochromocytoma	Flushing, palpitations, sweating, anxiety attacks, orthostatic hypotension
	Primary aldosteronism	Weakness, muscle cramps
Renal	Renal parenchymal disease	Nocturia, enlarged kidneys, edema
Drugs	Androgens	History of use
	Estrogens in birth control pills	History of use
	Glucocorticoids	History of use
	Cocaine	History of use
	Erythropoietin	History of use

2. Some patients will present with palpitations, lightheadedness, visual disturbances, or headaches. In many patients the symptoms will not correlate with an elevation in BP.

3. Symptoms suggestive of target organ damage may be present; thus patients should be asked about visual changes, chest pain, shortness of breath, edema, claudication, or focal weakness.

4. Symptoms suggestive of secondary causes of BP elevation may be present (Table 20-2).

F. Physical Examination

1. The objective is to assess for physical evidence of target organ damage, secondary causes, or concurrent diseases that may alter therapy.

2. Patient's general appearance should be assessed for a "buffalo" hump, "moon" facies, or truncal obesity that might suggest Cushing's syndrome/disease.

3. BP should be measured at each visit with the patient sitting comfortably and the arm supported at heart level. The patient should not have smoked, exercised, or consumed caffeine for 30 min before measurement. The proper

size cuff should be used, the bladder covering 80% or more of the arm's circumference. BP should be measured in both arms and in the supine and standing positions at initial evaluation.

4. Pseudohypertension due to calcification of arteries should be suspected in elderly patients with marked BP elevations. This may be detected with Osler's maneuver performed by inflating the BP cuff above the SBP and noting that the pulseless arteries distal to the cuff (brachial, radial) are still palpable.
5. Pulses should be assessed for strength of impulse and symmetry. It is important to listen for vascular bruits over the carotids, and renal and femoral vessels.
6. Thyroid size and configuration should be assessed.
7. Fundi should be examined to detect exudates, hemorrhages, papilledema, and arteriovenous compression.
8. Cardiac examination should evaluate for tachycardia, point of maximal impulse, precordial heaves, extra heart sounds, and murmurs to suggest valvular heart disease.
9. Pulmonary examination should include auscultation for rales, which may suggest pulmonary edema.
10. Abdominal examination should include assessment for aortic aneurysm, renal bruits, and enlarged kidneys.
11. Neurologic exam should focus on finding any deficits to suggest a cerebrovascular accident or intracranial process.

II. Diagnostic Approach

A. General

1. Assessment should be made for iatrogenic causes of elevated BP.
    a. Glucocorticoids
    b. Estrogens in birth control pills
    c. Androgens
2. Alcohol use should be evaluated because excess intake contributes to hypertension.
3. Assessment of other cardiac risk factors should be made on all patients and modifications recommended. (See chapters on hypercholesterolemia [39], smoking cessation [15], and exercise programs [23].)
4. Careful history of concomitant diseases should be obtained. Diseases that may have an impact on the treatment of hypertension include diabetes mellitus, hyperlipidemia, CHF, coronary heart disease, renal disease, asthma or chronic obstructive pulmonary disease, arrhythmias, impotence, gout, migraine headaches, and depression.

5. An ECG, complete blood count, urinalysis, serum electrolytes, and creatinine, glucose, calcium, cholesterol, and triglyceride levels should be obtained on all patients.

6. Serum uric acid should be checked when use of a diuretic is anticipated as treatment.

7. A chest x-ray may be helpful to assess for aortic dilatation or rib notching when coarctation of the aorta is suspected. Measurement of plasma renin activity serves as a crude screen for renovascular disease. Additional studies should be obtained to rule out possible secondary causes suspected based on history and physical examination.

8. Ambulatory BP monitoring is a useful modality to assess episodic hypertension, borderline hypertension with evidence of target organ damage, autonomic dysfunction, carotid sinus syncope, and pacemaker syndromes. It has been proposed as a means to provide better assessment of patients with "white coat" hypertension and mild hypertension so that unnecessary treatment of patients can be avoided.

III. Treatment

A. Goals

1. Lower BP to DBP < 90, SBP < 140. Additional decreases in morbidity and mortality occur as BP is lowered beyond these levels.

2. Correct other risk factors for cardiovascular disease.

3. Maintain long-term compliance with treatment.

B. Initial Management—Life-style Modification

1. These steps are appropriate for all stages of hypertension. They are the only treatment modalities suggested for high normal BP and are the initial therapies for stage 1 and 2 hypertension and ISH.

2. Weight reduction with goal to attain ideal body weight. Even small losses of weight may aid in BP control.

3. Decrease sodium intake to < 2 g/d. This is more effective as a treatment modality in African American patients and the elderly.

4. Increase physical activity: regular aerobic exercise such as brisk walking for 30 min three times weekly. In patients with stage 3 or 4 disease this should not be encouraged initially until BP is lowered pharmacologically.

5. Lower alcohol intake to moderate levels: 1 oz of hard liquor, 8 oz of wine or 24 oz of beer daily.

6. Tobacco cessation because smoking is a major risk factor for cardiovascular disease (see Chapter 15).

7. Reduction in elevated cholesterol is indicated because this is also a major risk factor for cardiovascular disease.
8. Increases in dietary potassium and calcium may be beneficial.
9. Allow 3–6 mo for response to these measures in patients whose hypertension is classified as stage 1 or 2.

C. Pharmacotherapy—General

1. Indicated in patients who have persistent elevation of BP despite 3–6 mo of well-attempted life-style modifications. May need to be instituted sooner if stage 3 or 4 hypertension present.
2. Goal is to achieve adequate control of BP with smallest number of agents at lowest possible doses with least side effects.

D. Pharmacotherapy—Individualization of Treatment

1. Loosely follows the guidelines developed by the Joint National Committee (JNC V) for the pharmacologic treatment of hypertension. It deviates from these recommendations by looking first at individual patient's characteristics such as age, race, or concurrent disease states and using these as the framework from which to select agents.
2. Generally treatment is started with an agent from one of five classes of medications: β blockers, diuretics, calcium antagonists, α_1 blockers, or angiotensin-converting enzyme (ACE) inhibitors.
3. The agent chosen is based on patient characteristics as well as knowledge of the agents in each class: their effectiveness in certain populations, side effects, drug interactions, contraindications, ability to treat/assist in treatment of concomitant disease and cost.
4. Because β blockers and diuretics are the only agents demonstrated to lower long-term morbidity and mortality and are readily available, they should be used as initial agents unless individual patient characteristics dictate otherwise. They are also less expensive than medications from the other classes.
5. A single agent should initially be instituted.
6. If after 3 to 6 months, BP remains elevated, consideration is given to increasing dose toward maximum *or* adding a second agent from a different class. Although single-agent treatment may improve compliance, side effects may be minimized with two agents from different classes at lower doses.
7. If BP remains elevated despite this intervention, the second drug is then added or the doses of both agents increased to maximum.
8. Because diuretics provide additional antihypertensive effect in combination with any of the other classes, they are frequently used as second agents.
9. It is not uncommon for patients with stage 3 or 4 hypertension to require two or three drugs at high doses.

E. Pharmacotherapy—Class Characteristics of Initial Antihypertensive Agents
See Table 20-3 for initial doses of commonly used agents.

Table 20-3. Doses of Commonly Used Oral Antihypertensives

Drug	Initial Daily Adult Dosage	Maintenance Dose
β Blockers		
Atenolol	25–50 mg qd	25–100 mg qd
Metoprolol	50 mg b.i.d.	50–250 mg b.i.d.
Propanolol	40 mg b.i.d.	60–120 mg b.i.d.
long-acting form	80 mg qd	120–160 mg
Diuretics		
Hydrochlorothiazide	12.5–25 mg qd	12.5–50 mg qd
Indapamide	2.5 mg qd	2.5–5.0 mg qd
Combination diuretics		
Hydrochlorothiazide 25 mg/triamterene 50 mg	1 tablet qd	1–2 tablets qd
Hydrochlorothiazide 50 mg/amiloride 5 mg	1/2–1 tablet qd	1/2–1 tablet qd
ACE inhibitors		
Benzapril	10 mg qd	20–40 mg qd
Captopril	12.5–25 mg b.i.d.	25–150 mg b.i.d.
Enalapril	2.5–5 mg qd	5–40 mg qd or split b.i.d.
Fosinopril	10 mg qd	20–40 mg qd
Lisinopril	5–10 mg qd	5–40 mg qd
Quinapril	10 mg qd	20–80 mg qd
Ramipril	2.5 mg qd	2.5–20 mg qd
Calcium antagonists (long-acting preparations)		
Amlodipine	5 mg qd	5–10 mg qd
Diltiazem	180–240 mg qd	240–480 mg qd
Felodipine	5 mg qd	5–20 mg b.i.d.
Isradipine	2.5 mg b.i.d.	2.5–5.0 mg qd
Nicardipine	30 mg b.i.d.	30–60 mg b.i.d.
Nifedipine	30 mg b.i.d.	30–120 mg qd
Verapamil	120–180 mg qd	120–480 mg qd/b.i.d.
α-β Blockers		
Labetolol	100 mg b.i.d.	200–400 mg b.i.d.
α-1 Adrenergic blocker		
Doxazosin	1 mg qd	1–8 mg qd
Prazosin	1 mg b.i.d./t.i.d.	1–10 mg b.i.d.
Terazosin	1 mg qhs	1–5 mg qhs

1. β Blockers
   a. Long-term studies demonstrate a decrease in morbidity and mortality in hypertensive patients treated with these agents. Provide mortality benefit in patients after myocardial infarction.
   b. Have been shown (in combination with diuretics) to decrease incidence of stroke in patients with isolated systolic hypertension
   c. Work well in younger patients and white patients
   d. Aid in concurrent treatment of angina or coronary artery disease, arrhythmias, migraine headaches, and diastolic dysfunction
   e. Contraindicated in reactive airways disease, bradycardia, and CHF with systolic dysfunction. Must be used cautiously when peripheral vascular disease or insulin-treated diabetes is present.
   f. Common side effects include fatigue, insomnia, bronchospasm, depression, and reduced exercise tolerance.
   g. The α-β blocker labetalol may be more effective in African Americans but is otherwise quite similar to the β-blocker class. It does have a higher incidence of postural hypotension and sexual dysfunction.

2. Diuretics
   a. Long-term studies demonstrate a decrease in morbidity and mortality in hypertensive patients treated with these agents.
   b. Have been shown to decrease the incidence of stroke in patients with ISH
   c. Work well in most patients but are especially effective in African American and elderly patients
   d. Require frequent laboratory monitoring of electrolytes
   e. Aid in concurrent treatment of CHF, renal insufficiency
   f. Contraindicated in gout
   g. Common side effects include electrolyte abnormalities, sexual dysfunction, weakness. They cause mild increase in cholesterol, but this is of unclear significance.
   h. Decreased calcium excretion may improve bone mass.

3. ACE inhibitors
   a. Work especially well in white patients with high renin state; work less well in African American patients as initial therapy
   b. Aid in concurrent treatment of CHF due to systolic dysfunction
   c. Preferred agent for treatment of hypertension in white diabetic patients because may reduce proteinuria and slow the progression of early renal disease associated with diabetes
   d. Contraindicated in hypertrophic cardiomyopathy with diastolic dysfunction, pregnancy, bilateral renal artery stenosis, or when significant stenosis exists in an artery to a solitary kidney. They must be used with caution in patients with an elevated serum creatinine level.
   e. Common side effects include cough (5–20% of patients), angioneurotic edema, rash, hypotension (especially if patient on concomitant diuretics), hyperkalemia.

4. Calcium antagonists
   a. Work well in almost all patients, especially African American

- b. Diltiazem, verapamil, and nifedipine are the best known agents in this class. They distinguish themselves by their differing sites of effective calcium blockade. Amlodipine, felodipine, isradipine, and nicardipine are newer agents in this class and as dihydropyridines have similar mechanisms of action and side effects as nifedipine.
- c. Diltiazem or verapamil aid in concurrent treatment of angina, coronary artery disease, and diastolic dysfunction. Raynaud's phenomenon and esophageal spasm may improve with nifedipine.
- d. Diltiazem or verapamil are contraindicated in bradycardia or heart block. Nifedipine must be used cautiously in systolic CHF because of its vasodilating effect.
- e. Common side effects for nifedipine and the other dihydropyridines include tachycardia, peripheral edema, dizziness, and headaches; constipation with verapamil; atrioventricular block or bradycardia with verapamil or diltiazem.

5. α_1-Adrenergic blockers
   - a. This class includes terazosin, doxazosin, and prazosin.
   - b. May aid in concurrent treatment of benign prostatic hypertrophy by lowering sphincter pressure
   - c. Contraindicated in diastolic dysfunction
   - d. Common side effects include orthostatic hypotension, weakness, syncope, and headache.

F. Pharmacotherapy—Supplemental Agents

1. Generally not used as initial agents, rather added to other agents that have been ineffective alone
2. Often used for more resistant hypertension
   - a. Centrally acting α_2 agonists
     1) This class includes clonidine, methyldopa, guanabenz, and guanfacine hydrochloride.
     2) Abrupt withdrawal of these agents may cause rebound hypertension.
     3) Methyldopa from this class is commonly used to treat hypertension in pregnancy.
     4) Methyldopa is contraindicated in liver disease.
     5) Common side effects include orthostasis, drowsiness, sedation, and fatigue.
   - b. Peripheral-acting adrenergic antagonists
     1) This class includes guanadrel, guanethidine, rauwolfia alkaloids, and reserpine.
     2) Side effects are not class specific but related to each drug.
     3) Rauwolfia alkaloids and reserpine are contraindicated in depression or peptic ulcer disease.
   - c. Direct vasodilators
     1) This class includes hydralazine and minoxidil.
     2) Often lead to tachycardia and fluid retention mandating simultaneous treatment with a diuretic and a β blocker

3) Hydralazine is useful in treatment of preeclampsia and hypertension in pregnancy.
4) Contraindicated in angina, hypertrophic cardiomyopathy.
5) Common side effects include headache, tachycardia, and fluid retention. Hydralazine may cause a lupus syndrome and minoxidil may cause hirsutism.

G. Treatment for ISH
1. Treatment is initiated with life-style modifications outlined above.
2. Pharmacotherapy is indicated if life-style modification fails to lower BP adequately and is individualized in the same manner presented above.
3. β Blockers and diuretics remain favored initial agents because they have been demonstrated to be effective in lowering the incidence of stroke in this population.

IV. Treatment of Hypertensive Crisis

A. Hypertensive crises have been traditionally divided into urgencies and emergencies, sometimes based on level of BP elevation, but this classification is awkward in clinical use.

B. There clearly are hypertensive emergencies when rapid reduction of BP within a short period of time is essential. This is the case when marked elevations of BP occur accompanied by encephalopathy, subarachnoid or intracerebral hemorrhage, unstable angina, acute myocardial infarction, acute left ventricular failure, or aortic dissection. Such patients should be referred immediately for admission to the hospital and therapy instituted as soon as possible.

C. Marked elevations of BP, which are unaccompanied by the concomitant conditions above or by azotemia, may be treated less acutely. These urgencies may be evidenced by retinal changes or papilledema. However, unless there is evidence of new or ongoing target organ damage, they may be treated on an outpatient basis. Treatment in these patients is generally instituted orally with the goal of reducing SBP to 170 mm Hg and DBP to 110 mm Hg within hours. Patients should then be continued on oral agents and reevaluated in 24 h to assess BP control and the possibility of secondary causes.

V. Inadequate Response to Treatment

A. Causes
1. Noncompliance, which can be due to many causes
    a. Patient's poor understanding of need for treatment
    b. Patient's misunderstanding of medication dose or frequency

c. Patient's poor motivation to comply or inability to comply due to dementia or concurrent illness
   d. Cost of medications
   e. Side effects of medications
2. Weight gain
3. Ethanol use or abuse
4. Unidentified or inadequately treated secondary cause of hypertension
5. Inadequate dose of medication
6. Concomitant drug therapy such as nasal decongestants, cold preparations, steroids, nonsteroidal anti-inflammatory agents

B. Once a cause is identified, it should be corrected.

C. If BP remains elevated despite correction of these factors or if no cause is found and BP remains elevated despite three drugs used at near maximal doses, a thorough search for a secondary cause of hypertension is indicated.

VI. Patient Education

A. Is important because many patients have no symptoms and feel well

B. Can improve compliance, BP control, and help decrease long-term complications

C. Should include defining the disease, explaining its short- and long-term consequences and how this could affect them individually

D. Needs to emphasize life-style modification

E. Includes information regarding the specific medications chosen to treat the patient

VII. Long-term Management

A. Patients should be seen approximately 1–2 mo after pharmacotherapy is instituted to assess for adequacy of response.

B. Once the BP is stabilized patients can be followed every 3–6 mo.

1. Monitor/measure BP.
2. Reinforce compliance with and assess for side effects of drugs.
3. Provide ongoing patient education.
4. Reinforce life-style modifications.

C. Annually patients should be assessed for target organ damage.

1. Urinalysis to assess for proteinuria
2. Serum creatinine to assess renal function
3. Fundoscopic examination to assess for retinal changes

D. Ambulatory BP monitoring may be helpful to assess drug resistance or hypotensive symptoms associated with antihypertensive medications.

E. If a patient's BP has been well controlled on therapy for 1 y, it is appropriate to make attempts to reduce the dosage of or eliminate drugs, especially if ongoing attempts at life-style modification have been successful.

VIII. Indications for Referral

A. Patients should be referred for admission if they have a marked elevation of BP with acutely progressive target organ damage.

1. Acute myocardial infarction or unstable angina
2. Acute aortic dissection
3. Encephalopathy
4. Intracerebral bleeding
5. Acute left ventricular failure
6. Rapidly declining renal function

B. Acute changes in vision indicative of possible retinal hemorrhage

C. Rapidly progressive renal insufficiency

D. Identification of a secondary cause requiring surgical intervention

1. Renal artery stenosis
2. Pheochromocytoma
3. Coarctation of aorta
4. Cushing's disease
5. Isolated adrenal adenoma

IX. Annotated Bibliography

Cunningham GF, Lindheimer MD. Hypertension in pregnancy. N Engl J Med 1992;326:927–932. A good overview of hypertension in pregnancy.

Gifford RW. Management of hypertensive crises. JAMA 1991;266:829–835. Provides a concise and detailed review of the evaluation and treatment of hypertensive crisis.

Report of the Fifth Joint National Committee on Detection, Evaluation and Treatment of High Blood Pressure (JNC V). Arch Intern Med 1993;153:154–183. This is a concise overview of the evaluation and treatment of hypertension. It has been criticized for maintaining the recommendation of diuretics and β blockers as best initial pharmacologic agents for hypertension.

SHEP Cooperative Research Group. Prevention of stroke by antihypertensive drug treatment in older persons with isolated systolic hypertension: final results of the Systolic Hypertension in the Elderly Program (SHEP). JAMA 1991;265:3255–3264. This five year study demonstrated the benefit of treatment of ISH with diuretics and β blockers in the elderly.

Stein PP, Black HR. Drug treatment of hypertension in patients with diabetes mellitus. Diabetes Care 1991;14:425–448. An excellent review of the use of drugs in patients with both hypertension and diabetes mellitus.

Williams GH. Hypertensive vascular disease. In: Wilson JD, Braunwald E, Isselbacher KJ, eds. Harrison's Principles of Internal Medicine, 12th ed. New York: McGraw-Hill;1991:1001–1015.

Chapter 21: Angina Pectoris

Rosemarie A. Leuzzi

I. Clinical Presentation

A. General Information

1. Angina occurs when the oxygen demand of the heart exceeds the supply. This occurs usually in the setting of coronary artery disease.
2. Types of angina
   a. Classic angina—transient, substernal discomfort typically provoked by exertion and relieved by rest or nitrates
   b. Atypical angina—involves similar symptoms but with the absence of one or more of the criteria for classic angina, ie; not consistently related to exertion
   c. Unstable angina—defined as a new onset of angina or a change in an established anginal pattern (such as the development of angina at rest; more severe, more frequent, or more prolonged episodes; nocturnal episodes)
   d. Prinzmetal's angina—thought to be caused by coronary artery vasospasm that may occur with or without underlying coronary artery disease

B. Symptoms

1. Location
   a. Angina usually begins in the substernal region and may radiate to the neck, jaw, epigastrium, shoulder, or arms; most commonly, the ulnar aspect of the left arm.
   b. When jaw pain occurs, it is usually mandibular rather than maxillary.
2. Quality
   a. Quality may vary and patients may have difficulty describing the sensation.
   b. Characteristics may include a sensation of constriction, pressure, squeezing, burning, heaviness, ache, or discomfort in the chest.
   c. Sensation is usually dull rather than sharp (due to the visceral innervation).
   d. The chest pain is not influenced by respiration.

3. Duration
   a. Angina usually begins gradually and lasts only a few minutes.
   b. A longer duration, especially at rest, may imply severe ischemia, myocardial infarction, or coronary spasm.
   c. Symptoms lasting for many hours or days are unlikely to be angina.
4. Severity—Angina varies from a slight discomfort to a disabling pain.
5. Frequency
   a. Frequency may vary from several episodes per day to once a month, and the frequency may fluctuate in an individual patient.
   b. New York Heart Association (NYHA) Functional Classification System
      1) Class I—angina with unusual activity with minimal or no functional impairment
      2) Class II—angina with prolonged or slightly more than usual activity with mild functional impairment
      3) Class III—angina with usual activity of daily living with moderate functional impairment
      4) Class IV—angina at rest and severely incapacitated
6. Aggravating factors
   a. Exercise or physical exertion
   b. Exposure to heat, humidity, or cold weather
   c. Emotional stress
   d. If pain occurs at rest, consider myocardial ischemia/myocardial infarction, or coronary artery spasm (Prinzmetal's angina).
7. Relieving factors
   a. Symptoms are usually relieved by rest or stopping activity within 5 min; chest pain lasting longer than 30 min may signify myocardial infarction.
   b. A history of relief noted within 1–3 min after sublingual nitroglycerin may be helpful indicating ischemic heart disease; however, the patient must be told that nitroglycerin will also relieve other causes of chest pain including esophageal spasm.
8. Associated symptoms or signs
   a. Diaphoresis
   b. Anxiety
9. Risk factors for atherosclerotic coronary artery disease include a history of
   a. Hypertension
   b. Diabetes mellitus
   c. Hypercholesterolemia
   d. Smoking
   e. A family history of premature coronary disease

C. Physical Examination

1. Blood pressure
   a. Hypertension is common during an episode of chest pain and also has important diagnostic and therapeutic implications because it accelerates atherosclerosis.
   b. Hypotension during an episode of chest pain is an ominous finding because it may indicate global ischemia produced by severe coronary artery disease and left ventricular failure.

2. Cardiac examination
   a. No findings on cardiac examination are clearly diagnostic of ischemic heart disease.
   b. An S_3 gallop is associated with increased left ventricular end-diastolic pressures and may suggest left ventricular systolic failure.
   c. The presence of S_4 gallop reflects decreased left ventricular compliance and is associated with long-standing hypertension.
   d. A mitral insufficiency murmur may be associated with papillary muscle dysfunction or dilatation of the mitral valve apparatus due to a dilated left ventricle; if transiently occurring during an episode of chest pain, this may imply ischemia.
   e. A paradoxically split S_2 in the absence of left bundle branch block generally reflects severe global left ventricular dysfunction.

3. Evidence of peripheral vascular disease with carotid artery bruits, femoral artery bruits, or diminished peripheral pulses indicates the presence of atherosclerosis and a higher likelihood of coronary artery disease.

4. Xanthomas or xanthelasma may suggest the possibility of familial hypercholesterolemia or premature coronary artery disease.

5. Fundoscopic changes may reflect long-standing hypertension or diabetes mellitus.

6. Pale oral mucosa or conjunctiva may be indicative of anemia, which may exacerbate angina due to decreased myocardial oxygen delivery.

II. Diagnostic Approach

A. Considering that chest pain is a very common complaint and that the differential diagnosis can be extensive, the initial evaluation should aim to distinguish cardiac from noncardiac chest pain.

1. Cardiac causes must be excluded before evaluating for possible noncardiac causes of the chest pain.
2. A careful history-taking should include location of the pain, quality, onset, duration, aggravating/relieving factors, and associated signs and symptoms.
3. During the examination, the clinician should try to elicit the chest pain by palpation or arm movement.

4. A patient's response to medication can also be helpful in the differential diagnosis, ie; pain from peptic ulcer disease being relieved by antacids.
5. Be sure to exclude the possibilities of hyperthyroidism or anemia in patients presenting with angina-like chest pain.

B. ECG

1. A standard 12-lead ECG should be obtained immediately in any patient with chest pain and suspected ischemic heart disease.
2. The ECG should then be repeated after the resolution of symptoms and compared with the ECG during the episode of chest pain.
3. A normal ECG is frequently found in patients without a history of previous infarction and may be found at rest or following the resolution of symptoms.
   a. A normal ECG is *not* good evidence against the possibility of coronary artery disease.
   b. 50% of all patients with known coronary artery disease will have a normal resting ECG.
4. Interpretation
   a. Q waves—infarcted myocardium
   b. ST depression—subendocardial ischemia
   c. ST elevation—may suggest transmural ischemia with or without coronary artery spasm indicating myocardial infarction
   d. T wave inversion—nonspecific finding that may be present after infarction or as a transient finding in a patient with ischemia.
   e. Nonspecific ST-T changes and conduction system abnormalities do not clearly establish the diagnosis of myocardial ischemia.
   f. Cardiac arrhythmias and intraventricular conduction delays are nondiagnostic findings.
5. ECG changes that appear with pain or exertion and resolve with rest are strongly indicative of myocardial ischemia.
6. A patient with a baseline abnormal resting ECG may develop only minor subtle ECG changes during an episode of angina; therefore, the ECG should be carefully compared to an old previous ECG (evaluate for "pseudonormalization" of previously inverted T waves).

C. Chest X-ray

1. Although not routinely indicated when evaluating a patient with typical anginal symptoms, a chest x-ray may be useful to evaluate the patient with atypical symptoms and may help to rule out other possible causes of chest pain, ie; pneumonia, pneumothorax, etc.
2. The presence of cardiomegaly on chest x-ray, as well as the presence of pulmonary edema, can be correlated with reduced left ventricular ejection

fraction, congestive heart failure, or previous myocardial infarction and may be associated with an adverse prognosis.

D. Stress Testing

1. By inducing a controlled, temporary ischemic state, stress testing can be useful in diagnosing myocardial ischemia, assessing the efficacy of antianginal therapy, and determining the extent of myocardium at risk.

2. Indications
   a. To clarify the etiology of chest pain and to provide reassurance that chest pain is not due to coronary ischemia
   b. To assess prognosis in patients with known ischemic heart disease and after myocardial infarction
      1) Submaximal stress test in patients following myocardial infarction.
      2) Positive stress test after minimal exertion may indicate severe triple-vessel disease or left main coronary artery disease.
      3) The physiologic significance of an anatomic lesion noted during catheterization can be evaluated.
   c. To evaluate the effects of medical or surgical management of coronary artery disease.
   d. To identify patients with positive stress tests after minimal exertion, or those who develop a hypotensive response to exercise, that should undergo early cardiac catheterization.
   e. To evaluate the functional capacity of patients to recommend appropriate activity and assess their ability to return to work. Some physicians also recommend stress testing in an apparently healthy middle-aged person who wishes to undertake a new physically stressful activity, ie; an exercise program.

3. Exercise ECG stress testing
   a. Method
      1) Patient is monitored with a 12-lead ECG while walking on a treadmill at workloads that can be progressively increased by increasing the speed and inclination of the device.
      2) A bicycle ergometer, using the arms, may be substituted for the treadmill for patients who are unable to exercise using their legs.
   b. Interpretation
      1) If during exercise, the patient develops anginal-type chest pain associated with downsloping or horizontal ST depression > 1 mm, the likelihood of coronary artery stenosis is high.
      2) Marked ST segment depression at a low level of exercise raises the possibility of left main coronary artery disease or multivessel disease.
      3) Overall, the sensitivity of routine exercise treadmill testing is 60–70%, with a specificity of up to 80%; the sensitivity is lowest in individuals with single-vessel disease and significantly higher in the presence of three-vessel coronary artery disease.

c. Contraindications to stress testing
   1) The recent onset of unstable angina
   2) Uncontrolled hypertension
   3) Patients with severe, uncontrolled congestive heart failure
   4) Significant ventricular arrhythmias are a relative contraindication.
4. Thallium 201 perfusion scintigraphy
   a. Because of the relative insensitivity of treadmill exercise testing to detect coronary artery disease, the exercise stress test can be modified by combining it with nuclear imaging agents.
   b. Method
      1) The patient is encouraged to exercise at maximal effort and 30–60 sec prior to termination of walking, the radionuclide is injected.
      2) Imaging begins 5–10 min following termination of exercise and is compared to a subsequent image obtained 4 h after exercise.
      3) Further scanning can be done 24 h later to improve sensitivity.
   c. Interpretation
      1) Areas of infarcted myocardium have no thallium uptake and hence show diminished or absent activity—a "fixed defect."
      2) Perfusion defects are also seen in transiently ischemic myocardium; however, these defects disappear as the ischemic episode resolves, ie; during the reperfusion scan (taken 4 h after the initial scintigraphy)—a "reperfusion defect."
      3) If the imaging procedure shows multiple zones of reduced perfusion, the patient has severe coronary artery disease.
      4) With this method, the sensitivity of thallium imaging is 82–98% depending on the extent of coronary artery disease: single-vessel disease (75%), double-vessel disease (89%), and triple-vessel disease (96%).
   d. Indications
      1) Patients whose baseline ECG readings indicate such abnormalities as left ventricular hypertrophy, repolarization disturbances, and left bundle branch block
      2) Patients with atypical symptoms and ambiguous ECG readings
      3) Elderly, female, and hypertensive patients who have a high likelihood of false positive ECG readings.
   e. For patients incapable of performing treadmill stress testing such as the elderly or patients with degenerative joint disease, pharmacologic methods may be used to increase coronary blood flow.
      1) Perfusion imaging can be performed after the IV injection of dipyridamole or adenosine, both potent vasodilators.
      2) Adverse effects
         a) *Dipyridamole—chest pain, hypotension, and headache*
         b) *Adenosine—chest pain, headache, flushing, and dyspnea; contraindicated in patients with asthma or severe chronic obstructive pulmonary disease*

5. Exercise echocardiography
   a. Another modality that is potentially useful to evaluate the cardiac response to exercise is the exercise echocardiogram, which analyzes wall motion abnormalities and failure of the ejection fraction to increase with exercise.
   b. The postexercise echocardiogram is compared with the resting study for regional wall motion abnormalities.
   c. The sensitivity and specificity are comparable to thallium scintigraphy.

E. Holter Monitoring
1. Useful for the detection of cardiac arrhythmias, 24-h Holter monitoring has no role in the routine evaluation of chronic stable angina.
2. 24-h ECG monitoring may be useful in detecting myocardial ischemia with ST segment elevation or depression observed during periods of ischemia in patients with exertional angina or Prinzmetal's angina; however, the sensitivity and specificity are less than that obtained with treadmill exercise testing.

F. Echocardiogram
1. Although not routinely used specifically for the evaluation of angina, an echocardiogram is useful to evaluate wall motion abnormalities as well as resting regional and global left ventricular systolic function.
2. Assessment of the cardiac valves, pericardium, ventricular wall thickness, and the presence of left ventricular thrombus and aneurysm can also be done.

G. Cardiac Catheterization
1. Coronary angiography can be used to confirm or exclude the diagnosis of coronary artery disease when the results of clinical examination and noninvasive tests are equivocal.
2. Coronary angiography is useful in identifying the anatomic extent of coronary artery disease. This information can be applied to the proper selection of medical therapy, angioplasty, or coronary artery bypass grafting in managing myocardial ischemia.
3. The administration of ergonovine during cardiac catheterization may be helpful in diagnosing coronary vasospasm in patients with Prinzmetal's angina.
4. Indications
   a. Exercise or dipyridamole stress test demonstrates low aerobic capacity, reduced heart rate response to exercise, hypotension or no increase in blood pressure, early or persistent ST segment depression or elevation, or multiple/large perfusion defects.
   b. This procedure may also be used when coronary artery bypass grafting or percutaneous transluminal coronary angioplasty is being contemplated as therapy for patients with chest pain unresponsive to standard medical therapy.

5. The decision to proceed to cardiac catheterization should be made in conjunction with a cardiologist.

III. Differential Diagnosis

A. Cardiac Disorders

1. Pericarditis
   a. Sharp chest discomfort in the center of the chest aggravated by deep breathing
   b. Worse with lying down and improved when sitting forward
   c. Pericardial friction rub heard on physical examination

2. Aortic dissection
   a. Sudden severe discomfort that may radiate to the back
   b. Symptoms prolonged and no prodromal symptoms
   c. Physical examination may reveal a disparity of peripheral pulses or an aortic insufficiency murmur.

B. Pulmonary Disorders

1. Pulmonary embolism
2. Pneumonia with pleurisy
3. Pneumothorax
4. Pulmonary hypertension

C. GI Disorders

1. Esophageal reflux/spasm (see Chapter 50)
2. Peptic ulcer disease (see Chapter 48)
3. Pancreatitis
4. Biliary disease/gallstones (see Chapter 51)

D. Musculoskeletal Disorders

1. Rib fracture
2. Costochondritis
3. Ruptured cervical disc
4. Degenerative joint disease of shoulder/spine
5. Muscle strain

E. Psychiatric—Anxiety Reaction

F. Herpes Zoster

IV. Treatment

A. Identification and Management of Risk Factors for Coronary Artery Disease

1. Obesity—weight loss program, nutrition counseling, exercise program
2. Tobacco abuse—smoking cessation program
3. Hypercholesterolemia—dietary counseling and treatment with antilipid medications, if indicated
4. Hypertension—antihypertensive medications should be used to control patients with elevated blood pressure.

B. Pharmacologic Therapy

1. No antianginal drug has been clearly shown to improve survival in patients with chronic stable angina.
2. Individual drugs or combination regimens may be chosen on the basis of specific desired pharmacologic effects and dosages should be adjusted according to the patient's clinical response.
3. Goal of therapy
   a. Increase blood flow to ischemic myocardium and/or decrease myocardial oxygen demand.
   b. Minimize the frequency and severity of angina and improve a patient's functional capacity with as few side effects as possible.
4. Angina may occur in patients who have various concomitant medical disorders, ie; diabetes mellitus, peripheral vascular disease, and so forth; therefore no one drug regimen is ideal for all patients under all circumstances (Table 21–1).
5. Patient convenience/compliance and cost of the drugs should be considered in selecting an antianginal medication.

C. Medications (Table 21–2)

1. Nitrate preparations
   a. Mechanism
      1) Acting as vasodilators, nitrates decrease venous return and, in turn, lower left ventricular diastolic volume and pressure.
      2) By decreasing preload, myocardial oxygen demand is also decreased.
   b. Preparations
      1) Sublingual/spray
         a) *Peak plasma levels are obtained within 2 min after dissolution of the tablet with sublingual administration or orally administered nitroglycerin spray.*
         b) *If the chest pain is not relieved after 3 sublingual nitroglycerin tablets or sprays taken 5 min apart, the patient should be instructed to call the physician or to immediately go to the closest emergency facility.*

Table 21-1. Treatments for Patients Who Have Angina in Conjunction With Other Medical Conditions*

Clinical Condition	Recommended Drug (Alternative Drug)
Cardiac arrhythmias and conduction abnormalities	
Sinus bradycardia	Nifedipine
Sinus tachycardia (not due to cardiac failure)	β Blocker
Supraventricular tachycardia	Verapamil or β blocker
Atrioventricular block	Nifedipine
Rapid atrial fibrillation	Verapamil or β blocker
Ventricular arrhythmias	β Blocker
Left ventricular dysfunction	
Congestive heart failure	
Mild-moderate (LVEF 35-50%)	Nifedipine or diltiazem (verapamil or β blockers cautiously)
Severe (LVEF < 35%)	Nitrates
Left-sided valvular heart disease[†]	
Aortic stenosis (mild)[‡]	β Blocker, calcium entry blocker, or nitrates
Aortic insufficiency	Nifedipine
Mitral regurgitation	Nifedipine
Mitral stenosis[§]	β Blocker or verapamil
Miscellaneous	
Systemic hypertension	β Blocker or calcium entry blocker
Headaches	β Blocker (verapamil or diltiazem)
COPD with bronchospasm or asthma	Nifedipine, verapamil, or diltiazem (low dose $β_1$-selective blocker or β-ISA)
Hyperthyroidism	β Blocker
Raynaud's syndrome	Nifedipine
Claudication	Calcium entry blocker (low-dose $β_1$ blocker or β-ISA)
Depression	Calcium entry blocker
Neurasthenia or fatigue states	Calcium entry blocker
Insulin-dependent diabetes mellitus	Calcium entry blocker (low-dose $β_1$ blocker or β-ISA)

* β-ISA, β blocker with intrinsic sympathomimetic activity (such as pindolol); COPD, chronic obstructive pulmonary disease; LVEF, left ventricular ejection fraction.
† Consideration should be given to surgical therapy for patients with severe valvular heart disease.
‡ Vasodilators might increase aortic valve gradient, and β blockers or verapamil could cause left ventricular failure. Any of these drugs can cause hypotension and should be used with caution in patients with severe aortic stenosis.
§ If congestive heart failure (associated with normal left ventricular function) occurs in a patient with angina, severe mitral stenosis, and rapid atrial fibrillation, a β blocker or verapamil (in combination with digitalis) may be used to decrease the heart rate.

SOURCE: Reproduced by permission from Shub C. Stable angina pectoris: 3. Medical treatment. Mayo Clin Proc 1990;65:256-273.

Table 21-2. Selected Drugs Used in the Treatment of Angina*

Class	Brand Name	Usual Starting Dose	Usual Maximum Dose	Onset	Duration
Nitrates*					
Nitroglycerin					
Sublingual[†]	Nitrostat and others	1 tablet (0.4 mg) at time of, or in anticipation of pain	2–3 tablets total at time of pain	30 sec	3–5 min
Topical					
Ointment	Nitro Bid, Nitrol	1/2 inch q 4–6 h	4–5 inches q 3–4 h	30–60 min	3–6 h
Patch[‡]	Transderm Nitro, Nitro-Dur and Nitrodisc	5 mg qd	2–3 patches that deliver 15 mg/24 h	30 min	24 h
Long-acting					
Erythrityl[†] tetranitrate	Cardilate	5 mg sublingually in anticipation of pain or 10 mg orally or chewed t.i.d.	100 mg/d in divided doses	5 min (sublingual and chewed)	4 h
Isosorbide[†] dinitrate	Isordil, Sorbitrate and others	10 mg q 4–6 h	60–80 mg q 4h	15–30 min	4–6 h
β-Adrenergic Blockers[†]					
Propranolol[†]	Inderal	10–20 mg t.i.d. or q.i.d.	320 mg/d in divided doses	1–1.5 h	4–6 h
Nadolol	Corgard	40 mg qd	240 mg	1–2 h	24 h
Tenormin	Atenolol	50 mg qd	100–150 mg	1–2 h	24 h

(continued)

* Due to the development of nitrate tolerance, a daily "nitrate-free" interval of 10–12 h is recommended.

Table 21-2. Selected Drugs Used in the Treatment of Angina* (continued)

Class	Brand Name	Usual Starting Dose	Usual Maximum Dose	Onset	Duration
Calcium Channel Blockers					
Nifedipine	Procardia	10 mg t.i.d. or q.i.d.; 10 mg at time of pain if sublingual	40 mg q 6 h	20–30 min	8 h
Verapamil	Calan, Isoptin	80 mg t.i.d. or q.i.d.	120 mg q.i.d.	30–45 min	6–8 h
Diltiazem	Cardiazom	30 mg q.i.d.	60 mg q 6h	30–45 min	6–8 h
Nicardipine	Cardene	20 mg t.i.d.	40 mg t.i.d.	30–120 min	8 h

* Other drugs, other doses of the drugs listed, and combinations of different drugs are marketed. The drugs and dosages shown are the ones most often used.

† Generic available.

‡ The brand name of these preparations is followed by a number (5, 10, 15, 20). It is important to know whether that number refers to milligrams per 24 hours (Transderm-Nitro) the patch (Nitro-Dur)

SOURCE: Reproduced with permission from Chandra NC. Angina pectoris. In: Barker LR, Burton JR, Zieve PD; eds. Principles of Ambulatory Medicine. Baltimore: Williams & Wilkins; 1991. © 1991, the Williams & Wilkins Co., Baltimore

  c) Patients should be encouraged to carry a fresh supply of sublingual nitroglycerin tablets because tablets more than 4–6 mo old may have reduced potency.
 2) Topical nitrates—transdermal patch/ointment
  a) The duration of action of nitroglycerin ointment is 6–8 h or more, due to the slow continuous uptake through the skin.
  b) Transdermal preparations allow for predictable, nonfluctuating plasma levels of nitrate and can be used once daily.
 3) Oral nitrate preparations—isosorbide dinitrate
c. Adverse effects
 1) Transient hypotension
  a) Especially noted in hot weather or after a hot bath
  b) Avoid hypovolemia
 2) Headache
  a) Start at low dosage and gradually increase as necessary.
  b) Transient side effect and subsides in 1–2 wk
  c) A mild analgesic may be useful when beginning therapy.
d. Nitrate tolerance
 1) Development of tolerance is variable and unpredictable.
 2) A daily "nitrate-free" interval of 10–12 h is advocated to restore nitrate responsiveness.

2. β-adrenergic blockers
 a. Mechanism
  1) Bind to myocardial β-adrenergic receptors (predominantly β_1) and competitively inhibit the binding of catecholamines.
   a) Decreased heart rate
   b) Decreased myocardial contractility, thereby decreasing myocardial oxygen demand
  2) In vascular smooth muscle, blockade of the β-adrenergic receptors (predominantly β_2) allows relatively unopposed α-adrenergic receptor stimulation.
   a) Increased vascular smooth muscle tone
   b) Peripheral vasoconstriction
 b. Preparations
  1) Therapy should be initiated with a low dosage, with the specific agent chosen depending on side effect profile, relative cardioselectivity, and coexistent diseases.
  2) The dosage must then be individualized to achieve the desired pharmacologic effects.
 c. Goals of therapy
  1) Reduction in the frequency and severity of angina attacks
  2) Resting heart rate of 50–60 beats/min
  3) Resting systolic blood pressure of 100–120 mm Hg
  4) Blunting of exercise heart rate and blood pressure response
  5) Absence of significant side effects

d. Adverse effects
   1) May worsen left ventricular systolic function and result in congestive heart failure if used in patients with poor left ventricular function, ie; ejection fraction < 30%.
   2) CNS effects—fatigue and depression
   3) Effects on peripheral circulation—worsening of claudication
   4) Pulmonary effects—worsening or precipitating bronchospasm
   5) Endocrine effects—masking of symptoms of hypoglycemia in patients with diabetes mellitus
   6) Genitourinary effects—impotence
   7) Withdrawal syndrome may rarely occur with abrupt termination of therapy—aggravation of angina, ventricular tachycardia, and precipitation of myocardial infarction

3. Calcium channel antagonists
   a. Mechanism
      1) Inhibit the entry of extracellular calcium into the cell through cell membrane channels
      2) Cardiovascular effects
         a) *Decreased myocardial contractility*
         b) *Depression of automaticity and conduction of the sinoatrial and atrioventricular (AV) nodes*
         c) *Decreased peripheral and coronary vasomotor tone*
   b. Preparations (Table 21-3)

Table 21-3. Comparative Clinical Effects of Calcium Entry Blockers*

Effect	Nifedipine	Verapamil	Diltiazem
Coronary vasodilation	+++	++	+++
Peripheral vasodilation	+++	++	+
Myocardial contractility†	↑↓‡	↓	↑↓
Heart rate	↑ (reflex)	↑↓	↑↓
Atrioventricular nodal conduction	NC	↓↓	↓
Side effects (incidence)	9–39%	10–14%	0–3%
Use with β blocker	Yes	Caution	Yes

* NC, no significant change is induced with commonly used clinical doses; ↑, increase; ↓, decrease; ↑↓, effect may either increase or decrease slightly; +, causes effect. The number of plus signs or arrows indicates the relative magnitude of the effect.

† A *direct* negative inotropic effect, which is dose-dependent, can be demonstrated with each calcium entry blocker (in decreasing order of potency: nifedipine, verapamil, and diltiazem) in the isolated heart preparation.

‡ Although the *direct* effect of nifedipine on isolated ventricular muscle is to decrease contractile function, in the intact heart this usually is compensated for by its salutary indirect effect on afterload and by reflex-mediated increases in left ventricular contractility (the latter can be blocked by propranolol).

SOURCE: Reproduced with permission from Shub C. Stable angina pectoris: 3. Medical treatment. Mayo Clin Proc 1990; 65:256–73.

1) Nifedipine (dihydroperidine)
   a) *Reflex sympathetic activation may occur with increased heart rate and speeding conduction through the AV node.*
   b) *Daily dose varies from 30–120 mg/d.*
2) Diltiazem—Daily dose varies from 120—360 mg/d.
3) Verapamil
   a) *Daily dose varies from 240–480 mg/d.*
   b) *Should be avoided in patients with overt congestive heart failure*

c. Adverse effects
   1) Flushing, hypotension, peripheral edema, and headaches occur more frequently with nifedipine; the slow release form tends to cause fewer side effects.
   2) Constipation occurs in approximately 10% of patients taking verapamil and can be a significant side effect especially in the elderly.
   3) Combination therapy of β-adrenergic blocker with either diltiazem or verapamil as calcium channel antagonists can result in severe bradycardia and AV conduction delay with AV block.

4. Other therapies in patients with coronary artery disease
   a. Angiotensin-converting enzyme (ACE) Inhibitors
      1) Mechanism
         a) *Decrease the coronary vasoconstrictor influences of angiotensin II*
         b) *As the blood pressure is lowered, ventricular wall stress is affected and myocardial oxygen demand is reduced.*
      2) The administration of ACE inhibitors after myocardial infarction has been shown to decrease mortality, episodes of heart failure, and recurrence of infarction in patients with impaired ventricular function.
   b. Aspirin
      1) Dosage: aspirin 325 mg/d or every other day
      2) No consistent antianginal effect
      3) Advantages—reduces mortality in patients with unstable angina and may prevent myocardial infarction; safe; inexpensive
      4) Disadvantages—increased bleeding complications

V. Indications for Referral to a Specialist

A. Patients with a markedly positive stress test should be referred to a cardiologist for cardiac catheterization to further evaluate the anatomy of the coronary arteries.

B. If medical therapy is ineffective or not tolerated, referral to a cardiologist is indicated for further evaluation as well as for consideration of revascularization either by percutaneous transluminal coronary angioplasty or bypass grafting.

VI. Indications for Hospitalization

A. Due to the risk of myocardial infarction and sudden death, any patient with unstable angina should be immediately evaluated and admission to the hospital is recommended for cardiac monitoring and aggressive medical therapy.

B. Patients with a history of angina presenting with acute congestive heart failure should be admitted for diuresis and aggressive medical therapy for left ventricular dysfunction.

VII. Annotated Bibliography

Chandra NC. Angina pectoris. In: Barker LR, Burton JR, Zieve PD, eds. Principles of Ambulatory Medicine. Baltimore: Williams & Wilkins 1991. Good review of diagnosis of angina in the ambulatory care setting with an extensive discussion of the indications and contraindications to exercise stress testing as well as the indications and complications of cardiac catheterization.

Gorlin R. Treatment of chronic stable angina pectoris. Am J Cardiol 1992;70: 28G–31G. Discussion of risk stratification and algorithm for therapeutic decision-making in patients with coronary artery disease and description of studies analyzing angioplasty versus bypass grafting.

Hackshaw BT. Excluding heart disease in the patient with chest pain. Am J Med 1992;92 (suppl 5A):46S–51S. Concise review covering the evaluation of a patient with the complaint of "chest pain" with a discussion of the diagnostic modalities available.

Shub C. Stable angina pectoris: 1. Clinical patterns, 2. Cardiac evaluation and diagnostic testing, and 3. Medical treatment. Mayo Clin Proc 1990;64:233–273. From the Symposium on Myocardial Ischemia, these articles review the current recommendations regarding the evaluation of anginal chest pain.

Chapter 22: Valvular Heart Disease

Gregg Fromell

22A Aortic Stenosis

I. Clinical Presentation

A. General Information

1. Represents the most common valvular lesion in the elderly
2. Patients with aortic stenosis (AS) are often asymptomatic for years.
3. Causes
   a. Progressive calcification of previously normal valve (senile calcification)
      1) Most common overall cause of AS
      2) In early and mid-1900s rheumatic valvular disease was a more common cause.
   b. Aortic congenital malformation
      1) Unicuspid
      2) Bicuspid
   c. Rheumatically damaged valve
      1) Now an uncommon cause of AS
      2) When it does occur is almost always associated with mitral valvular disease
4. Age and etiologies
   a. Stenosis before age 30—usually from aortic congenital valve abnormality
   b. Stenosis age 30–70—usually 50:50% congenital/rheumatic abnormality
   c. Stenosis after age 70—usually from degenerative calcification of normal aortic valve

B. Symptoms

Patients generally have no symptoms for many years. The classic triad of symptoms is dyspnea on exertion, angina, and syncope, although symptoms can occur individually. As expected, patients with symptoms have a decidedly worse prognosis than those without symptoms.

1. Exertional dyspnea
   a. Most common associated symptom. Often comes on insidiously with patients slowly decreasing involvement in physical activities.
   b. Thought to be secondary to increased pulmonary artery pressure
   c. Can occur as anginal equivalent
   d. Without valve replacement, average time of occurrence of symptoms to death is 2 y.

2. Angina
   a. The most common presenting symptom with a prevalence of 49–80% (except in the elderly where left ventricular failure is the most common presenting symptom).
   b. Usually develops somewhat later than exertional dyspnea
   c. Can have angina without coronary artery disease due to marked left ventricular hypertrophy (LVH) and resultant increased oxygen demands
   d. Angina can be atypical, in that it may occur *after* exertion
   e. Without valve replacement, average time of occurrence of symptoms to death is 3–4.5 y.

3. Syncope
   a. Often occurs during or just after exertion, but can also occur while supine
   b. Causes
      1) Evidence indicates that this is due to inappropriate left ventricular baroreceptor response in some patients.
      2) Inadequate blood flow across the aortic valve
      3) Arrhythmia—supraventricular tachycardia (SVT), atrial fibrillation/flutter, ventricular tachycardia
   c. Seizures and incontinence can occur with syncope of long duration.
   d. Sudden death (presumably secondary to arrhythmia) is common: 10–20% of deaths in patients with AS.
   e. Without valve replacement, average time of occurrence of symptoms to death is 3 y.

4. Left-sided heart failure
   a. In the elderly, this is the most common presenting complaint
   b. Severe dyspnea, orthopnea, paroxysmal nocturnal dyspnea
   c. Pulmonary edema
   d. Has been reported as the cause of death in one half to one third of patients with aortic stenosis
   e. Without valve replacement, average time of occurrence of symptoms to death is 1.5–2 y.

C. Physical Examination

1. Vital signs
   a. Usually not hypertensive
   b. Pulse pressure usually 30–40 mm Hg
   c. Heart rate usually slow

2. Palpation
   a. Except for advance AS, apical impulse is usually within left midclavicular line due to concentric hypertrophy.
   b. Advanced AS usually results in displacement of apical impulse inferiolaterally.
   c. Ventricular heave is often present.
   d. Thrill very often present; palpable at base of heart, jugular notch, and along carotids
      1) Occasionally only palpable during exhalation while patient leans forward
      2) In patients without abnormal chest wall, emphysema or congestive heart failure (CHF), absence of a thrill generally signifies mild disease.
   e. Delayed carotid upstrokes (may be absent in mild AS)
3. Auscultation
   a. Systolic click as result of forceful opening of aortic valve
      1) Generally occurs in congenital and rheumatic aortic stenosis
      2) Generally absent in calcified AS
   b. Systolic ejection murmur
      1) Usually 3/6 or greater
      2) Loudest at second intercostal space parasternally
      3) Usually radiates to base and carotids, although can sometimes radiate to apex
   c. Paradoxical splitting of S_2
      1) In normal heart, the aortic sound is usually heard first followed quickly by the pulmonic sound; this is normal splitting of the S_2.
      2) In AS this interval narrows, and as the stenosis progresses, the sounds may be superimposed on one another. In that case, exhalation causes later closure of the aortic valve resulting in the pulmonic sound occurring first, followed quickly by the aortic sound—paradoxical splitting.
   d. Diastolic murmur—In pure AS, can occur due to valve stenosis not allowing complete closure of the aortic valve. This results in an insignificant aortic insufficiency with an associated diastolic murmur

II. Diagnostic Approach

A. ECG

1. Is not helpful in assessing the severity of AS; can be normal in early AS
2. Left ventricular hypertrophy
   a. The most common ECG abnormality
   b. Absence of LVH does not exclude severe AS
3. ST segment can be depressed, T waves are often inverted with a strain pattern in leads I, aVL and the lateral precordial leads in advanced AS.

4. Conduction system disease
   a. Atrioventricular (AV) block
   b. Left anterior hemiblock
   c. Right bundle branch block
   d. Left bundle branch block
   e. QRS prolongation

5. Arrhythmias—usually occur late in the course of the disease and can be any of a variety of complex arrhythmias
   a. Superventricular tachycardia (SVT)
   b. Premature ventricular contractions (PVCs)
   c. R-on-T phenomenon
   d. Ventricular tachycardia
   e. Atrial fibrillation—not often seen in isolated pure AS; most commonly in association with rheumatic mitral valve disease or coronary artery disease (CAD) and when seen, should alert the clinician to these underlying diseases.

B. Echocardiogram with Doppler flow studies

1. The procedure of choice for the routine evaluation of aortic valvular disease

2. Accurately assesses aortic valve area and gradient with a high correlation to cardiac catheterization

3. Useful in differentiating congenital from rheumatic from calcification of valve

4. Useful in differentiating aortic sclerosis from aortic stenosis, which can be indistinguishable on general examination

5. Assesses LVH and overall ventricular function, which can start to deteriorate before symptoms

6. A peak systolic pressure gradient of ≥ 50 mm Hg (in the presence of a normal cardiac output) or an aortic valve area of ≥ 0.7 cm^2 is indicative of critical obstruction.

7. Echocardiogram may underestimate the severity of AS if the highest velocity jet is not parallel to the transducer. If symptoms suggest severe AS or if left ventricular dysfunction exists, cardiac catheterization should be performed.

C. Chest X-ray

1. May show no enlargement of cardiac silhouette for many years

2. Often see rounding of the ventricular silhouette due to concentric hypertrophy

3. Calcification can usually be assessed. Absence of aortic valve calcification in an adult usually suggests that severe AS is not present.

4. Poststenotic dilatation of the aorta is frequently seen.

D. Exercise Tolerance Testing

1. Generally should *not* be done until after the severity of stenosis and general left ventricular function can be assessed with Doppler echocardiography because exercise can worsen gradient and lead to syncope, arrhythmia, and possibly sudden death.
2. Other than assessing exercise tolerance (after Doppler echocardiography) it is of limited value in the evaluation of a patient with AS.

E. Cardiac Catheterization

1. Although is the most accurate means of assessing valvular gradient, and therefore valve surface area, is most often of little additional value over Doppler echocardiography in the routine evaluation of the patient with AS
2. Useful in evaluating comorbid conditions
    a. Suspected underlying CAD
        1) *Especially in men > 40 y of age and women > 50 y of age*
        2) Risk factors for CAD
        3) Symptoms consistent with angina
    b. Patients with multivalvular disease
    c. Assessment of aortic root prior to surgical valve replacement

III. Differential Diagnosis

A. Aortic sclerosis

B. Subaortic stenosis (idiopathic hypertrophic subaortic stenosis, asymmetrical septal hypertrophy)

C. Supraaortic stenosis

IV. Treatment

A. Endocarditis Prophylaxis (see Appendix B)

1. Should prescribe antibiotic prophylaxis for any type of aortic stenosis prior to dental procedures and genitourinary procedures

B. Risk Factor Intervention

1. Should always attempt to eliminate treatable risk factors
    a. Careful blood pressure control in hypertensive patient
    b. Careful diabetic control
    c. Smoking cessation
    d. Lipid evaluation and appropriate treatment
    e. Weight reduction in obese patients

C. Severe AS—no strenuous physical exertion, even in asymptomatic patients.

D. Medications—Patients requiring medical treatment of symptoms carry a worse prognosis than those not requiring treatment.

1. CHF—digoxin, oxygen, diuretics with gentle diuresis
   a. Avoid intravascular volume depletion, which can worsen the aortic gradient.
   b. Try to avoid nitrates, unless angina present because they can also decrease afterload and worsen the aortic gradient.

2. Angina—sublingual nitrates useful, but avoid long-term nitrate therapy due to reasons noted above. Calcium channel blockers useful, but avoid those with significant vasodilatory properties (afterload reducers) because they worsen aortic gradient.

3. Hypertension—avoid vasodilating medications (α blockers, angiotensin-converting enzyme [ACE] inhibitors, vasodilating calcium channel blockers such as nifedipine)

E. Indications for Valve Replacement

1. Symptomatic patient

2. Significant aortic valve gradient: gradient $\geq$ 50 mm Hg or valve area $\geq$ 0.7 cm^2/m^2 body surface area (even without symptoms).

3. Previously the mortality rate for aortic valve replacement in the elderly was 15–20%, although with improved surgical technique, postoperative care, and possibly better patient selection, the mortality rate for valve replacement in this age group has declined to 5–15%.

F. Aortic Balloon Valvuloplasty (Table 22A-1)

1. Not useful in the average patient because rapid restenosis (within 6 mo) is the rule in patients with degenerative AS. Also there is usually a significant residual stenosis remaining after the procedure.

2. May be appropriate in certain patients as a temporizing maneuver before valve replacement or as a palliative maneuver in patients with other significant comorbid diseases.

V. Patient Education

A. In severe aortic stenosis—no strenuous physical exertion

B. Risk factor intervention

C. Stress importance of at least yearly follow-up with physician and serial echocardiograms (however, senile AS may progress rapidly, and more frequent follow-up may be required).

Table 22A–1. Indications for Aortic Balloon Valvuloplasty in Elderly Patients with Symptomatic Aortic Stenosis

Limited life span secondary to noncardiac illness
Cardiac surgery undesirable
    Patient refusal
    Dementia
    Severe cachexia
    Surgical high risk: coexistent nonrevascularizable coronary artery disease, severe pulmonary hypertension, "egg-shell aorta"
"Bridge" before future surgery
    Valve replacement (cardiogenic shock or severe congenital heart failure secondary to AS)
    Urgent noncardiac surgery
Assessment of AS severity in patient with left ventricular dysfunction and low cardiac output and gradient

SOURCE: Reproduced with permission by Frankl WS, Brest AN Valvular heart disease: comprehensive evaluation and treatment. In: Brest AN, ed. Cardiovascular Clinics. Philadelphia: FA Davis; 1993:187.

D. Alert patient to report symptoms of dyspnea, angina, and syncope or presyncope immediately.

VI. Long-term Management

A. Endocarditis prophylaxis

B. Risk factor intervention

C. Continued follow-up of risk factor interventions

D. At least yearly follow-up examination and echocardiography (more frequently as clinically indicated).

E. Yearly ECG to assess conduction system disease

F. Surgical risk to noncardiac surgery

1. Asymptomatic patients are at slightly higher risk to noncardiac surgery, although this risk is generally not serious and the postoperative problems are usually easily treated. General cardiac function is the best indicator of risk in this population of patients.

VII. Indications for Referral to a Cardiologist

A. Anyone who is symptomatic generally should undergo cardiac catheterization

B. Valvular gradient ≥ 50 mm Hg or valve area ≥ 0.7 cm²/m² body surface area (even without symptoms)

C. Patients with multivalvular disease

VIII. Bibliography

See end of chapter

22B Aortic Insufficiency

I. Clinical Presentation

A. General Information
1. Definition—Aortic insufficiency (AI) is a condition of the aortic valve that results in incomplete closure of the aortic valve leaflets. This leads to the pathologic condition of regurgitation across the aortic valve during diastole—aortic regurgitation (AR).
2. Isolated AI is more common in men.
3. AI associated with mitral valve disease is more common in women.
4. Common causes of AI (Table 22B-1)
    a. Rheumatic fever—46% (not as common in isolated AI)
        1) Fibrous tissue infiltration of valve can lead to improper closure of the valve. Can also cause combined AI and aortic stenosis (AS).
        2) Often associated with rheumatic mitral valve disease
    b. Aortic root disease—21%
        1) Dilatation of the aortic root prevents full co-optation of the valve leaflets.
    c. Congenitally bicuspid valve—20%
        1) Although more likely to cause AS, can also cause AI due to prolapse of the larger valve
        2) Associated with ventricular septal defect 15% of time
    d. Infective endocarditis—9%
        1) Valvular insufficiency due to vegetation interfering with closure or valve perforation
    e. Trauma
        1) Tear in the ascending aorta with loss of valve leaflet support can lead to prolapse of the aortic valve
5. Resultant cardiac pathology
    a. Dilation and marked hypertrophy of the left ventricle due to large aortic regurgitation (AR)
    b. Endocardial pockets in the left ventricle at site of regurgitant jet
    c. Dilation of the mitral valve annulus
        1) May lead to mitral regurgitation
6. Natural history
    a. May be asymptomatic for years (as many as 7-10 y) but once symptoms develop, further cardiac dysfunction progresses fairly rapidly
    b. Mild to moderate AR carries a 10-y mortality rate of 5-15%
    c. Severe AR carries a 10-y mortality rate of 30%
    d. Associated angina and congestive heart failure (CHF) carry a much worse prognosis
        1) With angina, average time to death from onset of symptoms is 4 y
        2) With CHF average time to death from onset of symptoms is 2 y

Table 22B–1. Etiologies of Aortic Insufficiency

Aortic Valve Abnormalities	Aortic Root Abnormalities
Postrheumatic	Noninflammatory dilatation
Infective endocarditis	Ehlers-Danlos
Congenital anomaly	Pseudoxanthoma elasticum
Bicuspid valve	Familial aortopathy
Quadricuspid valve	Dissecting aorta
AI associated with ventricular septal defect	Marfan's syndorme
Tetrology of Fallot	Infectious
Subaortic stenosis	Syphilis
"Floppy" aortic valve	Aortitis
Trauma	Systemic lupus erythematosus
Spontaneous tear	Rheumatoid arthritis
Idiopathic	Nonspecific familial aortitis
	Annular ectasia of the aorta
	Aneurysm of the sinus of Valsalva

SOURCE: Adapted from Gaasch WH, Levine HJ, eds. Chronic Aortic Regurgitation. Boston: Kluwer Academic Publishers; 1988:3.

B. Symptoms

1. Chronic AR

   a. Patients are generally asymptomatic until late in the progression of the disease. Often there is significant left ventricular dilatation and dysfunction without significant symptoms.

   b. Can be symptom free for many years, depending on cause. Common symptoms when they do develop are:
      1) Exertional dyspnea
         a) *probably the most common symptom. Thought secondary to increased left ventricular end-diastolic pressure resulting in pulmonary venous congestion*
      2) Orthopnea
      3) Paroxysmal nocturnal dyspnea
      4) Increased cardiac awareness, particularly when lying down
      5) Tachycardia with exertion or emotional stress
      6) Angina
         a) *Common in the elderly although less frequent than with AS*
         b) *Can occur as nocturnal angina*

   c. Syncope
      1) Unlike in AS, syncope is rare

2. Acute AR

   a. Usually as a result of endocarditis, trauma, or dissection

b. Presentation is significantly different from chronic AR because there is not time for left ventricle to adapt; depending on the degree of AR, can be catastrophic
c. Usually patients markedly symptomatic
   1) Tachycardic
   2) Dyspneic
   3) Often cyanotic

C. Physical Examination

1. Chronic severe AR
   a. Vital signs
      1) Widened pulse pressure—elevated systolic pressure, with lower than average diastolic pressure
         a) *Generally not seen in mild AR or acute AR*
         b) *The degree of decreased diastolic pressure correlates with severity of AR better than increased systolic pressure.*
         c) *The normal finding of increased femoral systolic pressure is accentuated with AR.*
   b. Palpation—a host of physical findings can often be discerned (Table 22B–2) including:
      1) Water-hammer pulses (abrupt, strong pulse with sudden diastolic collapse)
      2) Diffuse apical impulse displaced laterally and inferiorly
      3) Hyperdynamic precordium with palpable ventricle filling wave
      4) Systolic thrill often palpable
   c. Auscultation
      1) S_1 usually normal or reduced slightly
      2) A_2 often accentuated but sometimes diminished and P_2 often obscured by diastolic murmur
      3) S_3, when present signifies increased left ventricular end-diastolic volume and is a poor prognostic sign
      4) Often a systolic ejection click
      5) Often a systolic flow murmur at base
      6) Diastolic AR murmur—high frequency murmur, thus best heard with diaphragm of stethoscope
         a) *Timing*
            i) Occurs immediately after A_2 component of S_2
            ii) In mild AR, usually early diastolic
            iii) In moderate/severe AR, usually holodiastolic
            iv) Generally quickly crescendos, then decrescendos roughly after the first third of diastole
            v) Duration rather than intensity of murmur correlates better with severity of AR
         b) *Location*
            i) Third left parasternal interspace—lower sternal border (often indicates primary valve disease)
            ii) Second right parasternal interspace (often indicates aortic root disease)

c) *Patient position*
      i) Milder murmurs best heard with patient leaning forward and in full expiration
      ii) Murmur accentuated with interventions raising blood pressure—isometric exercise, squatting
      iii) Murmur reduced by interventions lowering blood pressure—Valsalva maneuver, amyl nitrate inhalation
7) Austin Flint murmur
   a) *Caused when large regurgitant flow impinges on the mitral valve partially obstructing flow. Low-pitched, rumbling murmur, best heard with bell of stethoscope*
      i) Mid and late diastole
      ii) Can be confused with mitral stenosis (MS) murmur, but: no opening snap or loud S_1 (which is often heard in MS) and murmur diminished with amyl nitrate (which would be increased in MS)
8) Systolic murmur
   a) *Short mid systolic murmur may be heard*
      i) Often preceded by an opening snap

Table 22B–2. Peripheral or Nonauscultatory Signs of Severe Aortic Regurgitation: A Glossary of Terms

Bisferiens pulse	A double or bifid systolic impulse felt in the arterial pulse
Corrigan's Sign	Visible pulsation of the supraclavicular and carotid arteries
Pistol shot of Traube	A loud systolic sound heard with the stethoscope lightly placed over the femoral arteries
Palmar click	A palpable, abrupt flushing of the palms in systole
Quincke's pulse	Exaggerated sequential reddening and blanching of the fingernail beds when light pressure is applied to the tip of the fingernail. A similar observation can be made by pressing a glass slide to the lips.
Duroziez's sign	A to-an-fro bruit heard over the femoral artery when light pressure is applied to the artery by the edge of the stethoscope head. This bruit is caused by the exaggerated reversal of flow in diastole.
De Musset's sign	Visible oscillation or bobbing of the head with each heartbeat.
Hill's sign	Abnormal accentuation of leg systolic blood pressure, with popliteal pressure 40 mm HG or higher than brachial artery pressure
Water-hammer pulse	The high-amplitude, abruptly collapsing pulse of AR. This term refers to a popular Victorian toy comprised of a glass vessel partially filled with water, which produced a slapping impact on being turned over.
Muller's sign	Visible pulsation of the uvula

source: Reproduced with permission from Abrams J. Essentials of Cardiac Physical Diagnosis. Philadelphia: Lea & Febiger; 1987.

ii) Best heard at base of heart
  iii) Grade of murmur can vary
  iv) Often with palpable thrill

2. Acute AR

   The examination is significantly different from that for chronic AR. The "classic" findings noted above, such as water-hammer pulses, displaced apical impulse, and thrill are absent. Blood pressure does not exhibit widened pulse pressure. Austin Flint murmur is either briefer or absent. Also, S_3 and S_4 are often present.

II. Diagnostic Approach

A. ECG

1. Chronic AR, often see

   a. Left axis deviation
   b. Prominent Q waves leads I aVl and V3–V6
   c. Left ventricular hypertrophy (LVH) with increased amplitude of QRS
   d. Inverted T waves with ST segment depression
   e. Intraventricular conduction delay late in disease process, usually in the setting of left ventricular dysfunction.

2. Acute AR

   a. In the absence of other cardiac pathology, generally not significantly abnormal
   b. Nonspecific ST-T changes are common.

B. Chest X-ray

1. Chronic AR

   a. Early in course of disease, heart size usually appears normal.
   b. In long-standing disease, there may be a markedly increased size of cardiac silhouette
   c. Aortic calcification uncommon in pure AR, may be seen in AS/AR
   d. Dilatation of aorta in aortic root disease
   e. In bicuspid aortic valve there is sometimes an associated aortic coarctation, so should look for rib notching.

2. Acute AR

   a. In the absence of other cardiac disease, cardiac silhouette is often normal.
   b. If severe, pulmonary engorgement and pulmonary edema may be present.

C. Echocardiography with Doppler Flow Studies

1. Most reliable noninvasive test to evaluate AR

2. May underestimate regurgitant stream if velocity of jet is not parallel to transducer.
   a. Chronic AR
      1) Increased left ventricular end-diastolic dimensions
      2) Increased septal and posterior wall motion
      3) Anterior leaflet of mitral valve exhibits diastolic high-frequency fluttering (in both acute and chronic AR and even in mild disease)
      4) End-systolic left ventricular dimension of > 55 mm and fractional shortening of < 25% usually indicates irreversible left ventricle dysfunction.
      5) Findings dependent on cause of AR
         a) *Bicuspid valve*
         b) *Prolapsed valve*
         c) *Flail leaflet—more often seen in acute AI due to acute disruption of the valve from endocarditis*
         d) *Valve thickening*
         e) *Valvular calcification (rare in pure AR, not uncommon in AR/AS)*
         f) *Valve vegetation*
         g) *Aortic root dilatation*
   b. Acute AR
      1) Very little increase in left ventricular end-diastolic dimensions
      2) Delayed mitral valve opening
      3) Premature closure of mitral valve
      4) Anterior leaflet of mitral valve exhibits diastolic high-frequency fluttering.

D. Radionuclide Testing

1. Very helpful in noninvasively determining regurgitant fraction (although accuracy affected by other associated valvular disease)
2. Generally, Doppler echocardiography and gated radionuclide angiography are adequate to follow disease process and to make a decision on timing of surgical valve replacement.

E. Cardiac Catheterization

1. Use is generally reserved for additional assessment (assessment of coronary arteries and aorta, assessment of other associated valvular lesions)
2. Should likely be performed in the elderly patient with symptoms due to the high incidence of associated coronary artery disease in this population.

F. Exercise Tolerance Testing

1. May be useful in assessing exercise capacity, otherwise adds little to the work-up of AI.

III. Differential Diagnosis

A. Early or Holodiastolic Murmur

1. Pulmonic regurgitation—Murmur begins later, after P_2 rather than after A_2, and there is no widened pulse pressure.
2. Reverberation of S_2 sometimes is heard in patients with significant systemic hypertension.

B. Mid to Late Diastolic Murmur

1. Mitral stenosis (see also section I, Clinical Presentation—part C. Physical Examination—Austin Flint murmur)

IV. Treatment

A. Acute AR

1. Patients are often hemodynamically unstable and require emergent valve replacement.
2. In infective endocarditis, if stable can postpone surgery for at least 1 wk of antibiotic therapy, although may progress to emergent valve replacement as well.

B. Chronic AR

1. Antibiotic prophylaxis for endocarditis (see Appendix B)
2. Regular follow-up with echocardiography
3. Serial ECGs and chest x-rays
4. Consider serial radionuclide studies
5. Mild to moderate AR (asymptomatic with minimal cardiac enlargement)
   a. Other than antibiotic prophylaxis, no medical therapy
6. Severe AR, symptomatic AR, or asymptomatic AR with left ventricular dilation
   a. Salt restriction
   b. Vasodilators/afterload reducing agents—some evidence that these agents may slow the progression of disease
   c. Diuretics
   d. Digoxin (assuming no contraindication)
7. Surgical intervention—Timing of aortic valve replacement remains controversial.
   a. Generally not for asymptomatic patients with good exercise tolerance (even with severe AR)
   b. Generally for symptomatic patients with left ventricular dysfunction

c. Difficulty in deciding on those who lie between these extremes of clinical presentation

V. Patient Education

A. With left ventricular dysfunction, no vigorous sports or heavy exertion

B. Stress need for regular follow-up and serial testing (thought exact frequency of testing is debatable)

C. Risk factor education

VI. Indications for Referral to a Cardiologist

A. Any patient with
1. Symptoms
2. LVH or enlarged cardiac silhouette on chest x-ray
3. Evidence of left ventricular dysfunction even if asymptomatic
4. Questionable etiology of valvular disease
5. AR with an unclear etiology

VII. Bibliography

See end of chapter

22C Atrial Septal Defect

I. Clinical Information

A. General Information

1. One of the most common congenital cardiac anomalies in adults (occurring more frequently in women than men)

2. May be of three types

   a. Persistent ostium primum atrial septal defect (ASD)
      1) This form usually diagnosed and treated in childhood
      2) Actually a form of atrioventriculoseptal defect
      3) May be associated with mitral valve prolapse (MVP)
      4) One form or primum defect occurs commonly in Down syndrome
   b. Persistent ostium secundum ASD
      1) Most common type of ASD
      2) Associated MVP—less common than ostium primum defects, but still has been reported in as many as 8–37% of cases
   c. Sinus venosus ASD
      1) Often associated with anomalous connection of right lung pulmonary veins

3. Lutembacher's syndrome

   a. A rare combination of ASD and mitral stenosis thought secondary to rheumatic valve disease
   b. Left-to-right shunting that occurs in ASD depends on size of defect as well as impedance of pulmonary circulation as well as diastolic properties of both ventricles.
   c. As patient ages (usually over fourth decade) pulmonary hypertension from a chronically overloaded right ventricle causes bidirectional flow, then ultimately a right-to-left shunt—an Eisenmenger's syndrome (Eisenmenger's syndrome is far more common in ventricular septal defect and patent ductus arteriosus)

4. Pulmonary hypertension is not common, but when present, progression is the natural history. Rate of progression is quite variable.

B. Symptoms

1. Symptoms are not common in pediatric population.

2. May be asymptomatic in adults if defect is small.

3. Dyspnea

   a. Most common associated symptom
   b. Likely result of pulmonary hypertension

4. Congestive heart failure can develop in severe cases

C. Physical Examination

1. Vital signs
   a. Usually normal blood pressure and pulse
2. Inspection
   a. In ostium primum defects, often rounded chest
   b. Generally no cyanosis or nail clubbing; however in the small percentage with significant pulmonary hypertension and Eisenmenger's syndrome, can see cyanosis and nail clubbing
3. Palpation
   a. Prominent apical, right ventricular impulse
   b. May have systolic thrill along sternal border
4. Auscultation
   a. S_1 normal, occasionally split
   b. Fixed, split A_2, P_2 during inspiration and expiration
   c. Systolic murmur
      1) Auscultation: holosystolic, peaking slightly before mid-systole
      2) Location: left second and third interspaces parasternally
      3) Occurs from high-velocity flow through pulmonary artery from overfilled right ventricle.
      4) When associated with MVP, may hear classic mitral regurgitation murmur as well.
   d. Diastolic murmur
      1) Usually indicative of large shunt; occurs from increased blood flow across tricuspid valve. Usually associated with significant pulmonary hypertension
         a) *Auscultation: short, rumbling*
         b) *Location: left sternal border*

II. Diagnostic Approach

A. ECG

1. Ostium primum defects
   a. Incomplete or complete right bundle branch block (RBBB)
   b. Counterclockwise rotation of precordial leads
   c. PR prolongation
2. Ostium secundum defects
   a. Borderline right axis deviation and incomplete or complete RBBB is the most common ECG finding.
   b. Right ventricular hypertrophy is common in children but not in adults.
   c. Atrial fibrillation
      1) Generally occurs later in the course of the disease
      2) Very common in older patients (20–30% of cases)

3. Sinus venosus defect
   a. Ectopic atrial pacer
   b. First-degree atrioventricular block

B. Chest X-ray

1. Increased right atrium and right ventricle
2. Dilated pulmonary arteries
3. Left atrium not commonly enlarged

C. Echocardiography with Doppler Flow Studies

1. Diagnosis is possible for most patients by Doppler echocardiography, and therefore has all but replaced cardiac catheterization in the assessment of the patient with suspected ASD
2. Many cases can go to surgery without cardiac catheterization.
3. Findings
   a. Right atrial, right ventricle, and pulmonary artery dilatation
   b. Paradoxical septal motion if significant right ventricular overload.

D. Cardiac Catheterization

1. Reserved for instances when quality of echocardiography in question or inconsistencies of clinical information
2. Important in assessing suspected coronary artery disease
3. Important in evaluating patient with suspected pulmonary hypertension
4. Important in assessing other associated valvular lesions.

III. Differential Diagnosis

A. Other findings that also have a fixed sound after the S_2 mimicking fixed splitting of the second heart sound

1. Opening snap of mitral valve
2. High-pitched S_3
3. Pericardial knock

B. Other causes of holosystolic murmurs

1. Mitral regurgitation (generally can be distinguished by the location and classic radiation of murmur)
2. Tricuspid regurgitation

a. Best heard at the lower left sternal border
b. May radiate to the sternal border and the left mid-clavicular line but not into the axilla

IV. Treatment

A. Antibiotic Prophylaxis for Endocarditis (see Appendix B)

B. Surgical Repair

1. Ostium primum defects

    a. Diagnosis and repair are usually accomplished in childhood.

2. Ostium secundum defects

    a. If small and asymptomatic, simply follow.
    b. If large or symptomatic, surgical repair is recommended.

3. Pulmonary hypertension

    a. Increases risk to surgical valve replacement
    b. On cardiac catheterization, if pulmonary resistance is
        1) < 10 U/m2—repair valve
        2) > 15 U/m2—surgery is high risk
        3) from 10–15 U/m2—probably should be repaired

4. Atrial fibrillation

    a. Medication as appropriate for rate control
        1) Calcium channel blockers (avoid those that may worsen conduction deficits or cardiac ionotropy)
        2) Digoxin

V. Indications for Referral to a Cardiologist

A. Any patient with diagnosis confirmed by Doppler echocardiography

B. Any patient with suspected diagnosis but equivocal echocardiography (eg, poor quality echo due to body habitus)

VI. Bibliography

See end of chapter

22D Mitral Valve Prolapse

I. Clinical Presentation

A. General Information

1. Definition: prolapse of mitral leaflets back into left atrium above the level of the mitral annulus
2. The majority of patients are asymptomatic.
3. A common syndrome reported in both men and women, although it is more common in women. May affect as many as 3–4% of the general population.
4. Seen over a wide age range but more common in ages 14–30 y
5. Autosomal dominant inheritance with variable expression
6. Other names given mitral valve prolapse (MVP) include:
   a. Barlow's syndrome
   b. Systolic click-murmur syndrome
   c. Billowing and ballooning mitral valve syndrome
   d. Floppy mitral valve syndrome
   e. Overshoot or hooded mitral valve
   f. Myxomatous or mucinous degeneration of mitral valve
7. Myxomatous proliferation within valve is common but myxomatous degeneration can occur.
   a. Usually idiopathic
   b. May occur in association with connective tissue disorders
8. Mitral regurgitation (MR) may or may not be present and can range from mild to severe.
9. Conditions associated with MVP (Table 22D-1)
10. Complications associated with MVP
    a. Increased risk of endocarditis (although actual risk not known)
    b. Rupture of chordae
       1) Although fibrosis, ischemia, myocardial infarction, and endocarditis can lead to rupture of chordae with resultant MVP, MVP itself is a common cause of chordae rupture through fibrotic changes and "wear and tear" on chordae.
    c. Calcification of mitral annulus
    d. MR

Table 22D-1. Conditions Associated with Mitral Valve Prolapse

Connective tissue disorders—genetic
- Mitral valve prolapse—isolated
- Marfan syndrome
- Ehlers-Danlos syndrome—types I, II and IV
- Pseudoxanthoma elasticum
- Osteogenisis imperfecta
- Polycystic kidneys

Connective tissue disorders—inflammatory
- Systemic lupus erythematosus
- Relapsing polychondritis
- Rheumatic endocarditis
- Polyarteritis nodosa

Other genetic disorders
- Duchenne's muscular dystrophy
- Myotonic dystrophy
- Fragile X syndorme
- Mucopolysaccharidoses
- Cutis laxa
- Menke's kinky hair syndrome
- Homocystinuria

Other associated disorders
- Atrial septal defect—primum and secundum type
- Hypertrophic obstructive cardiomyopathy
- Wolff-Parkinson-White syndrome
- Papillary muscle dysfunction
    - Ischemic heart disease
    - Myocarditis
- Cardiac trauma
- Following mitral valve surgery
- Von Willebrand's disease
- Carcinoid tumor
- Alcoholism
- Acromegaly

SOURCE: Modified from Fontana ME, Sperks FA, Boudoules H, Wooley CF. Mitral valve prolapse and the mitral prolapse syndrome. Curr Prob Cardiol 1991;16:309–375 and Boudoulas H, Kolibash AJ, Beker P, King BD, Wooley CF. Mitral valve prolapse and the mitral valve prolapse syndrome: a diagnostic classification and pathogenisis of symptoms. Am Heart J 1989;118:797.

B. Symptoms

1. The vast majority of patients are asymptomatic. When symptoms do appear, the presentation can be variable.
2. Many have suggested that patients be divided into two groups:
   a. MV Prolapse
      1) Symptoms related to associated cardiac lesions (eg, associated MR with atrial fibrillation or pulmonary congestion)
   b. MVP syndrome (MVPS)
      1) Symptoms unassociated with structural abnormality, with some evidence suggesting a relationship to neuroendocrine and autonomic dysfunction:
         a) Measurable increased levels of epinephrine and norepinephrine compared to normal population
         b) β-Adrenergic receptor abnormality
            i) increased receptor responsiveness (may help to explain certain arrhythmias)
         c) Parasympathetic abnormalities
            i) Hypervagal
         d) Increased atrial natiurectic factor (usually in older patient)
         e) Subnormal rennin-aldosterone response to volume depletion
            i) May help explain common finding of decreased intravascular volume
3. Commonly reported associated symptoms (MVPS)
   a. Palpitations
      1) Along with chest pain, the most commonly reported complaint
      2) A wide variety of arrhythmias can be seen in association with MVP (see ECG section), but most often there are no abnormal rhythms on Holter monitor associated with symptoms.
   b. Chest pains
      1) Along with palpitation, the most commonly reported complaint (the most common complaint in men)
      2) Usually atypical in nature, often short and stabbing, but can have attributes that are difficult to distinguish from angina
      3) Cause is unknown
   c. Postural orthostasis
   d. Fatigability
      1) In 50% of women and 30% of men with MVPS
   e. Anxiety and increased cardiac awareness
   f. Panic attacks
      1) 30% of patients with panic attack have associated MVP
   g. Dyspnea
      1) Most commonly not associated with cardiac failure (usually no associated pulmonary rales, S_3, or abnormal apical impulse)
      2) Be wary, congestive heart failure (CHF) can result from MVP, though generally in elderly patient.

h. Lightheadedness
   1) May be result of common finding of decreased intravascular volume in patients with MVP
   2) May be associated with syncope, although when occurs has poor correlation with ECG findings
4. Increased incidence of migraine
5. Neurologic complaints
   a. Transient ischemic attack, cerebrovascular accident, amarosis fugax, and retinal artery occlusion are not common, but may be associated with MVP—cause is not known (though possibly embolic, generally seen in older patients with underlying atherosclerotic disease).
6. Arrhythmias
   a. Paroxysmal supraventricular tachycardia most common sustained tachyarrhythmia in MVP
      1) May be secondary to high incidence of atrioventricular bypass tracts noted in MVP patients
      2) Electrophysiologic testing suggested
   b. Atrial fibrillation
      1) When seen, usually in the setting of associated coronary artery disease (CAD).

C. Physical Examination

1. General appearance
   a. Often slender body habitus
   b. Weight often less than predicted by height
   c. Arm span often greater than height

2. Vital signs
   a. Usually normotensive
   b. May detect irregularity in pulse due to atrial or ventricular premature contractions

3. Palpation
   a. May have palpable thrill if associated with MR

4. Auscultation
   a. Classic findings: early systolic click and a late systolic murmur. Findings in a given patient may vary from examination to examination—one or both findings and even no obvious auscultatory abnormalities
      1) Systolic click—close to S_1
         a) *0.14 sec after S_1*
         b) *Distinguished from a systolic ejection click because begins after start of carotid upstroke*

2) Mid to late systolic crescendo murmur continuous to A_2
   a) *Severity of murmur often related to duration of murmur (ie, late systolic murmurs usually indicative of mild regurgitation)*
   b) *When MVP is substantial, classic MR murmur is apparent with radiation to the axilla.*
b. Maneuvers that decrease left ventricular end-diastolic volume will move the click and onset of the murmur closer to S_1 (ie, earlier click and murmur)
   1) Sudden standing
   2) Valsalva maneuver—strain phase of maneuver
   3) Inhalation of amyl nitrate
c. Maneuvers that increase left ventricular end-diastolic volume will move the click and onset of the murmur away from S_1 (ie, delay click and murmur)
   1) Squatting
   2) Isometric exercise
   3) Position change from standing to supine
   4) Valsalva—after release (will increase venous return and decrease heart rate)
d. Generally most important to note effect of above maneuvers on timing of the click and/or murmur rather than effect on intensity of murmur
e. Change of intensity of murmur does prove helpful in distinguishing click and murmur of MVP from similar sounds sometimes heard in hypertrophic cardiomyopathy (HCM):
   1) Valsalva increases intensity of murmur in HCM but not in MVP where murmur is only prolonged.
   2) Amyl nitrate increases intensity of murmur in HCM but not in MVP.
   3) Following a premature beat, the murmur is increased in HCM but unchanged or diminished in MVP.

II. Diagnostic Approach

Best approach is to combine physical findings with echocardiographic findings.

A. Physical Examination (see above)

1. The presence of both the systolic click and murmur is the most predictive physical finding in diagnosing MVP (although as many as 33% of patients with this finding can have a normal echocardiogram). Dynamic auscultation is often key to making the diagnosis.

B. Electrocardiogram (ECG)

1. The resting ECG is usually normal in asymptomatic patients.

2. In many symptomatic patients, and few asymptomatic patients:

   a. Inverted or biphasic T waves and nonspecific ST-T changes in leads II, III and aVf.

b. ST-T changes often improve on β blockers
   c. Atrial premature beats
   d. Ventricular premature beats
3. QT prolongation
   a. There is an increased association between MVP and QT prolongation.
   b. More important when associated with significant MR and ventricular arrythmias.
4. Q waves are not common but can be seen when MVP is associated with CAD.
5. Paroxysmal supraventricular tachycardia
   a. The most common sustained tachyarrhythmia in MVP
   b. Many patients exhibit accessory pathways or dual atrioventricular nodal pathways.
6. Atrial fibrillation
   a. Generally only in patients with moderate to severe MVP with progression to significant MR, and left ventricular and atrial enlargement
   b. More common in elderly patient with associated CAD
7. Ventricular tachycardia and ventricular fibrillation
   a. More frequent in patients with T wave and ST segment abnormalities on resting ECG
   b. More frequent in patients with significant MR

C. **Echocardiogram with Doppler Flow Studies**

1. Echocardiography is not a useful screening test in patient with serial negative dynamic auscultations.
2. An inherent problem in the Doppler echocardiographic diagnosis of MVP is the fact that the mitral valve is not planar throughout the cardiac cycle (actually saddle shaped during systole)
   a. This allows for mitral valve to appear to prolapse in one two-dimensional plane though not in another.
   b. Although careful three-dimensional assessments can help to avoid this problem, they are somewhat time consuming and cumbersome and therefore are not yet widely used.
   c. Is useful in assessing thickening of the valve leaflets
3. Color Doppler echocardiography
   a. Helpful in assessing MR if present
   b. Can discover MR in patients without a murmur on examination
   c. Useful in follow-up serial evaluations of patients with MR

D. **Chest X-ray**

1. Usually normal cardiac silhouette and lung findings

2. If progressive MR present:
   a. Left atrial and ventricular enlargement with or without pulmonary venous congestion
   b. May also see calcified mitral annulus

E. Exercise Tolerance Testing

1. Generally not useful in the patient with MVP
2. False positive tests have been reported in up to 50% of patients.
3. False positive findings often resolve with β-blocker therapy
4. If conducted to assess anginal symptoms, should use exercise thallium testing

F. Angiography

1. Physical examination and Doppler echocardiography generally obviate the need for cardiac catheterization.
2. When done, usually for the purpose of:
   a. Assessing suspected underlying CAD
   b. Assessing severe MR
   c. Assessing multiple valve disease
   d. Assessing other associated underlying cardiac disease

III. Differential Diagnosis

A. Mid-Systolic Clicks (Table 22D–2)

1. Aortic valvular disease
   a. Can be distinguished from mitral valve clicks by the timing of the click. The mitral valve click occurs after the carotid upstroke, whereas the aortic valve click occurs before the carotid upstroke.
2. Tricuspid valve click
3. Atrial septal aneurysms can cause clicks.
4. HCM
   a. Can have systolic click as well as systolic murmur. (See physical examination above for ways to distinguish between the two.)

B. Systolic Murmurs

1. Although not common, aortic stenosis murmur can radiate to the left axilla.
2. Although chronic aortic insufficiency can lead to retrograde flow across the mitral valve, this occurs during diastole.
3. HCM (as noted above)

Table 22D-2. Auscultatory Mimics of Mitral Valve Prolapse

Nonejection Click	Late Systolic Murmur
Pericardial knock of constrictive pericarditis	Mitral and tricuspid valve prolapse
Opening snap of mitral or tricuspid stenosis	Papillary muscle dysfunction
Widely split S_2 of RBBB	Hypertrophic cardiomyopathy
Fixed split of atrial septal defect	Ventricular septal defect
Mechanical prosthetic valve sounds	Severe valvular or infundibular pulmonic stenosis
Ebsteins's anomaly of the tricuspid valve	
Ejection clicks of semilunar valve stenosis	Coarctation of aorta
Ejection clicks of aortic or pulmonary artery dilatation	
Atrial sounds in compete heart block	
Ventricular septal aneurysm	
Pleuropericardial adhesions	
Left-sided pneumothorax	
Mediastinal emphysema	
Xiphosternal crunch	
Splenic flexure syndrome	

SOURCE: Fontana ME, Sperks EA, Boudoules H, Wooley CF Mitral valve prolapse and the mitral prolapse syndrome. Curr Prob Cardiol 1991;16:309–375.

IV. Treatment

A. Prophylaxis for Endocarditis (see Appendix B)

1. No definitive data regarding the need for prophylaxis, although it is recommended to give prophylactic antibiotics in patients with this diagnosis and an auscultatory murmur before certain surgical or dental procedures.

B. Asymptomatic Patient

1. "Normal life-style"

2. Exercise

3. Remove/treat underlying cardiovascular risk factors

C. Patients with Mild MVP and Mild Symptoms

1. As noted for normal patients

2. Eliminate potential exacerbating factors

    a. Caffeine
    b. Adrenergic stimulating drugs (decongestants, etc.)
    c. Avoid diuretic use
    d. Encourage adequate, daily hydration

D. Tachycardia, Chest Pain, and Anxiety

1. Eliminate potential exacerbating factors as above
2. If unsatisfactory response to above, consider β-blocker therapy.
   a. Small amounts of this class of drug are often all that are needed for control of sinus tachycardia and increased cardiac awareness.
   b. If side effects develop, it is worth trying another agent in this class.

E. Orthostatic Symptoms

1. Eliminate potential exacerbating factors as above
2. Adequate, daily hydration
3. Support stockings to prevent venous pooling in lower extremities
4. In severe cases may require salt-retaining steroids such as fludrocortisone (Florinef®).

F. Neurologic Events

1. Although etiology of acute neurologic events associated with MVP is not known, daily aspirin is often recommended despite lack of evidence of efficacy. Often one tablet (325 mg) daily is recommended.

V. Patient Education

A. Stress the need for antibiotic prophylaxis.

B. Advise regular exercise when appropriate.

C. Eliminate potential exacerbating factors as noted.

D. Educate patient regarding risk factors.

E. Avoid competitive sports or weight lifting in patients with

1. Left ventricular enlargement
2. Left ventricular dysfunction
3. Uncontrolled tachyarrhythmia
4. Unexplained syncope
5. Prior sudden death
6. Increased QT interval
7. Enlargement of aortic root

VI. Long-term Management

A. Asymptomatic Patients

1. Examine q 2–3 y
2. Doppler echocardiography q 5 y

B. Patients with MR
1. Yearly examination and Doppler echocardiography if symptomatic

C. Patients with Moderate to Severe MR
1. Generally should be followed by a cardiologist

VII. Indications for Referral to a Cardiologist

A. Left ventricular enlargement and/or dysfunction

B. Tachyarrhythmias (may need electrophysiologic studies)

C. Syncope or near syncope

D. Significant ECG abnormalities

E. Significant neurologic symptoms as noted above

F. Suspected associated CAD

G. Moderate to severe MR

H. Multivalvular disease or other important associated cardiac defect

VIII. Bibliography

Abrams J. Essentials of Cardiac Physical Diagnosis, Philadelphia: Lea and Febiger, 1987.

Braunwald E. Aortic Stenosis. In: Braunwald E, ed. Heart Disease, A textbook of Cardiovascular Medicine, 4th edition. Philadelphia: WB Saunders Inc., 1992.

Braunwald E. Valvular Heart Disease. In: Wilson JD, Braunwald E, Isselbacher KJ, et al, eds, Harrison's Principles of Internal Medicine, 12th edition. New York: McGraw-Hill Inc., 1991.

Frankl WS, Brest AN. Valvular Heart Disease: Comprehensive Evaluation and Treatment. In: Brest AN, ed. Cardiovascular Clinics. Philadelphia: FA Davis Co., 1993.

Gaasch WH, Levine HJ, ed. Chronic Aortic Regurgitation, Boston: Kluwer Academic Publishers, 1988.

Rackley CE. Valvular Heart Disease. In: Wyngaarden JB, Smith SH Jr, Bennett JC, eds. Cecil Textbook of Medicine. 19th edition. Philadelphia: WB Saunders Co., 1992.

Chapter 23: Prescribing Safe Exercise

Karen G. Kelly

I. Benefits of Exercise

A. Reduction in Cardiovascular Risk Factors

1. Lipids—Regular exercise increases high-density lipoproteins.
2. Diabetes—Regular exercise decreases the risk of type II diabetes mellitus. It also improves insulin sensitivity and reduces glucose production by the liver.
3. Hypertension—People who exercise regularly have a decreased risk of hypertension. Exercise training modestly reduces elevated blood pressure (5–10 mm Hg).
4. Obesity—Exercise improves weight loss and minimizes lean body mass lost during dieting.

B. Reduction in Cardiovascular Morbidity and Mortality

1. Primary prevention—Numerous population studies have found reductions in cardiovascular morbidity and mortality in active versus sedentary individuals. The Centers for Disease Control and Prevention (CDC) states that physical inactivity is a significant risk factor for coronary artery disease with a relative risk of 1.9.
2. Secondary prevention—Small studies of patients after myocardial infarction also suggest a beneficial effect of aerobic exercise in preventing recurrent cardiovascular events.

C. Improvement in strength, endurance, and maximum oxygen consumption.

D. Increased bone density—Exercisers have higher bone density than sedentary individuals.

E. Exercise may diminish the age-related decline in maximum O_2 consumption. Elderly individuals can increase strength and endurance and this may significantly improve functional capacity.

II. Risks of Exercise

A. Causes of Sudden Death During Exercise

1. In exercisers under the age of 35, most sudden death is caused by congenital heart disease.

2. In people over age 35, sudden death during exercise is largely caused by coronary artery disease.

B. Risk of Sudden Death During Exercise

1. The risk of sudden death is increased during exercise periods compared to while sedentary, particularly in previously sedentary exercisers. Overall, however, regular exercise decreases one's risk of cardiovascular death.

2. The magnitude of the risk of death during exercise is unclear. Estimates range from one per 300,000–900,000 man hours of exercise.

3. Even in patients after myocardial infarction, the risk of recurrent infarction due to sudden death during supervised exercise is low.

4. One study found most sudden deaths to occur during golf (23%), jogging (20%), and swimming (11%).

C. Orthopedic Injuries

1. Relatively common in joggers. A CDC study of 2500 runners in a 10K road race found a 35% annual injury rate. The knee was the most common site of injury and high mileage increased the injury rate.

2. The overall pattern and frequency of injuries will depend on the activity done and its frequency and intensity.

III. Evaluation of the Patient Who Wants to Exercise

A. All patients should have a complete history taken before being given a recommendation for vigorous exercise.

1. To elicit symptoms of cardiovascular or respiratory disease

2. To identify risk factors for coronary artery disease

3. To identify orthopedic problems or functional limitations that may limit or prevent exercise

B. Physical examination should focus on identifying existing cardiovascular or respiratory diseases as well as orthopedic problems.

Table 23-1. Contraindications to Exercise

Unstable angina
Uncontrolled hypertension (> 200 systolic or > 100 diastolic)
Significant orthostatic hypotension
Moderate to severe aortic stenosis
Uncontrolled arrythmia or heart block
Uncontrolled sinus tachycardia (> 100)
Symptomatic congestive heart failure
Recent or current thrombosis
Uncontrolled diabetes
Active myocarditis or pericarditis

C. The history and physical examination should attempt to identify contraindications to beginning an exercise program (Table 23-1).

D. Further evaluation will depend on the physician's assessment of the likelihood of underlying cardiac disease. A cholesterol value may help identify those at higher risk.

1. Both the American Heart Association and the American College of Sports Medicine recommend that exercise stress testing be performed in certain people who plan to begin more than moderate exercise.

2. Moderate exercise is defined as that which is well within the individual's current capacity, can be sustained comfortably for a long period, and is usually within 40-60% of maximal heart rate.

3. Vigorous exercise is exercise that is more than moderate.

4. An exercise stress test prior to vigorous exercise should be considered in men over 40, women over 50, and in younger individuals felt to be at increased risk for coronary artery disease because of risk factors or suggestive symptoms.

IV. The Exercise Prescription

A. Motivation

1. Physicians should encourage all appropriate patients to increase their level of activity.

2. Inquire as to what activities the patient does, what is enjoyable, and whether he or she would like to increase activity level.

3. Encourage reasonable goals and lifelong changes.

B. Exercise Program—Three Components

1. Begin with a warmup of 5–10 min with stretching
2. Aerobic component of 20–40 min, preferably low impact
3. Cooldown of 5–10 min
4. Activities to recommend might include walking, biking, swimming, or any other activity that can lead to a sustained increase in heart rate.
5. Weight lifting. Circuit weight training can be used to improve muscle strength.

C. Patient should aim for a target heart rate of 60–70% of age-predicted maximum (220–age).

D. Monitored Exercise Programs

1. Should be considered for those with
    a. Known coronary artery disease
    b. Congestive heart failure
    c. Arrhythmias
    d. Unexplained syncope

V. Patient Education

A. Patient should be told to stop exercising if chest pain or severe dyspnea occur.

B. The physician should follow-up with the patient regarding the success or failure of the program and any problems encountered.

VI. Annotated Bibliography

Levine GN, Balady GJ. The benefits and risks of exercise training: the exercise prescription. Adv Intern Med 1993;38:57–79. A detailed review of the physiology, risks, and benefits of exercise.

Peterson DM. Exercise and physical activity in the adult population: a general internists perspective. J Gen Intern Med 1993;8:149–159. A review of exercise risks, benefits, and recommendations for preexercise evaluation and exercise prescription.

Chapter 24: Office Management of Arrhythmias

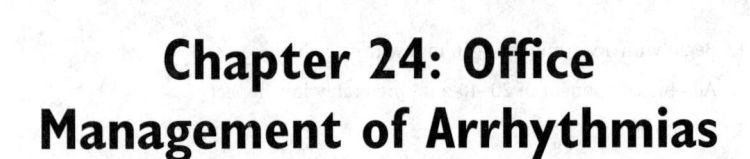

Arnold J. Greenspon

24A Palpitations

I. Clinical Presentation

A. General Information

1. Palpitation is defined as an unpleasant awareness of the forceful or rapid beating of the heart.

2. It may be brought on by a variety of disorders causing a change in heart rate including tachycardias, ectopic beats, compensatory pauses, or the sudden onset of bradycardia.

3. The clinical history obtained from the patient is critical in determining whether further diagnostic studies and treatment are indicated. It is important to remember that the symptoms of palpitations are not always related to an arrhythmia.

B. Symptoms
Clues to the etiology of palpitations are frequently uncovered by taking a careful clinical history.

1. Almost any cardiac arrhythmia may be associated with palpitations.

    a. Slow forceful beating—sinus bradycardia, atrioventricular (AV) block, periods of sinoatrial (SA) block
    b. Skipped or missed heart beat—ectopic beats such as premature atrial or ventricular contractions
    c. Sustained pounding—paroxysmal atrial tachyarrhythmias such as AV node reentry supraventricular tachycardia (AVNRT), atrial fibrillation, or paroxysmal ventricular tachycardia

2. Diagnosis of the arrhythmia cannot be made from the history alone.

    a. Anxiety and other medical conditions such as fever or sepsis are often associated with sinus tachycardia and the sensation of palpitations.
    b. ECG confirmation of the arrhythmia is required.

3. Patient-related symptoms often suggest the mechanism of the cardiac arrhythmia.
   a. Slow heart beat—periods of AV block or sinus bradycardia
   b. Abrupt onset/offset—paroxysmal atrial tachycardia or paroxysmal junctional tachycardia
   c. Chaotic heart action—atrial fibrillation
   d. Offset associated with breath holding, induced gagging, or vomiting—AVNRT.
4. Associated symptoms suggest the presence or absence of heart disease.
   a. Angina—During paroxysmal atrial tachycardias such as AVNRT or atrial fibrillation the presence of angina suggests significant coronary artery disease.
   b. Presyncope or syncope—Poor cerebral perfusion during the palpitations is generally related to the increased heart rate and resulting fall in cardiac output caused by an atrial or ventricular tachyarrhythmia.
   c. Nausea, vomiting, diaphoresis—When these precede palpitations they suggest vasodepressor syncope and not a cardiac arrhythmia.

C. Physical Examination
1. Search for clues to the presence of organic heart disease
   a. Hypertension
   b. Heart murmurs suggesting valvular heart disease
   c. Rales, jugular venous distention, peripheral edema associated with congestive heart failure

II. Diagnostic Approach—Document the Arrhythmia

A. Resting ECG—The office ECG is an ineffective test because it provides only a small snapshot of the daily cardiac rhythm.

B. Ambulatory monitor—The 24-h ambulatory monitor (Holter monitor) is the most frequent method for documenting cardiac arrhythmias.

1. Requires the patient to wear a tape recording monitor for 24–48 h.
2. Patient initiative not required except for logging symptoms in a diary.
3. Symptoms must be frequent (ie, daily).
4. All cardiac events during the monitoring period are recorded.

C. Cardiac event recorder—Patient-activated system records heart rhythm.

1. Continuous loop recorders—The monitor is attached to patient via an ECG cable and continuously monitors heart rhythm. The patient presses a button whenever the symptoms begin. This activates the system so that the heart rhythm that occurred 15–30 sec before the event is stored and recording continues for 15–30 sec after the event. The recording is transmitted, usually over the telephone, for analysis.

2. Patient-activated recorders—A monitor is carried by the patient. When the patient feels symptoms, the monitor is placed on the chest or attached to ECG cables and a button is pressed, which activates the system. The ECG is recorded for 15–30 sec following the event and then transmitted over the telephone for analysis.
3. Patient-activated event recorders require patient initiative.
4. Good for recording infrequent but symptomatic events.

III. Treatment

A. The treatment of the symptoms requires documentation of the arrhythmia.

B. Arrhythmias usually require treatment with antiarrhythmic drugs to suppress symptoms. Sinus tachycardia is not a symptom but generally a sign of an underlying medical problem or anxiety.

C. Sinus tachycardia requires no specific treatment. Search for the associated medical or psychological problem.

IV. Patient Education

A. Patients who have no arrhythmia documented during reports of palpitation or only have isolated premature beats should be assured they do not have heart disease and that no treatment is indicated.

V. Indications for Referral to a Cardiologist

A. Patients who continue to have episodes of sustained palpitations with a negative evaluation should be referred for possible electrophysiologic studies.

VI. Annotated Bibliography

Braunwald, E. Heart Disease: A Textbook of Cardiovascular Medicine, 4th ed. Philadelphia: WB Saunders; 1992. The "bible" of cardiovascular medicine. This is a comprehensive textbook with good chapters on the clinical evaluation of patients with suspected cardiac disease.

Cheitlen MD, Sokolow M, McIlroy MB. Clinical Cardiology, 6th ed. East Norwalk, CT: Appleton & Lange; 1993. A smaller textbook of cardiovascular medicine; comprehensive yet concise. Excellent review of the appropriate clinical evaluation of patients with cardiac symptoms.

Ruffy R, Roman-Smith P, Barbey JT. Palpitations: evaluation and treatment. Prog Cardiol 1988;1/2:131. Good clinical review of the appropriate differential diagnosis of patients with palpitations.

24B Paroxysmal Supraventricular Tachycardia (PSVT)

I. Clinical Presentation

A. Symptoms
The symptoms relate to the rate of the tachycardia and the presence and severity of underlying cardiac disease.

1. Palpitations
2. Lightheadedness or dizziness
3. Angina
4. Syncope
5. Dyspnea

II. Diagnostic Approach

A. Method for ECG diagnosis: see diagnostic approaches for palpitations (Chapter 24A)

B. ECG diagnosis

1. Narrow QRS tachycardia with regular ventricular response
2. Rate will vary between 150 and 250 beats/min.
3. P wave may occur either before, within, or after the QRS complex.

III. Differential Diagnosis

A. Mechanism for tachycardia—In each case the atrioventricular (AV) node is used as the final common pathway for conduction to the ventricle.

1. AV node reentry (AVNRT)—due to two pathways for AV nodal conduction (dual AV node physiology); responsible for up to 60% of all PSVT
2. AV reentry due to an accessory pathway—either manifest as in Wolff-Parkinson-White syndrome (WPW) or concealed; responsible for approximately 30% of all PSVT
3. Atrial or sinoatrial (SA) node reentry—rare causes of PSVT
4. Automatic atrial tachycardia—occur in patients with lung disease (eg, multifocal atrial tachycardia, MAT) or digitalis toxicity

B. Diagnosis of mechanism can sometimes be made from the surface ECG. Knowledge of mechanism often helpful in designing treatment plan.

IV. Treatment

Treatment is directed at slowing conduction through the AV node.

A. Acute Management

1. Continuous ECG monitoring during acute treatment
2. Vagal maneuvers—carotid massage, Valsalva maneuver alone and in combination. Dive reflex may be helpful (place an ice water towel on face covering the nose). Eyeball pressure not recommended.
3. Drug therapy
   a. Adenosine 6-mg IV bolus over 5 sec. Repeat within 5 min 12-mg IV bolus if first dose ineffective.
   b. Verapamil 5–10-mg IV bolus. If second bolus of 10 mg ineffective, patient should go to emergency room for more aggressive therapy.
4. Drug therapy should not be administered in the office to patients who have severe symptoms including hypotension, angina, or dyspnea.

B. Chronic Therapy

Drug therapy is given to patients with frequent or very symptomatic arrhythmias. Those with rare episodes and mild symptoms may be followed clinically.

1. β blockers—All β blockers appear to be effective for treating PSVT. Decisions influencing drug selection include presence of lung disease or heart failure and importance of dosing interval. Generally, drugs that are administered once daily are recommended.
   a. Nadolol (Corgard) 40–80 mg PO daily
   b. Atenolol (Tenormin) 50–100 mg PO daily
   c. Inderal LA 80–360 mg PO daily
   d. Metoprolol (Lopressor) 50–100 mg b.i.d. for patients with a history of bronchospasm
2. Calcium channel blockers—These drugs are generally used in patients who are either intolerant to β blockers or cannot take them due to pulmonary disease or heart failure.
   a. Verapamil 240–360 mg PO daily in divided doses q 8 h. Long-acting single daily dose may be used.
   b. Diltiazem 240–360 mg PO daily in divided doses
3. Type I antiarrhythmic drugs (quinidine, procainamide, disopyramide) may be added for patients with refractory symptoms. However, these patients should be referred to a cardiologist.

V. Patient Education

A. PSVT is not a life-threatening arrhythmia. Therefore, reassure the patient that treatment is directed toward the control of symptoms only.

B. Train the patient in the performance of various vagal maneuvers because these are often effective in terminating the tachycardias. Instruct the patient to lie down after the tachycardia has started and perform the Valsalva maneuver or dive reflex. If these fail to terminate the arrhythmia within 30 min, instruct the patient to go to the ER.

C. Come to the hospital if tachycardia is associated with the symptoms of chest pain, dyspnea, lightheadedness, or loss of consciousness.

VI. Indications for Hospitalization

A. Severe symptoms such as angina, dyspnea, lightheadedness, and syncope

B. These symptoms suggest that the rate of the tachycardia is very rapid, causing hemodynamic compromise. Patients should be admitted to the hospital for observation and further management if their PSVT is associated with these symptoms.

VII. Indications for Referral to a Cardiologist

A. Drug refractory PSVT—Refer patients for further evaluation if PSVT no longer responds to AV nodal blocking agents such as β-blockers or calcium channel blockers.

B. Patients with more than one ER visit per year for PSVT should be referred for further evaluation.

C. Women who wish to become pregnant and do not wish to be on life-long therapy for PSVT

D. Patients who are intolerant to antiarrhythmic medications

E. There are now good nonpharmacologic options for treating patients with PSVT. Radiofrequency catheter ablation is frequently effective in curing the vast majority of patients with PSVT. Therefore, referral of these patients is indicated in any case where cure of the arrhythmia by nonpharmacologic means seems appropriate.

VIII. Annotated Bibliography

Gallagher JJ, Pritchett ELC, Sealy WC, Kasell J, Wallace AG. The pre-excitation syndromes. Prog Cardiovasc Dis 1978;20:285–327. Simply the best review of this topic ever written.

Gursoy S, Schluter M, Kuck KH. Radiofrequency current catheter ablation for control of supraventricular arrhythmias. J Cardiovasc Electrophysiol 1993;4:194–205.

Josephson ME, Kastor JA. Supraventricular tachycardia: mechanisms and management. Ann Intern Med 1977;87:346–358. A classic review of the pathophysiology of supraventricular tachycardia. Treatment of this disorder is much easier once the mechanisms of this common arrhythmia are understood.

Morady F, Scheinman MM. Paroxysmal supraventricular tachycardia. Mod Concepts Cardiovasc Dis 1982;51:107–112. A concise review of the pathophysiology and treatment of the most common supraventricular tachycardias.

24C Atrial Fibrillation

I. Clinical Presentation

A. General Information

1. Atrial fibrillation is a common arrhythmia found in 2% of the population.
2. The incidence of atrial fibrillation increases with age with an incidence of 5% in those over the age of 60.
3. Atrial fibrillation is almost always the consequence of underlying heart disease. In the past atrial fibrillation was most often associated with rheumatic heart disease and mitral stenosis. Today, nonvalvular atrial fibrillation resulting from coronary artery disease or hypertension is most common.
4. Risk factors for the development of atrial fibrillation include smoking, hypertension, diabetes, left ventricular hypertrophy, and mitral valve disease.
5. The major risks from atrial fibrillation include hemodynamic changes and embolic stroke.
   a. Hemodynamic changes
      1) The loss of atrial systole, or "atrial kick," causes a drop in left ventricular preload with a resultant fall in cardiac output.
      2) The increased heart rate seen in atrial fibrillation leads to a decrease in diastolic filling time and therefore decreased coronary perfusion.
      3) Both of these changes lead to a fall in cardiac output and blood pressure. Sometimes a rise in pulmonary capillary wedge pressure also occurs. Symptoms of dyspnea, angina, or a fall in exercise tolerance may result depending on the patient's clinical condition.
   b. Risk of embolic stroke
      1) The risk of thromboembolic stroke is increased 5–9-fold in those with atrial fibrillation (1.6–5%/y).
      2) The risk of thromboembolic stroke is three times more likely in those who also have mitral valve disease.
      3) Patients with paroxysmal atrial fibrillation are just as likely to have embolic events as those patients with persistent atrial fibrillation.
      4) Patients with lone atrial fibrillation (under the age of 50 with no organic heart disease) are at low risk for cerebral emboli.
      5) Low-dose anticoagulation with warfarin decreases the risk of thromboembolic stroke in patients with atrial fibrillation.

B. Symptoms

1. The severity of symptoms resulting from atrial fibrillation depends on the hemodynamic consequences of the arrhythmia.
2. Symptoms might include palpitations, lightheadedness, syncope, angina, dyspnea, or fatigue.

3. Patients without heart disease who develop atrial fibrillation may be totally asymptomatic.

C. ECG Diagnosis
Atrial fibrillation is characterized by an irregular ventricular (QRS) response and a wandering or undulating baseline. No P wave activity is seen because the atria are beating at an extremely rapid rate.

II. Diagnostic Approach

A. Evaluate the Patient for Cardiac Disease.

1. History
    a. Risk factors for coronary disease including smoking, hypertension, family history of coronary disease or myocardial infarction
    b. History of rheumatic fever or heart murmur
    c. Alcohol or drug abuse
    d. Presence of pleuritic chest pain that might suggest pericarditis or pulmonary infarction

2. Physical examination
    a. Presence of hypertension
    b. Systolic heart murmurs suggesting either mitral valve regurgitation or prolapse or obstructive hypertrophic cardiomyopathy (IHSS).
    c. Diastolic heart murmur of mitral stenosis
    d. Signs of hyperthyroidism

3. Laboratory studies
    a. Thyroid function studies: 20–30% of patients with hyperthyroidism develop atrial fibrillation.
    b. Electrolytes

4. Chest x-ray or echocardiogram to assess cardiac chamber size

III. Treatment Options

A. Prevention of Thromboembolic Stroke

1. In patients under the age of 50 without structural heart disease (lone atrial fibrillation), anticoagulation is not necessary. Treatment with low-dose aspirin (325 mg/d or less) is low risk and may be of some benefit.

2. All other patients should receive low-dose warfarin unless anticoagulation is contraindicated.

3. Warfarin (coumadin) should be titrated until the INR is 2.0–3.0.

B. Improvement in Hemodynamic Performance

1. Control of heart rate—The primary goal of therapy is to control the heart rate in atrial fibrillation to minimize symptoms. A ventricular response between 60 and 100 beats/min is desirable. Treatment consists of drugs that act primarily at the atrioventricular (AV) node such as digoxin, β blockers, and calcium channel blockers. Titration of these agents may be safely done as an outpatient provided the patient does not have serious symptoms while in the arrhythmia. Patients should be evaluated in the office within 1 wk of any change in oral therapy.

    a. Digoxin—Oral digitalization may be safely performed as an outpatient. A dose of 0.25 mg is given twice the first day followed by a maintenance dose of 0.25 mg daily. A maintenance dose of 0.125 mg daily is used in patients over the age of 70 or those with a serum creatinine > 1.0 mg/dL. Digoxin should not be administered to patients with significant renal impairment.
    b. β Blockers—Oral β blockers are effective in controlling the ventricular response. No β blocker has been shown to be clearly superior to the others.
    c. Calcium channel blockers
        1) Verapamil 80–120 mg t.i.d. The sustained-release preparation is also effective once the dose of the drug is stabilized.
        2) Diltiazem 60–90 mg q 6–8 h. As with verapamil, the sustained-release preparation may be utilized.

2. Restoration of sinus rhythm—either DC cardioversion or chemical cardioversion

    a. The risk of embolic stroke following cardioversion (either DC or chemical) is approximately 9% in non-anticoagulated patients.
    b. Patients with atrial fibrillation of > 3 d duration should be anticoagulated for 3 wk before attempted cardioversion. Anticoagulation with oral warfarin (coumadin) may be done as an outpatient.
    c. Sinus rhythm should be restored in the hospital setting. Antiarrhythmic agents such as the type I drugs quinidine, procainamide, and disopyramide or the type III drugs amiodarone and sotalol should be first administered while the patient's ECG is being monitored in the hospital. Drug-induced proarrhythmia is most common during the initiation of a new antiarrhythmic drug.

3. Control of paroxysmal atrial fibrillation—In patients who are predominantly in sinus rhythm the goal is to prevent symptomatic recurrences.

    a. Use of an AV nodal blocking agent (see discussion above)
    b. Use of an oral agent to maintain sinus rhythm
        1) Quinidine sulfate or gluconate 1200–1800 mg daily in divided doses. Serum levels should be checked within 3 d of initiating therapy and following each change in dose.

2) Procainamide: Procan SR 2–4 g daily in divided doses
3) Disopyramide regular release or continuous release 300–600 mg daily in divided doses
4) Flecainide 100–200 mg b.i.d.
5) Propafenone 150–300 mg t.i.d.
6) Sotalol 80–160 mg b.i.d.

IV. Indications for Hospitalization or Referral

A. Atrial fibrillation associated with a rapid ventricular response (rate > 120 beats/min) often causes severe symptoms. These patients are best managed in the hospitalized setting.

B. Patients with new onset atrial fibrillation and structural heart disease who have symptoms of increased dyspnea, fatigue, orthopnea, or other complaints that suggest congestive heart failure

C. Atrial fibrillation associated with angina

D. Patients with preexcitation (Wolff-Parkinson-White syndrome) who develop atrial fibrillation

E. Patients with valvular heart disease and new onset of atrial fibrillation should be referred for further evaluation.

F. Patients with chronic atrial fibrillation who have continued problems with heart rate control despite treatment with two oral agents (usually digoxin combined with either a β blocker or a calcium channel blocker)

V. Annotated Bibliography

Cairns JA, Connolly SJ. Non-rheumatic atrial fibrillation: risk of stroke and role of anti-thrombotic therapy. Circulation 1991;84:469–479. An excellent review of the major clinical trials involving antithrombotic therapy in patients with nonvalvular atrial fibrillation.

Falk RH, Podrid PJ. Atrial Fibrillation: Mechanisms and Management. New York: Raven Press; 1992. An excellent monograph that comprehensively reviews the topic.

Halperin JL, Hart RG. Atrial fibrillation and stroke: new ideas, persisting dilemmas. Stroke 1988;19:937–941. A review of the risk of embolic stroke in patients with atrial fibrillation. Excellent review of the literature on this topic.

The Stroke Prevention of Atrial Fibrillation Investigators. The stroke prevention in atrial fibrillation study: final results. Circulation 1991;84:527–539. The largest double blind, placebo-controlled trial of antithrombotic agents in patients with nonvalvular atrial fibrillation. The data demonstrate that antithrombotic agents significantly reduce the risk of embolic stroke.

24D Ventricular Arrhythmias Including Premature Ventricular Contractions (PVCs) and Ventricular Tachycardia

I. Clinical Presentation

A. Premature ventricular contractions can be identified in a large proportion of asymptomatic individuals, even those with normal hearts. Up to 40–75% of healthy individuals may have PVCs detected if continuously monitored for 24–48 h.

B. It has been shown that patients with heart disease and PVCs, particularly coronary artery disease and recent acute myocardial infarction, are at increased risk for sudden cardiac death. However, no studies have demonstrated that drug suppression of ventricular ectopy improves survival. In fact, in the Cardiac Arrhythmia Suppression Trial (CAST) patients whose ventricular ectopy after myocardial infarction was treated with either flecainide or encainide did worse than those treated with placebo. Therefore, treatment of asymptomatic PVCs is not indicated.

C. PVCs may be associated with a variety of symptoms including palpitations, chest discomfort, a sensation of a skipped or dropped heart beat, and occasionally lightheadedness.

D. More complex ventricular ectopy such as nonsustained ventricular tachycardia (more than 3 PVCs in a row continuing for < 30 sec) may be totally asymptomatic. These patients may also present with symptoms of dizziness, lightheadedness, or syncope.

E. Further evaluation and management of ventricular ectopy is indicated for the relief of symptoms.

F. In patients with structural heart disease and abnormal left ventricular function (left ventricular ejection fraction < 40%), the presence of ventricular ectopy may be a poor prognostic sign.

II. Diagnostic Approach

A. Patients without structural heart disease

1. Asymptomatic patients require no further diagnostic studies because their prognosis is excellent.
2. If patients are symptomatic, then 24-h ambulatory monitoring may be useful to confirm the diagnosis.

B. Patients with structural heart disease

1. Determine the degree of left ventricular dysfunction.
   a. Echocardiogram
   b. Multiple gated analysis (MUGA) scan
2. If the left ventricular ejection fraction is > 40% no further diagnostic studies are required. In these patients treatment is directed against symptoms only.
3. If the left ventricular ejection fraction is < 40%, this suggests that there is left ventricular dysfunction. Patients with complex ventricular ectopy and left ventricular dysfunction are at risk for sudden cardiac death.
   a. Ambulatory monitoring for 24 h—Those patients with complex ventricular ectopy (PVC frequency > 10/h, multifocal PVCs, couplets, nonsustained ventricular tachycardia) should be referred to a cardiologist.
   b. Signal-averaged electrocardiogram—The absence of a ventricular late potential suggests that the patient is in a low-risk group.

III. Treatment Plan

A. In patients who are at low risk (normal hearts, patients with heart disease but simple ventricular ectopy), treatment is directed at the control of symptoms.

1. β Blockers—The best agents for the control of symptomatic ventricular ectopy are the β blockers. No single β blocker has been shown to be superior to the others. Agents that are given once daily are preferable, as outlined in Chapter 24B.
2. Reassurance—Most patients with normal hearts and symptomatic ventricular arrhythmias are concerned that they have a life-threatening condition. The physician should reassure the patient that these arrhythmias may cause symptoms but they do not place them at higher risk for sudden cardiac death.
3. Dietary counseling—Smoking, alcohol consumption, and caffeine should be avoided.
4. Antiarrhythmic drugs—These drugs should be avoided because the risk of drug-induced proarrhythmia outweighs the benefit to the patient.

B. High-risk patients with complex ventricular ectopy

1. Referral to a cardiologist is indicated.
2. Antiarrhythmic drugs should not be started as an outpatient.
3. Patients with significant symptoms associated with their ventricular arrhythmias (lightheadedness, syncope, angina, dyspnea) should be hospitalized and referred to a cardiologist.

IV. Annotated Bibliography

Anderson JL. Clinical implications of new studies in the treatment of benign, potentially malignant, and malignant ventricular arrhythmias. Am J Cardiol 1990;65:36B–42B. A short review of the rationale for classifying ventricular arrhythmias into risk categories.

Barrett PA, Peter CT, Swan HJC, et al. The frequency and prognostic significance of electrocardiographic abnormalities in normal subjects. Prog Cardiovasc Dis 1981;23:299–319. An extensive review of the frequency and clinical significance of ECG abnormalities and asymptomatic arrhythmias in healthy subjects.

Greenspon AJ, Waxman HL. Contemporary Management of Ventricular Arrhythmias. Cardiovasc Clin 1992;22(1). This monograph reviews most of the current trends in the management of patients with ventricular arrhythmias.

The Cardiac Arrhythmia Suppression Trial (CAST) Investigators. Preliminary report: effect of encainide and flecainide on mortality in a randomized trial of arrhythmia suppression after myocardial infarction. N Engl J Med 1989;321:406–412. The results of this trial demonstrated that the treatment of asymptomatic PVCs with the class IC drugs encainide and flecainide was associated with excess mortality. Sometimes the treatment is worse than the disease.

Chapter 25: Congestive Heart Failure

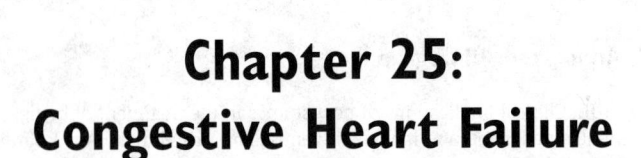

Karen G. Kelly

I. Clinical Presentation

A. General Information

1. Congestive heart failure (CHF) is a common clinical syndrome affecting about 2% of the U.S. population.
2. In the elderly it is even more common, with a prevalence of 10% by age 75. It is the most common discharge diagnosis in the Medicare population.
3. Its prognosis is poor with a 50% 5-y mortality rate; 40% of the deaths from CHF occur suddenly.
4. Therapy can improve symptoms and prolong life but must be based on an accurate diagnosis and a clear understanding of the pathophysiology.
5. CHF is a syndrome and in each patient the cause must be established.
6. Coronary artery disease (CAD) and hypertension are the two most common underlying causes.
7. CHF may be classified according to etiology
    a. Left ventricular systolic dysfunction
        1) Myocardial ischemia and/or infarction
        2) Cardiomyopathy
            a) *Idiopathic*
            b) *Postviral*
            c) *Drugs*
            d) *Hypertensive*
            e) *Alcohol*
    b. Left ventricular diastolic dysfunction
        1) Hypertension
        2) CAD
        3) Infiltrative disease such as amyloid, sarcoid
        4) Hypertrophic cardiomyopathy
    c. Right heart failure—cor pulmonale
    d. Valvular heart disease (see Chapter 22)
    e. Arrhythmias, such as rapid atrial fibrillation, bradyarrhythmias (see Chapter 24)
    f. Pericardial—constriction, tamponade

g. Extra cardiac
   1) Renal failure
   2) Anemia
   3) Thyroid disorders

B. Symptoms

1. Patients typically present with one or more of the following

   a. Dyspnea, which may be on exertion, at rest, or at night (orthopnea or paroxysmal nocturnal dyspnea)
   b. Dependent edema
   c. Fatigue

2. These symptoms reflect lowered cardiac output, high filling pressures, and salt retention by the kidneys.

3. Other symptoms will depend on the underlying etiology. Ask about:

   a. Chest pains suggestive of angina or myocardial infarction either currently or in the past
   b. History of ischemic heart disease
   c. Risk factors for CAD
   d. Hypertension
   e. History of rheumatic fever, previous endocarditis, and heart murmurs or congenital heart disease
   f. Excessive alcohol use or IV drug use
   g. Smoking or chronic respiratory disease
   h. History or symptoms of known systemic diseases that may cause cardiac disease
   i. History of malignancy, radiation to the chest, or chemotherapy

4. In addition to identifying the underlying etiology the physician should look for precipitating factors such as:

   a. Increased consumption of salt
   b. Factors increasing cardiac demand such as
      1) Uncontrolled hypertension
      2) Fever
      3) Infections
   c. Palpitations or lightheadedness that might suggest arrhythmias
   d. Chest pain, suggestive of ischemia or pulmonary embolus

C. Physical Examination

Focus on identifying the etiology and possible precipitating factors.

1. Vital signs

   a. Blood pressure—Hypertension is both an underlying etiology and a precipitating factor. Hypotension suggests severe CHF and may complicate therapy.

b. Pulse—Any sustained arrhythmia that causes decreased cardiac output may precipitate CHF. Sinus tachycardia suggests anemia, infection, hyperthyroidism, or hypoxia, although CHF alone may cause a sinus tachycardia.
   c. Respiratory rate—Severe respiratory distress mandates immediate hospitalization and therapy.
   d. Fever suggests infection. Endocarditis must be ruled out if no other source of infection is obvious.
2. A thorough cardiovascular examination will often clarify the cause of the CHF, identify the pathophysiology, and help to guide appropriate therapy. The physician should identify the following signs:
   a. Neck vein distention
   b. S_3 gallop
   c. Murmurs–for evidence of valvular heart disease (see Chapter 22)
   d. pericardial friction rub
   e. Paradoxical pulse (drop in systolic pressure of more than 10 mm Hg during normal inspiration), which could indicate pericardial tamponade
   f. Vascular bruits, which would suggest underlying atherosclerotic disease
3. Lung examination—Crackles, though nonspecific, may indicate pulmonary edema.
4. Other—Signs of systemic diseases that may cause heart failure should be sought.

II. Diagnostic Approach

A. ECG to identify rhythm abnormalities, evidence of ischemic heart disease, or may demonstrate signs of chamber enlargement.

B. Chest x-ray to identify chamber enlargement and look for signs of pulmonary edema. It may also be useful in identifying primary respiratory problems, which could be the cause of some of the patient's symptoms.

C. Cardiac echocardiogram to assess cardiac chamber size and ventricular systolic function as well as valvular anatomy. Cardiac Doppler can identify and quantitate valvular stenosis and regurgitation. This noninvasive assessment of ventricular function is useful to establish diagnosis and guide therapy in all patients.

D. Radionuclide angiography is an alternative technique to assess left ventricular function and ejection fraction.

E. Blood work should include complete blood count, electrolytes, blood urea nitrogen, and creatinine. Other tests should be guided by clinical suspicion.

F. Other tests may be useful in certain situations.

1. Exercise or pharmacologic stress tests may be useful to look for evidence of CAD.

2. Holter monitor in patients with syncope or significant arrhythmias.
3. Cardiac catheterization in patients in whom noninvasive and clinical evaluation suggest the need for valve replacement or coronary artery revascularization

III. Differential Diagnosis

A. Will depend on the symptom complex

B. Dyspnea

1. The major differential is with primary pulmonary diseases such as chronic obstructive pulmonary disease (COPD), interstitial lung disease, or acute and chronic pulmonary emboli.
2. A chest x-ray may be useful in identifying primary lung diseases.
3. Orthopnea and paroxysmal nocturnal dyspnea (PND) may occur in both COPD and CHF.
4. Dyspnea may also be a manifestation of anemia

C. Edema

1. Chronic venous stasis is distinguished from the edema of CHF by the lack of neck vein distention and the absence of other signs and symptoms of CHF.
2. Nephrotic syndrome and cirrhosis may cause edema when albumin is reduced. Look for nephrotic range proteinuria and signs of liver dysfunction. Severe CHF can cause liver dysfunction, but in this case neck veins will be distended.

D. In the elderly some signs of CHF may be misleading. Chronic venous disease leading to edema is common. Many elderly have systolic murmurs that are not hemodynamically significant. Basilar crackles may be normal. The clinician may thus have difficulty determining whether CHF is present.

IV. Treatment

A. Will depend on the cause of the CHF as determined by history, physical, and laboratory evaluation.

B. Medications

1. Digoxin
   a. Is beneficial in cases with left ventricular enlargement and decreased left ventricular function
   b. Indicated for rate control in atrial fibrillation
   c. No benefit in patients with normal left ventricular systolic function and normal sinus rhythm
   d. Blood levels should be monitored and hypokalemia avoided.

2. Diuretics
    a. For pulmonary congestion and peripheral edema
    b. Most commonly used agent is furosemide. Usual starting dose is 20–40 mg. In renal failure, the dose may need to be significantly increased.
    c. Other useful diuretics include ethacrynic acid 50–100 mg, and bumetanide 1–5 mg.
    d. Metolazone (2.5–5.0 mg) often potentiates the effect of furosemide in the end-stage CHF.
3. Angiotensin-converting enzyme (ACE) inhibitors
    a. Have been shown to prolong life in patients with symptomatic heart failure with left ventricular dysfunction
    b. May also have benefit in asymptomatic patients with reduced left ventricular ejection fraction
    c. Up to 25% of patients may get cough.
    d. Hyptotension and renal dysfunction may limit use.
    e. Alternative to ACE inhibitors is the combination of nitrates and hydralazine.
    f. See Table 20–3 for agents and doses.
4. β Blockers
    a. Potential benefit for heart failure secondary to reversible ischemia, diastolic dysfunction, and atrial arrhythmias
    b. May have benefit in cases with systolic dysfunction but use in this setting is controversial
    c. See Tables 20–3 and 21–2 for agents and doses.
5. Calcium channel blockers
    a. As with β blockers, may have benefit in cases due to reversible ischemia, diastolic dysfunction, and atrial arrhythmias.
    b. Verapamil, diltiazem, and nifedipine generally are not indicated for systolic dysfunction but newer calcium blockers are being studied for this indication.
    c. See Tables 20–3, 21–2, and 21–3 for agents and doses.
6. Nitrates and other vasodilators
    a. Nitrates reduce preload and may have symptomatic benefit in CHF.
    b. Hydralazine and nitrates improve survival in advanced CHF but are less effective than ACE inhibitors.
    c. See Table 21–2 for agents and doses.
7. Antiarrhythmics (See Chapter 24)
    a. Potentially indicated for documented sustained atrial and ventricular arrhythmias
    b. Patients may benefit from prior electrophysiologic study.

8. Anticoagulants
   a. Indicated in patients with atrial fibrillation
   b. Indicated in the presence of left ventricular or left atrial thrombi, especially if accompanied by embolic event
   c. May be useful in patients with a dilated cardiomyopathy and significant left ventricular dysfunction who are at high risk for emboli

C. Diastolic Dysfunction

1. Therapy of patients with CHF secondary to diastolic dysfunction should be approached somewhat differently from those with systolic dysfunction.

2. β Blockers or calcium channel blockers should be used in low doses.

3. Diuretics may be used in low doses.

4. There is no indication for digoxin if the patient is in sinus rhythm.

5. There is no indication for ACE inhibitors if the patient is normotensive.

D. Supportive Measures

1. Low-salt diet

2. Exercise

3. Blood pressure control

V. Indications for Referral to a Cardiologist

A. Refractory CHF

B. Question of significant valvular heart disease

C. Presence of sustained ventricular arrhythmias or syncope due to the high risk of sudden death

VI. Indications for Hospitalization

A. Significant respiratory distress

B. Rapid atrial fibrillation

C. Bradycardia requiring therapy

D. Syncope

E. Failure to respond to outpatient therapy

VII. Annotated Bibliography

Feldman AM. Can we alter survival in patients with congestive heart failure? JAMA 1992;267:1956–1961. A review of existing studies.

Shah PM, Pai RG. Diagnostic heart failure. CWR Probs Cardiol 1992;12:787–868. A thorough review.

SOLVD Investigations. Effect of enalapril on survival in patients with reduced left ventricular ejection fractions and congestive heart failure. N Engl J Med 1991;325:293–302. Mortality and hospitalizations for CHF were often reduced by the use of enalapril.

Weintraub NL, Chaitman BR. Newer concepts in the medical management of patients with congestive heart failure. Clin Cardiol 1993;16:380–390. A review.

Part V:
Consultative Medicine

Chapter 26: Outpatient Preoperative Evaluation

Barry Ziring

I. General Considerations

A. The goal of preoperative evaluation is to identify risk factors for surgery. The management of patients with preexisting medical problems is beyond the scope of this text.

B. Extensive research has focused on risk factors for perioperative cardiac complications. Criteria have been developed to evaluate patients for cardiac risk factors prior to general surgery (eg, Goldman Risk Assessment Scale) as well as specifically for peripheral vascular disease.

C. In addition, other systemic diseases influence surgical outcome and should be identified preoperatively.

D. A scheme for evaluation is presented in Table 26-1.

E. In this era of medical cost containment, attempts should be made to use laboratory testing only when these tests have proven benefit.

Table 26-1. Approach to Evaluation of Patient before Surgery

Evaluate for Cardiac Risk Factors	
General Surgery	**Peripheral Vascular Surgery**
Goldman criteria (Table 26-2)	Eagle criteria (Figure 26-1)
Take steps to decrease cardiac risk	
General Surgery	**Peripheral Vascular Surgery**
Correct above risk factors if possible	If patient has 1-2 risk factors listed above, consider exercise thallium stress testing for further risk stratification.
Delay or cancel elective surgery if the physician, patient, and surgeons agree that the risk factors for surgery outweigh the benefits.	Proceed as for General Surgery.
Identify and correct noncardiac risks for surgery		
History of bleeding	Adrenal insufficiency	Carotid stenosis
DVT prophylaxis	Hypertension	Diabetes
Endocarditis prophylaxis	Cancer and chemotherapy	Poor nutritional state
Thyroid disease	Alcohol and drug use	Pulmonary insufficiency

II. Identifying Risk Factors for Surgery

A. Risk Factors for Cardiac Complications as a Result of General Surgery
1. Goldman Risk Assessment Scale (Table 26–2)
   a. In 1977, a risk factor index defined by Goldman and associates was developed to identify patients at high risk for developing cardiovascular complications associated with noncardiac surgery.
   b. Nine clinical or historical features were found to be associated with an increased incidence of perioperative cardiac complications. Using the scale, the risk of developing a cardiac complication could be estimated.
   c. These risks may be lower in 1993 than in 1977 when the original study was published (Table 26–3) due to better anesthetic technique and invasive monitoring.
   d. The utility of this risk index has been validated, although other scales by different authors now exist.

Table 26–2. Multifactorial Index of Cardiac Risk in Noncardiac Surgery

Risk Factor	Points
History	
Myocardial infarction within six months	10
Age older than 70 years	5
Physical Examination	
S_3 or jugular venous distension	11
Significant aortic stenosis	3
ECG	
Rhythm other than sinus or sinus plus atrial premature beats on preoperative electrocardiogram	7
More than five ventricular premature contractions per minute at any time prior to surgery	7
Medical Status	
Poor general medical status (potassium < 3 mEq/L or HCO_3, < 20 mEq/l or BUN > 50 mg/DL or creatinine > 3 mg/dL or pO_2 < 60 mm Hg or pCO_2 > 50 mm Hg) Evidence of abnormal liver function Patient bedridden	3
Surgical Procedure	
Abdominal, thoracic, or aortic surgery	3
Emergency operation	4
Total	**53**

SOURCE: Reprinted by permission of the New England Journal of Medicine, from Goldman L. Caldera DL. Nussbaum SR, et al: Multifactorial index of cardiac risk in noncardiac surgical procedures. N Engl J Med 1977; 297:845–850.

Table 26-3. Complication Rates Determined by the Multifactorial Risk Index

Class (points)	Goldman* (%)	Zeldin† (%)	Detsky‡ (%)
I (0-5)	1	1	6
II (6-12)	7	3	7
III (13-25)	14	15	20
IV (>25)	78	30	100

*Goldman L, Caldera D, Southwick F, et al. Multifactorial index of cardiac risk in noncardiac surgical procedures. N Engl J Med 1977;297:845.
†Zeldin R. Assessing cardiac risk in patients who undergo noncardiac surgical procedures. Can J Surg 1984;27:402.
‡Detsky AS, Abrams HB, McLaughlin JR, et al. Predicting cardiac complications in patients undergoing noncardiac surgery. J Gen Intern Med 1986;1:211.

SOURCE: Reprinted by permission of the New England Journal of Medicine, from Goldman L: Multifactorial index of cardiac risk in noncardiac surgery: ten year status report. J Cardiothorac Anesth 1987;1:237-244.

2. History (features that increase cardiac risk)
   a. Myocardial infarction within 6 mo
   b. Angina
      1) Chronic stable angina (class I and II) is not a cardiac risk factor during noncardiac surgery.
      2) Canadian Cardiovascular Society class III patients (angina when walking two blocks or one flight of stairs) and class IV patients (angina with any activity and unstable angina) have been associated with an increased risk of cardiac complications during noncardiac surgery.
   c. Age older than 70
   d. Patient bedridden
   e. Emergency operation
   f. Abdominal thoracic or aortic surgery

3. Physical examination (features that increase cardiac risk)
   a. Clinical evidence of congestive heart failure (S_3 or jugular venous distention)
   b. Significant aortic stenosis

4. Laboratory (features that increase cardiac risk)
   a. Potassium < 3 mEq/L
   b. HCO_3 < 20 mEq/L
   c. Blood urea nitrogen > 50 mg/dL
   d. Creatinine > 3 mg/dL
   e. PO_2 < 60 mm Hg
   f. PCO_2 > 50 mm Hg
   g. ECG rhythm other than sinus
   h. Sinus rhythm plus atrial premature beats on perioperative ECG
   i. More than five ventricular premature contractions per minute at any time prior to surgery

B. Risk Factors for Cardiac Complications as a Result of Peripheral Vascular Surgery
1. Peripheral vascular surgery has been demonstrated to be a special situation with respect to evaluation for cardiac risk. This is due to the high prevalence of concommitant coronary artery disease in this group and due to the procedures involved in peripheral vascular surgery.
2. Eagle and colleagues have recommended a scheme for preoperative evaluation of these patients based on the presence of five preexisting risk factors.
    a. The presence of a Q wave on preoperative ECG
    b. Age > 70
    c. Ventricular ectopy
    d. Angina
    e. Diabetes
3. A patient who cannot perform any activity due to other medical problems may be considered at risk for having angina in the setting of severe peripheral vascular disease.
4. The scheme for evaluating these patients is outlined in Figure 26-1.

C. Factors That Increase Risk for Noncardiac Complications During Surgery
1. History or family history of problems with anesthesia
2. Episodes of unusual bleeding
    a. A history of unusual bleeding has been shown to be the most sensitive and cost-effective predictor of hemorrhagic complications.
    b. Coagulation studies should be used to confirm and better define a suspected coagulopathy.
    c. Also coagulation studies should be done before surgery when there is a chance of major blood loss. These tests are not indicated for screening.
3. Bacterial endocarditis prophylaxis (see Appendix B)
4. Deep vein thrombosis (DVT) prophylaxis
    a. Patients having surgery have a 10–80% change of developing a DVT and a 0.01–5% change of developing a pulmonary embolism. The chance of developing a DVT depends on preexisting factors.
    b. Factors that increase risk of developing a DVT include
        1) Age > 40
        2) Surgery > 30 min
        3) Orthopedic surgery (especially hip and knee replacement)
        4) Pelvic or abdominal surgery
        5) Hereditary or acquired hypercoagulable states
    c. Recommendations for DVT prophylaxis
        1) General surgery
            a) *Heparin 5000 units SQ beginning 2 h before surgery and continuing q 12 h postoperatively*
            b) *External pneumatic compression sleeves*

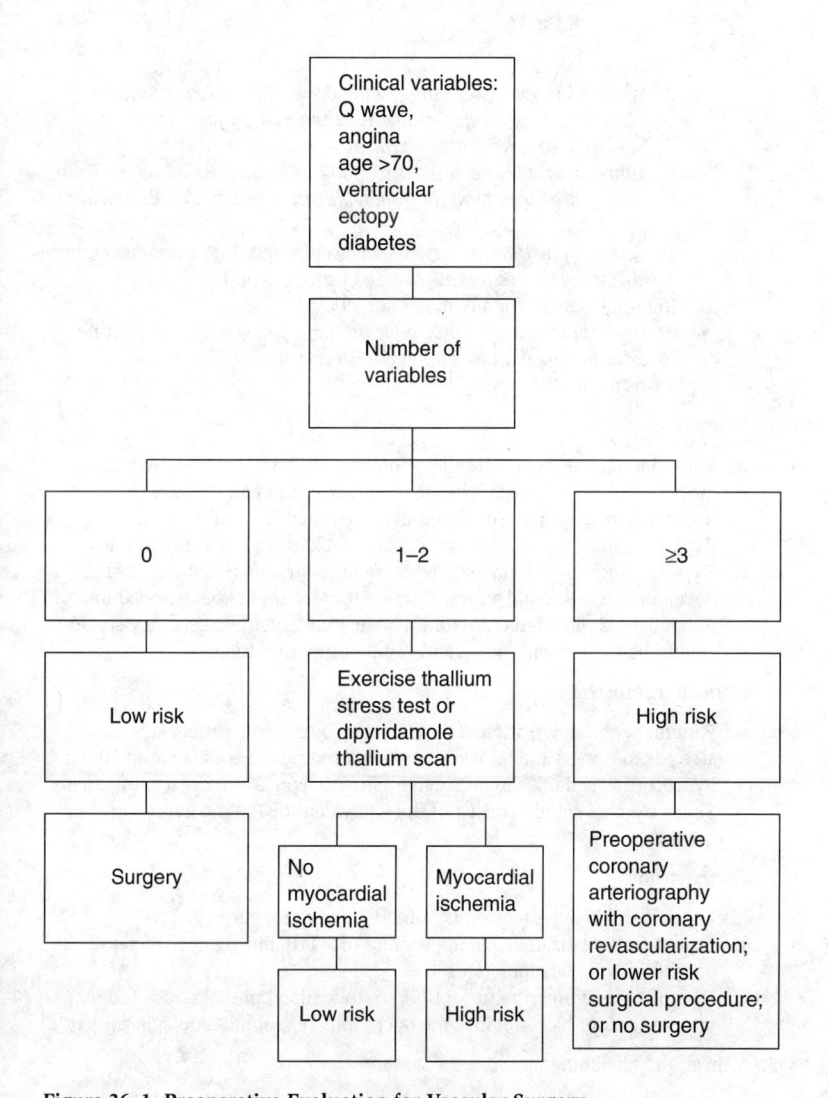

Figure 26–1. Preoperative Evaluation for Vascular Surgery
Reproduced by permission from Eagle K, Coley C, Newell J, et al. Combining clinical and thallium data optimizes preoperative assessment of cardiac risk before major vascular surgery. Ann Intern Med 1989, 110:859-866.

2) Orthopedic surgery
   a) *Warfarin prophylaxis using 10 mg evening prior to surgery, 5 mg evening of surgery, and adjusting afterward for prothrombin time 16–18 sec (or alternative warfarin regimen).*
   b) *adjusted dose SQ heparin using 3500 units SQ q 8 and adjusting dose to achieve a partial thromboplastin time 6 h after dosing of 41–45 sec.*
   c) *External pneumatic compression sleeves (less data available on the efficacy of this technique in orthopedic patients)*
3) High-risk patient for any major surgery
   a) *Use regimens listed for orthopedic surgery or consider combining external pneumatic compression sleeves with a pharmacologic regimen.*

5. Thyroid disease
   a. Mild to moderate hypothyroidism conveys minimal perioperative risk.
   b. Moderate to severe hypothyroidism may result in risk for intraoperative hypotension, gastrointestinal and neuropsychiatric complications. Replacement to a euthyroid state is preferable prior to elective surgery.
   c. Hyperthyroidism—All patients who are hyperthyroid are at risk for the development of thyroid storm. Elective surgery should be canceled until the patient is rendered euthyroid. Patients undergoing emergency surgery should be treated with β blockade and antithyroid drugs.

6. Adrenal insufficiency
   a. Patients with known adrenal insufficiency or patients using exogenous steroids for longer than 2 wk in doses exceeding the equivalent of 30 mg hydrocortisone daily should receive "stress steroids" on the day of surgery. Stress steroids should consist of the equivalent of 100 mg hydrocortisone q 8 h.

7. Hypertension
   a. Chronic stable hypertension is not a risk factor for surgery.
   b. A preoperative diastolic blood pressure of > 110 mm Hg does increase risk of cardiac complications.
   c. Diastolic blood pressure of > 110 or systolic blood pressure of > 160 may increase risk of bleeding in some operations (eg, ophthalmologic surgery).

8. Cancer and chemotherapy
   a. Systemic effects of malignancy include:
      1) Neuromuscular disorders
      2) Hematologic disorders—erythrocytosis, anemia, leukocytosis, leukopenia, eosinophilia, thrombocytosis, thrombocytopenia
      3) Endocrine disorders—ectopic adrenocorticotropic hormone, syndrome of inappropriate antidiuretic hormone
      4) Hypercalcemia

b. Systemic effects of cancer treatment include:
      1) Chemotherapy—cardiac, pulmonary, renal, CNS, GI, and hematologic toxicity
      2) Radiation—hematologic, GI, and endocrine effects.
9. Alcohol and drug use
   a. The medical consultant must be aware of potential drug interactions and the possibility of withdrawal in the perioperative period.
   b. Acute intoxication with cocaine is associated with increased risk of cardiac arrhythmias, hyperpyrexia, seizures, intestinal ischemia, and abruptio placenta, and other complications.
10. Carotid stenosis
    a. Most studies support a benign course for patients with asymptomatic carotid bruits undergoing surgery, although bruits may be a marker of other vascular disease.
11. Diabetes
    a. Stable blood glucose of ≤ 250 mg/dL should be achieved preoperatively. Levels above this increase risk of infection and poor wound healing.
    b. Potassium, sodium, and phosphate abnormalities should be corrected.
    c. Patients with diabetes are at significantly higher risk of having concommitant and sometimes silent coronary artery disease and peripheral vascular disease.
12. Large weight loss in preceding 6 mo (especially > 10% body weight).
    a. Poor nutritional status results in a several fold increase in surgical complications.
    b. It is not clear if preoperative nutritional support improves outcome.
13. Pulmonary insufficiency
    a. The incidence of complications increases for procedures close to the diaphragm.
    b. Patients with chronic obstructive pulmonary disease should have pulmonary function testing prior to major surgery. A forced vital capacity (FVC) lower than 70% of predicted and a forced expiratory volume in 1 sec FEV/FVC ratio lower than 50% of predicted have been associated with an increased risk of postoperative pulmonary complications.
    c. The high-risk patient should have an arterial blood gas determination. If the $PaCO_2$ is > 45 mm Hg, the incidence of surgical complications is very high and delay or cancellation of surgery should be considered.

III. Obtain Appropriate Studies

A. For routine nonblood loss surgery in healthy patients, there are few laboratory tests required.

1. Age under 40—A complete blood count and pregnancy test might be considered for women.

2. Age 40-59—An ECG should be done. Creatinine and glucose measurement may be useful.

3. Over age 60—An ECG and complete blood count should be done due to the higher prevalence of disease in this age group. Creatinine, glucose, chest x-ray, and nutritional values may be considered.

B. Tests should be ordered to quantitate risk in patients who have disease processes identified by the history and physical.

IV. Attempt Correction of Risk Factors

A. Surgery should be reconsidered where risks are considered to be very high and cannot be corrected.

B. Examples of correction of risks include:

1. Preoperative coronary bypass grafts or angioplasty for patients with high cardiac risk undergoing major surgery (especially vascular surgery).

2. Antihypertensive therapy

3. Bronchodilators, chest physiotherapy, and postural drainage

4. Nutritional support to reverse catabolism

5. Preoperative treatment of Grave's disease

6. Synthetic thyroid hormone for hypothyroidism

7. DVT prophylaxis

8. Bacterial endocarditis prophylaxis

9. Correct fluid and electrolyte abnormalities

V. Coordinate Surgical and Subspecialty Services

This role will vary according to the wishes of the attending surgeon. The goal is to minimize duplication of testing and help assign priorities in the patient's care.

VI. Encourage Communication with Patient and Family

A. Consider discussion of advance directives.

B. Encourage autologous blood donation for patients undergoing procedures that may require transfusion.

VII. Annotated Bibliography

Goldman L, Caldera D, Nussbaum SR, et al. Multifactorial index of cardiac risk in non-cardiac surgical procedures. N Engl J Med 1977;297:845. One of the original and still valid study of factors affecting preoperative risk.

Eagle KA, Colez CM, Newell JB, et al. Combining clinical and thallium data optimizes preoperative assessment of cardiac risk before major vascular surgery. Ann Intern Med 1989;110:859–866. Excellent paper that explores preoperative risk assessment in patients specifically undergoing vascular surgery.

Sax HC, ed. Common Diagnostic Tests: Use and Interpretation. Philadelphia: American College of Physicians; 1987. The exhaustive work covers the use and effectiveness of preoperative test ordering.

Ziring B. Preoperative testing. In: Merli G, Weitz H, ed. Medical Management of the Surgical Patient. Philadelphia: WB Saunders;1992:1–15. A summary of the current recommendations on routine ordering of preoperative tests for nonblood loss surgery. The text of this book deals with the broader issues of perioperative care.

Part VI:
Dermatology

Chapter 27: Acne

Guy F. Webster

I. Clinical Presentation

A. General Information

1. Disease usually begins at or near puberty.
2. Lesions may persist well into adulthood.
3. Acne should not be thought of as fundamentally an infectious process.
4. Lesion distribution parallels sebaceous gland size and density.

B. Symptoms—Lesions on face, upper back and chest

C. Physical Examination

1. Primary lesion is the *comedo*, an impaction of the pilosebaceous unit. If the follicular orifice is distended, a blackhead or open comedo is seen. Undistended orifices cover closed comedones or whiteheads.
2. Inflammation may occur producing a spectrum of lesions from superficial pustules and papules to deep-seated, scarring nodules.
3. Sinus tracts may form between neighboring nodules producing *conglobate acne*.
4. Scarring and sinus tracts may form in axillae and groin, termed hidradinitis supperitiva.

II. Evaluation

A. Check for evidence of virilization in females. Irregular menses, hirsuitism, or age > 25 should prompt check of testosterone and dehydroepiandrosterone sodium.

III. Differential Diagnosis

A. Rosacea—especially in the older age range and fairer skinned. Comedones are absent and predominant feature is a malar erythema.

B. Tuberous sclerosis—especially at younger ages. Red papules occur on malar and perinasal skin.

IV. Treatment

A. Topical

1. Tretinoin 0.025–0.1% cream. Apply daily. An effective treatment for comedones. Skin may become dry and irritated. Sunscreens should be used.

2. Benzoyl peroxide, clindamycin, or erythromycin (solution or cream). Apply b.i.d. Reduces inflammatory lesions. All preparations are of roughly equivalent efficacy.

B. Systemic—for widespread or refractory disease

1. Erythromycin or tetracycline 250 mg b.i.d.–q.i.d.

2. Doxycycline or minocycline 50–100 mg q.i.d.–b.i.d.

3. Isotretinoin—reserved for severe, treatment-resistant acne. It is a *potent teratogen*. The usual dose is 0.5–1 mg/kg/d.

V. Patient Education

A. Don't overwash—dirt has no role in acne.

B. Don't manipulate lesions.

C. Diet has no role in acne.

VI. Indications for Referral to a Dermatologist

A. Disease resistant to oral antibiotic therapy

B. If Isotretinoin treatment is considered

VII. Bibliography

See end of Part VI

Chapter 28: Alopecia

Guy F. Webster

I. Clinical Presentation and Differential Diagnosis

A. Telogen Effluvium

1. Sudden hair fall perhaps prompted by illness, pregnancy, medication, or trauma
2. Generalized scalp condition

B. Alopecia Areata

1. Localized complete hair loss usually in small circumscribed areas of face or scalp
2. No scarring evident
3. Fingernails rarely involved but may be pitted or atrophic

C. Hormone-related

1. Androgenetic alopecia
2. May begin as early as late teens, more usually in the 20s and 30s

D. Discoid Lupus Erythematosus

1. Localized hair loss with hyperpigmentation, hypopigmentation, scarring, and follicular plugging
2. Usually not accompanied by systemic lupus erythematosus

II. Diagnostic Approach

A. Determine

1. Distribution of alopecia
2. Presence of scarring and pigment disease

B. Hair loss counts—may help in borderline telogen effluvium in which counts exceed 100–200/d or androgenetic alopecia. In general, hair counting is more confusing than helpful.

C. Scalp biopsy—valuable for diagnosing discoid lupus, telogen effluvium (in which loss is high eg, > 100–200/d), or androgenetic alopecia, but often is more confusing than helpful

D. Thyroid function tests—both hyper- and hypothyroidism may be linked with alopecia areata

E. Androgen levels—In women with androgenetic alopecia, high androgens may contribute to process.

F. Antinuclear antibody—Is elevated in approximately 15% of discoid lupus patients

III. Treatment

A. Telogen Effluvium

1. Remove causative agent if present.
2. Topical 2% minoxidil may be of benefit.
3. Usually spontaneously resolves.

B. Alopecia Areata

1. May spontaneously resolve.
2. Topical corticosteroids eg, fluocinolone b.i.d. (see Appendix C)
3. Topical anthralin 0.1–1% b.i.d.
4. Intralesional triamcinolone acetonide 1–2 mg/mL, injected to entire area of alopecia
5. Psoralen and ultraviolet A
6. Cyclosporin A

C. Hormone-related

1. Topical 2% minoxidil b.i.d. for months to years
2. Hair transplant and scalp reduction

D. Discoid Lupus

1. Topical or intralesional steroids (see Appendix C)

2. Limit sun exposure
3. Consider course of oral corticosteroid
4. Consider hydroxychloroquine 200–400 mg qd.

IV. Patient Education

Alopecia has no relation to diet.

V. Indications for Referral

A. Patient's reassurance

B. Treatment-resistant alopecia areata or discoid lupus (eg, when psoralen and ultraviolet A or systemic medication is considered).

VI. Bibliography

See end of Part VI

Chapter 29: Pruritis

Guy F. Webster

I. General Description

A. Pruritus is always secondary to some other diagnosis but is a frequent presenting symptom.

B. Most inflammatory skin diseases itch.

C. Yeast, bacterial, and viral infections rarely itch.

D. Dermatophyte infections usually itch.

E. Several diseases may provoke intense pruritus with minimal apparent skin disease.

II. Diagnostic Approach

Search for identifiable skin or internal disease.

III. Differential Diagnosis

A. Causes listed in I. above

B. Scabies

1. Intense itch, especially waking from sleep frequently to scratch

2. Papules distributed widely on body. Classical distribution is groin (especially penis) hands, umbilicus, and axillae.

3. *BUT*—classical distribution is rare

4. Patients may have few lesions.

5. Mites are microscopic and hard to find, even in florid cases.

C. Cutaneous T Cell Lymphoma

1. Trivial appearing pigment or skin texture changes accompanied by marked itching

2. Diagnosis by skin biopsy

D. Dermatomyositis

1. May itch intensely, especially on the upper back
2. Some presentations do not manifest a detectable myositis.
3. Collaboration between dermatology and rheumatology usually will establish a diagnosis.

E. Metabolic Derangement

1. Renal impairment, liver disease, and thyroid disease frequently cause pruritus, but pruritus only rarely leads to an initial diagnosis of these diseases.

IV. Treatment

A. General Measures

1. Minimize bathing, especially before bedtime.
2. Antihistamines eg, astemazole or hydroxyzine, may be helpful.
3. Ultraviolet B irradiation is an effective antipruritic.

B. Scabies

1. Lindane lotion (Kwell) or permethrin cream applied *once* to the entire body surface.

C. Cutaneous T Cell Lymphoma

1. Topical mechlorethamine
2. Corticosteroid ointments
3. Psoralen and ultraviolet A phototherapy

D. Dermatomyositis

1. Systemic corticosteroids and/or cytotoxic agents (eg, cyclophosphamide or azathoprine).

E. Metabolic

1. Correction of underlying disease.
2. Hydroxyzine 25–50 mg 2–5 times/d
3. Ultraviolet B phototherapy

V. Bibliography

See end of Part VI

Chapter 30: Dermatitis

Guy F. Webster

30A Atopic Dermatitis (Eczema)

I. Clinical Presentation

A. History

1. May begin at any age although nearly all patients have some history of childhood disease. Patients may have a personal or family history of other atopic manifestations, eg, allergic rhinitis and asthma.

B. Physical Examination

1. The hallmark of atopic skin disease is epidermal edema that produces clinical or subclinical vesiculation.

2. Lichenification, a thickening of the skin due to chronic scratching/rubbing, is common in atopic dermatitis and may obscure classic diagnostic features.

3. Classic/juvenile atopic dermatitis—flexor accentuated patches and flat plaques. Lichenification on back of neck may be prominent.

4. "Dyshidrotic" eczema—palmar/plantar vesiculation, scale, and fissuring. May be triggered in some by tinea pedis; in others by chronic irritation (eg, handwashing).

5. Nummular eczema—coin-shaped patches and plaques of microvesiculation and scale. It is usually provoked by xerosis or frequent bathing and is more common on the legs.

II. Diagnostic Approach

Based on physical examination above

III. Differential Diagnosis

A. Psoriasis—sharply demarcated extensor plaques with tightly adherent white scale.

B. Contact dermatitis—especially chronic contact dermatitis. The linear distribution of lesions is often a key differential point favoring contact dermatitis.

C. Cutaneous T cell lymphoma—vesicles not present and papery atrophy is.

D. Tinea pedis—may be hard to differentiate from atopic dermatitis and may actually coexist.

IV. Treatment

A. Removal of irritants, eg, decrease handwashing

B. Topical steroids—ointments more effective than creams. Class 1 or 2 for hands, 2–4 for body, and 5 or 6 for face and groin (limit use; see Appendix C).

C. Systemic steroids—for acute exacerbations prednisone 20–40 mg/d tapered over 1–3 wk. Intramuscular depot steroids are fraught with risk and should be avoided.

D. Antihistamines—of some value in reducing itch. Newer, longer-acting preparations, eg, astemozole 10 mg/d may be of greater benefit.

E. Phototherapy—Ultraviolet A and B may be of benefit for long-term management of severe disease.

F. Systemic antibiotics—secondary infection with *Staphylococcus aureas* is common and is indicated by crusting and purulence. Appropriate staphylococcal coverage for 1–2 wk may be of great benefit.

V. Indications for Referral

Disease refractory to conservative topical therapy

VI. Bibliography

See end of Part VI

30B Contact Dermatitis

I. Clinical Presentation

A. Itchy papules and plaques, scale, and vesiculation or bullae

B. Lesions are often *linear* or are in an unusual distribution.

C. Chronic, low-grade reactions may closely resemble atopic dermatitis.

II. Diagnostic Approach

A. Contact dermatitis is best identified by physical examination.

B. Patch testing to likely allergens is valuable to confirm a suspected diagnosis. A significant degree of experience is needed to properly interpret patch tests.

III. Differential Diagnosis

A. Atopic dermatitis—usually is less acute in onset.

B. Tinea pedis—Bullous tinea may be mistaken for a contact dermatitis.

IV. Treatment

A. Avoidance of allergen is foremost.

B. Topical steroids—class 1–3 for hands and feet, 2–4 for trunk and extremities, and 5–6 for face and groin (see Appendix C)

C. Systemic steroids—30–40 mg prednisone PO tapered over 2–3 wk for severe to extensive disease. Shorter courses often produce rebound of disease when treatment ends.

D. Drying agents—Astringents are of some small value in the beginning of disease but are vastly overused and may actually prolong symptoms due to irritation.

V. Bibliography

See end of Part VI

Chapter 30C Seborrheic Dermatitis

I. Clinical Presentation

A. Erythema and fine scale around the ala nasi, eyebrows, hairline, ears

B. Seborrheic dermatitis is mildly pruritic in some patients.

C. Particularly in black patients, seborrheic dermatitis may extend to the malar region.

II. Diagnostic Approach

Although biopsy is occasionally of use, diagnosis is usually made on clinical grounds.

III. Differential Diagnosis

A. Rosacea—usually not scaly

B. Lupus erythematosus—The malar rash of systemic lupus erythematosus may be closely mimicked by seborrheic dermatitis, especially in African Americans. The absence of fine scarring in seborrheic dermatitis is a valuable diagnostic point.

C. Dandruff—In contrast to seborrheic dermatitis, dandruff is noninflammatory and is not accentuated at the hairline.

D. Psoriasis—Scalp psoriasis scale is tightly adherent, more coarse, and overlying well-defined plaques.

IV. Treatment

A. Topical steroids—class 4–6 applied daily, sparingly (see Appendix C)

B. Topical antifungals—(eg, ketoconazole cream b.i.d.), effective in > 50% of patients with seborrheic dermatitis

C. Selenium sulfide—2% or 3% selenium sulfide shampoo is of great value in scalp seborrheic dermatitis.

Chapter 31: Xerosis (Dry Skin)

Guy F. Webster

I. Clinical Presentation

A. General Description

1. It is important to discriminate between skin that lacks moisture or emollients and skin that *appears* dry and scaly due to an underlying dermatosis such as eczema or seborrheic dermatitis.

B. Clinical Features

1. Pure dry skin usually occurs on the extremities, especially the hands and feet.
2. Xerosis *rarely* occurs on the upper trunk and head.
3. Involved skin may show fine scale and/or fissures.
4. Xerotic skin *rarely* has a sharp border with normal skin.
5. Patient may have mild to moderate itching.

II. Differential Diagnosis of Scaling Disorders

A. Head—dandruff, seborrheic dermatitis, atopic dermatitis, contact dermatitis, tinea, psoriasis

B. Trunk—tinea, atopic dermatitis, psoriasis, contact dermatitis, cutaneous T cell lymphoma, parapsoriasis, sarcoidosis, icthyosis

C. Extremities—icthyosis, chronic edema/stasis dermatitis, psoriasis, cutaneous T cell lymphoma, tinea, atopic dermatitis, contact dermatitis

III. Treatment

A. Greasy preparations—eg, petrolatum or Eucerin, apply twice daily and after bathing

B. Lactic acid lotions—apply twice daily and after bathing

C. Corticosteroids—use only when evidence of inflammation is present. Use should be minimized in purely dry skin.

IV. Patient Education

A. Minimize washing and use mild soap (eg, Dove).

B. Use emollients liberally.

C. Minimize exposure to irritants at home or work.

V. Indications for Referral

Dry skin persists after several weeks of therapy.

VI. Bibliography

See end of Part VI

Chapter 32: Fungal Infections

Guy F. Webster

I. Clinical Presentation

A. Tinea corporis and cruris—annular plaque with raised scaly border

B. Tinea capitis—edematous scaly area of partial alopecia

C. Tinea pedis

1. Athlete's foot—macerated, itchy toe webs

2. Dry tinea—fine scale on plantar surface

D. Onychomycosis—invasion and destruction of nail. Plate may be dry and dystrophic, or opaque.

E. Tinea versicolor—largely asymptomatic hyperpigmented or hypopigmented fine scaly patches on trunk and proximal extremities.

F. Candidiasis

1. Intertriginous—bright pink minimally scaly patch with peripheral tiny pustules

2. Paronychia—distal onycholysis with periungual inflammation. In contrast to dermatophytic onychomycosis, the involved nail is often tender and suppurative.

II. Diagnostic Approach

A. Diagnosis usually made by clinical appearance (above)

B. KOH preparation

C. Fungus culture

D. Biopsy as indicated by clinical appearance

III. Differential Diagnosis

Atopic dermatitis: is KOH negative.

IV. Treatment

A. Dermatophyte Infections

1. Topical therapy—Azole antifungals (eg, ketoconazole cream or ciclopirox cream). Nystatin is inactive for dermatophytes. Consider topical therapy for most superficial infections.

2. Systemic therapy

   a. Griseofulvin 250–500 mg/d. Deep follicular infections and nail infections. Treat until cleared for at least 2–3 wk. Griseofulvin has no activity against *Candida* species.
   b. Azoles—Ketoconazole (200 mg), fluconazole, itraconazole given qd for 2–3 wk until clearing.

B. Tinea Versicolor

1. Topical antifungals of any pharmacologic class for 2–3 d
2. Selenium sulfide 2–3% lotion for 3 d

C. Candidal Infections

1. Topical antifungals—twice daily application appropriate for intertrigo
2. Systemic antifungals—Azoles (eg, ketoconazole 200–400 mg qd–b.i.d.) for *Candida* species. Candidal onycholysis and paronychia may require 3–6 wk of therapy.

V. Bibliography

See end of Part VI

Chapter 33: Psoriasis

Guy F. Webster

I. Clinical Presentation

A. Psoriasis vulgaris—pink plaques with well-defined margins and a tightly adherent silvery scale. Lesions may or may not itch and heal without scarring. Distribution is primarily on extensor surfaces.

B. Pustular psoriasis—plaques are deeper red with a yellow scale-crust. Pustules may be sparse or numerous. Distribution may be generalized or predominantly acral. More common in patients infected with HIV.

C. Psoriatic arthritis—occurs in about 5–10% of psoriatics.

II. Diagnostic Approach

A. Diagnosis usually made mainly on clinical grounds.

B. Skin biopsy is useful in equivocal cases.

III. Differential Diagnosis

A. Atopic dermatitis—may mimic mild psoriasis, has evidence of microvesicles.

B. Cutaneous T cell lymphoma (mycosis fungoides)—pruritic, often subtle rash. Usually initially misdiagnosed as "dermatitis" for several years. Major diagnostic point is subtle atrophy of skin.

C. Chronic cutaneous (discoid) lupus—may be a striking mimic of psoriasis; lesions, however, heal with scarring.

D. Tinea corporis—raised border, furiously itchy, KOH positive.

IV. Treatment (roughly in order of potency)

A. Emollients—eg, Eucerin, petrolatum twice daily, used liberally

B. Topical Steroids

1. Ointments are superior to creams.

2. Beware steroid atrophy with chronic use. Class 1 or 2 preparations must not be overused (see Appendix C).

C. Anthralin—0.1–1% cream applied to plaques for 10–20 min and washed off. Good for resistant plaques.

D. Phototherapy—ultraviolet B or ultraviolet A + psoralen (PUVA). Major adverse effect is risk of burning. There is a minor risk of low-grade skin cancers with PUVA.

E. Oral agents for severe disease

1. Methotrexate 7.5–15 mg/wk is typical dosage. Drug is given weekly. Generally not suitable for patients with renal impairment. Liver damage, cirrhosis, and marrow toxicity are potential major side effects.

2. Etretinate—vitamin A analog. Typical dosage is 25–100 mg/d. Major adverse reactions include hypertriglyceridemia and dry skin. Because of a *very* long half-life and the guarantee of birth defects, this drug is *not suitable for reproductive-age women.*

3. Cyclosporin A 1–2 mg/kg/d. Major risk is renal dysfunction and hypertension.

F. Long-term Management

1. The major strategy is to minimize drug side effects in this lifelong disease.

2. Vigorous use of emollients will aid in steroid or cytotoxic sparing.

V. Patient Education

A. Psoriasis is only *weakly* inherited and is not contagious.

B. Skin irritation (eg, excess washing, scratching) will trigger psoriasis.

C. It is frequently stated that β blockers or nonsteroidal anti-inflammatory agents will trigger psoriasis. Although this is clearly possible, studies document the extreme rarity of this phenomenon.

VI. Indications for Referral to a Dermatologist

A. Patients who do not have sufficient improvement in response to topical therapy should be referred for evaluation of diagnosis and treatment.

VII. Indications for Hospitalization

Erythrodermic or pustular psoriasis in the elderly or debilitated

VIII. Bibliography

See end of Part VI

Chapter 34: Benign and Malignant Growths

Guy F. Webster

I. Clinical Presentation and Differential Diagnosis

A. General Information

1. Many lesions are found on sun-damaged skin.
2. Magnification, eg, 5 or 10 times is often valuable in diagnosis.

B. Symptoms

1. May be asymptomatic, pruritic, tender, or show signs of growth.

C. Physical Examination

1. Actinic keratosis

    a. Pinkish/red flat patches with a sandpaper-like feel.
    b. On legs and hands may be raised and warty appearing

2. Angiomas

    a. Sharp-bordered red papules or macules
    b. Usually will blanch with pressure

3. Basal cell carcinoma—may have any one of the following appearances

    a. Pearly or translucent papule
    b. Erythematous red macule
    c. Gray-black pigmented papule
    d. Fluid-filled papule
    e. Ulcer
    f. Telangiectases may be prominent.

4. Keloids and hypertrophic scars

    a. Firm to hard brick-red nodule at site of trauma/infection

5. Melanoma

    a. Melanocytic lesion with varying shades of pink, brown, and black
    b. Borders are irregular, often indistinct in some areas.
    c. May ulcerate
    d. May be flat or raised

6. Melanocytic nevi
    a. Tan to black in color
    b. Borders usually smooth and distinct
    c. May be flat or raised

7. Seborrheic keratosis
    a. Superficial flat to hyperkeratotic papule
    b. Sharp borders
    c. Tan to black color
    d. May have visible microcysts

8. Squamous cell carcinomas
    a. Usually on sun-exposed skin
    b. Pink to red
    c. Scaly or crusted surface
    d. Borders may be indistinct.

9. Warts
    a. Sharp bordered
    b. May grow rapidly
    c. Surface is finely papillated.

II. Treatment

A. Actinic Keratosis

1. Many will progress to squamous cell cancer.

2. Destruction with liquid nitrogen

3. Topical 5-fluorouracil cream (2% or 3% qd for 2 wk). *BEWARE:* This will produce a markedly unpleasant but effective response.

4. Curettage usually leaves a residual scar.

B. Angiomas

1. Treatment is indicated if individual lesions are troublesome.

2. Curettage and light electrodessication

3. Tunable dye laser destruction

C. Basal Cell Carcinoma

1. Rarely metastatic but locally aggressive; treatment is therefore important.

2. Excision with microscopic check of margins

3. Curettage and dessication—about 90% effective for long-term care, *but* this technique is very operator-dependent and not appropriate for periorificial or recurrent lesions.

4. Radiation therapy—costly and time-consuming but effective

D. Keloids and Hypertrophic Scars

1. Intralesional triamcinolone acetonide 10–40 mg/mL given *monthly* until improvement ceases

2. Excision may trigger a new keloid. Pretreatment with intralesional steroids may be of benefit.

E. Melanoma

1. Highly metastatic tumor whose only effective treatment is surgical

2. Wide excision—excision of the lesion and a > 1 cm border of normal skin is sufficient for "moderate thickness" lesions.

3. All but the tiniest melanomas (< 0.15 mm thick) should have a thorough physical examination and diagnostic tests as indicated.

4. Skin examinations should be performed q 4–6 mo to identify new primary tumors or cutaneous metastases in patients with "moderate thickness" melanoma.

5. Referral—The physician should be very confident of own ability to diagnose early melanoma or refer to a dermatologist.

F. Nevi

1. Nevi not suspected to be melanoma need only be treated if they are individually troublesome.

2. Excision—Shave excision or full-thickness excision are both valuable.

3. Q-switched ruby laser will destroy thin or superficial nevi.

G. Seborrheic Keratoses

1. Treatment is indicated if individual lesions become troublesome.

2. Curettage—an ideal therapy for these superficial lesions.

3. Cryotherapy—Liquid nitrogen will also remove these lesions.

H. Squamous Cell Carcinoma

1. All are potentially metastatic (overall rate is about 2% for sun-induced squamous cells) and should be removed. Tumors on mucosa, genitals, and sites of chronic inflammation (eg, burn scars) are more invasive (30% become metastatic) and should be treated aggressively.

2. Excision with microscopic control of margins

3. Radiation therapy may be useful for particularly large lesions.

I. Warts

1. Topical salicylic acid preparations (eg, 12% salicylic acid) applied daily and covered with an adhesive dressing
2. Curettage
3. CO_2 laser destruction

III. Indications for Referral to a Dermatologist

A. Uncertainty of diagnosis

B. Need for surgery of known malignancy

C. Lack of expertise in excision techniques

IV. Annotated Bibliography

Fitzpatrick TB, Eisen AZ, Wolff K, Freedberg IM, Austen KF. Dermatology in general medicine, Fourth ed., New York: McGraw-Hill, 1993. An excellent general dermatology text with a good atlas attached.

Hurwitz S. Clinical pediatric dermatology, a textbook of skin disorders of childhood and adolescence. Philadelphia: WB Saunders, 1981. A good general dermatology reference book.

Braverman IM. Skin signs of systemic diseases. Second ed, Philadelphia: WB Saunders, 1981. A little old, but still a classic.

Part VII:
Endocrinology/Metabolism

Chapter 35: Adrenocortical Hyperfunction

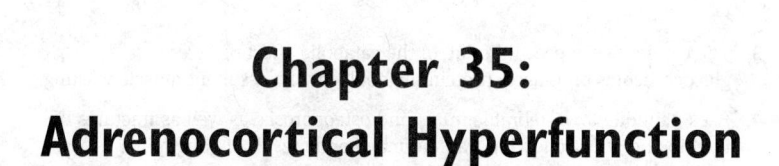

Rosemarie A. Leuzzi

35A Cushing's Syndrome

I. Clinical Presentation

A. General Information

1. All cases of endogenous Cushing's syndrome are due to increased production of cortisol by the adrenal gland.

2. Causes

   a. Hypersecretion of ACTH usually by a pituitary microadenoma ("Cushing's disease")—70% of cases of Cushing's syndrome
   b. Autonomous adrenal overproduction of cortisol due to an adrenal adenoma, adrenal carcinoma, or bilateral nodular adrenal hyperplasia—10% of cases
   c. Ectopic production of ACTH
      1) Small cell (oat cell) carcinoma of the lung
      2) Nonpituitary tumors such as tumors of the thymus, pancreas, ovary, or bronchial carcinoid tumors
      3) Medullary carcinoma of the thyroid

3. Incidence

   a. Pituitary causes of excessive ACTH occur more commonly in women (female:male is 5:1); however, ectopic ACTH production occurs more frequently in men.
   b. In adults, pituitary microadenomas and ectopic ACTH production occur more frequently than adrenal neoplasms; however, in children, adrenal neoplasms (particularly adrenal carcinoma) occur more frequently.

B. Symptoms

1. Obesity/weight gain is the most common feature presenting as truncal obesity with the characteristic increased abdominal girth.

2. Muscle weakness and fatigue from "steroid myopathy" are usually most prominent in the shoulder and pelvic girdle areas.

3. The extremities appear thin due to the catabolic effect of excess glucocorticoids on muscle protein metabolism with resultant muscle wasting.

4. Back pain due to vertebral features and osteoporosis, as well as fractures of the hip and wrist following trauma, may be the result of bone mineral loss.

5. Skin changes due to weakening and rupture of the collagen fibers in the dermis include

   a. Facial flushing or "plethora"
   b. Talengiectasias
   c. Easy bruisability
   d. Violaceous striae and thin paperlike skin

6. Psychological disturbances are present in two thirds of patients with confusion, irritability, depression, and emotional lability; severe depression, psychosis, and mania may also occur.

7. Androgenic effects are mostly noted in women with hirsutism, acne, menstrual abnormalities, and virilization; androgen excess varies depending on the etiology of the Cushing's syndrome.

8. Decreased libido and impotence in men may be noted.

9. Check if the patient is taking any medications and always check for steroid use.

10. Weight loss may suggest ectopic ACTH production from a tumor.

C. Physical Examination

1. Characteristic physical changes noted include

   a. Deposition of adipose tissue resulting in the typical "moon facies"
   b. Increased dorsal and supraclavicular fat pads—a "buffalo hump"
   c. Truncal obesity that is accentuated by the thin extremities

2. Hypertension reflects the increased mineralocorticoid activity.

3. A palpable abdominal mass may be found in patients with adrenal carcinoma.

II. Diagnostic Approach

A. In patients manifesting several of the above signs and symptoms, a diagnosis of Cushing's syndrome should be considered by the primary care physician.

1. The severity of signs and symptoms depends on the magnitude of the steroid excess, the rapidity with which it develops, and the degree to which androgen production is increased.

2. The most discriminating findings include objective weakness, ecchymoses, osteoporosis, central obesity, and hypokalemia.

3. Some of the most common clinical findings such as hypertension, impaired glucose tolerance, obesity, and oligomenorrhea are the least diagnostic and only helpful if absent.

4. Ectopic ACTH production by nonendocrine tumors usually does not present with the classic signs and symptoms but instead patients present with an abrupt onset of the biochemical abnormalities (hypokalemic metabolic alkalosis and glucose intolerance) and weight loss.

B. Electrolyte Abnormalities

1. Fasting hyperglycemia is found in 10–15% of patients; impaired glucose tolerance or frank diabetes mellitus is due to impaired hepatic gluconeogenesis and insulin resistance.
2. A hypokalemic, metabolic alkalosis may be present due to the excessive mineralocorticoid effects.

C. Screening Tests

1. To minimize the frequency of false positives, screening tests should be performed following resolution of any acute medical or psychiatric illness; because both cortisol and ACTH are stress hormones, patients with an acute illness may appear chemically to have Cushing's disease.
2. Overnight dexamethasone suppression test
    a. Dexamethasone is a potent glucocorticosteroid that inhibits the normal pituitary corticotroph cells so that no ACTH is released, resulting in a decrease in the serum cortisol level, urinary cortisol levels, and urinary 17-hydroxycorticosteroid (17-OHCS) levels.
    b. Very useful in the outpatient setting, this test has a low incidence of false negatives (< 2%).
    c. Method
        1) Administer 1 mg dexamethasone PO between 11 PM and 12 midnight.
        2) Draw a plasma cortisol level at 8:00 the following morning.
    d. Interpretation
        1) Normal patients will show suppression of cortisol to < 5 mg/dL.
        2) If the 8 am plasma cortisol level is < 5 mg/dL (< 140 nmoles/L), this excludes the diagnosis of Cushing's syndrome of any type.
    e. Limitations—10% false positives (8 AM plasma cortisol level is > 5 mg/dL)
        1) False positives found if patient is obese, stressed during the night, or rushed to get to the lab in morning, did not take the dexamethasone, has an acute/chronic illness or primary affective disorder.
        2) Oral contraceptives and anticonvulsants also may cause false positive results due to increased metabolism of dexamethasone.
    f. Serum cortisol values are not helpful unless coupled with dexamethasone testing.
3. 24-h urinary free cortisol excretion
    a. 24-h urine collection is the best screening test because all Cushing's patients will display elevations of urinary cortisol.
    b. There is a low false positive rate and obesity is less likely to affect the results

c. Method
   1) Instruct the patient to collect all urine for a 24-h period in a plastic container.
   2) Check simultaneous urinary creatinine to assess adequacy of the sample due to the question of reliability in outpatient collections.
d. Interpretation
   1) 24-h urinary free cortisol > 100 µg/dL (275 nmoles)/24 h is suggestive of Cushing's syndrome.
e. Limitations
   1) False negatives if renal failure/renal insufficiency
4. High clinical suspicion with a negative screening test
   a. About 5–10% of patients with Cushing's syndrome have intermittent or periodic secretion; therefore, they will have negative results if tested during a nadir.
   b. If a patient's symptoms are strongly suggestive of Cushing's syndrome and the initial tests are negative, the patient should have repeat testing.

D. Definitive Diagnosis

1. Once the screening test is abnormal, proceed with further testing to confirm the diagnosis of Cushing's syndrome and to determine whether the hypercortisolism is the result of adrenal overstimulation by excess ACTH or is ACTH independent.
2. Dexamethasone suppression test
   a. Method
      1) On days 1 and 2, collect baseline 24-h urine for free cortisol, 17 OHCS, and creatinine.
      2) On days 3 and 4 administer dexamethasone 0.5 mg (low dose) PO q 6 h × 8 doses.
      3) On day 4, collect 24-h urine for free cortisol, 17-OHCS, and creatinine.
      4) On days 5 and 6, administer dexamethasone 2 mg (high dose) PO q 6 h × 8 doses.
      5) On day 6, collect 24-h urine for free cortisol, 17-OHCS, and creatinine.
   b. Interpretation
      1) Normal patient
         a) *Urinary 17-OHCS < 3 mg/24 h*
         b) *Urinary cortisol < 30 mg/24 h*
         c) *Plasma cortisol at the end of the suppression period should be suppressed to < 5 µg/dL.*
      2) Diagnosis of Cushing's Syndrome is *confirmed* if:
         a) *Failure to suppress with low-dose dexamethasone*
         b) *24-h urinary free cortisol on day 4 is > 20 mg/24 h*
         c) *17-OHCS is > 2 mg/24 h*
      3) Pituitary hypersecretion of ACTH is *suggested* by:
         a) *Suppression on high-dose dexamethasone without suppression on low-dose dexamthasone*
         b) *24-h urinary free cortisol/17 OHCS on day 6 < 50% of baseline value from days 1 and 2*

4) Ectopic ACTH production or a functioning adrenal tumor is *suggested*:
   a) *Failure to suppress on high-dose dexamethasone*
   b) *24-h urinary free cortisol/17-OHCS on day 6 > 50% of baseline value*

3. Plasma ACTH levels
   a. An immunoradiometric assay for ACTH levels is commercially available and is very useful in distinguishing the various etiologies of Cushing's syndrome.
   b. Interpretation
      1) Low or undetectable ACTH levels (< 5 pg/mL) are found with functioning adrenal tumors.
      2) Normal/high ACTH levels are consistent with ectopic ACTH production.
   c. The combination of the dexamethasone suppression test and ACTH level is generally helpful for diagnosis.

4. Radiologic imaging
   a. Once the initial screening tests are suggestive of Cushing's syndrome, wait to perform imaging studies until biochemical evaluation points to the tumor's location. (This is important considering the frequency of benign adrenal incidental tumors and incidental pituitary abnormalities.)
   b. Abdominal CT scanning
      1) Thin tomographic cuts on CT scanning can identify adrenal masses < 1 cm as well as localize small ACTH producing tumors in the lung, pancreas, and mediastinum.
      2) Adrenal adenomas usually can be found because the suppression of ACTH by cortisol from the tumor leads to atrophy of the surrounding adrenal cortex and the contralateral adrenal gland.
      3) Adrenal carcinomas are usually extremely large (> 6 cm) by the time of diagnosis.
   c. MRI of the head
      1) MRI of the sellar region is abnormal in only 30–50% of pituitary-dependent Cushing's syndrome because most are microadenomas.
      2) In addition, false positive pituitary abnormalities may be noted in patients with ectopic ACTH production.

5. Bilateral inferior petrosal sinus (IPS) sampling
   a. Venous drainage of the anterior pituitary is sampled bilaterally to measure ACTH gradients as well as drawing a peripheral venous sample for an ACTH level.
   b. If pituitary-dependent Cushing's syndrome is suspected but CT or MRI scanning does not reveal any abnormality, this may help to localize a microadenoma and to exclude the diagnosis of ectopic ACTH production.
   c. When the gradient ACTH level (IPS to peripheral) is > 3.0, the patient likely has pituitary disease.
   d. Considering the invasiveness of this study, it should only be used in selective patients and following consultation with an endocrinologist.

III. Differential Diagnosis

A. Pseudo-Cushing's can be found in hypercortisol states and may cause confusion when interpreting the tests due to false positive results.

1. Obesity
   a. Obesity is frequently associated with hypertension and diabetes mellitus.
   b. Rapid weight gain can result in the appearance of striae.
   c. Obesity can also cause increased cortisol production; however, urinary cortisol levels are usually normal or mildly increased.
   d. The adiposity is usually generalized as opposed to truncal obesity.

2. Chronic alcoholism/depression—elevated morning plasma cortisol and insufficient dexamethasone suppression with absence of a diurnal rhythm

3. Acute or chronic illness—fail to suppress with dexamethasone because major stress (fever, pain) interrupts the normal regulation of ACTH secretion

B. Iatrogenic Cushing's syndrome due to long-term glucocorticoid treatment

IV. Treatment

A. Adrenal Neoplasms

1. Surgical exploration with excision of the tumor

2. Due to the potential atrophy of the contralateral gland, stress dose steroids are given.

3. Cure rate for benign adenomas is 100%.

4. Prognosis for adrenocortical carcinoma is poor despite surgery and chemotherapy (survival < 50% at 3 y).

5. Mitotane, a cytotoxic agent, is used to suppress cortisol production and for treatment
   a. Adrenal carcinoma that cannot be totally removed
   b. Metastatic adrenal carcinoma

B. Pituitary Hypersecretion of ACTH

1. Transsphenoidal exploration of the pituitary is treatment of choice.

2. Remission 60–90%

3. Radiation therapy may be useful as adjunctive therapy if not cured by surgery

4. Bilateral total adrenalectomy is reserved for failed pituitary surgery; however, the drawbacks include permanent adrenal insufficiency and the risk of developing Nelson's syndrome (enlarging pituitary adenoma with hyperpigmentation) as well as the operative morbidity/mortality.

C. Ectopic ACTH Production

1. Treat the underlying malignancy.
2. Prognosis is usually poor.
3. Medical therapy with adrenolytic agents that act as adrenal enzyme inhibitors blocking steroidogenesis
   a. Aminoglutethimide 250 mg q.i.d.
   b. Metyrapone 250–500 mg q.i.d.

V. Indications for Referral to a Specialist

A. Once the diagnosis of Cushing's syndrome is confirmed following a positive screening test, detailed evaluation usually requires the expertise of an endocrinologist. Due to the potential for false positive results on the screening tests, equivocal results may require further endocrinologic evaluation.

B. If screening tests are negative and the clinical features are strongly suggestive, referral to an endocrinologist for further evaluation may be appropriate.

C. Selection of the further diagnostic studies and therapy should be made in conjunction with an endocrinologist.

VI. Annotated Bibliography

Burch WM. Endocrinology for the House Officer. Baltimore: Williams & Wilkins 1988. Concise brief review of diagnostic studies and work-up for Cushing's syndrome.

Findling JW. Cushing syndrome—an etiologic workup. Hosp Pract 1992;27:59–74. A very thorough case management study reviewing the possible etiologies of Cushing's syndrome with a diagnostic approach. A discussion of modifications regarding the dexamethasone suppression test based on recent National Institutes of Health studies is included in the commentary.

Gregerman RI. Selected endocrine problems: disorders of pituitary, adrenal, and parathyroid glands; pharmacologic use of steroids; hypo- and hypercalcemia; osteoporosis, water metabolism; hypoglycemia. In: Barker LR, Burton JR, Zieve PD, eds. Principles of Ambulatory Medicine. Baltimore: Williams & Wilkins 1991. Ambulatory management of patients suspected to have Cushing's syndrome and modalities for screening are briefly discussed.

Williams GH, Dluhy RG. Diseases of the Adrenal Cortex. In: Wilson JD, Braunwald E, Isselbacher KJ, et al, eds. Harrison's Principles of Internal Medicine, 12th ed. New York: McGraw-Hill, 1991. In-depth review of physiology with thorough discussion of causes of Cushing's syndrome, available diagnostic biochemical tests, and algorithm for diagnostic evaluation.

35B Hyperaldosteronism

I. Clinical Presentation

A. General Information

1. Hyperaldosteronism is a rare cause of hypertension, < 1% of cases.
2. Types of hyperaldosteronism
   a. Primary hyperaldosteronism is due to increased intra-adrenal aldosterone production.
      1) Aldosterone-producing adrenal adenoma—80% of primary hyperaldosteronism cases (Conn's syndrome)
      2) Bilateral idiopathic nodular adrenal hyperplasia
      3) Aldosterone-producing adrenal carcinoma
      4) Glucocorticoid-suppressible hyperaldosteronism
      5) Congenital adrenal enzymatic defect (very rare)
   b. Secondary hyperaldosteronism due to an extra-adrenal stimulus for aldosterone secretion (reflecting the normal adrenal response to increased stimulation by the renin-angiotensin system) is responsible for the majority of cases of hyperaldosteronism.
      1) Decreased effective blood volume—diuretic therapy, cirrhosis, congestive heart failure, nephrotic syndrome
      2) Decreased renal perfusion—renal artery stenosis or malignant hypertension
      3) Estrogen-induced increases in renin due to pregnancy or oral contraceptive pills
      4) Juxtaglomerular hyperplasia—Bartter's syndrome

B. Symptoms

1. Patients are usually asymptomatic.
2. Fatigue, weakness, paralysis, and tetany may be present due to the effect of the hypokalemia at the membrane level.
3. Polyuria may result from impairment of renal concentrating ability and is often associated with polydipsia.
4. Patients may complain of headaches due to the hypertension.

C. Physical Examination

1. Hypertension is usually present due to increased sodium reabsorption and extracellular volume expansion.
2. Edema is absent in primary hyperaldosteronism but often present in secondary hyperaldosteronism.

II. Diagnostic Approach

A. Always measure the potassium level in a hypertensive patient before medical therapy is begun and suspect hyperaldosteronism if a patient has hypokalemia and hypertension and is not taking diuretics.

B. If a nonedematous patient with a normal sodium intake presents with persistent hypokalemia and is not taking potassium-wasting diuretics, evaluation for primary hyperaldosteronism should be done.

C. If a hypokalemic patient is taking potassium-wasting diuretics, the diuretic should be discontinued, potassium supplementation administered, and electrolytes repeated in 2 wk. If the patient remains hypokalemic, further evaluation for an excess mineralocorticoid state should be done.

D. Electrolyte Abnormalities

1. Hypersecretion of aldosterone stimulates the reabsorption of sodium and the renal wasting of potassium resulting in hypokalemia.
2. Hypokalemia
   a. Hypokalemia is present in both primary and secondary forms of hyperaldosteronism.
   b. Almost all patients with primary hyperaldosteronism have a serum potassium level < 4.0 mEq/L
   c. Although most patients with primary hyperaldosteronism have spontaneous hypokalemia, as many as 25% of patients may have serum potassium levels > 3.5 mEq/L.
   d. The development of severe hypokalemia after the initiation of potassium-wasting diuretics should be a clue to a hypermineralocorticoid state.
   e. These patients usually manifest hypokalemia after starting potassium-wasting diuretics or following large intakes of sodium chloride (4–5 g sodium) and may develop severe hypokalemia and metabolic alkalosis.
3. Hypernatremia may result from both sodium retention as well as the water loss from polyuria.
4. Serum magnesium levels are also reduced if the hypokalemia is severe.

E. 24-h Urine for Potassium

1. If a patient is hypertensive and hypokalemic, check a 24-h urine collection for potassium excretion.
2. Suspect hyperaldosteronism, either primary or secondary, if urinary potassium excretion > 30 mEq/ 24 h.
3. If urine potassium excretion < 30 mEq/ 24 h, primary aldosteronism is excluded and consider use of diuretics or GI potassium losses.

F. Plasma Renin Activity

1. Renin levels are affected by diurnal variation and are usually increased with the patient in an upright position; furthermore, renin secretion will be increased in patients following a sodium restricted diet.

2. A normal or elevated plasma renin level excludes the diagnosis of primary hyperaldosteronism; one must then consider secondary forms of hyperaldosteronism including renovascular hypertension, malignant hypertension, salt wasting disease, or rarely a renin-producing tumor.

3. If the renin level is low, the plasma renin level should be remeasured along with a plasma aldosterone level.

4. A low plasma renin level is consistent with the diagnosis of primary hyperaldosteronism; however, a low renin level alone does not make the diagnosis since 15% of hypertensive patients may have a suppressed renin level.

G. Plasma Aldosterone Level (or 24-h Urine for Aldosterone)

1. Plasma aldosterone levels are becoming more available and are more reliable than 24-h urinary aldosterone collections.

2. If the plasma renin level is decreased and the aldosterone level is elevated, this confirms the diagnosis of primary hyperaldosteronism; one must then distinguish between an aldosterone-producing adrenal mass and bilateral adrenal hyperplasia.

3. If the aldosterone level is decreased, then consider causes of pseudohyperaldosteronism with excessive licorice ingestion or other causes of excessive mineralocorticoid activity.

H. Radiologic Imaging for Localization

1. CT scanning of the abdomen

    a. High-resolution imaging can be used once the diagnosis of hyperaldosteronism is made to localize an adrenal or evaluate for bilateral adrenal hyperplasia.

2. If the CT scan is nondiagnostic, further imaging and interventional studies should be undertaken for localization following consultation with a specialist; further evaluation may include percutaneous transfemoral adrenal vein catheterization with aldosterone determinations and adrenal venography for lateralization and localization of an aldosterone-producing mass.

III. Differential Diagnosis

A. Pseudoaldosteronism may present with similar clinical manifestations of excessive mineralocorticoid activity but aldosterone levels are low.

1. Excessive licorice intake—Licorice (glycyrrhizinic acid) has mineralocorticoid activity and excessive intake may mimic hyperaldosteronism causing hypertension and hypokalemia.
   a. Licorice eaters > 1 lb/wk
   b. Chewing tobacco may also contain large amounts of licorice for flavoring.

B. Endogenous mineralocortiocoid excess (other than aldosterone) may be seen in patients with Cushing's syndrome and also in patients with congenital adrenal hyperplasia.

C. Liddle's syndrome—excessive renal sodium conservation due to a rare familial disorder characterized by hypertension, hypokalemia, and decreased renin and aldosterone levels. This disorder does not respond to therapy with aldosterone antagonists but does respond to triamterene.

IV. Treatment

A. Pharmacologic Therapy

1. Spironolactone (25–100 mg q 8 h) blocks the renal tubular effect of aldosterone and weakly inhibits aldosterone synthesis.
   a. A trial of spironolactone may be useful in all patients.
   b. Failure of the spironolactone to correct the blood pressure while correcting the hypokalemia strongly suggests that regardless of the anatomic cause of the excess aldosterone, surgery would not correct the hypertension; this may be seen in patients with secondary hyperaldosteronism.
   c. Chronic spironolactone therapy in men is limited by the development of gynecomastia, loss of libido, and impotence.

2. Amiloride (40 mg/d) and triamterene (100–300 mg daily) are other potassium-sparing diuretics that act by inhibiting potassium excretion by a direct effect on the renal tubules.
   a. May be useful for patients who cannot tolerate spironolactone
   b. May be considered the drug of choice for sexually active men due to the potential for impotence with chronic spironolactone therapy

B. Surgical Treatment

1. Adrenal adenomas are usually treated by surgical excision.

2. Hypertension due to bilateral adrenal hyperplasia responds poorly to surgery and, therefore, surgery is not indicated because it is seldom curative.

C. Treatment for Specific Etiologies of Hyperaldosteronism

1. Aldosterone-producing adrenal adenoma

a. Surgical removal is recommended if the patient is a good surgical risk because this procedure usually cures the hypertension and the hypokalemia.
   b. If not, pharmacologic treatment and sodium restriction may be used.

2. Bilateral adrenal hyperplasia
   a. Spironolactone is the recommended first-line therapy; however, other antihypertensive agents may also be used with potassium supplementation.
   b. Normalization of blood pressure may require the addition of another diuretic.
   c. Surgery is indicated only when significant symptomatic hypokalemia cannot be controlled with medical therapy; subtotal adrenalectomy is preferred over total adrenalectomy due to the long-term risks of adrenal insufficiency.

3. Secondary forms of hyperaldosteronism
   a. Control the underlying disease, eg, congestive heart failure, cirrhosis
   b. Sodium restriction and diuretics to reduce the retaining effects of aldosterone
   c. Potassium replacement if indicated
   d. Aldosterone antagonists, such as spironolactone

V. Indications for Referral to a Specialist

A. When a patient has hypokalemia, suppressed plasma renin activity, and an elevated aldosterone level, the patient should be referred to either an endocrinologist or a nephrologist with expertise in this area.

B. Localization procedures may then be discussed with the consultant.

VI. Annotated Bibliography

Burch WM. Endocrinology for the House Officer. Baltimore: Williams & Wilkins; 1988. Concise description of work-up for hyperaldosteronism.

Spital A. Hypokalemia. In: Barker LR, Burton JR, Zieve PD, eds. Principles of Ambulatory Medicine. Baltimore: Williams & Wilkins; 1991. General overview of evaluation of hypokalemia including GI losses, diuretic-induced hypokalemia with brief discussion of primary hyperaldosteronism.

Williams GH, Dluhy RG. Diseases of the Adrenal Cortex. In: Wilson JD, Braunwald E, Isselbacher KJ, et al, eds. Harrison's Principles of Internal Medicine, 12th ed. New York: McGraw-Hill; 1991. In-depth review of adrenal hormones with algorithm for diagnosis of hyperaldosteronism including rare endocrine abnormalities.

35C Pheochromocytoma

I. Clinical Presentation

A. General Information

1. Pheochromocytoma is quite rare, occurring in 0.1% of the hypertensive population.
2. Pheochromocytomas (which produce, store, and secrete catecholamines) arise from
   a. Chromaffin cells of the adrenal medulla in approximately 90% of cases
   b. Chromaffin cells in or about the sympathetic ganglia in approximately 10% of cases
3. It is usually curable if properly diagnosed and treated; however, it may be fatal if misdiagnosed or treated inappropriately.
4. Pheochromocytomas are inherited as an autosomal trait either alone or in combination with other disorders in 10% of cases.
   a. Multiple endocrine neoplasia type IIa (Sipple's syndrome) includes
      1) Pheochromocytoma—frequently bilateral, benign, and occasionally extraadrenal
      2) Medullary carcinoma of the thyroid
      3) Parathyroid hyperplasia
   b. Multiple endocrine neoplasia type IIb (mucosal neuroma syndrome) includes
      1) Pheochromocytoma—frequently bilateral and benign
      2) Medullary carcinoma of the thyroid
      3) Mucosal neuromas—usually of the tongue, gastrointestinal tract, conjunctiva, labia, and buccal mucosa
      4) Marfanoid habitus
   c. von Recklinghausen's neurofibromatosis includes
      1) Neurofibromas
      2) Cafe au lait spots
      3) Vertebral abnormalities
   d. von Hippel-Lindau's retinal cerebellar hemangioblastomatosis
5. The "10% rule"
   a. 10% occur bilaterally in the adrenal gland.
   b. 10% are extraadrenal.
   c. 10% are familial.
   d. < 10% are malignant.
6. Extra-adrenal pheochromocytomas are usually located in the abdomen in association with the celiac, superior mesenteric, or inferior mesenteric ganglia.

B. Symptoms

1. Pheochromocytomas usually present in the young or during midadult life; presentation during pregnancy carries a high risk of maternal and fetal mortality.

2. Paroxysmal attacks

    a. Paroxysmal or symptomatic attacks occur due to increased catecholamine secretion in 50–75% of patients.
    b. The characteristic triad includes headache, palpitations, and diaphoresis.
    c. Attacks occur abruptly and subside slowly usually lasting < 1 h in most patients; however, episodes may last several hours or longer.
    d. In an individual patient, the symptoms are often similar with each attack; with time, the paroxysms usually increase in frequency, duration, and severity.
    e. The hypercatecholaminemia may be precipitated by palpation of the tumor, exertion, anxiety, postural change, ingestion of foods or beverages containing tyramine (cheeses and wines) while being treated with monoamine oxidase inhibitors, use of certain drugs, and anesthesia.

3. Headaches usually have a rapid onset over minutes and may occur in any part of the head; they are usually described as severe, throbbing, and bilateral.

4. Episodes may be accompanied by abdominal pain with nausea and vomiting.

5. Generalized, profuse sweating may be noted.

6. Pallor occurs more frequently than flushing during paroxysms.

7. Acute anxiety, nervousness, and panic with fear of death are often noted.

8. Palpitations with tachycardia occur frequently and some patients may complain of chest pain or exertional angina.

9. Mild to moderate weight loss may be noted due to the increased metabolic rate.

10. Due to the potential for hereditary disorders, a thorough family history should be obtained.

C. Physical Examination

1. Hypertension

    a. The hypertension is occasionally episodic and severe; however, sustained hypertension is present in the majority of patients.
    b. In 60% of cases the hypertension is sustained although significant blood pressure lability is usually evident and patients have distinct crises or paroxysms.
    c. The hypertension is usually severe, occasionally malignant, and usually resistant to standard antihypertensive medications.
    d. Paradoxic blood pressure increases may occur during treatment with β blockers, guanethidine, or ganglionic blockers.

- e. Rarely hypertension will be absent. This is most common with familial pheochromocytoma.
- f. A marked change in blood pressure or heart rate in response to minor injury, general anesthesia, or during pregnancy at the time of delivery should raise one's suspicion of pheochromocytoma.

2. Orthostatic hypotension
   a. Orthostasis may occur due to a diminished plasma volume and blunted sympathetic reflexes.
   b. This may predispose the patient with unsuspected pheochromocytoma to hypotension or shock during surgery or major trauma.

3. Cardiac manifestations
   a. Angina and acute myocardial infarction may occur even in the absence of coronary artery disease due to the catecholamine-induced increase in myocardial oxygen consumption and perhaps coronary artery vasospasm.
   b. Arrhythmias may include sinus tachycardia/bradycardia, supraventricular arrhythmias, and premature ventricular contractions.

4. Ocular manifestations
   a. Hypertensive retinopathy
   b. Dilated pupils

5. Tremor with or without shaking may be noted on examination.

6. A slight temperature elevation is common.

II. Diagnostic Approach

A. In patients with a history of hypertensive crisis, paroxysmal symptoms suggestive of anxiety attacks, or hypertension that responds poorly to conventional treatment, a diagnosis of pheochromocytoma should be considered.

B. Adverse drug interactions may cause the initial presentation

1. Opiates, histamine, ACTH, and glucagon can precipitate severe and potentially fatal paroxysms by stimulating the release of catecholamines directly from the tumor.

2. Tricyclic antidepressants, guanethidine, and other drugs that block the neuronal uptake of catecholamines may enhance the physiologic effects of circulating catecholamines (these should be avoided in patients with known pheochromocytomas).

C. Screening Tests

1. 24-h urine collection for catecholamines, metanephrines, and vanillyl mandelic acid (VMA)

a. A 24-h urine collection for catecholamines, metanephrines, and VMA is used to detect increased pressor synthesis and is 70–80% sensitive for pheochromocytoma.
b. Due to a false positive rate of 2–5%, only screen patients in whom there is a high degree of clinical suspicion.
c. Method
  1) The patient is given a plastic container and asked to collect all urine output for a 24-h period.
  2) Creatinine should also be determined to ensure adequacy of the specimen.
  3) Warn patients to avoid strenuous exercise during the period of collection. No dietary limitations are necessary during the collection.
  4) Drugs that specifically interfere with the assay should be avoided (see below).
d. Interpretation
  1) Total metanephrines in the urine are normally < 1.3 mg/24 h and urinary VMA is normally < 7 mg/24 h.
  2) Excretion of the metabolites is usually three times the normal range in a patient with pheochromocytoma.
  3) If results are borderline, remeasurement is suggested and proceeding with clonidine suppression test.
e. In the rare patient who is normotensive between paroxysms, repeat testing may be necessary to document the elevated catecholamines. The urine specimen should be taken during a paroxysm or hypertensive crisis.
f. Effect of medications on test results
  1) Catacholamine levels may be affected by methyldopa, L-dopa, theophylline, hypoglcemia, and isoproterenol.
  2) Metanephrine levels may be increased by monoamine oxidase inhibitors, methyldopa, and phenothiazines.
  3) VMA levels may be decreased by monoamine oxidase inhibitors and clofibrate.

2. Clonidine suppression test
  a. Clonidine, a centrally acting α_2-adrenergic agonist, inhibits sympathetic outflow and decreases plasma catecholamine levels in normal and hypertensive patients; because catecholamine release is not under central neural control, patients with pheochromocytomas will not have suppressed catecholamine levels.
  b. For the clonidine suppression test, the criterion for a positive test is a plasma catecholamine level > 500 ng/L, 3 h after clonidine administration.
  c. This test is reserved for patients with borderline 24-h urine studies and is not used routinely due to the expense, time required, and potential risks of hypotension following administration of clonidine.
  d. β-Blockers should be discontinued 48 h before testing because they can prevent significant suppression of plasma catecholamine concentrations by clonidine in patients with neurogenic hypertension and falsely suggest the presence of a pheochromocytoma.

3. Provocative testing with histamine, tyramine, or glucagon is not advised because there are significant hazards to this mode of testing and the results are unreliable.

D. Localization Tests

1. Patients with positive screening tests, ideally on more than one occasion, should undergo further testing for localization of the tumor after being started on α-blockade therapy.

2. Imaging studies
   a. CT imaging
      1) Identifies 95% of pheochromocytomas
      2) Reveals adrenal lesions > 1 cm in size and extra-adrenal lesions > 2 cm
      3) Reliably demonstrates intrathoracic lesions
   b. MRI scanning
      1) Most reliable method of identifying pheochromocytomas with a characteristic high intensity signal
      2) Superior to CT at detecting extra-adrenal tumors
   c. Metaiodobenzylguanidine I^{131} (MIBG) scintigraphy
      1) Because MIBG is trapped by neural crest tissue, scintigraphy is used with radiolabeled I^{131}-MIBG to localize the lesion and to detect metastases.
      2) Highly specific test for diagnosing pheochromocytoma and locating tumors, especially very small tumors and tumors in unusual locations
      3) Drugs such as labetelol, calcium antagonists, tricyclic antidepressants, sympathomimetics, and tranquilizers may inhibit uptake and should be discontinued one week before scintigraphy.
   d. Central venous blood sampling
      1) Venous sampling for catecholamine concentration at different levels of the inferior and superior vena cava may be necessary for localization when all attempts at localization have failed.
   e. Abdominal aortography may be helpful to identify intra-abdominal tumors if the MRI/CT scans are not revealing because these lesions are often supplied by a large aberrant artery.

E. Further Evaluation for Familial Pheochromocytomas

1. Medullary carcinoma of the thyroid and hyperparathyroidism should be excluded in all patients diagnosed with pheochromocytoma and in all relatives of patients with familial pheochromocytoma.

2. Diagnosis and treatment of these disorders should be delayed until after the pheochromocytoma is removed.

III. Differential Diagnosis

A. All cases of hypertension when the cause is unknown

B. Hyperthyroidism

C. Reactive hypoglycemia

D. Panic attacks or other anxiety disorders

E. Sympathomimetic drugs (phenylpropanolamine), cocaine, amphetamines

F. Vasodilating headaches (migraine or cluster type)

G. Seizure disorder

H. Eclampsia in pregnant women

I. Carcinoid syndrome

J. Acute porphyria

K. Intracranial lesions, particularly posterior fossa tumors or subarachnoid hemorrhages, may be associated with hypertension and the increased release of catecholamines.

IV. Treatment

A. Pharmacologic Management

1. Indications

   a. Preoperative management—Phenoxybenzamine should be administered for at least 10–14 d prior to surgery to restore a contracted plasma volume back to normal.
   b. Cases of metastatic or locally invasive tumors
   c. Patients who are a poor surgical risk

2. Phenoxybenzamine (Dibenzyline)

   a. Used for α-adrenergic receptor blockade
   b. Initial dose is 10 mg b.i.d. and the dose is increased over several days (up to 40 mg t.i.d.) until the blood pressure stabilizes and symptoms abate.
   c. Most patients require 40–80 mg/d.
   d. Urine determinations for VMA and metanephrines are not affected by this medication.

3. Phentolamine

   a. Used to treat acute hypertension episodes and paroxysms before adequate α blockade is achieved with phenoxybenzamine.
   b. Hypertensive crises are usually aborted by a rapid intravenous bolus of 5 mg.

c. If there is no response, the dose can be repeated q 2 min until the blood pressure is adequately reduced.

d. Because phentolamine's effect is transient, repeated hypertensive crises are best controlled by infusing phentolamine 100 mg in 500 mL of D5W at a rate that normalizes and cautiously lowers the blood pressure.

4. Nitroprusside

   a. Only other antihypertensive agents that reliably reduces blood pressure in patients with pheochromocytoma
   b. Prolonged infusion can result in thiocyanate toxicity.

5. β-Blocking agents

   a. Should be given only after α blockade is ensured due to the potential for causing a paradoxical increase in blood pressure by antagonizing β-mediated vasodilatation.
   b. Initiated when tachycardia develops during α blockade or to treat catecholamine-induced arrhythmias.
   c. Dose—propranolol 10 mg t.i.d.–q.i.d. increased as needed to control heart rate.

B. Surgery

1. Surgical removal of the catecholamine-producing tumor is best performed at centers with expertise in the perioperative and anesthetic management of these patients.

2. Hypertension and cardiac arrhythmias are most likely to occur during induction of anesthesia, intubation, and manipulation of the tumor.

V. Indications for Referral to a Specialist

A. Once the screening test results are positive or borderline, consultation with an endocrinologist is recommended to help guide the rest of the evaluation for localization of the tumor especially if the CT or MRI scan failed to detect the lesion.

B. Following localization, referral to a surgeon with expertise in the resection of pheochromocytomas is recommended.

VI. Annotated Bibliography

Burch WM. Endocrinology for the House Officer. Baltimore: Williams & Wilkins; 1988. Concise brief review of diagnostic studies and work-up for pheochromocytomas.

Landsberg L, Young JB. Pheochromocytoma. In: Wilson JD, Braunwald E, Isselbacher KJ, et al, eds. Harrison's Principles of Internal Medicine, 12th ed. New York: McGraw-Hill; 1991. In-depth review of pathology as well as clinical features and biochemical testing with discussion of preoperative management and prognosis for malignant tumors.

Manger WM, Gifford RW. Pheochromocytoma: current diagnosis and management. Cleveland Clin J Med 1993;60:365–378. Excellent review article including tables of reported symptoms, signs, extensive differential diagnosis, and indications for screening. A diagnostic algorithm reviews the recommended evaluation for localization and preoperative and operative management guidelines are clearly presented.

Stein PP, Black HR. A simplified diagnostic approach to pheochromocytoma. Medicine 1990;70:46–52. Review of the literature including stratification of patients into low-risk and high-risk groups based on presenting symptoms and signs. Biochemical testing is extensively described in relation to patients with and without a diagnosed pheochromocytoma.

Chapter 36: Adrenocortical Insufficiency (Addison's Disease)

Rosemarie A. Leuzzi

I. Clinical Presentation

A. General Information

1. Inadequate adrenal function results from destruction of the adrenal cortex (primary adrenal insufficiency) or from adrenocortical atrophy due to ACTH deficiency (secondary adrenal insufficiency).
2. Primary adrenocortical insufficiency (Addison's disease)
   a. Addison's disease is either due to anatomic destruction of the adrenal gland or metabolic failure of hormone production.
   b. 90% of the adrenal gland must be destroyed before Addison's disease is clinically apparent.
   c. Addison's disease can occur at any age and both sexes are affected with equal frequency.
   d. Etiology
      1) Autoimmune destruction of the adrenal glands—80% of cases
         a) *Polyendocrinopathies—Addison's disease may be associated with any of the following: primary ovarian failure, thyroid disorders (thyrotoxicosis or hypothyroidism), diabetes mellitus, vitiligo, pernicious anemia, and hypoparathyroidism*
         b) *Schmidt's syndrome—the association between Addison's disease and hypothyroidism*
         c) *Polyglandular autoimmune syndrome type 1—association between Addison's disease, chronic mucocutaneous candidiasis, and hypoparathyroidism*
         d) *Polyglandular autoimmune syndrome type 2—association between Addison's disease and diabetes mellitus*
      2) Granulomatous disease such as tuberculosis, histoplasmosis, or sarcoidosis
      3) Infiltrative disease such as amyloidosis, lymphoma, hemochromatosis, or metastatic disease
      4) Adrenal hemorrhage may be associated with the use of anticoagulants or related to coagulopathy, sepsis, pregnancy, trauma, or surgery.

5) Infarction of the adrenal gland due to thrombosis, embolism, or arteritis
6) Adrenogenital syndromes due to a variety of enzyme failures resulting in cortisol deficiency, which is partially or completely compensated by an increase in ACTH.
7) Cytomegalovirus, *Mycobacterium avium intracellulare, Cryptococcus*, and Kaposi's sarcoma involvement of the adrenal glands have all been reported in patients with AIDS.

3. Secondary adrenal insufficiency
   a. Secondary adrenocortical insufficiency is due to decreased or suppressed ACTH secretion by the pituitary gland.
   b. Secondary adrenocortical insufficiency is relatively common due to the use of exogenous steroid preparations (via suppression of ACTH).
   c. Mineralocorticoid function is preserved because the predominant regulator of aldosterone synthesis is the renin-angiotensin system, not ACTH.

B. Symptoms

1. The patient may complain of gradually increasing weakness, slowly progressive fatigue, anorexia, irritability, and depression.
2. GI complaints may include nausea, vomiting, diarrhea, ill-defined abdominal pain, and weight loss.
3. Darkening of the skin may be noted.
4. Salt craving is present in 20% of patients.
5. The patient may also note mental sluggishness, excessive irritability, or restlessness.
6. Enhancement of the sensory modalities of taste, olfaction, and hearing is often present.
7. The patient may present in "addisonian crisis" with abdominal pain mimicking an acute abdomen, profound hypotension, volume depletion, and possibly fever.
   a. Adrenal crisis is a potentially life-threatening situation and occurs when adrenal gland destruction is rapid.
   b. Adrenal crisis may be precipitated by any stressful situation including fever, infection, radiographic studies, or surgery.
   c. Fasting hypoglycemia symptoms may also occur especially during crisis situations because of lack of glucocorticoid effect.
8. Patients on anticoagulant therapy may present with symptoms of back or flank pain and manifest crisis symptoms due to bilateral adrenal hemorrhage.

C. Physical Examination

1. Hyperpigmentation may precede the onset of other symptoms and is usually generalized but is accentuated in sun-exposed areas, skin creases, new scars,

the scrotum and perineum, nipple areola, and areas subjected to trauma such as elbows, knuckles, and knees.

   a. Pigmentation of the buccal mucosa is a pathognomonic finding in white patients.
   b. The increased pigmentation results from increased melanin stimulation associated with the increased ACTH levels; therefore, hyperpigmentation is noted only in primary adrenal insufficiency and not secondary forms.

2. Arterial hypotension is frequent and postural hypotension often occurs due to mineralocorticoid insufficiency.
3. Loss of axillary and pubic hair may occur in women and is an important finding when present.
4. The presence of vitiligo may signal an autoimmune etiology.

II. Diagnostic Approach

A. Consider the diagnosis of adrenal insufficiency in any patient who presents with any of the above symptoms especially if the patient suddenly stopped taking glucocorticoids or if there was a precipitating cause to unmask insufficient adrenal reserve.

B. Remember, manifestations of secondary adrenal insufficiency are those of cortisol deficiency alone (including lethargy, abdominal pain, nausea), whereas primary adrenal insufficiency includes symptoms of cortisol deficiency as well as aldosterone deficiency (volume depletion, hypotension, hyponatremia).

C. Routine Laboratory Studies

1. Complete blood count
   a. A normochromic/normocytic anemia, a relative lymphocytosis, and a moderate eosinophilia are commonly present.
   b. If a macrocytic anemia is present, one should suspect a concomitant pernicious anemia.

2. Electrolytes
   a. A mild hyperkalemia may be accompanied by mild hyponatremia in the early stages as a result of associated mineralocorticoid insufficiency.
   b. An elevated blood urea nitrogen reflects the prerenal azotemia of salt wasting and volume contraction.
   c. Mild to moderate hypercalcemia occurs in 10–20% of patients with Addison's disease.
   d. With secondary adrenal insufficiency, fluid-electrolyte abnormalities are not as severe and usually patients do not present with hyperpigmentation.

D. Diagnostic Studies

1. If the diagnosis of adrenal insufficiency is suspected during a stress situation, blood for cortisol and ACTH determination should be drawn immediately and

the patient begun on hydrocortisone sodium succinate (Solu-Cortef) IV. If the diagnosis is suspected in a nonacute situation, then provocative testing with an ACTH stimulation test is indicated.

2. Serum cortisol level
   a. Serum cortisol measurement without ACTH stimulation has many limitations including diurnal rhythm and a high degree of variability; in addition, this measurement may fail to detect mild cases or yield indeterminate values.
   b. Plasma cortisol can be measured at any time of the day and a normal value (15–25 µg/dL) will exclude the diagnosis of adrenal insufficiency. Any subject with normal adrenal glands should have serum cortisol levels > 18 µg/dL during severe stress.
   c. Values lower than 5 µmg/dL at any time are highly suggestive of adrenal insufficiency.

3. Serum ACTH level
   a. This measurement is useful in establishing a diagnosis of secondary or pituitary-related adrenocortical insufficiency.
   b. An elevated ACTH level will be seen in primary adrenocortical insufficiency.

4. Rapid ACTH stimulation test
   a. Evaluation of the low or borderline plasma cortisol value should be made using the rapid ACTH stimulation test, which is the best screening test for adrenal insufficiency (a deficient plasma cortisol response to exogenous ACTH administration).
   b. Method
      1) Synthetic ACTH, cosyntropin (Cortrosyn) 0.25 mg is administered IV or IM.
      2) The serum cortisol level is determined at baseline and at 30 min and 60 min following the injection.
   c. Under normal conditions, with a baseline serum cortisol > 7 µg/dL, the cortisol level should rise by at least 7 mg/dL or be > 18 µg/dL.
   d. A normal adrenal response excludes primary adrenal insufficiency.

5. Prolonged ACTH stimulation test
   a. Method
      1) A continuous IV infusion of 0.25 mg cosyntropin over 8 h/d is administered for 1–5 d.
      2) The plasma cortisol level is measured before the infusion and every 12 h.
      3) Daily 24-h urinary 17 hydroxysteroids levels are also collected.
   b. Interpretation
      1) Normal adrenal response—doubling of plasma and urine steroids on the first day
      2) Primary adrenal insufficiency—no response and never achieve doubling on any day

3) Secondary adrenal insufficiency—characterized by a stepwise or delayed response after the first day

E. In patients with autoimmune adrenal insufficiency, monitoring for signs and symptoms as well as evaluation of other forms of glandular failure (hypothyroidism, hypogonadism, and hypoparathyroidism) should be considered.

III. Differential Diagnosis

A. Because weakness and fatigue are common complaints, the diagnosis of adrenal insufficiency is frequently difficult; for example, depression and hypothyroidism may present with fatigue and decreased energy.

B. The combination of symptoms including weakness, nausea, anorexia, weight loss, and hyperpigmentation should raise the possibility of adrenal hypofunction and further evaluation should be undertaken to exclude this diagnosis.

IV. Treatment

A. Treatment of Addisonian Crisis

1. Adrenal crisis may occur as the initial presentation of adrenal insufficiency or in recognized cases of adrenal insufficiency with inadequate steroid therapy resulting from a precipitating stressor (infection, trauma, surgery) or noncompliance.
2. The management of adrenal crisis involves taking of blood for cortisol and ACTH levels, aggressive replacement of fluids and electrolytes to avoid hypotension and shock, cortisol administration, and treatment of any precipitating causes.
   a. Steroid administration—Hydrocortisone sodium succinate (Solu-Cortef) 100 mg is given IV immediately and then 100 mg IV q 6 h over the next 24 h (mineralocorticoids are not needed because cortisol at these large doses has enough salt-retaining activity).
   b. Volume repletion—5% dextrose/saline administered initially with 1–2 L over the first 2 h and with 3–5 L during the first 24 h.
   c. Careful monitoring of vital signs and electrolytes is essential.
   d. Serum cortisol/ACTH measurement—If the previously drawn cortisol returns low and the ACTH value is elevated, the work-up is simplified and the diagnosis of Addison's disease is confirmed. Any subject with normal adrenal glands should have serum cortisol levels > 19 µg/dL during severe stress.
   e. Treatment of precipitating causes should include evaluation for infection, especially if there is no obvious precipitating stressor.

B. Treatment of Stable Adrenal Insufficiency

1. Corticosteroid replacement therapy

   a. Under normal circumstances, patients are given 20–30 mg cortisol daily. Recommended dosages and preparations vary greatly. The simplest regimen is 12.5 mg cortisone twice a day. Cortisol (30 mg daily) or prednisone (7.5 mg daily) in divided doses may also be given.
   b. Some prefer to use a slightly higher AM dose to stimulate diurnal rhythm.
   c. Adequacy of glucocorticoid dosage is assessed by clinical response; however, overtreatment with glucocorticoids should be avoided because iatrogenic Cushing's syndrome is possible.
   d. During times of increased stress, the glucocorticoid requirement increases and, therefore, the steroid dosage needs to be adjusted with physician guidance.
      1) For a nonspecific, febrile viral illness unaccompanied by vomiting or diarrhea, the dosage of cortisol should be increased to 50–75 mg/d in divided doses.
      2) For a more severe infection such as pneumonia or bronchitis, the dose should be increased to 100 mg/d in divided doses.
      3) If vomiting or diarrhea are present, the use of parenteral steroids and hospitalization may be indicated depending on the circumstances.

2. Mineralocorticoid replacement

   a. Mineralocorticoid replacement with fludrocortisone (Florinef) 0.05–0.2 mg/d is usually administered following the diagnosis of primary adrenal insufficiency.
   b. The dosage is adjusted based on the serum sodium and potassium levels as well as normalizing the blood pressure without orthostasis or edema.
   c. The use of prednisone or another glucocorticoid for patients with Addison's diseases may require additional mineralocorticoid supplementation because they have less mineralocorticoid activity than cortisone or cortisol.
   d. Secondary adrenal insufficiency usually only requires glucocorticoid replacement and mineralocorticoid supplementation is unusual.

3. Patient education

   a. The patient must understand the importance of taking steroid replacements regularly and the necessary precautions required during times of increased stress with adjustment of the steroid dose.
   b. Every patient with adrenal insufficiency should have a syringe and vial of sterile dexamethasone carried at all times to be administered IM in case of an emergency (syringes containing dexamethasone phosphate 4 mg in 1 mL water can be conveniently carried).
   c. Patients should consume a diet with a liberal amount of sodium (100–150 mEq/d) and increase salt intake if diarrhea or profuse sweating occurs.
   d. Close contact with a physician is essential to avoid the potential risk of addisonian crisis and hospitalization.

e. Family members also need to be educated about the clinical symptoms and emergency care.
f. The patient should wear an identification or Medic Alert bracelet or carry documentation identifying the Addison's disease, instructions for therapy, and the physician's name and number.

C. Perioperative Management

1. Patients with known or suspected primary or secondary adrenocortical insufficiency including patients on current or recent exogenous steroid therapy require glucocorticoid supplementation in the perioperative period.
2. Any patient who has been treated with exogenous steroid preparations for > 3 wk over the past year is at risk for secondary adrenal insufficiency and should be either screened for adrenal insufficiency or given stress dose steroids when indicated.
3. Hydrocortisone sodium succinate 100 mg IV q 8 h should be begun the night before surgery and continued throughout the day of surgery.
4. The dosage should then be tapered depending on the extent of the surgery usually by decreasing the dose by 50% each day thereafter until the maintenance dose is achieved.

V. Indications for Referral to a Specialist

A. Once the diagnosis is made following an ACTH stimulation test, further evaluation and treatment by an endocrinologist is recommended.

B. Indeterminate results on the ACTH stimulation test may also require the expertise of an endocrinologist for further evaluation.

VI. Annotated Bibliography

Burch WM. Endocrinology for the House Officer. Baltimore: Williams & Wilkins; 1988. Excellent review of handling addisonian crisis with succinct style.

Gregerman RI. Selected endocrine problems: disorders of pituitary, adrenal, and parathyroid glands; pharmacologic use of steroids; hypo- and hypercalcemia; osteoporosis, water metabolism; hypoglycemia. In: Barker LR, Burton JR, Zieve PD, eds. Principles of Ambulatory Medicine. Baltimore: Williams & Wilkins; 1991. Good explanation of outpatient treatment of patients with Addison's disease including recommendations for increased steroid dosage during stress and febrile illness.

Williams GH, Dluhy RG. Diseases of the adrenal cortex. In: Wilson JD, Braunwald E, Isselbacher KJ, et al, eds. Harrison's Principles of Internal Medicine, 12th ed. New York: McGraw-Hill; 1991. Detailed description of adrenal hormones and testing as well as clinical presentation and treatment of Addison's disease.

Chapter 37: Management of the Patient on Glucocorticosteroids

Karen G. Kelly

I. General Information

A. Steroids are widely used for a variety of serious medical problems.

B. They have serious adverse effects and may lead to adrenal suppression.

C. Withdrawing patients from steroids can take a prolonged period of time.

II. Adverse Effects

A. Will depend on the dose, dosing schedule and potency of the steroid used as well as the length of time the patient has taken it.

B. The higher the dose and the longer the time the patient takes them the more likely adverse effects are to occur. Alternate day therapy will be associated with fewer adverse effects.

C. Metabolic

1. Negative nitrogen balance secondary to inhibition of protein synthesis and enhancement of catabolism
2. Glucose intolerance
3. Fat redistribution leading to cushingoid appearance (see Chapter 35A)
4. Weight gain

D. Infectious

1. Immunosuppressive—increased risk of a variety of infections including bacterial and viral pathogens
2. Can have reactivation of TB and herpes
3. Candidial infections are common.

E. Bone
1. Osteoporosis is common and may be severe.
2. Avascular necrosis is less common.

F. GI
1. Peptic ulceration probably occurs only with prolonged use or with high doses.

G. Psychologic—may be more common in elderly
1. May note increase in appetite, changes in sleep, and mild euphoria
2. Psychosis may occur.
3. Depression may occur.

H. Miscellaneous
1. Cataracts in 10–35% of patients
2. Hypertension and fluid retention, especially if agents with mineralocorticoid properties
3. Hypokalemia may occur.
4. Acute pancreatitis
5. Myopathy with normal muscle enzymes

III. Hypothalmic-Pituitary-Adrenal Axis Suppression

A. May occur after 2–4 wk of high-dose steroids

B. More severe with doses given at night, long-acting preparations, or when more than one dose a day are used

C. Alternate day therapy using short- or intermediate-acting preparations will not induce clinically significant suppression.

D. Nasal and inhaled steroids will not suppress the adrenal axis.

E. Full recovery of the adrenal axis once steroids are withdrawn may take up to a year, particularly when long courses have been given.

IV. Management of the Patient on Steroids

A. Use the lowest possible effective dose. In general a single dose of an intermediate-acting agent given once a day in the morning is preferred.

B. Consider alternate day steroids once the condition is controlled and while tapering.

C. Watch for adverse effects carefully, particularly during high-dose therapy and in high-risk patients.

D. Prior to Therapy

1. A purified protein derivative should be placed prior to initiation of steroid therapy. If positive a chest x-ray should be done.
2. Baseline glucose, electrolytes, and complete blood count should be obtained.
3. Baseline spine films should be obtained in patients at risk for osteoporosis.
4. Stool hemoccult should be done.

E. During Therapy

1. Monitor weight, blood pressure, glucose, electrolytes. Restrict calories and salt as necessary. Replace potassium.
2. It is not clear if estrogen therapy during steroid therapy will help minimize osteoporosis, but it should be considered in postmenopausal women.
3. Vitamin D and calcium supplementation should likewise be considered.
4. High-risk individuals such as those with history of peptic ulcer disease and those on high-dose steroids (> 15 mg prednisone a day or its equivalent) should receive antiulcer therapy either with antacids or H_2 blockers although the efficacy of this is uncertain.
5. In patients on chronic steroids, increase in dose should be given during periods of acute stress. Double the maintenance dose may be used. Perioperatively even higher doses are given (hydrocortisone 100 mg q 8 h).

V. Withdrawal from Steroids

A. Made problematic due to three factors that may occasionally be difficult to separate clinically

1. Flare of the underlying disease
2. Adrenal insufficiency secondary to adrenal axis suppression
3. Steroid withdrawal syndromes

B. A variety of tapering schedules have been proposed.

1. High-dose (> 40 mg) prednisone can be tapered at 10 mg q 1–3 wk.
2. < 40 mg slower tapering may be necessary, eg, 5 mg q 1–3 wk.
3. At 5–7.5 mg even slower taper may be necessary, eg, 1 mg prednisone at a time.
4. A change to alternate day therapy by tapering every other day may be successful. Alternatively, one day's dose may be increased, while the alternative day's is decreased.

5. Once the patient is taking the medicine every other day tapering can begin. Once the patient is down to 2.5 mg (5 mg every other day) of prednisone, steroids may be stopped.

C. Flare of Underlying Disease

1. If the symptoms of the underlying disease reappear during tapering, the dose may need to be increased and a slower taper tried at a later time. The physician should be sure maximal nonsteroid therapy is being used as well.

D. Adrenal Axis Suppression

1. Clinically symptomatic adrenal insufficiency is rare during slow tapers but is present chemically and may occur during periods of stress. Dose should be empirically increased as discussed above.

2. A Cortrisyn stimulation test can be done to document recovery from adrenal axis suppression.

   a. Draw a baseline cortisol
   b. Administer 0.25 mg cosyntropin IM and draw a repeat cortisol at 30 min and mg/dL 60 min afterward.
   c. An increase of 7 mg/dL or an absolute value of 18 mg/dL or above is normal.

E. Withdrawal

1. Patient coming off steroids may suffer an apparent steroid withdrawal syndrome during tapering. Lethargy, malaise, nausea, and vomiting may occur without evidence of adrenal insufficiency. Management requires increasing or reinstituting steroids and a slower taper.

VI. Patient Education

A. Knowledge of dangers of long-term steroid use including risk of osteoporosis and life-threatening infections

B. Need to know never to stop steroids abruptly and to notify physician of even minor infections

C. Need to inform other physicians of current and past steroid use

D. Use of Medic Alert bracelet

VII. Bibliography

Williams GH, Dluhy RG. Diseases of the adrenal cortex. In: Wilson JD, Braunwald E, Isselbacher KJ, et al., eds. Harrison's Principles of Internal Medicine, 12th ed. New York: McGraw-Hill; 1991.

Chapter 38: Diabetes Mellitus

Richard G. Paluzzi

38A Clinical Presentation and Diagnostic Approach

I. Clinical Presentation

A. General Information

1. Heterogeneous group of disorders characterized by hyperglycemia, affecting approximately 2–4% of the U.S. population
2. Abnormal metabolism of carbohydrates, fats, proteins, minerals, and electrolytes due to a deficiency of *biologically active* insulin (absolute or relative insulin deficiency or insulin resistance)
3. Leads to long-term sequelae of macro- or microangiopathy or both.
4. Can be classified by pathophysiology
   a. Type 1 or insulin-dependent diabetes mellitus (IDDM)
      1) About 10% of all cases of diabetes mellitus
      2) Virtually no native insulin secretion
      3) Lack of insulin leads to development of ketosis in untreated patients (defines insulin dependency)
      4) HLA-linked inheritance (DR3/DR4/B8/B15) probably of the susceptibility to develop diabetes mellitus following some triggering mechanism, which leads to the production of autoantibodies against pancreatic islet cells
      5) Typically occurs in younger patients (peak age 11–13); rare after age 40
   b. Type 2 or non–insulin dependent diabetes mellitus (NIDDM)
      1) Patients retain ability to secrete insulin and are often hyperinsulinemic when compared to nondiabetics.
      2) Pathophysiology is based on inappropriate insulin response to a carbohydrate load or failure of normal insulin receptor function (binding or postbinding failure).
      3) Presence of native insulin makes patient nonketosis prone and therefore insulin independent (may be insulin *requiring* to control hyperglycemia).

4) Typically later age of onset (generally past age 40)
5) 80% of patients are obese (may exacerbate insulin resistance).
6) 10–15% risk of developing NIDDM if a parent or sibling has the disease (100% in identical twins) but no clear HLA associations; more prevalent in females
7) Occasionally see patients who gradually lose the ability to secrete insulin and cross over to features of IDDM. These are typically thin, older patients (type 1 in evolution).

c. Secondary causes of diabetes
1) Pancreatic destruction—chronic pancreatitis, hemochromatosis, trauma, pancreatic resection, cystic fibrosis, pancreatic cancer, toxic drugs (streptozocin)
2) Excess counterregulatory hormones—glucagonoma, Cushing's syndrome, pheochromocytoma, acromegaly
3) Drugs—corticosteroids, oral contraceptives, thiazides, sympathomimetics, lithium, tricyclic antidepressants, phenothiazines, β blockers, phenytoin, clonidine, ethanol. Generally all inhibit synthesis or release of insulin. Hyperglycemia has also been reported to occur with use of isoniazid, cimetidine, heparin, nicotinic acid, marijuana, and many other drugs.
4) Metabolic abnormalities—hypokalemia (drug induced or due to hyperaldosteronism), hypocalcemia, hypochloremic metabolic alkalosis
5) Significant illnesses, stress, trauma infections, and burns, which can lead to catecholamine excess
6) Other syndromes—chromosomal abnormalities (Downs, Turner, Klinefelter), inborn errors of metabolism, neuromuscular diseases, lipodystrophy

d. Impaired glucose tolerance
1) Generally normal basal glucose levels with abnormal response to glucose loads
2) Unclear significance
3) Generally does not lead to serious sequelae and the majority of cases do not develop overt diabetes
4) Glucose intolerance increases with aging due to increased insulin resistance (postreceptor failure).

e. Gestational diabetes
1) Affects 1–2% of pregnant women, generally in the third trimester
2) Approximately 50% normalize following delivery but half of these develop diabetes mellitus later in life
3) Significant fetal morbidity—macrosomia, congenital heart defects, fetal demise

B. History

1. IDDM typically presents acutely with significant polyuria, polyphagia, polydipsia, weight loss, and fatigue. Ketoacidosis may be present at the time of diagnosis.

2. NIDDM typically has a more insidious onset with progressive polyuria, polydipsia, weight loss, fatigue, and weakness.
3. Dizziness, headache, and blurry vision (due to abnormalities in hydration of the lens) are frequent.
4. Vague symptoms such as pruritis (generalized or perianal/genital), leg cramps, nervousness, irritability, or paresthesias may occur and should prompt an investigation of diabetes mellitus if no other cause is apparent.
5. Recurrent, unexplained infections (ie, recurrent vaginal candidiasis) may occur.
6. Family history of diabetes mellitus or personal history of previous hyperglycemia may be useful.
7. Presentation in patients with secondary diabetes is variable based on severity or duration of the underlying illness as well as the resultant pathophysiologic defect.

C. Physical Examination
1. Most physical findings are not diagnostic but rather are a result of the disease.
2. Look for signs of dehydration, hypotension, and infection (particularly pulmonary, urinary, and skin).
3. Perform a thorough physical examination looking for elevated blood pressure, vascular bruits, retinal changes, skin changes, or other signs of end organ damage.

II. Diagnostic Approach

A. Diagnostic Criteria for Diabetes Mellitus in Nonpregnant Adults
1. Fasting blood suger (BS) > 140 mg/dL on more than one occasion
2. Unequivocal hyperglycemia (BS > 200 mg/dL when checked 2 h postprandially) with classic signs or symptoms
3. Abnormal glucose tolerance test
   a. Draw fasting BS then administer a standard 75-g oral glucose load. BS is then checked every 30 min for 2 h.
   b. Diagnostic of diabetes mellitus if the 2-h and one intermediate BS are > 200 mg/dL
   c. Generally not necessary as criteria noted above are simply performed
   d. Generally used to screen pregnant women
   e. Consistent with impaired glucose tolerance if only one intermediate BS is > 200 mg/dL

B. Other Testing
1. Based on concomitant symptoms and physical findings
2. Generally based on screening for complications

38B Potential Complications of Diabetes Mellitus

I. Acute

A. All acute complications are metabolic.

1. Diabetic ketoacidosis
   a. Due to insulin deficiency/glucagon excess
   b. Maximal gluconeogenesis associated with increased fatty acid and ketone formation
   c. Usually some inciting event—illness, intoxication, severe stress; can occur in type 2 diabetes during periods of profound metabolic stress
   d. Mortality 10%, usually due to complications of associated illnesses
   e. Treatment consists of insulin administration with fluid and electrolyte replacement—details are beyond scope of this book (see Bibliography).
   f. Occasionally see ketonuria without serum ketones or acidemia, which may respond to high-dose sulfonylurea therapy in newly diagnosed NIDDM

2. Hyperosmolar hyperglycemic nonketotic coma
   a. Presence of some endogenous insulin prevents ketogenesis.
   b. Unrestrained hyperglycemia leads to profound dehydration and hyperosmolarity with resultant CNS symptoms.
   c. Often triggered by associated illness or drug usage
   d. Mortality rate ranges as high as 50% with a high incidence of thromboembolic events, respiratory infection or failure, and other infections.
   e. Mainstay of treatment is rehydration. Insulin used as an adjunct to lower BS level and decrease osmolarity.

3. Hypoglycemia
   a. Generally due to overly aggressive treatment or poor planning (meals, exercise)
   b. Symptoms as well as level of BS at which symptoms occur are variable.
   c. Can be serious or fatal because glucose is the primary energy source for the brain
   d. Release of counterregulatory hormones can lead to rebound hyperglycemia (Somogyi phenomenon); typically presents as fasting hyperglycemia despite increasing therapy (due to a nocturnal hypoglycemia).

II. Chronic

A. Chronic hyperglycemia is associated with abnormal lipid metabolism and accelerated atherosclerosis as well as protein glycosylation with abnormalities in vascular basement membranes.

B. Macrovascular Complications
1. Premature atherosclerosis affecting coronary, cerebrovascular, and peripheral vascular systems
2. Risk is increased by smoking, uncontrolled hypertension, hyperlipidemia as well as other risk factors for atherosclerosis.
3. Incidence of vascular events is increased as is the morbidity and mortality of each event compared to that in nondiabetic patients.
4. Disease often involves distal, small vessel branches that are not amenable to surgical intervention.
5. Myocardial infarction is primary cause of premature death in diabetic patients. Painless myocardial ischemia can occur as can a primary cardiomyopathy.

C. Microvascular Complications
1. Retinopathy
    a. Occurs in 90% of type 1 patients and up to 60% of type 2 (of > 20 y duration)
    b. Primary cause of blindness in adults
    c. Simple retinopathy
        1) Begins as increased capillary permeability (reversible with good glycemic control)
        2) Leakage of lipid/protein containing fluid leads to hard waxy exudates.
        3) Retinal microinfarction due to capillary occlusion and microaneurysms leads to soft, cotton-wool exudates.
        4) Microhemorrhages can occur.
    d. Proliferative retinopathy
        1) Neovascularization due to retinal ischemia leads to hemorrhage and scarring.
        2) Visual loss and blindness are due to clouding of the vitreous and retinal detachment
        3) Up to 18% of patients will develop proliferative retinopathy after 10 y of diabetes and 50% of these will go blind within 5 y if untreated.
        4) Photocoagulation of neovascularized retina segments can prevent complications. Hemorrhage typically requires vitrectomy and repair of retinal detachments.
    e. Other visual complications include fluctuating visual acuity, early cataract formation, and an increased incidence of glaucoma.
    f. Baseline and yearly ophthalmologic examinations are mandatory.
    g. Refraction should not be corrected until BS is controlled for 6–8 wk.
2. Nephropathy
    a. Occurs in 40–50% of type 1 patients, 6% of type 2 (of long duration); often parallels retinopathy
    b. Begins as thickening of the glomerular basement membrane with protein leakage (can revert with intensive insulin therapy)

c. Once proteinurea becomes fixed, glomerular filtration falls by about 1 cc/min/mo.
   d. Approximately 70% of patients with nephropathy develop hypertension. If untreated, hypertension often heralds progression to renal failure within 5 y as does significant proteinurea (3–5 grams/d).
   e. Renal pathology varies but most often see nodular sclerosis (Kimmelstel-Wilson) or diffuse sclerosis; may also see atherosclerosis of the renal arteries.
   f. Progression of nephropathy can be slowed by control of hypertension as well as by institution of therapy with angiotension-converting enzyme (ACE) inhibitors before proteinurea exceeds 150 mg/d even in nonhypertensive patients.
   g. Should monitor blood pressure at every visit as well as creatinine and 24-h protein excretion yearly.
3. Neuropathy
   a. Pathogenesis is unclear. May involve vascular changes in the vaso-nervorum as well as buildup of sorbitol or deficiency in myoinositol
   b. Onset is variable. Typically progresses with duration of diabetes mellitus but can occur very early (even before overt hyperglycemia) and in the absence of other chronic complications
   c. Symmetrical distal polyneuropathy
      1) "Stocking-glove" distribution
      2) Painless paresthesias, burning pain, or significant hyperesthesia
      3) Generally progressive and irreversible
      4) Can see loss of deep tendon reflexes, loss of vibratory sense, and development of Charcot joints
      5) Loss of sensation can predispose to development of ulcerations over pressure points (heels, metatarsal heads, etc).
   d. Asymmetrical neuropathy
      1) Generally a dysfunction of nerves in the distribution of a single nerve trunk or more than one nerve trunk (mononeuritis multiplex)
      2) Can involve peripheral nerves leading to entrapment-like syndromes (foot drop, wrist drop, etc)
      3) Can involve cranial nerves, particularly III, VI, and IV
      4) Can involve nerve roots leading to radiculopathies, which can be mistaken for postherpetic neuralgia
      5) Often resolve over time (months)
   e. Amyotrophy
      1) Proximal muscle weakness with muscle wasting
      2) Often resolves over 1–2 y
   f. Autonomic neuropathy
      1) Can involve any part of the autonomic system
      2) Primarily GI (gastroparesis, diarrhea), orthostasis, and genitourinary (impotence, bladder dysfunction)
      3) Loss of normal variation in heart rate during respiration may be associated with an increased risk of sudden death.

4. Dermopathies
    a. Necrobiosis lipoidicum diabeticorum
        1) Pretibial plaques with elevated, hyperpigmented borders and depressed centers
        2) Can ulcerate with minor trauma
        3) Uncommon but can precede hyperglycemia in 20%
    b. Diabetic dermopathy
        1) Red papules that result in hyperpigmented atrophic areas
        2) Usually pretibial, also seen on forearms and thighs
        3) Occur in 60% of male diabetics and 30% of female diabetics
    c. Bullous diabeticorum
        1) Tense digital bullae
        2) Associated with neuropathies
5. Miscellaneous complications
    a. Increased risk of infection due to decreased leukocyte function (the risk is felt to increase when BS level is consistently > 250 mg/dL
    b. Poor wound healing
    c. Electrolyte abnormalities
        1) Hyperkalemia due to relative aldosterone insensitivity
        2) Pseudohyponatremia due to expansion of the water fraction of plasma during hyperglycemia

38C Treatment of Diabetes Mellitus

I. Rationale

A. Prevention of symptoms, acute complications, metabolic derangements, and early atherosclerosis

B. Intensive control of BS levels has now been shown to favorably influence the development of retinopathy, nephropathy, and neuropathy (only intensive insulin therapy was studied).

II. Goals

A. Normalization of blood sugar

1. Fasting BS < 140 mg/dL
2. 2-h postprandial BS < 180–200 mg/dL
3. Glycohemoglobin no more than 1.5 percentage points above the upper limit of normal

B. Avoidance of frequent or severe hypoglycemia

C. Prolongation of life—requires reduction of associated cardiovascular risk factors

D. Goals must be individualized based on concomitant diseases, compliance, and quality, as well as expected duration, of life.

III. Modalities

A. Diet and Exercise

1. Hypocaloric diet and exercise can enhance insulin release, insulin sensitivity at the receptor level, and glucose utilization.
2. 50% of calories should be complex carbohydrates, 35% polyunsaturated fat, and 15% protein, with no more than 450 mg cholesterol daily.
3. Calories should be evenly distributed through the meals or adjusted to coincide with the peak action period of exogenous insulin.
4. Total basal caloric intake should average about 30 Kcal/kg/d for sedentary patients, 35 Kcal/kg/d for active patients, and approximately 25 Kcal/kg/d for obese patients if maintenance of present weight is desired. Ideally, the patient should attempt to achieve a weight within 10% of ideal body weight.

B. Sulfonylureas

1. Act by initially enhancing insulin secretion and also by decreasing hepatic glucose formation, decreasing the insulin receptor defect, and increasing insulin receptor number

2. Differ in potency, pharmacokinetics, metabolism and to a minor degree, side effects
   a. Potency
      1) Does not imply difference in efficacy
      2) Glyburide and glipizide are the most potent. Tolbutamide is the least potent.
   b. Pharmocokinetics
      1) Glyburide and glipizide can be given once a day and act for up to 30 h. Chlorpropamide can be given once a day but can have a duration of action up to 60 h.
      2) Acetohexamide and tolazamide are given 1–2 times daily and act up to 24 h.
      3) Tolbutamide must be given 2–3 times daily and acts for 6–12 h.
   c. Metabolism
      1) Tolbutamide, glyburide, and glipizide are metabolized in the liver to inert products
      2) Acetohexamide and tolazamide are metabolized to active metabolites.
      3) Chlorpropamide is partly excreted intact by the kidneys and partly metabolized by the liver to a less active product.
   d. Side effects
      1) Common to all
         a) Nausea, vomiting, cholestasis, and abnormal liver enzymes occur in 1–3% of patients
         b) Rash, pruritis, exfoliative dermatitis, and erythema nodosum occur in 0–1% of patients.
         c) Small risk of allergy in patients allergic to other sulfa-containing compounds
      2) Drug specific
         a) Chlorpropamide can exhibit antidiuretic and disulfuram (Antabuse)-like effects.
         b) Tolbutamide can exhibit antidiuretic effects and in one study was associated with an increased risk of cardiac mortality.
      3) Drug interactions (common)
         a) Potentiate sulfonylurea action—alcohol, anabolic steroids, warfarin, monoamine oxidase inhibitors, β blockers, salicylates, sulfonamides, tetracycline
         b) Antagonize sulfonurea action—chronic alcoholism, corticosteroids, phenytoin, rifampin, thiazide diuretics
         c) Sulfonylureas may potentiate the action of warfarin or other protein-bound drugs.
   e. Administration
      1) Always start with lowest dosage and increase the dose q 5–7 d to maximum dose.
      2) Monitor postprandial glucose (PPG); once level is < 180–200 mg/dL can attempt to lower fasting BS to < 140 mg/dL if hypoglycemia can be avoided

3) About 10–20% of patients will fail to respond to the first agent used. A small percentage of these may respond to a different agent, which must again be instituted at the lowest dosage.
4) Approximately 5–10% of patients who initially respond to sulfonylureas will cease to respond over 1–2 y.
5) An evening dosage of intermediate-acting insulin may lower the fasting BS to a point that allows acceptable control.

C. Insulin

1. Promotes glucose uptake by cells and suppresses gluconeogenesis and lipogenesis. Action is antagonized by glucagon, growth hormone, cortisol, and catecholamines.

2. Rapid-acting insulins are modified by altering the pH (Lente, Ultralente) or by adding protamine (NPH, PZI) to increase the time to peak action as well as duration of action.

3. Insulin can be derived from beef or pork sources or genetically synthesized as human insulin.

4. Can administer in multiple different regimens
   a. Single daily dose of intermediate (I) or intermediate with regular (R) insulin (two thirds of total doses as I). Administer prior to morning meal.
   b. Two daily doses of I or I with R (two thirds of total dose in the morning and two thirds of each dose as I). This regimen should be considered in patients requiring more than 60 units of insulin daily. The second dose is given prior to the evening meal.
   c. Doses of R prior to each meal with a bedtime dose of I or a dinnertime dose of ultralong-acting insulin (U)
   d. Continuous SQ infusion of insulin via a pump that the patient can then activate to administer boluses of insulin prior to each meal

5. In each regimen, longer-acting insulin or continuous infusion is used to mimic the normal basal insulin secretion with short-acting insulin added to cover the glucose surges of meals.

6. There is little evidence that combining sulfonylureas with insulin is beneficial except perhaps in cases of extreme insulin resistance (requirements for > 200 units/d) or when insulin is used to enhance the response to the sulfonylurea.

7. Titration of dosage
   a. Ideally could monitor BS q 4–6 h and cover each result with R using approximately 1–2 units for every increase in BS of 30–50 mg/dL above 120 mg/dL. Once a total daily requirement is established, can either add evening long-acting insulin to control fasting BS or split total daily dose into I and R using rule of two thirds above.
   b. Nondiabetics produce approximately 25 units of insulin per day. NIDDM patients can typically begin with 20 units daily (25–30 units/d if obese) of I.
   c. IDDM patients can be started on physiologic replacement dosages.
   d. Can deliver entire daily dosage as I in the morning or two injections of I using the rule of two thirds above.

e. Adjust dosage q 2–3 d based on BS. Increase dosage by no more than 10% at a time.
   f. IDDM patients generally have a period of decreased insulin requirements (honeymoon period), which can last weeks to years.
   g. Injections should be given into area of abdominal wall with frequent rotation of sites. Injection into limbs should be avoided due to changes in absorption with physical activity.

8. Complications of insulin usage
   a. Hypoglycemia—can result in release of counterregulatory hormones with rebound hyperglycemia (Somogyi phenomenon), which often presents as persistent elevation in fasting BS despite progressive increases in insulin dose
   b. Local reaction—itching, local erythema and induration or SQ nodules at injection sites; often self-limited
   c. Systemic allergy, urticaria, and anaphylaxis generally occur following reinstitution of insulin.
   d. Lipoatrophy or hypertrophy at injection site
   e. Resistance—generally due to anti-insulin antibodies
   f. Allergic and immune type reactions can be minimized by usage of human insulin preparations.

D. Selection of Treatment Modality

1. All patients should be counseled regarding diet and exercise.
2. All patients with true IDDM require insulin therapy.
3. Patients with true NIDDM
   a. If mild or no symptoms, can initiate diet alone for 1–6 mo. If fasting BS normalizes then check PPG. If fasting BS does not normalize or PPG remains > 180–200 mg/dL, then initiate treatment with a sulfonylurea (agent selection based on half-life and side effect profile).
   b. If dietary therapy fails or patient has moderate symptoms, initiate drug therapy and increase the dose until fasting BS falls below 140 mg/dL, then measure PPG. If unable to satisfactorily control PPG, need to consider changing agent or initiating insulin. If intermediate results occur, then base decision on whether to continue or change treatment on the glycosylated hemoglobin level.
   c. Patients who are significantly symptomatic, have had marked weight loss, or who are presenting with preexisting chronic complications should receive insulin therapy. Therapy can then be changed once symptoms and hyperglycemia are controlled. Alternatively, in markedly symptomatic patients who have marked hyperglycemia with normal serum bicarbonate levels and negative serum ketone levels (even in the face of mild ketonuria) therapy can be initiated with maximum doses of a sulfonylurea (one half maximum dose in the elderly). Failure to achieve adequate symptom control and BS response should prompt initiation of insulin therapy.
4. Secondary causes of diabetes often respond poorly to sulfonylureas. Insulin should be considered for all but mild cases.

38D Monitoring of Therapy and Management of Complications

I. Blood Sugar Monitoring

A. Monitoring of urine glucose should always be avoided.

B. NIDDM patients on dietary or sulfonylurea therapy should have PPG monitored monthly and glycosylated hemoglobin checked q 3 mo.

C. All patients on insulin should be taught self-monitoring of BS, which should be checked fasting and at times that correspond to peaks of insulin action. Once glycemic control is achieved, monitoring need not strictly be daily but should be scheduled to produce a 24-h profile of glycemic control over time (ie, check BS daily or every other day, varying time of monitoring at each check). All symptoms suggestive of hypoglycemia should prompt a BS check.

D. Glycohemoglobin levels can be used to ensure glycemic control in NIDDM on diet or sulfonylurea therapy or to further assess control and compliance in patients whose random or daily glycemic control appears adequate, but who present with progressive symptoms or signs.

II. Other testing

A. Baseline and yearly ECG monitoring for silent ischemia

B. Baseline and at least yearly lipid profiles depending on intervention

C. Yearly 24-h urine collections for protein excretion and creatinine clearance. Spot urine checks for protein are useful but insensitive for microproteinuria.

D. At least yearly electrolyte evaluations to monitor for hyperkalemia, azotemia, and deteriorating renal function. Periodic electrolyte assessment may be necessary if hyperglycemia or symptoms raise the concern of hyponatremia, acidemia, or dehydration.

III. Physical Assessment

A. Periodic (q 1–3 mo) monitoring of vital signs including orthostatic blood pressure

B. Baseline and yearly ophthalmologic examinations

C. Periodic (q 1–3 mo) assessment of skin integrity especially of the skin of the soles of the feet, the interdigital spaces, and the toenails which are common portals of entry of infection

IV. Management of Complications

A. Acute complications are managed as discussed above.

B. Macrovascular complications require aggressive modification of cardiovascular risk factors (lipids, smoking, hypertension, etc.) as well as good glycemic control. Management of hypertension with β blockers or calcium blockers may add cardioprotective effects and ACE inhibitors may inhibit nephropathy.

C. Microvascular Complications

1. Aggressive insulin therapy has been associated with delayed onset and slowed progression of microvascular disease.
2. Proliferative retinopathy can be treated with photocoagulation.
3. Microproteinurea should prompt the institution of ACE inhibitors even in nonhypertensive patients. The maximum tolerated dose should be used.
4. Motor neuropathies often resolve with time.
5. Painful neuropathies respond poorly to treatment.
   a. First-line agents include topical capsaicin, tricyclic antidepressants, and carbamazepine beginning at low dosage and titrating upward as needed and tolerated.
   b. Second-line treatment includes combining the above or switching to or adding trazodone, phenothiazines, nonsteroidal anti-inflammatory drugs, acetaminophen, topical capsaicin or nonpharmacologic modalities (TENS units).
   c. Third-line agents include clonidine and mexilitine (contraindicated with heart block or history of myocardial infarction).
   d. Myoinisitol and aldose reductase inhibitors are being studied.
6. Gastroparesis may respond to metoclopramide or cisapride. Gastroparesis may be worsened by calcium channel blockers and narcotics.
7. Orthostasis may require the usage of abdominal binders, compression stockings, and volume expanders (fludrocortisone).
8. Diabetic diarrhea may be decreased by bulking agents or clonidine.

V. Indications for Hospitalization

A. Significant symptoms, dehydration, or serious infection

B. Initiation of therapy in the face of significant hyperglycemia. Defining reasonable levels of significant hyperglycemia is often dictated by third-party payers but are often in the range of 400–600 mg/dL.

C. Management of complications requiring IV insulin or fluids (diabetic ketoacidosis, hyperosmolar hyperglycemic nonketotic coma)

D. Possibly hypoglycemia in patients on sulfonylureas especially chlorpropamide with its extremely long half-life.

VI. Indications for Referral to Endocrinologist

A. All diabetic patients of physicians who are unfamiliar or uncomfortable with the disease

B. Possibly all patients with brittle or difficult to control diabetes, particularly those with rapidly progressive end organ damage

C. Patients with newly diagnosed diabetes mellitus in areas with inadequate dietary counseling or diabetic education

D. Motivated patients interested in aggressive methods of insulin delivery (pumps) or experimental therapies

E. Patients with severe insulin resistance or systemic insulin allergy

VII. Annotated Bibliography

Callaway CW, Rossini AA. Diabetes mellitus. In: Branch WT Jr, ed. Office practice of medicine, 2nd ed. Philadelphia: WB Saunders, 1987:764–793. A well written, easy to follow review of the subject with excellent tables.

Davidson MB: Diabetes mellitus: diagnosis and treatment; 3rd ed. New York: Churchill Livingstone; 1991. Good discussion on applying treatment methods to patients.

DCCT Research Group. The effect of intensive insulin treatment on the development and progression of long term complications in insulin-dependent diabetes mellitus. N Eng J Med 1993;329:977–986. Provides compelling evidence to justify tight glycemic control.

Olefsky JM. Diabetes mellitus. In: Wyngaarden JB, Smith LH Jr, Bennett JC eds, Cecil textbook of medicine, 19th ed, Philadelphia: WB Saunders;1391–1410. Somewhat disjointed but thorough review of pathophysiology, diagnosis, and complications. Treatment modalities are well described but text is weak on specific recommendations.

Chapter 39: Hypercholesterolemia

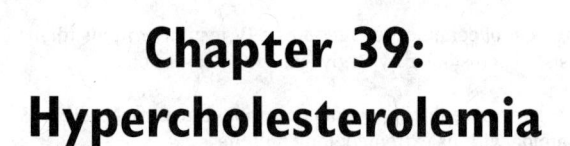

Barry Ziring

I. Clinical Presentation

A. General Information

1. The serum cholesterol identifies patients at risk for coronary artery disease. Values above 200 mg/dL (the upper 50th percentile) are associated with risk, which increases by four- to fivefold as the value approaches 300 mg/dL.

2. Randomized trials have proven that lipid-lowering medication and diet can diminish morbidity and mortality for symptomatic men with elevated cholesterol levels.

3. The benefit of treating elevated cholesterol in the elderly, women, and young persons is less well established.

4. Taken together elevated cholesterol, hypertension, lack of physical activity, and cigarette smoking explain two thirds of excess coronary deaths.

B. Symptoms

1. There are no symptoms directly referrable to hypercholesterolemia.

2. History-taking should be directed at identifying other cardiac risk factors including hypertension, age (men over 45 or women after menopause not taking estrogen replacement), cigarette smoking, male sex, a family history of premature coronary heart disease, diabetes mellitus, severe obesity, or a history of definite cerebrovascular or occlusive peripheral vascular disease.

C. Physical Examination

1. Xanthomas may be associated with hyperlipoproteinemia. When hyperlipoproteinemia is present xanthomas are particularly suggestive of type IIa, IIb, and III.

2. Premature corneal arcus suggests type IIa disease

3. Orange yellow deposits on palmar creases may indicate type III disease.

4. Examination should be directed at identifying potential secondary causes of dyslipidemia, including

   a. Diabetes mellitus

- b. Nephrotic syndrome
- c. Thyroid disease
- d. Obstructive liver disease
- e. Alcoholism
- f. Multiple myeloma
- g. Gaucher's, Neimann-Pick disease

II. Diagnostic Approach

A. General Evaluation and Screening

1. Screening recommendations differ but most authorities suggest measuring of total cholesterol and high-density lipoprotein (HDL) cholesterol in asymptomatic persons at least once q 5 y.

B. The recommendation of the National Cholesterol Education Program have been commonly adopted in practice.

1. Measure total serum cholesterol level and HDL cholesterol at least once q 3–5 y for all adults aged 20 y or older.
2. Repeat the test for any person whose cholesterol level exceeds 200 mg/dL.
3. Measure fasting HDL, triglyceride, and calculated low-density lipoprotein (LDL) level for all persons with borderline to high cholesterol 200–230 mg/dL who have two risk factors including
   - a. Men > 45 or women > 55 or premature menopause without estrogen replacement therapy
   - b. Hypertension
   - c. Cigarette smoking
   - d. Male sex
   - e. Diabetes mellitus
   - f. Severe obesity
   - g. History of definite cerebrovascular or occlusive peripheral vascular disease
   - h. Family history of premature coronary heart disease (myocardial infarction or sudden death in a parent or sibling < 55 y)
4. Measure fasting HDL, triglycerides, and calculated LDL for all persons with high cholesterol 240 mg/dL or higher.
5. Evaluate for familial hyperlipidemia
   - a. The majority of hyperlipoproteinemias are not familial.
   - b. The major classes of hyperlipoproteinemia are
     1) Type I
        - a) *Chylomicrons increased*
        - b) *Associated with abdominal crises and pancreatitis but generally not premature coronary heart disease*
     2) Type IIa
        - a) *LDL increased*

b) Approximately 0.1% of the population are heterozygotes for the congenital form of type IIa.
c) The congenital form is associated with serum cholesterol levels > 350 mg/dL.
d) The congenital form is almost invariably associated with premature coronary heart disease and should be aggressively treated.

3) Type IIb—increased LDL and very low-density lipoprotein (VLDL)
Type IV—increased VLDL
   a) These two forms can be congenital. The risk of coronary heart disease is increased but less than in other congenital forms

4) Type III—abnormal lipoprotein of the VLDL type
   a) This form is frequently congenital.
   b) The congenital form is associated with premature heart disease and premature peripheral vascular disease.

5) Type V—increased chylomicrons and VLDL
   a) Associated with painful abdominal crises and pancreatitis

III. Treatment Strategies

A. If there is a secondary cause of hyperlipoproteinemia, this should be treated.

B. **Primary Prevention in Patients without Known Coronary Heart Disease (Figures 39-1 and 39-2)**

1. Desirable blood cholesterol level of < 200 mg/dL and HDL > 35 mg/dL.

   a. Repeat cholesterol measurement within 5 y.
   b. Provide general dietary and risk factor education.
   c. If HDL is < 35, lipoprotein analysis should be done and treatment strategies described below.

2. Borderline high blood cholesterol level of 200–230 mg/dL and HDL > 35

   a. Without coronary heart disease or two coronary risk factors
      1) Provide information on step I diet, which reduces fat intake to < 30% of total calories, saturated fat intake to < 10%, and dietary cholesterol to < 300 mg/d.
      2) Reevaluate annually.
      3) Remeasure total cholesterol level
      4) Reinforce dietary education annually.

3. Borderline high blood cholesterol level 200–239 with two coronary heart disease risk factors or high blood cholesterol level > 240, or any total cholesterol value where HDL cholesterol is < 35.

   a. Base treatment decision on LDL cholesterol
      1) LDL < 130—provide dietary and risk factor counseling
      2) LDL 130–159—provide information on step I diet and physical activity.
      3) LDL > 160 or LDL level 130–159 with two coronary risk factors—begin step I diet. Proceed to step II diet if step I fails. This requires

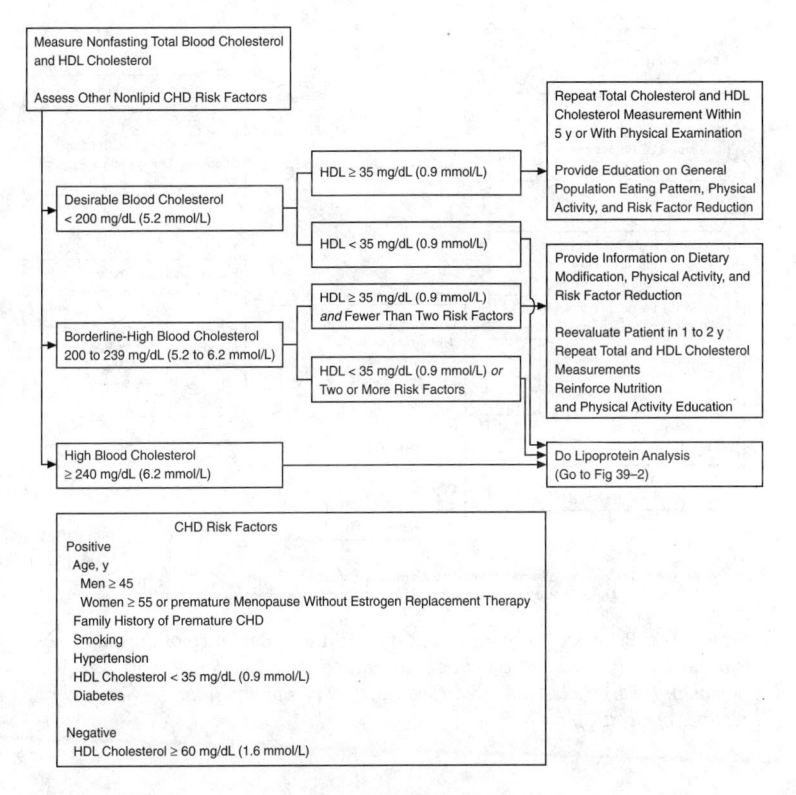

Figure 39-1. Primary Prevention in Adults Without Evidence of Coronary Heart Disease (CHD). *Initial classification is based on total cholesterol and high-density lipoprotein (HDL) cholesterol levels. (Reprinted by permission from the National Institutes of Health.)*

```
Measure Nonfasting Total Blood Cholesterol and HDL Cholesterol
Assess Other Nonlipid CHD Risk Factors
```

- Desirable Blood Cholesterol < 200 mg/dL (5.2 mmol/L)
  - HDL ≥ 35 mg/dL (0.9 mmol/L) → Repeat Total Cholesterol and HDL Cholesterol Measurement Within 5 y or With Physical Examination; Provide Education on General Population Eating Pattern, Physical Activity, and Risk Factor Reduction
  - HDL < 35 mg/dL (0.9 mmol/L)
- Borderline-High Blood Cholesterol 200 to 239 mg/dL (5.2 to 6.2 mmol/L)
  - HDL ≥ 35 mg/dL (0.9 mmol/L) *and* Fewer Than Two Risk Factors → Provide Information on Dietary Modification, Physical Activity, and Risk Factor Reduction; Reevaluate Patient in 1 to 2 y; Repeat Total and HDL Cholesterol Measurements; Reinforce Nutrition and Physical Activity Education
  - HDL < 35 mg/dL (0.9 mmol/L) *or* Two or More Risk Factors
- High Blood Cholesterol ≥ 240 mg/dL (6.2 mmol/L) → Do Lipoprotein Analysis (Go to Fig 39-2)

CHD Risk Factors
Positive
- Age, y
  - Men ≥ 45
  - Women ≥ 55 or premature Menopause Without Estrogen Replacement Therapy
- Family History of Premature CHD
- Smoking
- Hypertension
- HDL Cholesterol < 35 mg/dL (0.9 mmol/L)
- Diabetes

Negative
- HDL Cholesterol ≥ 60 mg/dL (1.6 mmol/L)

---

minimal cholesterol and fat intake while maintaining acceptable nutrition. Involvement of a registered dietitian may be helpful.
4) Consider medical management if diet fails.
5) The goals of therapy are outlined in Table 39-1.

C. Secondary Prevention in Adults with Known Coronary Heart Disease (Figure 39-3)

a. Optimal LDL cholesterol in this population is < 100 mg/dL.
b. Goal of treatment in patients with coronary heart disease is LDL cholesterol < 100 mg/dL.

IV. Pharmacologic Treatment

A. Goals of Therapy—see Table 39-1.

280 • Manual of Office Medicine

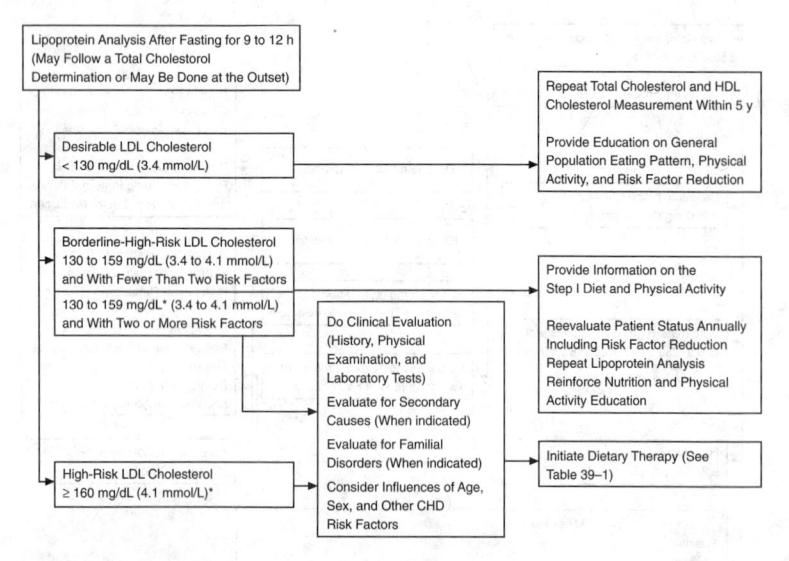

```
Lipoprotein Analysis After Fasting for 9 to 12 h
(May Follow a Total Cholesterol
Determination or May Be Done at the Outset)
    │
    ├──> Desirable LDL Cholesterol ──────────────> Repeat Total Cholesterol and HDL
    │    < 130 mg/dL (3.4 mmol/L)                  Cholesterol Measurement Within 5 y
    │
    │                                              Provide Education on General
    │                                              Population Eating Pattern, Physical
    │                                              Activity, and Risk Factor Reduction
    │
    ├──> Borderline-High-Risk LDL Cholesterol
    │    130 to 159 mg/dL (3.4 to 4.1 mmol/L)
    │    and With Fewer Than Two Risk Factors
    │
    │    130 to 159 mg/dL* (3.4 to 4.1 mmol/L)     Provide Information on the
    │    and With Two or More Risk Factors ──>     Step I Diet and Physical Activity
    │                                              
    │                          Do Clinical         Reevaluate Patient Status Annually
    │                          Evaluation          Including Risk Factor Reduction
    │                          (History, Physical  Repeat Lipoprotein Analysis
    │                          Examination, and    Reinforce Nutrition and Physical
    │                          Laboratory Tests)   Activity Education
    │                          Evaluate for
    │                          Secondary Causes
    │                          (When indicated)
    │                          Evaluate for Familial
    │                          Disorders (When indicated)   Initiate Dietary Therapy (See
    └──> High-Risk LDL Cholesterol ──────>         Table 39-1)
         ≥ 160 mg/dL (4.1 mmol/L)*                 
                                   Consider Influences of Age,
                                   Sex, and Other CHD
                                   Risk Factors
```

* On the basis of the average of two determinations. If the firs two LDL-cholesterol test results differ by more than 30 mg/dL (0.7 mmol/L), a third test result should be obtained within 1 to 8 weeks and the average value of the three tests used.

Figure 39–2. Primary Prevention in Adults Without Evidence of Coronary Heart Disease (CHD). *Subsequent classificaiton is based on low-density lipoprotein (LDL) cholesterol level. (Reprinted by permission from the National Institutes of Health.)*

Table 39–1. Treatment Decisions Based on LDL Cholesterol Level

Patient Category	Initiation Level	LDL Goal
Dietary Therapy		
Without CHD and with fewer than two risk factors	≥ 160 mg/dL (4.1 mmol/L)	< 160 mg/dL (4.1 mmol/L)
Without CHD and with two or more risk factors	≥ 130 mg/dL (3.4 mmol/L)	< 130 mg/dL (3.4 mmol/L)
With CHD	≥ 100 mg/dL (2.6 mmol/L)	≤ 100 mg/dL (2.6 mmol/L)
Drug Treatment		
Without CHD and with fewer than two risk factors	≥ 190 mg/dL (4.9 mmol/L)	< 160 mg/dL (4.1 mmol/L)
Without CHD and with two or more risk factors	≥ 160 mg/dL (4.1 mmol/L)	< 130 mg/dL (3.4 mmol/L)
With CHD	≥ 130 mg/dL (3.4 mmol/L)	≤ 100 mg/dL (2.6 mmol/L)

LDL, low-density lipoprotein; CHD, coronary heart disease
(Reprinted by permission from the National Institutes of Health.)

Part VII: Endocrinology/Metabolism • 281

```
Lipoprotein Analysis* After Fasting for 9 to 12 h
Average of Two Measurements
1 to 8 wk Apart†
    │
    ├──→ Optimal LDL Cholesterol ≤ 100 mg/dL (2.6 mmol/L)
    │         →  Individualize Instruction on Diet and Physical Activity Level
    │            Repeat Lipoprotein Analysis Annually
    │
    └──→ Higher Than Optimal LDL Cholesterol ≥ 100 mg/dL (2.6 mmol/L)
              →  Do Clinical Evaluation (History, Physical Examination, and Laboratory Tests)
                 Evaluate for Secondary Causes (When indicated)
                 Evaluate for Familial Disorders (When indicated)
                 Consider Influences of Age, Sex, and Other CHD Risk Factors
                 →  Initiate Therapy (See Table 39–1)
```

* Lipoprotein analysis should be performed when the patient is not in the recovery phase from an acute coronary or other medical event that would lower the usual LDL-cholesterol level.

† If the first two LDL-cholesterol test results differ by more than 30 mg/dL (0.7 mmol/L), a third test result should be obtained within 1 to 8 weeks and the average value of the three tests used.

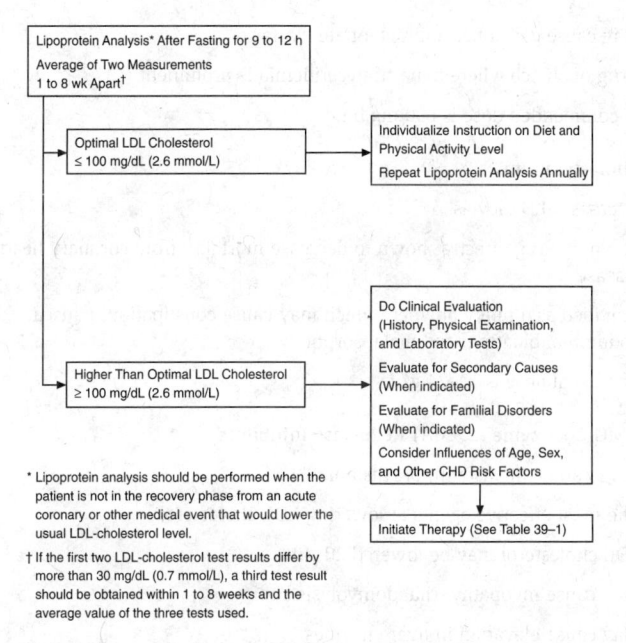

Figure 39–3. Secondary Prevention in Adults With Evidence of Coronary Heart Disease (CHD). *Classification is based on low-density lipoprotein (LDL) cholesterol level. (Reprinted by permission from the National Institutes of Health.)*

B. Nicotinic Acid

1. Decreases LDL and VLDL
2. Increases HDL
3. Minor side effects include flushing and pruritus.
4. Adverse effects include dyspepsia, hepatotoxicity, worsening glucose tolerance.
5. Dose starts at 100 mg t.i.d. and may be increased to 1.0 g t.i.d.
6. Valuable in treating high total cholesterol when low HDL or elevated triglyceride are present

C. Gemfibrozil

1. Increases HDL
2. Modest decreases in LDL
3. Substantial decreases in VLDL and triglycerides
4. Contraindicated in patient with hepatic or renal disease

5. May cause gallstones and potentiate warfarin
6. Drug of choice where hypertriglyceridemia is prominent
7. Recommended dose is 600 mg b.i.d.

D. Cholestyramine

1. Decreases LDL levels
2. The only drug directly shown to decrease mortality from coronary heart disease
3. Provided as a bulky powder, which may cause constipation, nausea, abdominal bloating, and malabsorption
4. The usual dose is 12–24 g/d.

E. HMG Coenzyme A (CoA) Reductase Inhibitors

1. Lovastatin, simvastatin, pravastatin
2. The most effective agents at lowering LDL cholesterol
3. LDL cholesterol may be lowered 20–40%
4. May cause myopathy, rhabdomyolysis
5. May cause elevation in liver enzymes
6. Contraindicated in patients with preexisting liver disease
7. Liver enzymes (including alanine aminotransferase) should be checked at regular intervals before treatment, q 6 wk during the first 3 months, q 8 wk during the first year, and q 6 mo thereafter.
8. The drug should be stopped if there is any clinical evidence of myositis.
9. The recommended starting doses are lovastatin 20 mg, simvastatin 5–10 mg and pravastatin 5–10 mg once daily with evening meal.

F. Other Agents Include

1. Colestipol
2. Probucol
3. Clofibrate

G. For postmenopausal women with high serum cholesterol consideration may be given to estrogen replacement therapy.

H. Combination therapy may be used but adverse reactions increase

1. The combinatin of a bile acid sequestrant with either nicotinic acid or an HMG CoA reductase inhibitor may lower LDL cholesterol 40–50%
2. Avoid combining HMG CoA reductase inhibitors with gemfibrizol due to the increased incidence of rhabdomyolysis.

V. Patient Education

A. Diet is always primary therapy.

1. Decrease saturated fat.
2. Reduce high-cholesterol foods.
3. Increase vegetable or fish oils.

B. Pharmacologic therapy should supplement (not substitute for) diet and exercise.

C. Exercise is an important part of weight reduction and may raise HDL levels.

VI. Indications for Referral to an Endocrinologist or Lipid Specialist

A. Consider referral of patients with congenital hyperlipoproteinemias if the physician is not comfortable with treatment in this high-risk group.

B. Consider referral of those with refractory hyperlipoproteinemias.

C. Consider referral for combined pharmacologic therapy where adverse reactions are increased.

VII. Annotated Bibliography

Consensus Conference. Lowering blood cholesterol to prevent heart disease. JAMA 1985;253:2080–2086. The recommendation and summary of the National Institute of Health Consensus Conference.

Expert Panel on Detection, Evaluation, and Treatment of High Blood Cholesterol in Adults. Summary of the Second Report of the National Cholesterol Education Program (NCEP). JAMA 1993; 269:3015–3023.

Jones PM. A clinical overview of dyslipidemias: treatment strategies. Am J Med 1992;93:187–198. A good review of treatment strategies with discussion of primary and secondary dyslipidemias.

Multiple Risk Factor Intervention Trial Research Group. Multiple risk factor intervention trial: risk factor changes and mortality results. JAMA 1982;248:1465–1477. One of the largest original trials showing the link between elevated cholesterol and coronary artery disease.

Report of the National Cholesterol Education Program Expert Panel on detection, evaluation and treatment of high blood cholesterol in adults. Arch Intern Med 1988;148:36–69. A thorough review of the subject with algorithms for treatment, which have become common clinical practice.

The Cholesterol Facts. A summary of the evidence relating dietary fats, serum cholesterol and coronary heart disease. Circulation 1990;81:1721–1733. The recommendations of the American Heart Association and the National Heart, Lung and Blood Institute.

Chapter 40: Hypercalcemia

Karen G. Kelly

I. Clinical Presentation

A. History

1. Often asymptomatic, especially if calcium is only mildly increased.
2. If patient is symptomatic look for
   a. Gastroenterologic—anorexia, nausea, vomiting, constipation, ulcers, rarely pancreatitis
   b. Renal—stones, decreased renal function, polyuria due to decreased concentrating ability
   c. CNS—fatigue, depression, confusion, headache, can lead to coma when severe
   d. Neuromuscular—weakness, bone loss
   e. Hypertension

B. Physical

1. There are no specific signs of increased calcium.
2. Physical examination should be directed to looking for signs of malignancy.

II. Diagnostic Approach

A. For All Patients

1. Repeat value, especially when only mildly increased
2. Correct calcium for abnormalities in albumin (0.8 mg for every gram albumin is below 4.0 g)
3. Discontinue drugs associated with increased calcium (see below)
4. Measure serum parathyroid hormone (PTH)
5. Measure Cl, PO_4, CO_2, and renal function
6. Other work-up as indicated by history and physical

7. Remember that a severe increase > 14 mg/dL (3.5 mmol/L) in calcium is usually secondary to malignancy.

B. Increased PTH

1. If nonsurgical therapy contemplated measure yearly:

   a. 24-h urine for creatinine clearance
   b. Kidney-ureter-bladder (KUB) looking for kidney stones
   c. 24-h urine for calcium
   d. Bone mass measurement

2. If parathyroidectomy surgery is planned, no further imaging need be done.

C. If PTH is not increased

1. Work-up for malignancy, sarcoidosis, thyrotoxicosis

2. Other causes (see differential diagnosis below)

3. Remember that most but not all malignancies in the presence of hypercalcemia are metastic.

III. Differential Diagnosis

A. Primary hyperparathyroidism—serum PTH increased or high normal with elevated calcium

1. Hyperparathyroidism increases in frequency with age.

2. It is the most common cause of mild hypercalcemia; associated with MEN I + II syndromes

3. Most cases are caused by parathyroid adenoma (80%) or hyperplasia (15%), occasional adenocarcinoma

B. Malignancy—serum PTH low with elevated calcium

1. Most common cause of severe hypercalcemia

2. Most commonly seen with metastatic disease

3. Several mechanisms

   a. PTH-related protein secretion
   b. Ectopic production of vitamin D
   c. Other ectopic factors
   d. Lytic bone metastases

4. Common tumors include

   a. Squamous cell carcinoma of lung, head, and neck

b. Breast
c. Myeloma
d. Lymphoma
e. Genitourinary
f. Other lung cancers
g. Adenocarcinoma of pancreas and other sources are less common.

C. Other Causes of Hypercalcemia

1. Endocrine

    a. Thyrotoxicosis
    b. Pheochromocytoma
    c. Adrenal insufficiency
    d. Vasoactive intestinal peptide (VIP)-producing tumors

2. Granulomatous diseases such as

    a. Sarcoid
    b. TB
    c. Mechanism is 1,25-dihydroxy vitamin D excess

3. Medications including

    a. Thiazide diuretics
    b. Lithium
    c. Estrogen
    d. Antiestrogens

4. Miscellaneous

    a. Milk alkali syndrome
    b. Vitamin A intoxication
    c. Vitamin D intoxication
    d. Immobilization
    e. Acute and chronic renal insufficiency
    f. Familial hypocalciuric hypercalcemia

IV. Treatment

A. Severe Symptomatic Hypercalcemia (calcium > 14 mg/dL [3.5 mmol/L])

1. Hospitalize

2. Hydration with IV isotonic saline

3. Once the patient is well hydrated, furosemide or ethacrynic acid can be used to increase calcium excretion. Hydration must be maintained during diuretic administration.

4. In patients with severe hypercalcemia and those whose calcium is still significantly elevated after hydration, specific therapy for hypercalcemia should be initiated with a biphosphate, mithramycin, or calcitonin. (See Bilezikian review for a fuller description of management.)
5. Glucocorticoids are only effective in patients with vitamin D excess or hematologic malignancies that respond to steroids.

B. Mild Hypercalcemia

1. Hyperparathyroidism
    a. If asymptomatic either refer to surgeon for neck exploration or provide medical follow-up.
    b. It is not clear if estrogen therapy is beneficial in postmenopausal women.
    c. Surgery is definately indicated for
        1) Serum calcium in the range of 11.4–12 mg/dL (2.85–3.0 mmol/L), given a normal range of 8.8–10.4 mg/dL (2.2–2.6 mmol/L)
        2) Declining creatinine clearance (particularly if there is a 30% decline)
        3) 24-h urine excretion of calcium > 400 mg
        4) Decreased bone mass or declining bone mass
        5) Presence of nephrolithiasis
        6) Symptoms consistent with hyperparathyroidism
        7) Hypertension alone is not an indication for surgery.
    e. Other causes of hypercalcemia such as thyrotoxicosis or sarcoidosis should be treated appropriately.

C. Patient Education

1. Patients should be told to avoid dehydration, know signs of increasing calcium, and follow-up appropriately.

V. Indications for Referral

A. Malignancy

B. Indications for parathyroidectomy above

VI. Indications for Hospitalization

A. Severe increase in calcium (> 14 mg/dL)

B. Less severe hypercalcemia if mental status changes are present

C. Dehydration

VII. Annotated Bibliography

Bilezikian JP. Management of acute hypercalcemia. N Engl J Med 1992; 326:1196–1203. A review of causes and management of acute hypercalcemia. Includes therapy of severe hypercalcemia

Consensus Development Conference Panel. Diagnosis and management of asymptomatic primary hyperthyroidism: consensus development conference statement. Ann Intern Med 1991;114:593–597.

Lafferty FW, Hubay CA. Primary hyperparathyroidism: a review of the long-term surgical and nonsurgical morbidities as a basis for a rational approach to treatment. Arch Intern Med 1989;149:789–796. Long-term follow-up in patients who underwent surgical and medical therapy.

Chapter 41: Osteoporosis

Kenneth R. Epstein

I. Epidemiology

A. Osteoporosis is responsible for over 1.5 million fractures per year, including 650,00 vertebral, 250,000 hip, and 200,000 Colles' fractures.

B. Annual costs referable to osteoporatic fractures exceed $10 billion per year in the United States.

C. The mortality rate in the first year following a hip fracture is 12–20%, and those who survive are often unable to live independently.

D. Any reduction in costs will depend on preventing osteoporotic fractures, not improving the care of persons who have suffered a fracture.

II. Characteristics of Osteoporosis

A. Osteoporosis is caused by a loss of bone mass.

1. In normal bone, resorption equals formation.
2. Osteoporosis results from an imbalance of bone remodelling, with the rate of bone resorption exceeding that of new bone formation.
3. Peak bone mass occurs at about age 35 y. Both genders lose bone mass continuously after age 40.
4. Women have accelerated bone loss for 1–7 y postmenopausally.

B. Two Types of Bone in Adult Skeleton

1. Cortical (compact) bone
    a. Is present on the surface of all bones and in the shafts of long bones
    b. 80% of skeletal mass is cortical bone.
2. Trabecular (cancellous) bone
    a. Predominant in the vertebrae, flat bones, and ends of long bones
    b. Is more metabolically active than cortical bone
    c. Trabecular bones are the main sites of osteoporotic fractures.

C. Types of Osteoporosis

1. Type I (postmenopausal) osteoporosis

    a. Is due to increased osteoclastic activity, resulting in accelerated bone loss
    b. The bone lost is predominantly trabecular, resulting in an increased incidence of vertebral fractures.
    c. Type I osteoporosis is more structurally damaging than is type II.

2. Type II (age-related) osteoporosis

    a. Occurs in both genders
    b. Is age dependent, occuring primarily in individuals > 70 y of age
    c. Is due to decreased osteoblastic activity, resulting in a slow, steady loss of trabecular and cortical bone
    d. Is potentiated by an age-related decrease in vitamin D absorption and hydroxylation, as well as decreased dietary calcium intake

III. Risk Factors for Osteoporosis

A. Risk Factors for Primary Osteoporosis

1. Age—incidence increases with increasing age
2. Race—incidence higher in whites and Asians
3. Gender—incidence higher in women than in men
4. Estrogen deficiency—incidence higher with menopause, oophorectomy, or anovulation
5. Body frame—incidence higher in thin, small boned individuals than in obese persons
6. Genetics—incidence higher with positive family history
7. Dietary—incidence higher with calcium deficiency or excessive alcohol use
8. Tobacco use—incidence higher in cigarette smokers

B. Secondary osteoporosis may result from the following conditions.

1. Medications

    a. Glucocorticoids
    b. Thyroid hormone
    c. Anticonvulsants
    d. Long-term heparin
    e. Aluminum-containing antacids

2. Endocrine causes

    a. Hypogonadism
    b. Hypercortisolism
    c. Hyperthyroidism

d. Hyperparathyroidism
3. Malignancy
   a. Metastatic carcinoma
   b. Multiple myeloma
4. Nutritional causes
   a. Malabsorption syndromes—affect vitamin D and calcium absorption
   b. Malnutrition—osteoporosis can result from both calcium deficiency and protein deficiency
5. Prolonged immobilization

IV. Diagnosis and Screening

A. Diagnostic Evaluation in Patients with Suspected Osteoporosis
1. Look for presence of risk factors.
2. Screen for presence of secondary osteoporosis.
   a. History and physical examination for diseases causing osteoporosis
   b. Order laboratory tests specific to suspected diseases.

B. Measurement of Bone Mineral Density
1. Bone mineral density (BMD) measurement is the best method of screening for osteoporosis.
2. Evidence supports a direct relationship between BMD and fracture risk.
3. Indications for screening with BMD measurement include
   a. Patient high risk for primary osteoporosis due to presence of risk factors
   b. Suspect secondary osteoporosis
   c. Postmenopausal woman who is considering hormonal replacement therapy only if BMD measurement places her at high risk for osteoporosis
4. Methods
   a. Skeletal x-rays
      1) Very poor sensitivity because need to lose 30–50% of bone mineral before can see demineralization on x-ray
      2) Only indicated if suspect a fracture, not to predict risk of fracture
   b. Single photon absorptiometry (SPA)
      1) Measures appendicular bone only; does not directly assess areas at most concern for fractures, such as spine or femur
      2) Cannot distinguish cortical from trabecular bone
      3) Is quick (10–20 min), inexpensive, and results in low radiation exposure
   c. Dual photon absorptiometry (DPA)
      1) Can measure axial bones, such as hip and spine

2) Cannot distinguish cortical from trabecular bone
3) Is longer (20–60 min) more expensive, and more radiation than SPA
d. Dual energy x-ray absorptiometry (DEXA)
1) Is the current method of choice for BMD measurement
2) Is the most precise method, with the best resolution
3) Can measure both axial and appendicular BMD
4) Very short scan time (10 min) with low radiation exposure
e. Quantitative CT
1) Usually used for lumbar spine; measures spine density against standards
2) Can distinguish cortical from trabecular bone
3) Is expensive, long, with a larger radiation dose
4) Is less accurate than DEXA; bone marrow fat can confound density.

V. Prevention and Treatment

A. Once bone mass is reduced to below the fracture threshold, it is difficult to increase the mass to above the threshold again. Therefore, it is important to prevent bone loss from ever progressing this far.

B. Exercise

1. Regular exercise increases bone formation and decreases resorption.

2. Regular exercise, particularly weight-bearing, is recommended for all patients.

C. Calcium

1. Recommended intake for all adults is 1000 mg/d. For adolescents and postmenopausal women is 1500 mg/d. Average daily dietary intake in United States is 450–550 mg.

2. Increasing calcium intake slows down rate of bone loss, but does not prevent loss.

3. Contraindications—hypercalcemia, hypercalciuria, calcium-containing renal stones

D. Vitamin D

1. Vitamin D is required for optimal calcium absorption. This requirement increases with age.

2. Recommended intake for older men and postmenopausal women is 600–800 IU daily. This amount is available in 1–2 multivitamins daily.

3. Overdose of vitamin D can be toxic and can induce hypercalcemia and hypercalciuria. This may be seen with doses > 2000 IU daily.

E. Estrogen Therapy (see Chapter 55 for details)

1. Is the most effective method of preventing bone loss in postmenopausal women
2. Reduces bone resorption by the osteoclasts, preventing progressive bone loss
3. Studies have demonstrated a 50% reduction in osteoporotic fracture risk.

F. Calcitonin

1. Acts directly on osteoclasts to suppress their activity, thereby decreasing bone resorption
2. Has been shown to increase vertebral bone mass, but its effect on cortical bone is unclear
3. Calcitonin must be administered parenterally. Usual dose is 50–100 U daily or every other day, either SQ or IM.
4. Is available either as human or salmon calcitonin. Salmon is more potent than human, but may lead to antibody production, which then causes resistance.
5. Side effects are flushing, nausea, vomiting, and irritation at the injection site.
6. Calcitonin's cost, side effects, and route of administration decrease its usefulness.

G. Biphosphonates

1. Biphosphonates such as etidronate are analogues of naturally occurring pyrophosphates that inhibit osteoclasts' ability to resorb bone.
2. The dose that is sufficient to inhibit bone resorption may also impair the mineralization of new bone matrix. Therefore, they cannot be used continually long term.
3. Etidronate is therefore given cyclically. Usual dose is 400 mg/d for 2 wk, followed by 11–13 wk of calcium supplementation.
4. Is very poorly absorbed and causes GI irritation
5. Etidronate is not presently recommended for the standard prevention or treatment of osteoporosis. Newer agents that are under investigation may allow normal mineralization, and could therefore be used continuously.

H. Fluorides

1. All the above regimens inhibit resorption. Fluoride directly stimulates bone formation.
2. The new bone formed has mineralization defects and is more fragile.
3. Flourides are not currently indicated for the treatment of osteoporosis.

VI. Annotated Bibliography

Aloia JF, Vaswani A, Yeh JK, et al. Calcium supplementation with and without hormone replacement therapy to prevent postmenopausal bone loss. Ann Intern Med 1994;120:97–103. A study demonstrating the superiority of hormone therapy plus calcium to calcium alone in the prevention of osteoporosis.

Ettinger G, Genant HK, Cann CE. Long-term estrogen replacement therapy prevents bone loss and fractures. Ann Intern Med 1985;102:319–324. Retrospective study demonstrating the protective effect of long-term estrogens on bone loss and fractures.

Melton LJ, Eddy DM, Johnston CC, et al. Screening for osteoporosis. Ann Intern Med 1990;112:516–528. A review of the evidence for and against unselective screening of post menopausal women for osteoporosis.

Riggs BL, Melton LJ. The prevention and treatment of osteoporosis. N Engl J Med 1992;327:620–627. An excellent review of these topics.

Wahner HW, Dunn WL, Brown ML, Morin RL, Riggs BL. Comparison of dual-energy x-ray absorptiometry and dual photon absorptiometry for bone mineral measurements of the lumbar spine. Mayo Clin Proc 1988;63:1075–1084. A study that demonstrates the advantages of DEXA scans over previous technologies.

Chapter 42: Thyroid Diseases

Richard G. Paluzzi

I. General Information

A. Thyroid Hormone Formation

1. Thyroid takes up iodine (I), oxidizes it, and incorporates it into tyrosine (organification).

2. Mono- and diiodotyrosine are combined via thyroid peroxidase to form 3,5,3',5'-tetraiodothyronine (T_4) and 3,5,3'-triiodothyronine (T_3) (coupling).

3. T_3 is the more active hormone and is formed by distal deiodination of T_4. Both T_3 and T_4 circulate primarily bound to plasma proteins (predominately thyroxine-binding globulin [TBG]).

4. Some T_4 is deiodinated proximally to form 3,3,5'-triiodothyronine or reverse T_3 (rT_3), which is metabolically inactive. rT_3 production is increased during acute and chronic illnesses.

5. All steps of thyroid hormone synthesis and release are stimulated by pituitary thyroid-stimulating hormone (TSH). TSH production is stimulated by hypothalamic thyrotropin-releasing hormone (TRH) and suppressed by both T_3 and T_4 in serum.

B. Thyroid Function Tests

1. Can measure total T_3 and T_4 as well as free T_3 and T_4; most cost efficient is total T_4

2. Can estimate free T_3 level by measuring the thyroid hormone binding ratio (T_3 resin uptake or T_3RU). An increased T_3RU suggests that TBG is saturated by an excess of circulating T_4. A decrease in T_3RU suggests that a lower than normal amount of circulating T_4 has left many open binding sites on TBG.

3. Typically measure T_4 and T_3RU as well as TSH. Ultrasensitive TSH assays make this the most useful assay to assess thyroid function.

4. Can multiply the total T_4 by the T_3RU to get the free T_4 index (FTI)

5. Can measure TSH following a TRH infusion if primary pituitary failure is suspected

6. Abnormal levels of circulating TBG will result in corresponding abnormalities of total T_3 and T_4 levels. Free levels remain unchanged. TBG can be increased

by pregnancy, estrogens, cirrhosis, and use of heroin, methadone, and clofibrate. TBG can be decreased by malnutrition, chronic illness, nephrosis, and with steroid usage.

7. Drug effects on thyroid function

   a. Decreased TSH—dopamine, L-dopa, steroids, iodide, lithium, sulfonylureas
   b. Decreased thyroid hormone synthesis or release—iodide, lithium, sulfonylureas
   c. Decreased T_4 binding to TBG—salicylates, phenytoin, furosemide
   d. Decreased T_4 to T_3 conversion—propylthiouracil, propranolol, steroids, amiodarone, some iodinated contrast media

C. Thyroid Imaging Studies

1. Radioactive iodine uptake (RAI uptake)—thyroid is scanned 24 h after a radioiodine injection. Normal glands take up 5%–30%. Contraindicated in pregnancy. Used to differentiate etiology of hyperthyroidism.

2. Thyroid scan—used to determine location of ectopic thyroid tissue or to determine the functional status of a thyroid mass. I^{123} or TcO_4 99m (pertechnetate) is injected and preferentially trapped by thyroid tissue.

3. Thyroid ultrasound—can identify nodules 1–3 mm in size. Can differentiate cystic from solid nodules and can be used to follow response of a nodule to therapy

II. Hyperthyroidism

A. General Information

1. Caused by sustained overactivity of the gland, hormonal leak during inflammation, or excess hormone levels form outside the gland

B. Symptoms

1. Primarily due to sympathomimetic action of T_4 and increased catabolism

2. Onset of symptoms may be gradual and nonspecific

3. May see nervousness, irritability, hyperhidrosis, heat intolerance, palpitations, weight-loss, dyspnea, fatigue, increased appetite, hyperdefecation, oligo- or amenorrhea, and eye problems (photophobia, tearing, diplopia)

4. In the elderly, may see nonspecific depression, anorexia and weight-loss (apathetic hyperthyroidism), or congestive heart failure associated with atrial fibrillation.

C. Physical Examination

1. Often nonconclusive

2. Palpate gland for enlargement (goiter) or nodules

3. Can auscultate neck for thyroid bruits or jugular venous hums
4. May see hyperkinesis, tremor, velvety skin, moist hands, onycholysis (Plummer's nails), hyperreflexia (rapid upstroke and release), and tachycardia (virtually required for diagnosis in the young)
5. May find new-onset atrial fibrillation and signs of high output heart failure
6. The elderly may lack all hyperadrenergic signs (apathetic hyperthyroidism).
7. Ocular signs are common (exophthalmos, lid lag, lid retraction).

D. Laboratory Studies

1. Increased T_4, T_3RU and FTI; TSH generally suppressed
2. Can see increased T_3 alone in T_3 toxicosis. Measure T_3 if clinical suspicion is high and other tests are normal
3. May see mild hypercalcemia, increased alkaline phosphatase (enhanced bone turnover), increased liver function test values, and mild anemia (macrocytic) or neutropenia
4. May see increased T_4 and T_3RU in euthyroid patients who are ill. Also seen with acute psychosis, hyperemesis gravidarum or following usage of oral cholecystogram dye or amiodarone). Effect is due to diminished conversion of T_4 to T_3, leading to an elevated TSH.

E. Differential Diagnosis

1. Graves's disease (Basedow's disease)
   a. Accounts for more than 85% of cases of hyperthyroidism.
   b. Female to male ratio is 7:1; primarily affects those 20 to 40 years old
   c. Triad of diffuse goiter, ophthalmopathy, and pretibial myxedema (brown plaquelike swelling of pretibial areas, ankles, and feet).
   d. Associated with long-acting thyroid stimulatory immunoglobulin in 50% of cases (binds to TSH receptor)
   e. Disease course may remit and exacerbate; approximately 30% of cases "burn out," leading to hypothyroidism.
   f. More than 50% of patients have eye findings (exophthalmos, easy tearing, photophobia, and possibly diplopia, which are uncommon in other forms of hyperthyroidism); also may see periorbital edema, lid lag and impairment of upward/outward gaze
   g. Tachycardia is common in younger patients. Systolic blood pressure is elevated (increased inotropy) and diastolic pressure is decreased (decreased peripheral resistance).
   h. Confirm that the TSH is suppressed in order to rule out TSH-secreting pituitary tumor.
   i. Radioiodine uptake and thyroid scanning are not necessary unless subacute thyroiditis (brief duration of symptoms or small, tender gland), nodular goiter, or factitious hyperthyroidism are suspected.
   j. Unilateral ophthalmopathy can occur but orbital pathology must be ruled out with CT scan or ultrasound.

k. Treatment is with medications or ablation.
   1) Medications
      a) *propylthiouracil (PTU)*
         i) Inhibits T_4 synthesis and conversion of T_4 to T_3.
         ii) 100–300 mg t.i.d. titrated to thyroid function tests
         iii) Must be given orally
         iv) Treatment of choice in pregnancy
      b) *Methimazole (Tapazol)*
         i) Inhibits T4 synthesis
         ii) 10–30 mg t.i.d.
         iii) Must be given orally
      c) *Treat until T_3 is normal (6–8 wk) then decrease to lowest dose that maintains normalcy*
      d) *Treat 1–2 y then try to taper*
      e) *Side effects*
         i) Primarily rash and agranulocytosis (0.5%)
         ii) May see fever, myalgias, or a lupus-like syndrome
         iii) No utility in routine monitoring of complete blood count but must watch for signs of infection
      f) *Drugs work best with early disease and small glands*
      g) *β blockers may help reduce adrenergic symptoms until antithyroid medications begin to work.*
   2) Ablation
      a) *Radioactive I^{131}*
         i) Primary treatment for most adults and for patients who fail drug therapy; contraindicated in pregnancy
         ii) Should first suppress the disease with drugs to reduce T_3 levels and minimize the thyroid hormone surge that can occur due to leakage following radiation injury
         iii) Dosage is 5–15 μCi given orally. Most patients become euthyroid in 6–12 wk, 40–70% become hypothyroid within 10 y.
      b) *Surgery*
         i) Subtotal thyroidectomy—primarily recommended for children, patients who fail treatment, and pregnant women
         ii) Should first suppress the gland with drugs or potassium iodide (SSKI) 5 drops orally to inhibit T_4 synthesis and release

2. Toxic nodular goiter (Plummers's disease)
   a. Nodular goiter is the most common thyroid abnormality and is usually associated with normal thyroid function tests.
   b. Occasionally areas can function autonomously, causing hyperthyroidism.
   c. Diagnosis
      1) Primarily women after age 60
      2) Symptoms often mild and vague
      3) Thyroid scan shows patchy uptake.
      4) Toxic symptoms may occur following iodine ingestion or early in treatment.
   d. Treatment
      1) Suppress the gland initially with drugs as above, may then perform radioactive I^{131} ablation.

2) Large bulky glands may require resection due to compressive symptoms.
3. Thyroiditis
   a. Subacute (deQuervain's granulomatous, or giant cell) thyroiditis
      1) Generally follows an upper respiratory infection
      2) Gland is tender and may be enlarged.
      3) 50% of patients are hyperthyroid due to follicilar disruption.
      4) Disease is generally self-limited.
      5) Treatment is with aspirin to control pain. Severe symptoms may require steroids.
      6) Hyperadrenergic symptoms can be reduced with β blockers.
   b. Painless thyroiditis
      1) Gland is slightly enlarged and nontender.
      2) Common in postpartum period and generally self-limited.
      3) Treat hyperadrenergic symptoms with β blockers
   c. Hashimoto's thyroiditis
      1) Gland is firm to "rock" hard
      2) Find high titers of antimicrosomal antibodies
      3) Can blunt symptoms with β blockers
      4) Often "burns out," leading to hypothyroidism after a variable period of euthyroidism
4. Other disorders
   a. Toxic adenoma
      1) Generally benign
      2) See rise in T_3 level before increases in T_4 occur
      3) Scan shows "hot" nodule with suppression of remainder of gland
      4) Treat with ablation by I^{131} or surgery
   b. Exogenous hyperthyroidism
      1) Generally occurs when treating hypothyroidism with T_3/T_4 combination but monitoring only T_4
   C. Factitious hyperthyroidism
      1) Self-administration of T_4
      2) T_3 and T_4 levels are increased with minimal symptoms.
      3) TSH and TRH stimulation are suppressed.
      4) Scan shows diminished uptake.
   d. TSH or T_4 producing tumors
      1) Rare, includes pituitary tumors, trophoblastic tumors, and struma ovarii
   e. Iodine ingestion (Jod-Basedow's disease)
      1) May be due to iodine retaining drugs—contrast dyes, amiodarone
      2) Stimulates function in multinodular goiter and adenomas

III. Hypothyroidism

A. General Information

1. Invariably due to diminished T_4 synthesis
   a. Loss of tissue—surgery, radiation ablation
   b. Antithyroid antibodies
   c. Defective iodine metabolism
   d. Blockade of hormone secretion (drugs)
   e. Pituitary disorders leading to decreased TSH
   f. Rarely, decreased TRH

2. Rarely due to peripheral resistance to hormonal action

B. Symptoms

1. Congenital (cretinism)—jaundice, hoarse cry, mental retardation

2. Juvenile—short stature due to epiphyseal degeneration

3. Adults—lethargy, constipation, cold intolerance, muscle cramps, weakness, mental slowing/dementia, anorexia/weight loss, hearing loss, paresthesias, hoarseness

C. Signs

1. Skin—pallor, sallow color (anemia, hypercarotenemia), coarse, dry, thinning hair that breaks easily

2. Cardiac—bradycardia, pericardial effusion (usually asymptomatic), hypertension

3. Gastrointestinal—decreased motility, ileus

4. Neurologic—hypokinesia, hyporeflexia with delayed relaxation phase

5. Myxedema—brawny thickening of skin over tibial area, hands, eyelids

6. Severe disease can lead to coma, anasarca, and respiratory arrest

D. Laboratory Findings

1. Classically see decreased T_4 and T_3RU (if TBG levels normal)

2. TSH is the most sensitive measure and is always elevated except in rare cases of isolated pituitary failure of TSH secretion. TSH may rise prior to the onset of T_4 decrease or symptoms. Levels > 10 mµ/L generally warrant treatment, particularly in the elderly.

3. Pituitary failure can be diagnosed by failure of TSH response to TRH stimulation.

4. 50% have normal T_3 levels.

5. May see antibodies to thyroid microsomes and thyroglobulin or other associated autoimmune disorders (diabetes, vitiligo, pernicious anemia)

6. Other findings
   a. Anemia
      1) Microcytic if the patient has menorrhagia
      2) Normocytic secondary to decreased erythropoietin
      3) Macrocytic if associated with pernicious anemia
   b. Elevated creatine phosphokinase, aspartate aminotransferase, lactic dehydrogenase, cholesterol
   c. May see enlarged sella tursica on CT
   d. Pericardial effusions can lead to cardiomegaly on chest radiography and low voltage on ECG.

E. Differential Diagnosis

1. Nongoiterous hypothyroidism
   a. Post-surgical or radioactive ablation
   b. Spontaneous thyroid atrophy affects females 6 times more often than males.
   c. Chronic autoimmune disorder leading to fibrosis (thyroiditis)
   d. Polyendocrine failure (diabetes, pernicious anemia, hypoparathyroidism, hypogonadism, hypoadrenalism)
   e. Pituitary or hypothelemic disease

2. Goiterous hyperthyroidism
   a. Hashimoto's thyroiditis
      1) Chronic autoimmune disorder that leads to lymphocytic infiltrates with acinar formation and follicular hypertrophy with oxyphillic (Hurthle) cells
   b. Drug associated
      1) $LiCO_3$—inhibits T_4 release
      2) Antithyroid treatment
      3) Iodine
   c. Iodine deficiency—endemic goiter
   d. Dysmorphogenesis
      1) Rare autosomal recessive disorder
      2) Decreased hearing, goiter, inability to organify iodine (Pendred's syndrome)

F. Treatment

1. L-Thyroxine
   a. Preferred therapy overall
   b. In young patients, can start 0.1–0.15 mg daily
   c. In elderly patients, start with 0.025 mg daily to avoid uncovering coronary insufficiency; increase by 0.025 mg every 2–3 wk
   d. Follow T_4 and TSH levels; aim for TSH level within normal limits but not < 0.05 U/mL

e. T_3 preparations are generally undesirable due to expense, t.i.d. dosing, and inconsistent levels.
f. In very severe illness can administer identical dosages of L-thyroxine intravenously

IV. Simple Nontoxic Goiter

A. General Information

1. Young women with asymptomatic thyroid enlargement that is not nodular

2. Often related to iodine deficiency, biosynthetic defect, or goiteragens (lithium, sulfonamides)

B. Clinical Presentation

1. Generally asymptomatic but can progress to hypothyroidism

2. Laboratory studies are generally normal.

C. Management

1. Generally can just follow clinically

2. Can attempt to suppress growth of the gland with L-thyroxine using replacement doses to bring TSH to lower end of normal range without excessive suppression

V. Euthyroid Sick Syndrome

A. Defined as nonthyroidal illness with decreased T_3, elevated rT_3 and normal or low TSH

B. Normothyroxinemic

1. Normal T_4, free T_4, and FTI

2. Clinically euthyroid

3. Seen in starvation, severe illness, perioperatively and in association with iodine-containing drugs, steroids, high-dose propanolol and PTU

C. Hypothyroxinemic

1. Decreased T_4 and FTI with normal free T_4

2. Patient often ill but not clinically hypothyroid

3. TSH/TRH stimulation normal

4. Probably adaptive to decreased catabolism

5. Treatment generally doesn't help, 80% mortality when T_4 is less than T_3

D. Euthyroid Hyperthyroxinemia

1. Increased T_4, FTI. TRH stimulation test is normal

2. Due to excessive TBG (estrogens, liver disease, porphyria). Also seen after iodinated contrast dyes (competition with 5'-deiodinase), high-dose propanolol, and with familial dysalbuminemic hyperthyroxinemia

3. T_4 often normalizes in 6–8 wk

E. Treatment

1. Generally treat the underlying illness

2. If seriously ill, give thyroxine for low T_4 syndromes or propanolol and PTU for high T_4 syndromes

VI. Thyroid Nodules

A. General Information

1. Thyroid nodules affect 1–5% of the population.

2. More frequent in women over age 50

3. Increased incidence in patients who received head and neck irradiation in childhood (2% incidence per year; 30% lifetime risk)

4. Incidence of thyroid malignancy in the general population is 1/25,000 with an increased incidence of 0.5% per year in patients who received head and neck irradiation (15% risk over 20 y).

B. History

1. Age < 20 or > 60 y significantly raises the suspicion of malignancy, especially in males.

2. Family history of thyroid cancer raises suspicion of familial medullary carcinoma of the thyroid.

3. Prior neck irradiation increases the overall risk of thyroid cancer, but the majority of thyroid nodules in these patients are benign.

4. Symptoms of thyrotoxicosis associated with "hot" nodules often represent benign disease; when associated with "cold" nodules, carries increased incidence of malignancy.

5. Local compressive symptoms, hoarseness, dysphagia, dyspnea, neck pressure, and hemoptysis often occur with thyroid cancers.

6. Rapid growth of nodule suggests malignancy but may occur with hemorrhage into a benign cyst.

C. Physical Examination

1. Firmness of nodule is nonspecific in judging benign versus malignant nature.

2. Regional adenopathy, fixation of the nodule to surrounding tissues, or evidence of vocal cord paralysis is often associated with malignancies, as are nodules > 4 cm.
3. Presence of one or more of the high-risk history or physical examination factors is associated with malignancy in 70% of cases (more than 50% of malignancies, however, are not associated with any of the factors).

D. Differential Diagnosis

1. Malignant nodules
    a. Papillary carcinoma
        1) 70% of all thyroid cancers, most common thyroid malignancy following irradiation
        2) 2–3 fold predilection for women
        3) Can be cystic but typically solid
    b. Follicular carcinoma
        1) 20% of all thyroid cancers
        2) Can be aggressive or show subtle growth with invasion of microvasculature
    c. Nodular carcinoma
        1) 5% of thyroid malignancies
        2) Preceded by C cell hyperplasia
        3) May be sporadic (generally after age 50) or familial, with or without multiple endocrine neoplasia type 2 (generally prior to age 40)
        4) Elevated calcitonin is a reliable marker in all forms.
    d. Thyroid lymphoma
        1) 3% of thyroid malignancies
        2) Generally occurs in older women who have Hashimoto's thyroiditis
        3) Many patients are hypothyroid
    e. Anaplastic carcinoma
        1) Generally aggressive
        2) Typically elderly patients with no gender predilection
        3) Often arises from one of the primary thyroid cancers
    f. Metastatic cancer to the thyroid
        1) Occurs in up to 25% of patients with disseminated cancer
        2) May occur as a manifestation of an occult renal or colonic cancer

2. Benign nodules
    a. Follicular adenoma
        1) Truly benign lesion when accurately diagnosed
        2) Grossly benign lesions may harbor microinvasive foci in 25% of cases
        3) The Hurthe cell variant may be even more difficult to identify as benign and should be excised.
    b. Colloid nodules
        1) Enlarged thyroid follicles
        2) Multiple colloid nodules make up a multinodular goiter, which is 8 times more common in women and may lead to thyrotoxicosis.

c. Thyroid cysts
   1) Lesion containing more than 1 mL fluid
   2) Can occur due to most benign or malignant lesions
   3) 5–25% harbor cancer, suspect if after aspiration the mass persists or lesion recurs
   4) 30–40% harbor follicular adenomas

E. **Diagnostic Testing**

1. All patients with high clinical suspicion for malignancy should undergo fine-needle aspiration.
2. Thyroid function tests should be done for all patients but work-up is based on *clinical* thyroid status.
   a. Euthyroid patients—fine-needle aspiration with cytologic evaluation
   b. Hyperthyroid patients
      1) ^{123}I scintigraphy
         a) "Hot" nodules
            i) Low risk of malignancy
            ii) Treat thyrotoxicosis with drugs or ablation
         b) *"Warm" or "cold" nodules warrant fine-needle aspiration due to increased risk of malignancy.*
         c) Hypothyroid patients
            i) Treat with thyroxine to correct functional status
            ii) Fine-needle aspiration if lesion persists after treatment
      2) Fine-needle aspiration
         a) *May be done with or without anesthesia, and blindly or with CT or ultrasound guidance*
         b) *Results*
            i) 10% malignant
            ii) 10% suspicious cytology—20% carcinoma at surgery; 30–40% adenomas
            iii) 70% benign cytology—5% may still harbor carcinoma and excision should be performed if clinical suspicion is high
            iv) 10% of aspirations yield insufficient material. Up to 50% of these turn out to be malignant and excision is warranted if repeat aspiration is inadequate.

VII. Indications for Hospitalization

A. **Clinical Signs of Thyrotoxicosis (20–40% mortality with untreated thyroid storm)**

1. Uncontrolled arrhythmia
2. Uncontrolled hypertension
3. Respiratory compromise, congestive heart failure
4. Mental status changes
5. Significant hyperthermia

B. Clinical Signs of Myxedema

1. Respiratory compromise, hypoxia, congestive heart failure
2. Mental status changes (myxedema madness or myxedema wit)
3. Severe bradycardia, hypotension
4. Hypothermia

VIII. Indications for Referral to Endocrinology

A. All patients of physicians who are unfamiliar or uncomfortable with the diagnosis and management of thyroid disorders.

B. Inability to interpret abnormal thyroid function test results.

C. Thyrotoxicosis requiring rapid treatment

D. Myxedema requiring rapid T_4 replacement, especially in patients who are at high risk for having complications of treatment (those with coronary artery disease, etc.).

E. Patients requiring I^{131} treatment

F. Patients who have suspicious nodules and those requiring fine-needle aspiration (this procedure is also frequently performed by ultrasonographers and surgeons).

IX. Annotated Bibliography

Cushing GW. Subclinical hypothyroidism. Postgrad Med 1993;94:95-107. Thorough review of topic. Easy to follow.

Hamburger JI. The various presentations of thyroiditis. Ann Intern Med 1986;104:219-224. A complete review of the various forms and presentations of thyroiditis.

Hammings JF, Goslings BM, vanSteenis GJ, et al. The value of fine-needle aspiration biopsy in patients with nodular thyroid disease divided into groups of suspicion of malignant neoplasms on clinical grounds. Arch Intern Med 1990;150:113-116. Review of risks for thyroid cancer and rationale for fine-needle aspiration.

Helfand M, Crapo LM. Monitoring therapy in patients taking levo thyroxine. Ann Intern Med 1990;112:840-849.

Helfand M, Crapo LM. Testing for suspected thyroid disease. In: Soc HC Jr, ed. Common diagnostic tests: use and interpretation, 2nd ed. Philadelphia: American College of Physicians, 1990:174.

Good, easy to read overview of disorders of the thyroid. Includes a good review of thyroid physiology.

Wool MS. Thyroid nodules. Postgrad Med 1993;94:111-122. Excellent flow chart on which to base patient selection for fine-needle aspiration.

Part VIII:
Foot Problems

Chapter 43: Hyperkeratotic Lesions (Corns and Calluses)

Arthur E. Helfand

I. Clinical Presentation

A. General Information

1. The primary hyperkeratotic lesions involving the foot are mechanically induced.

2. They can generally be classified as follows:

   a. Tyloma, or callus—a diffuse and broad based hyperkeratosis
   b. Heloma durum, or hard corn—hyperkeratosis with a deeper central core due to excessive pressure, either internal or external
   c. Heloma molle, or soft corn—an interdigital hyperkeratosis softened by excessive perspiration (since hyperkeratosis is hydrophilic)
   d. Heloma miliare, or seed corn—pin-point hyperkeratosis due to concentrated pressure
   e. Heloma vasculare, vascular corn—hyperkeratosis that contains minimal interstitial hemorrhage or hematomas due to intense trauma or pressure. Also common in diabetics due to angiopathy.
   f. Heloma neurofibrosum, or neurofibrous corn—hyperkeratosis containing a neural filament related to trauma and tissue herniation.
   g. Intractable plantar keratosis—hyperkeratosis with an encapsulated central core, verrucoid in character, as a result of intense long-standing microtrauma and pressure
   h. Onychophosis—callus in the nail grooves or periungual area

2. Hyperkeratotic lesions in the adult are usually related to tissue trauma. This trauma may be the result of

   a. Physiologic changes in the skin
   b. Morphologic variations in anatomic structure
   c. Inappropriate footwear
   d. Environmental factors, such as flat, hard surfaces
   e. Changes in gait
   f. Atrophy of foot musculature
   g. Any other form of repeated tissue trauma

3. Hyperkeratosis is a normal body defense and is found on other parts of the body. However, because of weight-bearing and ambulation, these lesions may become painful and gait may be altered to relieve pain.

B. Symptoms

1. The primary complaint is pain, particularly on ambulation. The pain varies with intensity and is related to the degree of keratotic buildup.

2. Ambulation is often altered as a compensation for associated atrophy and bony deformities, such as digity flexus, hallux valgus, and metatarsal prolapse.

C. Physical Examination

1. Tyloma (callus) are usually diffuse and generally involve the plantar surface of the foot. Primary locations include the ball, marginal heel, and distal toes. Tyloma may also be present dorsally as an early sign of heloma.

2. Heloma durum, or hard corns, usually present with a deeper central conical area. They may also be demonstrated with tyloma.

3. Heloma molle are soft lesions and are found interdigitally. They are soft due to maceration and are usually located at opposing bony surfaces where they are subjected to compressive stress.

4. Heloma miliare are small, circumscribed, seed-sized lesions at points of great stress. Often, this occurs due to some mechanical alteration in shoe construction.

5. Heloma vasculare and heloma neurofibrosum are somewhat circumscribed and invaded by a small vascular component or nerve fiber. They tend to be more painful and appear wartlike.

6. Intractable keratotic lesions are circumscribed, wartlike but devoid of bleeding points. They are cornified, painful, and well demarcated.

7. Onychophosis in the adult is a callus formation in the nail grooves and is associated with nail deformities such as onychauxis, onychogryphosis, pincer nails, and onychomycosis. Subungual heloma are keratotic areas that form as a result of a dorsal bony abnormality on the distal phalanx, which produces compression of the soft tissues under the nail plate.

II. Diagnostic Approach and Differential Diagnosis

A. The primary differential diagnosis with heloma is verruca.

1. With the exception of intractable keratoses, most hyperkeratotic lesions are not encapsulated, meaning that they do not have skin whirls or lines passing over the hyperkeratosis.

2. They also do not contain pinpoint bleeding.

3. Xerosis and keratotic tinea are also in the differential diagnosis.

B. Efforts should be made to identify the etiologic factors. If intrinsic morphologic variations and deformities are suspected, radiographic weight- and non–weight-bearing studies should be obtained.

C. The complications associated with hyperkeratotic lesions should be carefully looked for. These are of particular concern in the presence of systemic diseases such as diabetes mellitus, which may involve sensory deficits and vascular insufficiency. In these patients, the keratosis produces pressure and creates local avascularity. Primary concerns include:

1. Infection
2. Ulceration
3. Fibrosis
4. Bursal enlargement
5. Sinus formation
6. Dermal protrusions
7. Fissures
8. Furrowing

D. Painful keratotic lesions are not normal. They all have a complex set of etiologic factors that have as a common thread repeated microtrauma, diminished hydration and lubrication, morphologic variation, and environmental change.

III. Treatment

A. Initial Management

1. Debridement of the hyperkertotic tissue using either instruments or dermabrasive procedures. Initial debridement may uncover a shallow ulcer if the pressure has been long-standing.
2. The initial dressing should provide protection and help reduce pressure. Materials that can be used include moleskin, foam rubber, polyform, and tube foam, as well as weight diffusion and dispersion procedures to reduce pressure to painful areas.
3. Instruct the patient to use emollients to provide skin softening. Examples include 10–20% urea, 5–12% ammonium lactate, lanolin products. The emollients should be used following a bath or shower to increase both hydration and lubrication.
4. Depending on the location of the lesion, plantar padding is useful to diffuse and disperse weight from painful areas.
5. Shoe modifications may be required if the shoes are a causative factor.
6. If deformities exist, conservative management can also include orthotics to reduce stress.
7. Onychophosis requires management of the nail deformities and the use of emollients. Where the onychial deformity is severe, surgical revision of the nail plate may be required. Silicone molds and certain types of shoe padding also may be useful to reduce digital pressure.

B. Long-term Management

1. Long-term management depends on the patient response to initial and subsequent care.
2. Additional therapy is based on the etiologic factors, radiographic review, and degree of pain. Surgical revision may be necessary, especially when there is a clear osseous abnormality or deformity.

C. Patient Education

1. Warn the patient not to attempt any self-reduction of keratotic tissue with sharp instruments and not to use commercial corn or callus removers.
2. Many excellent booklets are available dealing with primary foot care (see Bibliography).

IV. Indications for Referral to Podiatrist

The patient should be referred to a podiatrist if the extent of debridement exceeds the physician's expertise and pressure-reducing measures are indicated.

V. Indications for Hospitalization

Hospitalization is not required unless complications such as infection develop, usually related to systemic diseases such as diabetes mellitus. Hospitalization may be required for surgical revision.

VI. Annotated Bibliography

Birrer RB, DellaCorte MP, Grisafi PJ, eds. Common Foot Problems in Primary Care. Philadelphia: Hanley and Belfus; 1992. A multidisciplinary textbook that addresses problems commonly seen in a primary care setting.

Harkless LB, Krych SM. Handbook of Common Foot Problems. New York: Churchill Livingstone; 1990. This text approaches foot problems from both a primary care and podiatric orientation.

Helfand AE, ed. Clinical Podogeriatrics. Baltimore: Williams & Wilkins; 1981. A multidisciplinary text with a primary focus on the older patient with foot problems.

Hefland AE. Feet First. Pennsylvania Professional Diabetes Academy, 7717 East Park Drive, Harrisburg, PA, 17105–8820. An excellent patient educational booklet on foot care.

Neale D, Adams IM, eds. Common Foot Disorders, 3rd ed. Edinburgh: Churchill Livingstone; 1989. A primary foot care text developed in the United Kingdom.

Yale JF. Yale's Podiatric Medicine, 3rd ed. Baltimore: Williams & Wilkins, 1987. The third edition of a textbook that comprehensively addresses primary foot care needs.

Chapter 44: Foot Pain

Arthur E. Helfand

44A Digital Deformities

I. Hallux Valgus (Bunion Deformity)

A. General Information

1. Mechanism of deformity—There is a progressive subluxation of the first metatarsal-phalangeal joint. This results in a lateral deviation of the hallux associated with and secondary to medial deviation of the first metatarsal, called metatarsus varus primus.

2. Enlargement of the first metatarsal head results in soft tissue inflammation, increasing the degree of deformity and symptoms. As the deformity progresses, the joint capsule contracts, tendons are displaced, and the plantar sesamoids deviate laterally.

3. As a result of chronic pressure, capsulitis and bursitis can occur. Where pressure is prolonged, hyperkeratosis may form, which can cause counterpressure, local tissue ischemia, atrophy, and ulceration.

4. The pain is usually inflammatory in origin, resulting in ambulatory dysfunction.

5. Other factors may be related to the development of hallux valgus or hallux abducto valgus. These include

   a. Morton's syndrome—a short first metatarsal
   b. Excessive pronation
   c. Contractures
   d. Varus deformity of the first metatarsal
   e. Cerebral palsy
   f. Rheumatoid arthritis
   g. Osteoarthritis
   h. Exostosis
   i. Incompatible footwear

B. Clinical Presentation

1. Evaluate for

   a. Degree of deformity
   b. Evidence of inflammation

c. Related hyperkeratotic lesions
d. Abnormalities in range of motion
e. Degree of pain
f. Radiographic appearance
g. The presence of other disease processes

2. With increasing deformity and subluxation, medial and plantar keratosis may result.

3. An overriding second toe may increase the degree of pain and deformity and increase pressure on the joints.

C. Therapy

1. Nonsurgical management

   a. Careful shoe selection to reduce direct pressure. Examples include shoes with soft, usually kid uppers, a wide and high toe box, and consideration of special lasts, such as bunion last. Thermold or custom-molded shoes can be modified to compensate for the deformity.
   b. Various forms of protective padding can be used such as felt, open and closed cell foam pads, or silicone molds to provide primary protection.
   c. Inflammation can be managed with oral anti-inflammatory agents, local steroid injection, and the use of physical therapy modalities such as ultrasound, phonophoresis, iontophoresis, and electrical stimulation.
   d. Orthotics can help compensate for dysfunction provided there is proper shoe selection.

2. Surgical management

   a. Should be based on the symptoms, primarily pain and a failure of conservative treatment
   b. The expectation of surgical revision, using any number of techniques and procedures, is to provide a foot that looks cosmetically correct.
   c. Repair of the deformity without appropriate consideration of the etiologic biomechanical factors will result in recurrence.

II. Hallux Limitus and Hallux Rigidus

A. General Information and Clinical Presentation

1. Hallux limitus and rigidus are essentially monoarticular degenerative arthritidies involving the first metatarsal-phalangeal joint.

2. If dorsal and dorsal-medial spurring is minimal to moderate and some motion is demonstrable, the term limitus is used. If the deformity is severe and motion is almost eliminated, the term rigidus is used.

3. Pain is the primary factor early, with limitation of motion increasing with the degree of joint change.

4. The etiology usually involves repetitive trauma to the joint related to extension.

5. Radiographs, particularly lateral, will demonstrate the degree of spurring.
6. As the spurring worsens on the first metatarsal head, a mechanical locking and irritation occurs, which creates inflammation and pain.

B. Therapy

1. Initial management includes
   a. Oral anti-inflammatory agents
   b. Local steroid injections
   c. Physical therapy modalities as mentioned in I.C. above

2. Efforts must be made to reduce the degree of extension of the joint. These include
   a. Padding
   b. Devices that bridge the joint, such as silicone molds and orthotics
   c. Shoe modifications such as a steel plate placed between the midsole and outsole, from sulcus to sulcus, to restrict motion.

3. Where pain becomes significant and the reduction of motion impairs function, surgical revision of the joint should be considered.

III. Hammer Toe, Claw Toe, and Mallet Toe

A. General Information

1. Hammer toe
   a. Is a flexion deformity involving the proximal interphalangeal joint of the lesser toes. Some rotational deformity is also usually noted, especially as lateral digits are involved.
   b. The middle and distal phalanges become increasingly plantar flexed and progressive enlargement of the head of the proximal phalanges results.

2. Claw toe—is a variation of hammer toe with a hyperextension at the metatarsal-phalangeal joint and a bow string appearance of the extensor tendons on the dorsum of the foot.

3. Mallet toe—is a flexion deformity of the distal interphalangeal joint, with the distal phalanx flexed on the middle phalangeal joint

B. Etiology and Clinical Presentation

1. Etiologies may be multifactorial
   a. Atrophy of the interossei may result in contracture of the lesser toes, with anterior displacement of the metatarsal fat pad and metatarsal head prolapse.
   b. Trauma and fractures
   c. Congenital anomalies
   d. Connective tissue diseases, eg, rheumatoid or psoriatic arthritis

e. Neurologic disorders, eg, cerebral palsy, muscular dystrophy, postpolio, and poststroke
f. Improper shoes—Cramping of feet into confined spaces may cause contracture.

2. Clinical Presentation

   a. Hyperkeratotic lesions and pressure ulcerations are usually the factors that cause the patient to seek care. Limited flexibility and deformity increase pain and restrict function.
   b. In mallet toe, hyperkeratosis and pain develop as a result of increased weight-bearing on the distal rather than ball of the toes. Pressure ulceration is again a factor.
   c. For all of these deformities, contracture of the dorsal tendons may occur, and with long-standing deformity, subluxation of the joint and restricted motion and rigidity result.
   d. The deformities are well demonstrated radiographically. Radiographs will demonstrate the degree of change, subluxation, and bony abnormality.

C. Therapy

1. Initial care involves supportive and protective measures and the management of any hyperkeratotic and/or ulcerative lesions.

   a. Shoes should have an adequate toe box and if needed, extra depth, soft uppers, and modifications to conform to the deformity. Any protective measures without adequate toe box area modification often exaggerate the condition.
   b. Metatarsal pads and soft Plastazote shoe liners add additional protection. Lamb's wool, tube foam, felt padding, silicone molds, and crest pads can provide comfort.
   c. Exercise should be suggested to maintain the maximum degree of mobility.
   d. Metatarsalgia, anterior metatarsal bursitis, and capsulitis are additional considerations in symptoms and management.
   e. Given the chronicity of these conditions, management must be considered long term.

2. Surgery

   a. Surgical considerations includes both tendon and joint revision, based on the degree of deformity, pain, rigidity, as well as consideration of all of the etiologic factors.
   b. Postoperative splinting and protective measures are essential to minimize recurrence.

3. If the factors that cause the deformity are not considered and managed or modified, recurrence is probable.

44B Anterior Foot Pain

I. Sesamoid Disorders

A. General Information and Clinical Presentation

1. Sesamoid disorders, involving the two sesamoids under the first metatarsal head usually include
   a. Inflammation resulting in sesamoiditis
   b. Related degenerative changes
   c. The possibility of fracture due to minor trauma

2. Pain, swelling, inflammation, and a podalgic gait are the most common findings.

3. With fracture, the symptoms reported are sudden pain that progresses, without any apparent history of acute trauma.

4. Radiographs and other imaging procedures can usually identify the site. Bilateral studies may be needed to also focus on bipartite sesamoids.

B. Therapy

1. Immobilization is important, depending on the degree of the patient's symptoms. Modalities include
   a. Casting
   b. Surgical shoes
   c. Felt padding

2. Inflammation, which is usually related to deformities and biomechanical and pathomechanical changes, as well as repetitive microtrauma usually responds to
   a. Analgesics
   b. Local steroid injections for inflammation
   c. Local physical modalities
   d. Weight redistribution with pads, such as the Dancer's pad or orthotics

3. Efforts to protect the area should continue to prevent recurrence.

4. True union of the sesamoid may not occur, but the residual fragments may not cause pain or limit function if weight redistribution can be achieved.

II. Metatarsalgia

A. General Information

1. Metatarsalgia is not a specific diagnostic category, but rather refers to pain in the plantar forepart or anterior segment of the foot, usually at or anterior to the metatarsal head area.

2. It best describes pain of nonsystemic origin associated with chronic disorders in weight-bearing that affect weight diffusion and weight dispersion.

3. These changes in weight-bearing may result in atrophy or anterior displacement of the plantar fat pad, and inflammation of the soft tissue structures, such as bursitis or capsulitis.

4. There is usually some digital contracture and prolapse of the metatarsal heads with possible change in the morphologic length pattern of the metatarsals.

B. Etiologic Considerations

1. Morton's syndrome—is an anatomic variation, with a short first metatarsal segment with hypermobility, and resulting increased weight-bearing on the second metatarsal head. Cortical thickening of the second metatarsal shaft results and pain is usually associated with anterior metatarsal bursitis.

2. Hallux valgus, limitus, and rigidus, as described above, may cause metatarsalgia.

3. Congenital structural deformities

4. Rheumatoid or osteoarthritis

5. Gout

6. Neuromuscular disorders such as multiple sclerosis and poststroke contractures

7. Sesamoiditis, stress fractures, and trauma also are contributing factors.

8. Excessive pressure from improper shoe protection and selection may result in weight maldistribution and misdistribution. Environmental factors such as walking on hard flat surfaces may be a factor as well.

9. Hammer toes

C. Therapy

1. Management should be directed at the etiology.

2. Pain can be controlled with nonsteroidal anti-inflammatory drugs, local steroid injections for acute pinpoint pain, physical modalities, and shoe modifications.

3. Anterior heels and metatarsal bars as well as rocker bottoms can be helpful, depending on the etiology of the metatarsalgia, symptoms, and response to initial measures.

4. Foot orthoses include metatarsal bands, digital splints, silicone molds, crest pads, weight diffusion and dispersion plantar molds, metatarsal pads, and cushioning material.

5. Physical modalities include heat, ultrasound, phonophoresis, iontophoresis, muscle-stimulating currents, and exercise.

6. When conservative management of the pain fails, surgical approaches should be considered. These should be directed to the specific etiology of the pain and deformity.

III. Tailor's Bunion

A. General Information

1. Tailor's bunion is described as a valgus deviation of the fifth metatarsal, with varus deviation of the fifth toe and enlargement of the head of the fifth metatarsal.

2. This condition is at times referred to as a bunionette.

3. Pain is associated with inflammatory changes that are exaggerated by shoe pressure.

4. There may be associated bursal formation. This can be large and with deformity and pressure, hyperkeratosis develops.

B. Therapy

1. Management should include radiographs, debridement of hyperkeratotic lesions, protective padding, local steroid injections, physical modalities, and shoe modification or change.

2. With persistent pain and limitation of mobility, as well as hypertrophy and deformity, surgical revision can be considered.

44C Posterior Foot Pain

I. Pes Cavus

A. General Information

1. Pes cavus is a deformity characterized by an excessively high medial longitudinal arch. There is an equinus relationship of the forefoot to the rearfoot.
2. With age, the symptoms and problem progress and discomfort increases. Contracture of the plantar aponeurosis with clawing of the toes becoming more fixed with time and distal migration of the plantar fat pad occurs.
3. These changes can result in a decreased total weight-bearing area of the foot and a decrease in flexibility.
4. Neurologic disorders may be the cause and should be explored.
5. Certain systemic diseases are present that place the patient at increased risk, such as diabetes mellitus. In these patients, plantar ulcerations are more common with their related complications.

B. Therapy

1. Management includes methods to prevent the progression of the deformity, support (shoes and orthoses), increasing muscle balance, and correcting painful bone deformities as indicated.
2. Physical modalities, cushioning inserts, metatarsal bars, shoe modifications, and rocker bottoms may all be of help.
3. Surgical revision may become necessary when conservative measures do not relieve symptoms

II. Pes Planus

A. General Information

1. Pes planus represents a lowering or flattening of the medial longitudinal arch.
2. There are multiple varieties. Examples include asymptomatic, flexible, peroneal spastic, congenital, and acquired due to pronation or the residual of direct trauma.
3. Symptoms may occur, including pain, tiredness, and recurrent sprains, although the deformity itself may be functionally normal.
4. Radiographs provide a clinical mechanism to correlate symptoms with measurements.

B. Therapy

1. Management depends on the symptoms rather than the physical finding associated with a lowering of the arch.

2. Excessive pronation can be managed with appropriate shoe modifications and the use of orthotics.
3. Cushioning inserts are helpful.
4. Anti-inflammatory medications may decrease pain.
5. Physical modalities such as whirlpool, ultrasound, and muscle-stimulating currents are useful.
6. Surgical repair depends on the nonresponse to conservative measures and radiographic findings that support the criteria for more definitive management.

III. Neuralgia, Neuritis, and Neuroma

A. General Information and Clinical Presentation

1. Neuralgia, neuritis, and neuroma generally produce similar symptoms, with the diagnosis based on nonresponse to therapy. Long-standing inflammation results in pain, which leads to neuralgia, then neuritis, and finally neuroma
2. Pain is usually reported as a tingling and lightning-like pain between the toes, extending from the metatarsal area to the end of the toes.
3. Compression is a key factor. Nerve entrapment is also felt to be a key mechanism that explains the clinical findings.
4. Disorders that need to be ruled out before labeling the symptoms idiopathic include
   a. Tarsal tunnel nerve entrapment
   b. Lumbar disc disease
   c. Localized inflammatory disorders such as synovitis or fasciitis
5. Before therapy, radiographs should be obtained, to determine metatarsal head position, particularly comparing weight-bearing with non–weight-bearing positions.

B. Therapy

1. Initial management includes
   a. A wide shoe last
   b. Local injections of anesthetics or steroids
   c. Physical therapy modalities
   d. A reverse metatarsal pad to change the position of the intermetatarsal head relationships
2. If the pain recurs shortly after injection with local anesthetic and steroids, then the potential for neuroma formation is greater.
3. If conservative therapy fails to relieve the symptoms and other diagnoses have been eliminated, then surgical excision should be considered. The removal of any nerve compression is an essential element in the treatment.

IV. Bursitis, Capsulitis, Tendonitis, and Tenosynovitis

A. General Information and Clinical Presentation

1. These disorders are the result of soft tissue inflammation due to repetitive trauma.
2. Bursal formation and capsulitis may occur in any joint area. Tendonitis and tenosynovitis produce pain and limitation of motion.

B. Therapy

1. Initial management includes local steroid injections, physical therapy modalities such as ultrasound, phonophoresis, and iontrophoresis, and the reduction of pressure.
2. Anti-inflammatory drugs are quite effective. Efforts then need to be made to prevent pressure areas.
3. If the etiology is shoe related, such as pressure from metal eyelets on the extensor hallucis tendon, eyelet removal can easily be accomplished and felt pads used.

44D Heel Pain

I. Haugland's Deformity, Albert's Disease, False Albert's Disease

A. General Information and Clinical Presentation

1. Haugland's deformity represents an enlargement of the osseous segment of the posterior-dorsal area of the calcaneus. It presents with pain due to from shoe counterpressure.

2. When a retro-Achilles bursa forms between the calcaneus and Achilles tendon, it is termed Albert's disease.

3. With bursal formation between the Achilles tendon and skin, the term is false Albert's disease. All are many times referred to as "pump bumps."

4. Radiographs should be obtained to identify any bone change.

B. Therapy

1. Management includes anti-inflammatory drugs, local steroids, and physical modalities to relieve inflammation.

2. Efforts should be made to change the relationship between the posterior shoe counter and the calcaneal area. Counter pads, heel pads, and orthotics as well as a change in shoe last or style are useful modalities.

3. These conditions can usually be managed without surgical revision.

II. Plantar Fasciitis and Calcaneal Spur

A. General Information and Clinical Presentation

1. These disorders represent a common painful complaint. The usual symptoms include a report of pain on arising and initial ambulation. There may be some lessening as the day progresses but within hours, discomfort, pain, and limited mobility usually return.

2. If bursitis is present, pain is usually acute and localized at the intersection of the plantar fascia along the medial aspect of the calcaneus.

3. The presence of periostitis and spur formation indicate chronic, long-standing inflammation.

4. Radiographs and occassionally bone scans are helpful both for diagnosis and to rule out etiologies for the pain such as fractures, infections, neoplasms, and arthritis.

B. Therapy

1. An important aspect of management is rest to minimize weight-bearing.

2. Physical therapy modalities such as ice, massage, ultrasound, and stretching exercises are also useful.

3. Changing the position of the calcaneus to a more superior, lateral, and posterior alignment is helpful to reduce stress on the medial calcaneal tuberosity. Orthotic devices include heel cups (soft and rigid), heel lifts, Plastazote inserts, and other means of changing the calcaneal position. Night splints may also be of value.

4. Choosing appropriate footwear or modification of shoes is essential given the stress-related etiology.

5. Anti-inflammatory oral drugs and local steroid injections, usually with local anesthetic, provide relief of the acute pain.

6. If the cause of stress on the heel is not addressed, symptoms will recur.

7. If symptoms persist for 8–12 mo and there is a failure to all conservative measures, surgical therapies are an option.

44E Assorted Other Foot Pain Disorders

I. Subungual Exostoses and Spurs

A. General Information and Clinical Presentation

1. Subungual exostosis and spurs produce significant pain and subsequent nail deformity.
2. Lateral radiographs of the distal phalanx should demonstrate an exostosis, spur, or deformity of the tufted end of the distal phalanx. The usual site is the hallux.

B. Therapy

1. Management consists of reducing nail plate pressure, the use of protection such as tube foam and lamb's wool, and a high toe box shoe.
2. If pain can not be resolved, excision of the bony abnormality is indicated.

II. Rheumatologic Diseases

A. General Information

1. Rheumatologic diseases, such as osteoarthritis, rheumatoid arthritis, gout, and psoriatic arthritis can produce acute and residual changes in the foot. Their diagnosis and management will not be addressed in detail here.
2. It is, however, important to be aware that with weight-bearing and repetitive trauma, in combination with existing pathomechanical and biomechanical changes in the foot, symptoms and findings can be potentiated.
3. In addition to appropriate medication and physical therapy measures, consideration should be given to the role of orthotics, footwear, and local care in relieving pain, restoring a maximum level of function, and maintaining that function so that the quality of life can be maintained.

III. Annotated Bibliography

Evans JG, Williams TF, eds. Oxford Textbook of Geriatric Medicine. Oxford: Oxford University Press; 1992. The first edition of a comprehensive geriatric textbook covering the primary care of foot problems.

Helfand AE, ed. The Geriatric Patient and Considerations of Aging. Clinics in Podiatric Medicine and Surgery, vol I, January 1993, vol II, April 1993. This double volume addresses the management of foot problems in the older patient.

Levy LA, Heatherington VJ, eds. Principles and Practice of Podiatric Medicine. New York: Churchill Livingstone; 1990. A comprehensive review of the management of foot problems and related issues.

Pathy MSJ, ed. Principles and Practice of Geriatric Medicine, 2nd ed. Chichester, United Kingdom: John Wiley & Sons; 1991. This text is from the United Kingdom, with some American contributors, and addresses foot care in the geriatric patient.

Chapter 45: Foot Care in the Diabetic Patient

Arthur E. Helfand

I. Clinical Presentation: History and Physical

A. General Information

1. Amputations are many times more common among patients with diabetes than among nondiabetic patients.

2. Preventive measures can result in a 50–75% reduction in the number of diabetic persons who require amputation.

3. Diabetic foot problems and complications usually result from peripheral vascular disease, resulting in a decreased blood supply, and neuropathy, resulting in loss of sensitivity of the feet. Changes related to use, abuse, and coexisting diseases are additional risk factors.

4. The loss of sensitivity results in deformity, which is magnified by pathomechanical and biomechanical changes. This fosters the development of foot ulceration due to pressure and local vascular ischemia.

5. Preventing amputation and providing primary foot care includes the identification of the at-risk diabetic patient, preventing ulcerations, treating ulceration, and preventing their recurrence.

6. Local tissue trauma contributes to the etiology of ulcer formation. Three primary areas of trauma include

   a. Mechanical—improper and incompatible shoes and inappropriate and improper home treatments
   b. Thermal—electric pads, hot foot baths, and hot water bottles
   c. Chemical—strong antiseptics and keratolytic agents found in most commercial "corn remedies"

B. Symptoms

1. Symptoms of vascular insufficiency may include

   a. Lower extremity claudication and foot pain, particularly on ambulation
   b. Decreased temperature and cyanotic appearance of the foot
   c. Sensory symptoms such as paresthesias and numbness
   d. Swelling of the foot
   e. Failure of wounds and superficial ulcers to heal

2. Symptoms of diabetic neuropathy may include

   a. Paresthesia
   b. Hyperesthesia or hypoesthesia
   c. Nocturnal cramps
   d. Reduction and/or loss of pain and temperature sensation

C. **Physical Examination**

1. The clinical findings associated with arterial impairment include

   a. Color changes (rubor or cyanosis)
   b. Xerosis
   c. Atrophy of the plantar fat pad
   d. Edema
   e. Absent pedal pulses
   f. Coldness associated with vasospasm
   g. Trophic skin changes such as a decrease or absence of hair growth or thin, shiny skin texture
   h. Dystrophic nail changes

2. The clinical findings associated with diabetic neuropathy include

   a. Decreased pain and temperature sensation
   b. Decreased vibratory sense
   c. Decreased proprioception
   d. Loss of deep tendon reflexes
   e. Anhidrosis
   f. Tendon contractures with claw or hammer toes
   g. Peroneal nerve involvement with drop foot

3. The primary dermatologic findings include

   a. Excoriations secondary to pruritis
   b. Bacterial and/or fungal cutaneous infections
   c. Dermal atrophy and loss of elasticity
   d. Hyperkeratosis due to pathomechanical and biomechanical changes from repetitive microtrauma
   e. Fissures
   f. Ulceration
   g. Necrobiosis lipoidica diabeticorum
   h. Idiopathic bullae

4. Many nail changes may occur in diabetic patients. Examples include

   a. Paronychia
   b. Onychomycosis
   c. Diabetic onychopathy with subungual hemorrhage
   d. Involution or pincer nails
   e. Thickening of the eponychium

5. Deformities may exist in relation to foot function. Examples include

   a. Hallux valgus

b. Hallux limitus
   c. Hammer toes
   d. Digital rotations
   e. Metatarsal prolapse

II. Diagnostic Approach

A. Assessment of the diabetic patient at risk for foot problems includes obtaining a detailed history to include

1. A history of foot problems and prior care

2. Pain, either at rest or with ambulation

3. Temperature changes, either cold or hot

4. Paresthesias—loss of pain perception

5. Weakness and a loss of position sense

6. Slow healing wounds

7. Any change in shoe size. Patients with diabetic neuropathy may purchase and wear tight footwear to have a feeling of shoes on their feet. A larger size may indicate recognized deformity and a smaller size might demonstrate a loss of sensation.

B. Radiographic examination of the foot may reveal changes in the diabetic patient. These include

1. Thin trabecular bone

2. Changes in bone growth

3. Decalcification

4. Arthropathy

5. Arthritic changes with destruction and deformity

6. Osteophyte formations

7. Osteolysis

8. Osteoporosis

C. Lower-risk diabetic patients are identified as those who

1. Maintain their protective sensation

2. Do not present with hammer toe deformities

3. Do not exhibit any signs of neuropathy, either motor or sensory

4. Maintain adequate skin tone

5. The lower-risk patient should be examined periodically with sensory testing and radiographs as indicated, Doppler studies as necessary, as well as notations of changes in skin and toe nail structures and deformities.

D. **The medium-risk diabetic patient is defined by**

1. The absence of ulceration
2. The presence of structural changes discussed above, such as hammer toes, hallux valgus, onychial abnormalities, and onychomycosis.
3. Gait changes or abnormal shoe wear
4. The higher-risk patient should be evaluated more frequently and at regular intervals for additional signs of vascular impairment and/or neuropathy. Knowledge of preventive measures should also be reinforced.

E. **The high-risk patient is defined by**

1. The presence of ulceration
2. The presence of neuropathy and arterial occlusive changes
3. Any patient with a history of prior ulceration should also be considered high risk.

III. Treatment

A. Lower-Risk Patient

1. Shoe selection, personal hygiene, and protective modalities form the basis for early care.
2. Treat hyperkeratotic lesions and nail dystrophies, deformities, and diseases.
3. Make appropriate modifications as required to manage early and existing deformities.

B. Medium-Risk Patient

1. Assess for neuropathic and arterial occlusive changes.
2. If ulcerations are not present, take necessary steps to minimize trauma, especially to contracted toes, deformities, and to the plantar surface. Materials such as Plastazote, PPT, and Spenco are examples of some of the modalities available.
3. Appropriate shoe selection is quite important. Special shoes such as the Thermold or Custom Molded shoes are alternatives.
4. Specialized orthotics can also be constructed to help reduce pressure to at-risk areas of the foot.
5. Appropriate emollients may be used for anhidrosis and/or xerosis. 10–20% urea compounds and 5–12% ammonium lactate compounds are reasonable approaches to management.

6. Tinea should be controlled with topical fungicides. Onychomycosis should be considered as evidence of residual tinea infection.

7. Silicone molds/braces can be used to help manage digital contractures.

C. Diabetic Foot Ulcers

1. Evaluate diabetic ulcers for
   a. Ulcer size—length, width and depth
   b. Tissue appearance—color and texture
   c. Exudate—amount, color, odor
   d. The condition of surrounding tissues
   e. The presence of necrotic tissue and eschar
   f. Evidence of infections such as cellulitis or abscess

2. Examine the base carefully, because it provides information on the vascular supply as well as infection.

3. Consider hospitalization if there are systemic signs of infection.

4. Obtain radiographic examination looking for bony changes, infection, gas, osteolysis, or osteomyelitis with frank bone loss. If plain films are nondiagnostic and infection is suspected, consider either bone scan or MRI.

5. Prevent excessive pressure on the ulcer and other areas of the foot. Modalities include
   a. Contact casts
   b. Crutches
   c. Walkers to limit weight-bearing
   d. Prescription shoes
   e. Orthotics
   f. Bed rest
   g. Heel and ankle protectors

6. Wound care includes
   a. Surgical debridement of necrotic and nongranulating tissue and callus tissue
   b. Incision and drainage of abscesses
   c. Sterile dressings
   d. Consideration of enzymatic debridement with growth factor application

7. Evaluate vascular adequacy with appropriate arterial studies. Consider need for arterial revascularization.

8. Patient education is essential

IV. Indications for Referral

A. Referral to a podiatrist—for primary foot assessment, ongoing care, and patient education

B. Referral to a vascular surgeon—if revascularization is potentially indicated

C. Referral to general or orthopedic surgeon—if surgical procedures, such as bone biopsy, debridement, or amputation, potentially indicated

D. Referral to physiatrist—for rehabilitation related to lower extremity deformity or amputation.

V. Indications for Hospitalization

A. If IV antibiotics are required for deep-seated infection or osteomyelitis

B. If extensive surgical debridement is necessary

C. If arterial revascularization is planned

VI. Annotated Bibliography

American Diabetes Association. Diabetic Foot Care. Alexandria, VA; 1990. This is the current basic guide of the ADA's Foot Care Council.

Department of Health and Human Services, Public Health Service. The Prevention and Treatment of Complications of Diabetes, A Guide for Primary Care Practitioners. Atlanta: Centers for Disease Control and Prevention, NCCDPHP; 1991. This information from the Public Health Service provides basic information on the major complications, including foot care, for primary care practitioners.

Frykberg RG, ed. The High Risk Foot in Diabetes Mellitus. New York: Churchill Livingstone; 1991. A multidisciplinary text addressing diabetic foot problems and their treatment.

Helfand AE. Feet First—A Booklet about Foot Care for Older People with Diabetes. Harrisburg: Pennsylvania Professional Diabetes Academy, Pennsylvania Medical Society; 1992. A patient education booklet designed to teach diabetic patients about foot health and care. (See Bibliography in Chapter 43 for address.)

Levin ME, O'Neal LW, Bowker JJ. The Diabetic Foot, 5th ed. St. Louis: CV Mosby; 1993. The fifth edition of a multidisciplinary text that addresses diabetic foot problems.

Part IX:
Gastroenterology

Chapter 46: Acute Nausea and Vomiting

David S. Weinberg and Christine Laine

I. Clinical Presentation

A. General Information

1. In the approach to the patient with acute nausea and vomiting, it is crucial to clearly define the nature of the patient's complaint. The physician must differentiate nausea and vomiting from

   a. Regurgitation
      1) Act by which ingested food is brought back to the mouth without the associated autonomic/motor findings of vomiting
      2) Suggests gastroesophageal reflux or esophageal obstruction
   b. Anorexia
      1) Loss of urge to eat
      2) Patients with nausea and vomiting may still experience urge to eat
   c. Early satiety
      1) Feeling of being full after eating small amount of food

2. History should cover the following points

   a. Acute versus chronic (≤ 2 wk of symptoms)
   b. Nature of vomitus
      1) Digested
      2) Undigested (achalasia, esophageal diverticulum)
      3) Bilious (suggests open pylorus)
   c. Timing of vomiting
      1) Immediately or soon after eating (gastric or esophageal obstruction or psychogenic causes)
      2) Several hours after eating (gastroparesis or intestinal motility disorder)
   d. Previous history of peptic ulcer disease or diabetes mellitus
   e. Potential pregnancy
   f. Time of day—nausea and vomiting in AM before eating (pregnancy, postgastrectomy, uremia, ETOH)
   g. Medications (see below)
   h. Pain
      1) Severe, noncramping (obstruction, peritoneal irritation)
      2) Crampy with diarrhea (infection)
      3) No pain (infection, toxin, drug)
   i. Fever, myalgia, history of questionable food ingestion (virus, toxin)

B. Physical Examination

1. Vital signs, evidence of orthostasis, volume depletion, weight change
2. Abdominal examination looking for clues to underlying pathology—tenderness, mass, bowel sounds, hernia, rebound, guarding, Murphy's sign (cholecystitis), succussion splash (gastric outlet obstruction)
3. Rectal examination looking for mass, tone, blood
4. Neurologic examination looking for signs of CNS etiology—photophobia, meningismus, papilledema, nystagmus

II. Diagnostic Approach

A. History and Physical Examination (as above)

B. Diagnostic Algorithm: Acute nausea and vomiting with

1. Associated systemic symptoms (fever, malaise, diarrhea)?
   a. Yes: viral (Norwalk/Hawaii), toxin, food poisoning, hepatitis (viral)
2. If no to above, could patient be pregnant?
   a. Yes: check pregnancy test
3. If no to above, is pain prominent?
   a. Yes: colic-like
      1) RUQ: Obtain abdominal ultrasound/DICIDA (HIDA) scan to rule out gallbladder or biliary disease
      2) Epigastric, lower abdominal: Obtain obstruction series to rule out small or large bowel obstruction
   b. Yes: constant-especially with radiation to back—Obtain amylase/lipase to rule out pancreatitis
   c. Yes: rebound/guarding/peritoneal signs—obtain obstruction series, potentially abdominal CT to rule out perforation with free air under diaphragm, abscess, or fluid collection
4. If no to above, inquire about complaints regarding vertigo or other CNS symptoms, or about drugs and medications.

C. Laboratory tests to consider on the basis of the history and physical findings

1. Pregnancy test
2. Liver function tests
3. Hepatitis serologies
4. Amylase/lipase
5. Stool cultures, clostridium difficile toxin

D. Imaging studies to consider

1. Abdominal radiographs (kidney-ureter-bladder) if suspicious of obstruction (dilated loops of bowel, air/fluid levels), perforation (free air under diaphragm), or pancreatitis (pancreatic calcification)

2. RUQ ultrasound if suspicious of biliary pathology

3. Upper GI series with small bowel follow-through if suspicious of gastro-esophageal obstruction, esophageal pathology, or decreased gastric emptying

4. Abdominal CT, DICIDA, lumbar puncture, or head CT may be indicated for further evaluation of intra-abdominal, biliary, or CNS pathology, respectively.

III. Differential Diagnosis

A. Infectious Etiologies

1. Suspect if associated with systemic symptoms (fever, myalgia)
   a. Nonspecific viral (Norwalk, Hawaii)
   b. Salmonella
      1) Nausea/vomiting with bloody diarrhea
   c. Food poisoning
      1) Similar symptoms in others who have ingested same food
      2) Onset of symptoms several to 24 h after ingestion
   d. Hepatitis
      1) Nausea/vomiting can occur days prior to abdominal pain and icterus. Need to consider hepatitis A, B, and C viruses, and delta superinfection in patients with either new hepatitis B or chronic hepatitis B with delta superinfection.

B. CNS Etiologies

1. Head trauma—usually evident by history

2. Meningitis—associated with fever and headache

3. Labyrinthitis—associated with vertigo

4. Migraine headache—usually evident by history

C. Visceral Pain

1. Suspect nausea and vomiting due to intra-abdominal pathology if pain is the predominant feature, pain is unusual if nausea/vomiting is due to infection, drugs, or toxins

   a. Consider peritonitis if tender abdomen with rebound or guarding
   b. Consider obstruction if waves of pain separated by pain-free periods
   c. Consider pancreatitis if epigastric pain radiating to back particularly with a history of alcohol abuse or cholelithiasis

d. Consider obstruction due to adhesions if patient has a history of abdominal surgery or inflammatory bowel disease
e. Consider cholelithiasis/cholecystitis if waxing and waning right upper quadrant pain or if positive Murphy's sign

D. Drugs

1. Oral antibiotics (particularly erythromycin)
2. Opiates
3. Digitalis
4. Theophylline
5. Chemotherapeutic agents (including the doses used to treat rheumatologic disease)
6. Dopamine agonists

The above is a list of major offenders, most drugs have been reported to cause nausea and/or vomiting in some patients.

E. Psychogenic

1. This particularly refers to eating disorders, depression, and major psychoses.
    a. Consider if inappropriate attitude toward the symptoms or if weight loss present
    b. Consider if vomiting (chronic or intermittent) is present for years
    c. Consider if vomiting begins within several bites of meal or just after conclusion of eating
    d. Despite nausea and vomiting, appetite often normal

IV. Treatment

A. General Points

1. If there is specific pathology, that pathology should be treated.
2. If infection is causing the nausea and vomiting, supportive care with fluids and electrolytes is usually sufficient. This may be in the form of clear liquids or may require IV administration, depending on level of illness and degree of dehydration.
3. If pregnancy is the cause
    a. 80% of women will have nausea without emesis, which resolves in 50% by the 15th week of gestation with no adverse pregnancy outcomes.
    b. 0.3% of women will develop hyperemesis gravidarum, which usually resolves by the end of the first trimester, but if persistent or severe may warrant IV fluids/nutrients.

4. If drugs are causing the nausea and vomiting, discontinuation of the offending medication is advocated. If drug must be continued, antiemetics can be prescribed after other causes of nausea/vomiting are ruled out.

B. Pharmacologic Therapy

1. Central-acting agents
   a. Anticholinergics (scopolamine) not recommended unless nausea and vomiting is due to motion sickness.
   b. Prochlorperazine (Compazine) 5–10 mg PO 30–60 min before meals or 25 mg per rectum q 12 h PRN
2. GI-acting agents
   a. Prokinetic drugs are helpful when drug-induced, chemotherapy, or motility disorders are the cause of nausea/vomiting
      1) Metoclopramide (Reglan) 10 mg PO t.i.d.–q.i.d.
         a) *Works via central and peripheral antidopamine effects*
         b) *Side effects in 10–20% (anxiety, insomnia, dystonia, gynecomastia)*
         c) *Elderly are most prone to side effects*
      2) Domperidone 10–20 mg PO b.i.d.–q.i.d. before meals
         a) *Peripheral antidopamine, less central effect*
         b) *Avoid H_2 blockers or antacids*
      3) Cisapride 10–20 mg PO b.i.d.–q.i.d. before meals
         a) *Cholinergic stimulant*
         b) *Avoid H_2 blockers or antacids*

V. Indications for Referral

A. Hyperemesis gravidarum (obstetrics, nutrition)

B. Cholelithiasis (surgery and/or gastroenterology for endoscopic retrograde cholangiopancreatography)

C. Pseudo-obstruction (gastroenterology)

D. Eating disorders or other causes of psychogenic vomiting (psychiatry)

E. Labyrinthitis or other CNS disease (neurology)

VI. Indications for Hospitalization

A. Evidence of mechanical obstruction

B. Peritonitis

C. In any patient in whom dehydration is due to severe vomiting, hospitalization may be needed for IV fluid administration.

VII. Annotated Bibliography

Feldman M. Nausea and vomiting. In: Sleisenger MH, Fordtran JS, eds. Gastrointestinal Disease. Philadelphia: WB Saunders; 1989:222–238. Concise discussion of nausea and vomiting.

Ouyang A. Approach to the patient with nausea and vomiting. In: Yamada T, ed. Textbook of Gastroenterology. Philadelphia: JB Lippincott; 1991:647–670. A well referenced chapter discussing pathophysiology as well as the general diagnostic approach.

Chapter 47: Bowel Symptoms

Christine Laine and David S. Weinberg

47A Constipation

I. Clinical Presentation

A. General Information

1. Definition—Patients may complain of constipation when they experience a decrease in frequency of defecation, difficulty during defecation, a decrease in stool volume, hard stool, incomplete evacuation of the rectum, and/or a change in their usual bowel habits. Because bowel habits are subject to individual, geographic, and ethnic variability, no standard definition of constipation exists. Reports suggest that persons eating an average western diet will have at least three bowel movements per week.

2. Pathophysiology

   a. Constipation can be due to environmental, systemic, colonic, or rectal factors.
   b. Constipation results from an imbalance of nonpropulsive and propulsive colonic motility.

B. History

1. A thorough history is the first step in diagnosis of the etiology of constipation.

   a. Which symptoms does the patient report?
   b. How does the patient define constipation?
   c. What is the time course of the problem?
   d. Is the patient on medications that may cause constipation?
      1) Opiates
      2) Vitamin and mineral supplements
      3) Aluminum-containing antacids
      4) Sympathomimetic agents
      5) Nonsteroidal anti-inflammatory agents
      6) Anticholinergic agents
      7) Some antihypertensive agents (calcium channel blockers, clonidine)
      8) Some antiarrhythmic agents (disopyramide)
      9) Antispasmodic agents

10) Antiparkinson agents
11) Chronic laxative abuse
   e. What are the patient's toilet habits?
      1) Do patients allow adequate time during periods of high colonic motility (morning, after meals)?

2. Symptoms—Along with the previously mentioned symptoms, patients may report
   a. Weight loss
   b. Anorexia
   c. Abdominal discomfort
   d. Passage of small amounts of liquid stool

C. Physical Examination

1. GI examination should include
   a. Abdominal palpation looking for bowel distention, retained stool, or mass lesions
   b. Rectal examination looking for fecal impaction, mass lesions, anal fissures or fistulas, hemorrhoids, rectal tone, rectal prolapse and blood in stool

2. The physical examination should also include investigation for evidence of pathology of other body systems that may lead to constipation.
   a. Neurologic examination looking for autonomic dysfunction
   b. Pelvic examination in women looking for mass lesions that may interfere with bowel function
   c. Psychosocial evaluation looking for anxiety, depression, or other emotional disturbance
   d. Evidence of thyroid or adrenal disease

II. Diagnostic Approach

A. History and physical examination will suggest whether constipation is due to anorectal disease, colonic disease, structural abnormalities, extracolonic disease, psychological factors, diet, or medications.

B. In younger adults and in persons with a clear etiology to the constipation, conservative management can safely be instituted without further evaluation.

C. In refractory cases, in older adults, or when the etiology is unclear or suggestive of pathology, the following diagnostic studies may prove helpful.

1. Complete blood count to look for anemia
2. Chemical profile to assess metabolic or adrenal disorders
3. Thyroid-stimulating hormone to assess for hypothyroidism
4. Abdominal radiographs to assess for obstruction

5. Anoscopy and/or sigmoidoscopy to assess for pathology of the anus, rectum, or sigmoid colon
6. Colonoscopy or barium enema should be performed in cases where colonic malignancy is suspected such as patients older than 50 y, when weight loss is present, when there is evidence of blood in the patient's stool or anemia
7. Colonic transit studies may be useful in patients whose primary complaint is of infrequent bowel movements.
   a. Patient ingests radiopaque markers and a high-fiber diet (30 g/d) while abstaining from laxatives or other medications that can affect bowel function.
   b. Serial abdominal radiographs monitor transit through the colon until 80% of the marker has been evacuated or for a time period of 1 w.
   c. The upper limit of normal transit time is approximately 3 d.
   d. Delayed colonic transit times indicate a physiologic cause of the constipation; normal transit times indicate a psychological or behavioral cause.
8. Anorectal manometry supplies information about internal and external sphincter function, rectal sensation and compliance, and pattern of expulsion and is particularly useful to rule out adult Hirschsprung's disease.
9. Defecatography may be useful in patients who complain of difficulty or straining during defecation.
   a. Fluoroscopy is used to monitor the patient while evacuating barium media or a ball and chain device.
   b. It provides information about completeness of evacuation, puborectalis musculature, and anatomic abnormalities of the rectum such as rectocele.

III. Differential Diagnosis

A. Environmental/Behavioral

1. Inadequate fiber in diet
2. Inadequate physical activity
3. No allowance for defecation during periods of high colonic motility
4. Psychological disorders
5. Inadequate fluid intake

B. Drug Related

1. Laxative abuse
2. Medication induced (see above list of potentially constipating drugs)

C. Metabolic, Endocrinologic, or Systemic Disease

1. Hypothyroidism
2. Adrenal insufficiency

3. Hyperparathyroidism or other cause of hypercalcemia
4. Diabetes mellitus
5. Renal failure with uremia

D. Neurologic Disease

1. Cerebrovascular accident
2. Spinal cord injury
3. Multiple sclerosis
4. Parkinson's disease
5. Idiopathic autonomic dysfunction of the intestine
6. Amyotrophic lateral sclerosis
7. Hirschsprung's disease

E. Anatomic Conditions

1. Pregnancy
2. GI tumors
3. Pelvic tumors
4. Anorectal disease (fissures, fistulas, masses)

IV. Treatment

A. Acute and Long-term Management

1. When there is a specific cause of constipation, treatment should be directed at the offending etiology such as the discontinuation of a constipating medication, treatment of hypothyroidism, surgery for a neoplasm, etc.
2. When constipation is functional in etiology, management consists of dietary, behavioral, occasional pharmacologic, and rarely surgical intervention.

    a. Dietary intervention
    1) Increase dietary fluids
    2) Increase dietary fiber to 30 g/d
        a) *Grains and cereals are the optimal means of increasing dietary fiber (1.1 oz of wheat bran provides 10 g dietary fiber)*
        b) *Fruits and vegetables are high roughage but supply less dietary fiber than grains and cereals*
        c) *Fiber supplements such as psyllium (Metamucil) or methylcellulose (Citrucel) may be helpful, but need to be taken with adequate amounts of fluid (at least 1 L/d) or they can actually exacerbate constipation.*

b. Behavioral intervention
   1) Patients must be instructed to allow time for bowel movements during periods of high colonic motility (in the morning, after meals).
   2) Physical activity will help to promote regular bowel movements.
   3) Retraining of pelvic musculature may be helpful in patients whose primary problem is outlet delay as diagnosed by manometry or defecatogram.
c. Pharmacologic therapy—The majority of patients can be managed without laxatives and these agents, especially irritant/stimulant laxatives, should be used as infrequently as possible.
   1) Stool softeners
      a) *Stool softeners (docusate salts such as Colace 100–300 mg QD) help by maintaining fecal moisture.*
      b) *Avoid preparations where stool softener is combined with an irritant laxative.*
   2) Lubricants
      a) *Mineral oil 15–30 mL PO 1–2 times per day*
      b) *Avoid in patients at risk for aspiration.*
   3) Antispasmodics
      a) *These drugs can be constipating and may be dangerous in elderly patients, but can also be helpful in treating constipation when cramping, depression, or irritable bowel exists.*
      b) *Tricyclic antidepressants start at 25 mg PO qd and increase as necessary*
   4) Osmotic agents
      a) *Nonabsorbable sugars that increase water content of feces*
      b) *Agents of choice in chronic constipation*
      c) *Lactulose, sorbitol, or mannitol 15–30 mg PO 1–2 times per day*
   5) Local agents
      a) *Enemas and suppositories*
      b) *Work by distending the rectum and colon leading to reflex evacuation*
      c) *Glycerine or tap water enemas are preferred.*
      d) *Oil retention enemas can aid disimpaction.*
      e) *Enemas/suppositories with soap suds, saline, or bisacodyl are irritants and should be avoided.*
      f) *Chronic use can lead to incontinence.*
   6) Irritant laxatives
      a) *Chronic use leads to altered colonic motility and worsening of constipation.*
      b) *Should be reserved for refractory symptoms and used only on a PRN basis*
      c) *Several classes of these agents:*
         i) Phenolphthalein-related (Correctol, Feen-a-mint, Ex-Lax, Doxidan, Dulcolax, bisacodyl)
         ii) Magnesium salts (Milk of Magnesia)
         iii) Anthraquinone derivatives (cascara, senna, Peri-Colace)

7) Investigational agents
    a) *Cisapride*
    b) *Opiate antagonists*
8) Surgery—In very rare cases when chronic constipation is due to megacolon-like changes, partial or complete colectomy may be indicated

B. Patient Education

1. Patients must be advised that prevention is the mainstay of therapy (diet and behavior).
2. Patients must be informed about the potential adverse consequences of irritant laxatives, and that OTC treatments may be counterproductive
3. Many patients fear "autointoxication" if they do not move their bowels qd; patients should be educated that bowel patterns vary and that there is a wide range of normal and that they need not fear "autointoxication."

V. Indications for Referral to a Gastroenterologist

Patients with clinical presentations that raise the suspicion of GI pathology (blood loss, sudden change in bowel patterns, symptoms refractory to usual measures) should be referred for evaluation/endoscopy.

VI. Indications for Hospitalization

Fecal impaction with resulting bowel obstruction can lead to significant morbidity and if disimpaction not possible, if patient dehydrated, or if there is significant comorbidity patients may require hospitalization.

VII. Annotated Bibliography

Castel SC. Constipation: endemic in the elderly? Med Clin North Am 1989;73:1497–1509. A review of constipation, which focuses on the elderly, but is applicable to other patient groups as well. Discusses a "stop-care" approach to the management of constipation.

Divroede G. Constipation. In: Sleisenger MH, Fordtran JS, eds. Gastrointestinal Disease, 4th ed. Philadelphia: WB Saunders; 1989:1994–2006. This chapter contains a very complete discussion of constipation including epidemiologic information and descriptions of all possible etiologies for this symptom.

Donatelle EP. Constipation: pathophysiology and treatment. Am Fam Pract 1990;42:1335–1342. A concise review of constipation with a good review of pharmacologic therapy.

Wald A. Approach to the patient with constipation. In: Yamada T, ed. Textbook of Gastroenterology. Philadelphia: JB Lippincott; 1991:779–793. An overview of constipation from pathophysiology to treatment.

Wrenn K. Fecal impaction. N Engl J Med 1989;321:658–662. A complete review of fecal impaction from pathophysiology through prevention and treatment.

47B Diarrhea

I. Clinical Presentation

A. General Information

1. Definition—The formal definition of diarrhea is the passage of > 250 mL water in the stool/d or a daily stool weight of > 200 g. Patients will often call any increase in frequency or loosening of consistency from their normal pattern of bowel movements diarrhea.

2. Pathogenesis—Diarrhea develops as a consequence of abnormal motility, abnormal absorption, and/or abnormal intestinal secretion.

3. Epidemiology—Each year millions of people die of diarrheal illness. Most of these persons are infants and children residing in developing countries, but diarrheal illness is also a cause of significant morbidity and occasional mortality in developed countries.

B. Symptoms

1. The clinician must ask the patient to report specifically on the duration of symptoms and the frequency, volume, consistency, color, and timing of bowel movements.

2. The above information will enable the clinician to differentiate true diarrhea from

   a. Isolated increased frequency of defecation without associated increase in fluid content
   b. Incontinence, which is the involuntary passage of normal fecal material

3. In addition, the clinician should ask about associated symptoms

   a. GI symptoms
      1) Abdominal pain
      2) Nausea and/or emesis
      3) Perianal discomfort
      4) Evidence of GI bleeding
   b. Systemic symptoms
      1) Fever
      2) Chills
      3) Weight loss
      4) Arthritis
      5) Flushing

4. Other information that can be helpful in determining the etiology of diarrhea include

   a. Review of medications including OTC preparations
   b. Dietary history
   c. Sexual history

d. Travel history
e. Family history
f. Review of medical history looking for diabetes, vascular disease, connective tissue disease, or alterations in immunocompetence

C. Physical Examination

1. A complete physical exam should be performed with special attention to

    a. Vital signs checking for fever and orthostatic changes in blood pressure and pulse
    b. Abdominal examination checking for tenderness, organomegaly, and masses
    c. Rectal examination checking for rectal tone, mass, and occult blood

II. Differential Diagnosis

The differential diagnosis for diarrhea is extensive. It is most useful to consider acute and chronic diarrhea separately.

A. Acute Diarrhea

Acute diarrhea is the presence of diarrhea for up to 3 wk.

1. Infectious diarrhea

    a. Infection is the most common cause of acute diarrhea and is most often acquired by viral infection, fecal-oral contamination, or improperly cooked foods.
    b. Infection can cause diarrhea via several different mechanisms.
        1) Production of a toxin that stimulates intestinal secretion of fluid and electrolytes (ie, *Vibrio cholera*, some *Escherichia coli*)
        2) Invasion of the mucosa by organisms (ie, *Salmonella*)
        3) A combination of toxin production and invasion of the mucosa (ie, *Shigella*)
    c. Persons at risk for infectious diarrhea include
        1) Children or contacts of children (rotavirus)
        2) Persons residing or traveling in developing countries (*E. coli, Giardia lamblia, Salmonella, Shigella, Yersinia*)
        3) Persons who have been drinking unpurified ground water (*G. lamblia, Campylobacter*)
        4) Persons ingesting undercooked or poorly refrigerated foods (staphylococcal enterotoxin, *Salmonella*, parasites like fish tapeworm)
        5) Persons with AIDS (*Cryptosporidia, Isospora*, amoeba)
        6) Persons who engage in oral-genital or oral-anal sexual contact (ameba, *Neisseria gonorrhea*, herpes, cytomegalovirus)
        7) Persons residing in institutions (rotavirus, *Clostridium difficile*, cryptosporidia)
    d. Symptoms of infectious diarrhea include watery or bloody stools with associated abdominal pain, fever, and/or chills in a person with a risk

factor. However, it is important to remember that viral gastroenteritis is the most common cause of diarrhea and often occurs in persons without risk factors.

2. Medication/therapy-related—Any diarrhea that begins after a new medication/therapy is started may be due to the medication and a trial of withdrawing the medication should be considered. Some common culprits include
    a. Antacids
    b. Nonsteroidal anti-inflammatory agents
    c. Laxatives
    d. Diuretics
    e. Antibiotics
    f. Colchicine
    g. Quinidine
    h. Theophylline
    i. Cholinergic agents
    j. Cancer chemotherapeutic agents
    k. Radiation therapy

3. Paradoxical diarrhea—results from partial bowel obstruction or the passage of liquid stool around impacted stool. Should be suspected in persons with prior history of severe constipation.

4. Miscellaneous causes of diarrhea—usually evident from the history
    a. Diarrhea may result from vigorous physical activity, as during training for a marathon.
    b. Idiopathic diarrhea may occur during periods of high stress.

B. Chronic Diarrhea

Chronic diarrhea is diarrhea lasting > 3 wk. The first step in the evaluation of chronic diarrhea is trying to decide if the diarrhea is secretory, osmotic, malabsorptive, inflammatory, or functional.

1. Functional diarrhea
    a. Irritable bowel syndrome (see Chapter 47D)
    b. Suggested in a younger patient when symptoms are nonprogressive or fluctuating, do not occur at night, and occur in the absence of fever, bloody stool, anemia, or weight loss
    c. Other etiologies must be excluded, especially in older patients.

2. Inflammatory diarrhea
    a. Ulcerative colitis, Crohn's disease, prolonged infection, ischemia
    b. Suggested when blood or pus is present in stool

3. Malabsorptive diarrhea
    a. Pancreatic insufficiency, postsurgical, tropical and nontropical sprue, intestinal bacterial overgrowth, Whipple's disease, bile salt deficiency, lactase deficiency

b. Suggested when diarrhea resolves during periods of fasting
4. Hypersecretory diarrhea
   a. Laxative abuse, Zollinger-Ellison syndrome, medullary thyroid cancer, carcinoid
   b. Suggested when severe diarrhea persists during periods of fasting
5. Osmotic diarrhea
   a. Lactase deficiency, magnesium-containing laxatives, saline cathartics, disaccharidase deficiency
   b. Usually suggested by diet and medication history

III. Diagnostic Approach

The diagnostic approach should be guided by history, physical examination, and consideration of the differential diagnosis.

A. Acute Diarrhea

1. If no fever, no dehydration, no blood in stool, and symptoms present for < 10 days, then conservative therapy is indicated.
   a. Clear fluids by mouth
   b. No laboratory studies
   c. No antibiotics
2. If fever, dehydration, blood in stool, or if symptoms are present for > 10 days
   a. Supportive therapy with oral or IV fluids as necessary
   b. Stool stain for white blood cells
      1) No white blood cells present
         a) *Stool culture for* Salmonella, Yersinia, E. coli
         b) *Consider checking* C. difficile *toxin especially if patient recently on antibiotics*
         c) *Reconsider noninfectious causes*
      2) If white blood cells present
         a) *Stool culture (yield improves with multiple specimens)*
         b) *Stool for ova and parasites (yield improves with multiple specimens)*
3. Consider complete blood cell count looking for anemia, eosinophilia (seen with parasitic infections)
4. Barium enema should not be performed in cases of acute diarrhea
5. Flexible sigmoidoscopy is usually reserved for the work-up of chronic rather than acute diarrhea, but may be helpful in the following cases
      a) *When anal-rectal fissures, fistula, or abscess is suspected*
      b) *When inflammatory bowel disease is suspected*
      c) *When laxative abuse is suspected, flexible sigmoidoscopy will reveal melanosis coli.*

- d) When C. difficile *is suspected, flexible sigmoidoscopy will reveal characteristic pseudomembranes, but this diagnosis can usually be made by checking for toxin in the stool.*
- e) *When performed to evaluate acute diarrhea, the examination should be performed without prior patient preparation with enemas.*

B. Chronic Diarrhea

The evaluation of chronic diarrhea should include examination of the stool for white blood cells, stool culture, and stool ova and parasites to rule out a prolonged infectious etiology. Subsequent testing should be guided by clinical suspicion of etiology.

1. Functional diarrhea
   a. See Chapter 47D
2. Inflammatory diarrhea
   a. Rule out infection as described above
   b. Barium enema or flexible sigmoidoscopy
3. Malabsorptive diarrhea
   a. Fecal fat collection of > 6 g/d suggests fat malabsorption.
   b. Small bowel biopsy if sprue, Whipple's disease, or *Giardia* is suspected.
   c. Abnormal D-xylose absorption test suggests mucosal malabsorption.
   d. C-glycholate breath test will help detect bile salt deficiency.
   e. Calcium, vitamin B_{12}, and folate will be low in malabsorption.
   f. Plain abdominal film looking for calcification, secretin test, and amylase to evaluate for pancreatic insufficiency.
4. Hypersecretory diarrhea
   a. Gastrin level to evaluate for Zollinger-Ellison syndrome
   b. Thyroid function tests to evaluate for medullary thyroid cancer
   c. Phenolphthalein test to evaluate for laxative abuse
   d. 24-h urine 5-hydroxyindole acetic acid to evaluate for carcinoid
5. Osmotic diarrhea
   a. Lactose tolerance breath test to evaluate for lactase deficiency

IV. Treatment

A. A complete review of the treatment for every etiology of diarrhea is beyond the scope of this chapter. Therefore the discussion will be limited to the treatment of acute diarrhea.

B. Most patients with acute diarrhea can be appropriately managed with supportive therapy.

A. Fluids

1. Oral replacement is usually sufficient.
2. Beverages containing glucose and electrolytes (soda, Gatorade) should be used rather than free water because glucose facilitates the absorption of sodium and water.
3. IV fluids may be necessary when nausea and emesis make adequate oral replacement impossible; sometimes also necessary in infants or elderly patients.

B. Diet

1. When able to eat, patient should maintain a diet high in protein and calories.
2. Milk products should be avoided.

C. Antibiotics

1. Should be prescribed only when an enteric pathogen is identified or if there is a very high clinical suspicion of a particular pathogen
2. Most cases of the common infectious causes of diarrhea (*Salmonella*, *Shigella*, *E. coli*, and *Campylobacter*) are self-limited and can be appropriately managed without antibiotics.
3. Treating *Salmonella* infection with antibiotics prolongs the carrier state and should be avoided.
4. Regimens for specific infections include
   a. *C. difficile*—vancomycin 125 mg PO q.i.d. for 10 d or metronidazole 250 mg PO q.i.d. for 10 d
   b. *Giardia*—quinacrine 100 mg PO t.i.d. for 7 d or metronidazole 250 mg PO t.i.d. for 7 d
   c. *Shigella*—Bactrim DS 1 PO b.i.d. for 5–10 d or ciprofloxacin
   d. *Campylobacter*—erythromycin 500 mg PO q.i.d. for 5–10 d
   e. Traveler's diarrhea—some improvement seen with ciprofloxacin (variable doses used; 250–750 mg qd–b.i.d.)

D. Other Symptomatic Treatment Options

1. Opiates
   a. Reduce stool volume and frequency, but should be avoided in acute infection because they will slow elimination of the organisms
   b. If opiates are necessary to make the patient comfortable, appropriate regimens are
      1) Codeine 15–30 mg PO q.i.d. PRN
      2) Diphenoxylate (Lomotil) 5 mg PO q.i.d. PRN
      3) Loperamide (Imodium) 1–4 2-mg tablets PO b.i.d. PRN
2. Bulking agents (metamucil 4–6 g PO qd) help in mild cases of diarrhea.

3. Aluminum-containing antacids may help to bind bile salts and lessen diarrhea.
4. Bismuth preparations (Pepto-Bismol) help in viral and traveler's diarrhea. In prophylactic doses of 60 mL PO q.i.d. Pepto-Bismol will decrease the incidence of traveler's diarrhea.

E. Patient Education

1. Patient should be educated about the necessity of maintaining adequate hydration.
2. Patient should be educated about the disadvantages of taking antibiotics when antibiotics are not clearly indicated.
3. Patients in risk groups for diarrheal illness should be educated about hygiene, avoiding potentially contaminated food and water.

V. Indications for Referral to a Gastroenterologist

The evaluation of chronic diarrhea almost always requires endoscopic examination of the colon, so patients with chronic diarrhea should be referred to a gastroenterologist.

VI. Indications for Hospitalization

Hospitalization is required if intravenous fluid replacement is necessary to treat dehydration. Often intravenous fluids are necessary in very young or very old patients with severe diarrhea and/or associated electrolyte abnormalities.

VII. Annotated Bibliography

Bruckstein AH. Acute diarrhea. Am Fam Pract 1988;38:217–228. A comprehensive discussion of acute diarrhea from pathophysiology through treatment.
Powell DW. Approach to the patient with diarrhea. In: Yamada T, ed. Textbook of Gastroenterology. Philadelphia: JB Lippincott; 1991:732–778. A comprehensive discussion of diarrhea including a long discussion of the pathophysiology of diarrhea and an extensive review of chronic diarrhea.
Thorne GM. Diagnosis of infectious diarrheal diseases. Infect Dis Clin North Am 1988;2:719. A concise overview of infectious diarrhea.

47C Colonic Diverticulosis and Diverticulitis

I. Clinical Presentation

A. General Information

1. Colonic diverticulosis is an acquired condition characterized by the formation of multiple pseudodiverticula when the mucosal and submucosal layers of the colon herniate through the muscular layers.
2. Epidemiology
   a. Most common in developed, western countries, rare in developing countries
   b. 5% of adult Americans have diverticulosis by age 50, 65% have diverticulosis by age 85
   c. Affects men and women equally
   d. Diverticular disease of the left side of the colon is most common in the United States, whereas isolated right-sided diverticular disease occurs in only 0.1–2.5% of cases.
   e. Diverticular disease is 2–3 times more common in nonvegetarians as in vegetarians.
3. Pathogenesis
   a. Diverticulosis
      1) Low-fiber diets lead to hypertrophy of the muscular layers of the colon as the colon contracts to expel the small amount of fecal material; increased intraluminal pressure leads to herniation of the nonmuscular layers at weak points in the muscular layer near transversing blood vessels.
      2) May be related to irritable bowel syndrome
   b. Diverticular bleeding occurs when blood vessels are disrupted by diverticula.
   c. Diverticulitis
      1) Fecal material trapped in a diverticulum causes pressure necrosis of the mucosa and microperforation resulting in inflammation/infection (usually a single diverticulum is affected).
      2) May result in true abscess formation or peritonitis

B. Symptoms

1. Only 20–30% of persons with diverticulosis will develop symptoms secondary to the diverticula.
2. 10–25% of persons with diverticulosis will develop diverticulitis and its complications.
3. 5% of persons with diverticulosis will have significant diverticular bleeding.

4. Symptoms of diverticulosis

   a. Most common symptom is pain that is often colicky in nature
   b. Pain typically worsened by eating, relieved by bowel movement or flatus
   c. Constipation, diarrhea, and/or flatulence may occur.

5. Symptoms of diverticular bleeding

   a. Abdominal cramps, urge to defecate
   b. Passage of a large volume of bright red blood, clots, or melena
   c. Bleeding may be continuous or intermittent and will cease spontaneously in > 75% of patients after several days.

6. Symptoms of diverticulitis

   a. Pain often localized to left lower quadrant, may radiate to back
   b. Fever and/or chills
   c. Anorexia, nausea, emesis, and/or change in bowels may occur.

C. Physical Examination

1. Diverticulosis

   a. Often examination is completely unremarkable.
   b. Occasionally a firm or tender loop of colon may be palpable.

2. Diverticular bleeding

   a. Abdomen benign
   b. Evidence of lower GI bleeding

3. Diverticulitis

   a. Usually LLQ tenderness
   b. May have peritoneal signs
   c. Palpable mass sometimes present
   d. Abdomen often distended and tympanic

II. Diagnostic Approach

The diagnosis of diverticular disease is based largely on clinical grounds as described in the preceding sections on symptoms and physical examination. Yet, diagnostic tests are helpful.

A. Diverticulosis

1. Plain abdominal x-rays will be normal.
2. Barium enema study is the best way to document the presence of diverticulosis.

B. Diverticular bleeding

1. Plain abdominal x-rays will be normal.

2. Barium enema can help to document diverticulosis and to rule out malignancy as the cause of the bleeding.

3. Mesenteric angiography
   a. Is useful to localize the site of bleeding
   b. Permits therapeutic injection of vasopressin or embolization of bleeding vessel
   c. Should be done when surgery is considered

4. Technetium 99m-tagged red blood cells or sulfur colloid nuclear medicine scans are not specific enough for diverticular bleeding to be used to guide surgical intervention.

5. Sigmoidoscopy/colonoscopy is helpful to rule out malignancy and should be considered in patients > 40 y.

C. Diverticulitis

1. Plain x-rays may show local ileus or evidence of large bowel obstruction.

2. Barium enema is contraindicated during acute diverticulitis because of the potential of exacerbating symptoms or causing barium peritonitis if barium leaks through a perforation.

3. CT scan should be considered in the following situations
   a. Abscess suspected
   b. Uncertainty of the diagnosis
   c. Fistula suspected
   d. Patient immunosuppressed
   e. No improvement after empirical therapy
   f. Sigmoidoscopy/colonoscopy is contraindicated during the acute phase, but may be helpful later if colonic stricture is suspected.

III. Differential Diagnosis

The differential diagnosis of diverticular disease includes other diseases that cause abnormal gut motility, lower GI bleeding, or intra-abdominal inflammation.

A. Irritable bowel syndrome

B. Inflammatory bowel disease

C. Colon cancer

D. Appendicitis

E. Colitis (infectious, ischemic, or radiation-induced)

F. Intestinal arteriovenous malformations

G. Gynecologic pathology

IV. Treatment

A. Diverticulosis

1. Asymptomatic
   a. Theoretically, a high-fiber diet may be beneficial, but no empirical evidence exists that dietary changes prevents or delays the occurrence of symptoms/complications of diverticulosis.
   b. Maintain regular bowel movements, avoid irritant laxatives

2. Symptomatic
   a. Maintaining high-fiber diet
   b. Fiber supplements such as psyllium in doses of 4–6 g/d
   c. Anticholinergic agents may help to relieve pain during attacks (dicyclomine 10–20 mg before meals and qhs), but should not be maintained chronically.
   d. Widely held belief that patients with diverticulosis should avoid foods with seeds, but no conclusive evidence to prove that this is of true benefit

B. Diverticular Bleeding

1. Patients should be hospitalized to maintain hemodynamics with IV fluids and blood products.

2. 80% will stop bleeding spontaneously, so surgery can often be avoided.

3. The recurrence rate is approximately 20% after the first diverticular bleed and increases with subsequent bleeds, so surgery may be warranted for recurrent diverticular bleeding.

C. Diverticulitis

1. Most patients should be hospitalized.

2. Bowel rest

3. IV hydration

4. Analgesia

5. Antibiotics to cover both enteric aerobes and anaerobes

6. Patients with no comorbidity, mild tenderness, and low-grade fever may be treated as outpatients with oral broad-spectrum antibiotics as long as they are followed closely.

D. Patient Education

1. Patients should be instructed regarding a high-fiber diet and/or fiber supplementation.

2. Patients should be advised to avoid laxatives.

3. Patients should be educated about the variable and unpredictable course of diverticulosis and be made aware of the symptoms of the complications of diverticulosis.

V. Indications for Referral

A. Gastroenterology consultation should be obtained when endoscopy is necessary for diagnosis.

B. Surgery consultation should be obtained in all patients with diverticular bleeding or diverticulitis to facilitate surgical intervention if such intervention becomes necessary.

VI. Indications for Hospitalization

Most patients with suspected diverticular bleeding or diverticulitis should be hospitalized for monitoring and treatment.

VII. Annotated Bibliography

Cheskin LJ, Bohlman M, Schuster MM. Diverticular disease in the elderly. Gastroenterol Clin North Am 1990;19(2):391–403. An overview of special considerations regarding the diagnosis and treatment of diverticular disease in the elderly.

Dietzen CD, Pemberton JH. Diverticulitis. In: Yamada T, ed. Textbook of Gastroenterology. Philadelphia: JB Lippincott;1991:1734–1748. A discussion of the entire scope of diverticular disease from pathophysiology to treatment.

Ertan A. Colonic diverticulitis. Postgrad Med 1990;8:67–77. A discussion of colonic diverticulitis aimed at the primary care physician.

Naitove A, Almy TP. Diverticular disease of the colon. In: Sleisenger MH, Fordtran JS, eds. Gastrointestinal Disease, 4th ed. Philadelphia: WB Saunders; 1989:1419–1434. A review of diverticular disease with an extensive discussion of pathogeneses and a good summary of complications of diverticulosis.

Pohlman T. Diverticulitis. Gastroenterol Clin North Am 1988;17(2):357–385. A comprehensive review of diverticulitis including diagnosis, therapy, unusual presentations, and complications of the disease.

47D Irritable Bowel Syndrome

I. Clinical Presentation

A. General Information

1. Irritable bowel syndrome (IBS) is a common functional disorder of the intestinal tract thought to be caused by interaction of GI, psychological, and dietary factors.
2. Functional GI disorders are characterized by symptoms not attributable to anatomic or biochemical abnormalities.

B. Epidemiology

1. Surveys report that IBS is 2–30 times more prevalent in women than in men in the United States. Gender distribution differs in other cultures, suggesting that patterns of care-seeking may account for the apparent female predominance in the United States.
2. More common in whites than in nonwhites
3. 50% of patients with IBS will develop symptoms by age 35, 90% by age 50.

C. Symptoms

1. The clinical spectrum of IBS encompasses a diversity of symptoms and a wide spectrum of severity among patients, but particular patients will usually have a constellation of symptoms typical for them.
2. Patients with IBS may report
    a. Bloating
    b. Flatulence
    c. Alterations in bowel habits
        1) Characterized by alternating diarrhea and constipation, with either diarrhea or constipation predominating
        2) Small stool volumes whether diarrhea or constipation
        3) A sense of rectal urgency or incomplete evacuation
    d. Abdominal discomfort or pain
        1) More often lower than upper quadrant
        2) Often coincides with meals regardless of type of food consumed
        3) Often relieved with bowel movement
    e. Other symptoms occasionally reported in IBS include mucinous stools, dysmenorrhea, dyspareunia, headache, dysuria, urinary frequency (independent of somatization disorder).
3. Symptoms that suggest IBS
    a. Nonspecific abdominal distention
    b. Looser and more frequent bowel movements coincident with onset of abdominal pain

c. Relief of abdominal pain after bowel movement
d. Symptoms exacerbated by psychological stress

4. Symptoms that suggest organic disease (*not* IBS)
   a. Fever
   b. Weight loss
   c. Dehydration
   d. Blood per rectum
   e. Steatorrhea
   f. Symptoms that awaken patient from sleep
   g. Onset of symptoms after age 50

5. Important to determine whether symptoms interfere with patient's functional status (work, school, social function)

D. Physical Examination

1. No specific findings on physical examination, but may find
   a. Anxious-appearing patient
   b. Palpable sigmoid colon
   c. Abdominal tenderness

2. Should *not* find
   a. Fever
   b. Dehydration
   c. Heme-positive stool
   d. Rebound or guarding

II. Diagnostic Approach

IBS is a diagnosis of exclusion. The challenge is the cost-effective exclusion of other diagnoses when a functional disorder is suspected.

A. The following studies should be performed in all patients when considering the diagnosis of IBS.

1. Complete blood count with differential to rule out anemia, leukocytosis, or eosinophilia

2. Erythrocyte sedimentation rate to screen for inflammatory process

3. Stool for culture, ova, and parasites

4. Examination of stool smear for amoeba, leukocytes, and occult blood

5. Sigmoidoscopy or barium enema to rule out inflammatory bowel disease and anatomic abnormalities

B. In certain cases, the clinical presentation may warrant additional studies to rule out organic disease.

1. When diarrhea is the predominant symptom, patients should follow a lactose-free diet for 14 d or undergo a hydrogen breath test to rule out lactose intolerance.
2. When dyspepsia is part of the symptom complex
   a. Upper GI series or endoscopy
   b. Ultrasound of the gallbladder, biliary tree, liver, and pancreas
3. If diagnosis is uncertain after all of the above, manometric studies can be performed. Expect spastic response to rectosigmoid distention if IBS is present.

III. Differential Diagnosis

The differential diagnosis of IBS is broad and is somewhat dependent on the patient's predominant symptom.

A. When diarrhea predominates, the differential includes

1. Laxative abuse
2. Inflammatory bowel disease
3. Gastrinoma
4. Endocrine disease (Addison's disease, hyperthyroidism)
5. Pancreatic insufficiency
6. GI infection

B. When constipation predominates, the differential includes

1. Chronic laxative abuse
2. Drug-induced bowel dysfunction
3. Diverticulosis
4. Colon cancer (particularly in patients > 50 y old)

C. When pain predominates, the differential includes

1. Biliary tract disease
2. Porphyria
3. Heavy metal intoxication (lead)

IV. Treatment

A. Acute and Long-term Management

1. A good patient–physician relationship is of utmost importance in the safe, cost-effective management of IBS.

2. The manner in which the physician explains the diagnosis to patients can have a large impact on the way the patient handles the disorder.
3. All necessary diagnostic studies should be performed before diagnosis is assumed. Patients who believe they have had an incomplete evaluation will often change physicians and undergo repetitive and costly evaluations.
4. Treatment is multifactorial and optimal management is directed toward a given patient's symptoms.
   a. Diet
      1) High-fiber diet is thought to be beneficial.
      2) Fiber supplements such as psyllium (Metamucil 4–6 g/d) can be helpful.
      3) Patients should avoid foods that they find aggravate their symptoms (caffeine and legumes are examples of typical culprits).
   b. Psychologic factors
      1) Patients must be reassured that IBS does not put them at increased risk for cancer or colitis.
      2) Emphasis on decreasing symptoms rather than cure
      3) Data suggest that medical therapy in combination with behavioral therapy is more successful than medical therapy alone.
      4) Formal psychiatric evaluation/management may be beneficial in select cases.
      5) Sedatives, tranquilizers, and antidepressants may occasionally be necessary but should be used with caution.
   c. Medications
      1) To treat diarrhea
         a) *Diphenoxylate (Lomotil) 2.5–5 mg q 4–6 h*
         b) *Loperamide (Immodium) 2 mg q 6–8 h*
         c) *Opiates should be avoided due to addictive potential.*
         d) *Cholestyramine (Questran) 4 g PO 1–6 times per day has been found to be helpful to some patients.*
         e) *Antidiarrheal agents should be used as infrequently and sparingly as possible to avoid the development of constipation.*
      2) To treat constipation
         a) *Laxatives (see Chapter 47A)*
         b) *Laxatives should be used infrequently and sparingly to avoid the development of diarrhea following the use of these agents or worsening of constipation from chronic laxative use.*
      3) To treat pain
         a) *Anticholinergics (antispasmodic) may be helpful taken 30 min prior to meals*
            i) Dicyclomine (Bentyl) 20 mg
            ii) Propantheline 15 mg
   d. Other elements occasionally helpful in the management of IBS include
      1) Avoidance of chewing gum, artificial sweeteners, carbonated drinks, and legumes
      2) Simethicone
      3) Antacids

4) Metoclopramide
   5) Discontinuation of tobacco
   6) Increased exercise
   7) Behavioral therapy (meditation, biofeedback, hypnosis, psychotherapy, etc.)

B. Patient Education

1. Patients benefit from reassurance that no serious disease exists and that IBS does not require surgery nor increase their risk of cancer or premature mortality.

2. Physician should explain to the patient that IBS is a real disorder where the intestine is hypersensitive to various stimuli (food, hormones, psychological stress).

3. Patient should be educated about possible aggravating factors.

4. Patients should be made to understand that symptom management not cure is the goal of therapy.

5. Patients should be educated about the dangers of chronic medication use in IBS; pharmacologic therapy should be used PRN.

V. Indications for Referral

A. Referral to a Gastroenterologist

1. May be necessary if endoscopic procedures are required to exclude organic disease

2. May be necessary for patient reassurance that serious disease is not being overlooked

3. May be necessary if symptoms are recalcitrant to therapy

B. Referral to Pain Specialist

Some patients with IBS become functionally disabled by their symptoms and referral to a pain specialist may be beneficial in controlling the patient's symptoms allowing the return to work, school, or other activity.

VI. Indications for Hospitalization

Hospitalization is rarely indicated in IBS unless necessary to rule out serious organic pathology, for example, if patient's presentation is worrisome for appendicitis or other condition that would require hospitalization.

VII. Annotated Bibliography

Camilleri M, Prather CM. The irritable bowel syndrome: mechanisms and a practical approach to management. Ann Intern Med 1992;116:1001–1008. A review that combines features of diagnosis and treatment in a practical management algorithm.

Drossman DA, Thompson WG. The irritable bowel syndrome: a review and a graduated multicomponent treatment approach. Ann Intern Med 1992;116:1009–1016. A review of IBS that emphasizes a graduated and individual treatment plan tailored to each patient's clinical presentation.

Schuster M. Irritable bowel syndrome. In: Sleisenger MH, Fordtran JS, eds. Gastrointestinal Disease, 4th ed. Philadelphia: WB Saunders; 1989:1402–1418. This chapter contains a good review of irritable bowel disease with an emphasis on etiologic factors.

47E Lactose Intolerance

I. Clinical Presentation

A. General Information

Lactose intolerance is a cluster of symptoms resulting from lactose malabsorption due to lactase deficiency (hypolactasia). Three different types of lactase deficiencies have been described.

1. Congenital—lactase activity absent from birth

    a. Very rare autosomal recessive disorder
    b. Presents as watery stool, failure to thrive in infants

2. Primary delayed onset—genetically determined decrease in lactase activity that occurs throughout life beginning in late childhood

    a. The most common genetic enzyme deficiency. Delayed decrease in lactase activity may be the norm with retained lactase activity representing a selected mutation.
    b. Variation in adult prevalence
        1) 45–80% African Americans
        2) 10–25% American whites
        3) 90–100% Asians
        4) Lowest prevalence in northern Europeans

3. Secondary—decreased lactase activity due to other intestinal pathology (infection, inflammatory disease, surgical resection). Chronic alcoholics can have decreased lactase activity that improves with cessation of alcohol consumption.

B. Symptoms

1. The presence of unabsorbed lactose in the intestinal tract has osmotic and irritant effects. Following lactose ingestion the following may occur

    a. Abdominal discomfort
    b. Distention, bloating
    c. Flatulence
    d. Diarrhea (without blood or mucus)

2. Patients will exhibit great variability in symptoms and symptom severity.

3. Patients are often not aware that symptoms are associated with lactose ingestion.

C. Physical Examination

1. Nonspecific
2. The presence of fever, GI blood loss, mucus in stool, or frank abdominal findings should provoke an evaluation for other pathology and secondary lactose intolerance.

II. Diagnostic Approach

A. Eliminate lactose-containing products from diet for at least 5–7 d (some studies recommend up to 3 wk). If symptoms diminish, this is suggestive of hypolactasia. If diagnosis is still unclear, proceed with further testing.

B. Oral Lactose Tolerance Test

1. A 50-mg oral dose of lactose is given to patient and blood glucose levels are measured over 2 h.
2. A > 20 mg/dL rise in blood glucose and the lack of symptoms indicates adequate lactose absorption.
3. Results can be spurious in the setting of diabetes mellitus or delayed gastric emptying.

C. Alternate Oral Lactose Tolerance Test

1. Same procedure as above, but rather than measuring blood glucose you monitor the quantity of galactose in urine or blood following lactose ingestion
2. More reliable than the simple lactose tolerance test, but requires simultaneous administration of alcohol along with the lactose

D. Breath Test

1. Uses gas chromatography to measure the amount of hydrogen liberated during colonic fermentation of unabsorbed lactose
2. A > 20 ppm increase in exhaled hydrogen indicates decreased lactase activity.
3. Spurious results can occur when patient smokes or is taking oral antibiotics.
4. The preferred diagnostic test because it is noninvasive and simple to perform; not available in all institutions; usually done through gastroenterology division

E. Stool Test for pH and Reducing Substances

1. An infrequently performed test useful to indicate whether unabsorbed lactose is reaching the colon, but not sensitive enough to rule out lactose intolerance
2. To measure reducing substances place a small amount of fresh stool in a test tube and dilute 1:2 with water; place 15 drops in a second test tube and add a Clinitest tablet and compare with color chart for testing glycosuria; > 0.5% is positive, 0.25–0.5% is equivocal, < .25% is negative.
3. To measure stool pH, test with nitrazine paper into fresh stool; pH < 5.5 is consistent with lactose malabsorption.

F. Tissue Diagnosis

1. Biopsy of intestinal mucosa and assay for lactase is the gold standard method of diagnosis.
2. Rarely indicated unless tissue is required to rule out other disorders

III. Differential Diagnosis

Presentation and time course of symptoms helps to distinguish lactose intolerance from other disorders in the differential.

A. Irritable bowel syndrome

B. Tropical sprue

C. Celiac disease

D. Intestinal infection

IV. Treatment

A. Acute and Long-term Management
1. Diet
   a. Mainstay of treatment is to decrease dietary lactose.
   b. Not necessary nor prudent to eliminate all lactose-containing products from the diet because there is usually a threshold below which patients will remain symptom free, most lactose intolerant patients can tolerate at least 3 g lactose/d.
   c. Yogurt is the one lactose-containing product that is well-tolerated by individuals with hypolactasia because of lumenal digestion of lactose by bacterial lactase in the yogurt cultures.
   d. Lactose-containing foods may be better tolerated when gastric emptying is delayed by consuming lactose along with other foods with increased fat/calorie content.
   e. Calcium supplements may be necessary for patients on low-lactose diets, especially women.
2. Milk that has been 70–90% hydrolyzed by yeast enzyme preparation can be purchased in some food stores (Lact-Aid).
3. Enzyme preparations (Lact-Aid) can be added to regular, refrigerated milk, result in 70% hydrolysis in 24 h and 90% by 48–72 hours; milk prepared in this manner will taste sweet and may not be palatable to some patients.
4. Lactase enzymes can be purchased in tablets (Lactaid, Lactrase), 1–4 tablets taken with lactose-containing products.

B. Patient Education
1. Patient must be educated about dietary management.
   a. Foods that contain lactose
      1) High lactose—skim milk, whole milk, buttermilk, cream, ice milk, ice cream, milk chocolate, soft cheeses, butter

2) Lower lactose—yogurt, hard cheeses, sherbet
3) Many prepared and packaged foods contain lactose. Patients should be advised to read labels and avoid foods with the following ingredients: milk products, milk solids, casein, whey, lactose, milk sugar, curd, galactose, or skim milk powder.

2. Patients should attempt to determine their own threshold for lactose consumption and to supplement calcium if no milk products are ingested.
3. Patient should be aware that serious symptoms such as fever, hematemesis, or bloody diarrhea are not attributable to lactase deficiency and warrant medical attention.

V. Indications for Referral to a Gastroenterologist

A. Refractory symptoms despite dietary compliance may require referral to rule out other pathology with a tissue diagnosis.

B. When secondary lactose intolerance exists, the patient may require referral for treatment of the primary GI pathology.

VI. Indications for Hospitalization

Hospitalization is rarely indicated unless necessitated by severe primary GI pathology in secondary forms of lactose intolerance.

VII. Annotated Bibliography

Alpers DA. Dietary management and vitamin-mineral replacement therapy. In: Sleisenger MH, Fordtran JS, eds. Gastrointestinal Disease, 4th ed. Philadelphia: WB Saunders; 1989:1994–2006. This chapter contains a good description of dietary considerations in lactose intolerance.

Arola H. Hypolactasia: a normal condition for the adult. Dig Dis 1989;7:301–308. A review of hypolactasia that covers the genetics, ethnic variation, and pathophysiology of the syndrome.

Lloyd ML, Olsen WA. Specific mucosal protein deficiency states. In: Yamada T, ed. Textbook of Gastroenterology. Philadelphia: JB Lippincott; 1991:1520–1530. A complete overview of digestive mucosal protein deficiency states including a concise review of lactase deficiency.

Montes RG, Perlman JA. Lactose intolerance. Postgrad Med 1991;89:175–184. A review of lactose intolerance covering etiology, clinical presentation, diagnosis, and management of the disorder.

Chapter 48: Epigastric Pain

David S. Weinberg and Christine Laine

48A Peptic Ulcer Disease

I. Clinical Presentation

A. General Information
1. Epidemiology—Approximately 4 million people in the United States are affected by peptic ulcer disease (PUD) each year.
2. 5–10% of all persons will develop a peptic ulcer in their lifetime. The peak incidence for duodenal ulcer (DU) is age 40; for gastric ulcer (GU) it is age 50. DU is more common than GU.
3. Risk factors for PUD
   a. Tobacco use
      1) DU is 33–110% more frequent in smokers.
   b. Alcohol use
      1) Probable association
   c. Corticosteroids
      1) Considerable controversy about steroids alone and PUD
      2) Steroids in combination with nonsteroidal anti-inflammatory drugs (NSAIDs) significantly increase risk
   d. Aspirin or NSAIDs
      1) 10–30% of patients who regularly use aspirin/NSAIDs report dyspeptic symptoms, but the presence of symptoms does not correlate with endoscopic evidence of injury.
      2) Food and Drug Administration reports symptomatic PUD in 2–4% of patients treated with NSAIDs for 1 y.
      3) NSAIDs are clearly linked to GU and probably related to DU formation.
      4) The risk of PUD in NSAID users is increased when
         a) Patient age > 60 y
         b) Concomitant steroid use
         c) History of PUD
         d) High-dose or multiple NSAIDs
         e) Previous NSAID use discontinued secondary to dyspeptic symptoms
   e. *Helicobacter pylori* infection
      1) Spiral bacterium described in 1983
      2) Now recognized as an important, if not the critical, factor in PUD

3) Shown to infect the mucosal layer of nearly all patients with DU, most patients with GU, and almost all patients with antral gastritis
4) *H. pylori* has *not* been associated with nonulcerative dyspepsia.
  f. Zollinger-Ellison syndrome (gastrinoma)
   1) Non-beta islet cell, gastrin-secreting tumor
   2) Associated with multiple neuroendocrine neoplasia (MEN-1) in 20% of cases
   3) 70% of patients with Zollinger-Ellison will have associated diarrhea secondary to increased acid production.
  g. Stress/personality type
   1) Role is controversial in PUD.
   2) Not clearly linked to PUD

B. Symptoms

1. Patients with PUD will typically complain of burning, gnawing epigastric pain.
2. Other symptoms may include nausea, vomiting, anorexia, bloating.
3. Pain is episodic, lasting minutes rather than hours and occur in clusters lasting days to weeks. Recurrence is typical.
4. Pain is only variably relieved by food or antacids.
5. Attempts to differentiate GU from DU by symptoms is often fruitless.

C. History and Physical Examination

1. History should include questions regarding alcohol and NSAID use, smoking history as well as history of prior PUD.
2. Need to ask specifically about symptoms that may occur in complicated PUD
   a. Vomiting can occur with outlet obstruction.
   b. Diarrhea can occur with Zollinger-Ellison.
   c. Melena or blood per rectum indicates bleeding PUD.
   d. Significant weight loss indicates severe, complicated PUD or underlying carcinoma.
3. A complete physical examination should be performed with special attention to
   a. Vital signs, checking for orthostatic changes in blood pressure and pulse, which suggest significant blood loss
   b. Abdominal examination, checking for tenderness, bowel sounds, succussion splash
   c. Rectal examination, checking for occult blood
   d. Any evidence of significant weight loss

II. Diagnostic Approach

A. In the absence of complications, suspected PUD can be treated empirically for 4–6 wk without further diagnostic studies. If complications are present, disease is recurrent, or response to empirical therapy is inadequate, two major diagnostic modalities exist.

1. Barium swallow
    a. Advantages
        1) Inexpensive
        2) Nearly risk free
    b. Disadvantages
        1) Lower sensitivity and specificity than endoscopy (misses up to 20% of ulcers)
        2) Biopsy of lesions not possible
        3) Less able to evaluate competing diagnoses such as esophagitis or gastritis
2. Endoscopy
    a. Advantages
        1) Sensitive and specific for PUD
        2) Biopsy capability
        3) Direct visualization of lesions
    b. Disadvantages
        1) Expensive
        2) Small associated risk to the patient
        3) Requires sedation
        4) Requires referral to gastroenterologist

B. When there is clinical suspicion of *H. pylori* infection or Zollinger-Ellison syndrome, further diagnostic testing is indicated.

1. Testing for *H. pylori*—Availability of different testing methods varies widely.
    a. Widely available
        1) Endoscopic biopsy for culture and stains
        2) Endoscopic biopsy for "clo" test (a rapid urease test)
    b. Less widely available
        1) 13c or 14c breath test
        2) IgG serology or IgG enzyme-linked immunosorbent assay
2. Testing for Zollinger-Ellison syndrome
    a. Serum gastrin should be checked while patient is not on H_2 blockers to rule out Zollinger-Ellison when
        1) Multiple ulcers present
        2) Ulcers resistant to therapy with frequent recurrence
        3) Strong family history of PUD
        4) Ulcer recurrence after PUD surgery
    b. Normal serum gastrin is ≤ 100 pg/mL; patients with Zollinger-Ellison can have fasting gastrin > 1000 pg/mL.

III. Differential Diagnosis

A. Gastritis

B. Gastric carcinoma

C. Nonulcerative dyspepsia (see Chapter 48B)

D. Esophagitis

E. Pancreatitis

F. Cholecystitis (see Chapter 51B)

G. Irritable bowel syndrome (see Chapter 47D)

H. Myocardial infarction

IV. Treatment

Several drugs, as discussed below, are safe and effective as primary therapy for PUD. Because of their proven safety and efficacy, H_2 blockers remain standard first-line therapy. At this point, initial antibiotic or antibiotic + H_2 blocker/proton pump blocker to treat *H. pylori* cannot be advocated, because there are no data which specifically address this point. Because most ulcers recur, various strategies for either eradication or maintenance suppression are under investigation. Currently, low-dose H_2 blockers are standard, but as evidence mounts for the central role of *H. pylori* as well as long-term safety of proton pump blockers, treatment recommendations will likely change.

A. Acute Therapy

1. H_2 antagonists

    a. H_2 antagonists are effective in relieving ulcer symptoms, healing ulcers, and reducing frequency of ulcer recurrence.
    b. Healing rates for DU are faster and more complete than GU. For *DU*, healing rates and control of pain are comparable between all available drugs. Twice a day dosing has no advantage over once at night therapy. Symptoms are usually improved within 7 d. Duration of therapy is 6–8 wk. At that point approximately 95% of all DU will be healed.
    c. *GU* rates of healing at 8 wk are 80–90%. Unlike DU, GU healing should be documented endoscopically or radiographically to exclude malignancy.
    d. Side effect profile (nephrotoxicity, hepatic toxicity, bone marrow suppression) are identical for all agents. Very low overall.
    e. Relative dosing in PUD for H_2 antagonists
        1) Cimetidine (Tagamet) 400 mg PO b.i.d. or 800 mg PO hs (acute), 400 mg PO hs (maintenance)
        2) Ranitidine (Zantac) 150 mg PO b.i.d. or 300 mg PO hs (acute), 150 mg PO hs (maintenance)
        3) Famotidine (Pepcid) 40 mg PO hs (acute), 20 mg PO hs (maintenance)
        4) Nizatidine (Axid) 150 mg PO b.i.d. or 300 mg PO hs (acute), 150 mg PO hs (maintenance)

2. Proton pump inhibitors
   a. Omeprazole (Prilosec) is the first available of this new class of gastric acid inhibitors.
   b. 20 mg PO qd abolishes acid production in > 85% of patients. 20 mg PO b.i.d. or 40 mg PO qd, stops acid in all patients except those with Zollinger-Ellison (typically 40–80 mg qd).
   c. Omeprazole achieves comparable healing of GU and DU to H_2 blockers, at a faster rate. Symptom control is identical.
   d. Relapse rate at 1 y is similar.
   e. Safety profile short term (months) well documented.
   f. Long-term maintenance (10 mg or 20 mg qd) appears effective. Side effects long term are less well known.

3. Sucralfate (Carafate)
   a. Multiple mechanisms of action that enhance mucosal defense
   b. Can be used as acute (1 g PO q.i.d., pill or slurry) or maintenance (1 g PO b.i.d.) therapy for PUD.
   c. Safety well documented; drug of choice in pregnancy because of low absorption
   d. Frequent dosing is inconvenient relative to other therapies.
   e. Constipation is most frequent side effect.

4. Therapy for *H. pylori*
   a. Therapy should not be given unless a diagnostic test for *H pylori* is positive.
   b. First-line therapy
      1) Pepto-bismol 2 tablets PO q.i.d.
      2) Metronidazole (Flagyl) 250 mg PO q.i.d.
      3) Tetracycline 500 mg PO q.i.d.
      4) 80–90% eradication with 14 d therapy (no advantage to longer)
      5) Amoxicillin 500 mg PO q.i.d. can be substituted for Pepto-bismol or tetracycline.
   c. Success of therapy is based on symptom relief and a negative diagnostic test for *H pylori* 1 mo after treatment initiated.
   d. If no success or a contraindication to first-line therapy, there are numerous second-line combinations with 70–80% eradication rates (all used for 14 d).
      1) Amoxicillin 500 mg PO q.i.d. + omeprazole (Prilosec) 40 mg PO qd
      2) Clarithromycin (Biaxin) 500 mg PO b.i.d. + omeprazole 40 mg PO qd
   e. Patients who continue to have symptoms after documented eradication of *H pylori* usually have gastroesophageal reflux and should be treated with H_2 blockers.

5. Antacids—In sufficient dose antacids control symptoms of PUD as well as other agents. However, because of inconvenience of frequent large dosing as well as greater efficacy in healing by other drugs, they cannot be recommended as first-line therapy.

B. Maintenance Therapy

1. Maintenance therapy decreases annual recurrence from approximately 70% to 30%.
2. Patients with a single episode of uncomplicated PUD, who do not smoke, can be treated with a second full course of therapy if there is recurrence.
3. Patients with multiple episodes, or those who smoke, need maintenance therapy. Alternatively, documentation of *H. pylori* as etiology may be pursued, and if present treated.
4. Duration of maintenance therapy is at least 1-2 y.

V. Indications for Referral to a Gastroenterologist

A. Complicated PUD (bleeding, perforation, obstruction)

B. Endoscopic diagnosis including biopsy for *H. pylori*

C. Follow-up of gastric ulcer in most circumstances (endoscopic biopsy needed to rule out malignancy)

D. No response to therapy

E. Zollinger-Ellison syndrome

VI. Patient Education

A. Patient must be advised to discontinue tobacco, alcohol, and NSAIDs.

B. Diet should consist of small, frequent meals to buffer gastric acid.

VII. Indications for Hospitalization

Active, complicated PUD (bleeding, perforation, obstruction)

VIII. Annotated Bibliography

Clearfield HR. *Helicobacter pylori*: aggressor or innocent bystander? Med Clin North Am 1991;75(4):815-829. Comprehensive review of *H. pylori* with emphasis on epidemiology and relationship to PUD.

Freston JW. Overview of medical therapy of peptic ulcer disease. Gastroenterol Clin North Am 1990;19(1):121-140. Extensively referenced discussion of PUD therapy.

Rubin W. Medical treatment of peptic ulcer disease. Med Clin North Am 1991;75:981-999. A detailed discussion of natural history and current therapy for PUD, both acute and maintenance.

Silverstein F. Nonsteroidal anti-inflammatory drugs and peptic ulcer disease. Postgrad Med 1991;89(7):33–40.

Walsh J. *Helicobacter pylori*: selection of patients for treatment. Ann Intern Med 1992;116(9):770–771. Editorial accompanying one of the first studies reporting the eradication of *H. pylori* and resultant decreased recurrence rate of PUD. Good overview of when to treat.

48B Nonulcerative Dyspepsia

I. Clinical Presentation

A. General Information

1. Definition—a constellation of GI symptoms that prompts a physician to believe an ulcer may be present, but no ulcer is found on evaluation.

2. Epidemiology

    a. Prevalence is 20–30% in large population surveys.
    b. Nonulcerative dyspepsia is at least twice as common as peptic ulcer disease (PUD).

3. Pathogenesis is unclear, but several hypotheses exist.

    a. Abnormal acid secretion (most studies have found normal acid secretion)
    b. Duodenitis (seen in < 20% of patients with nonulcerative dyspepsia)
    c. Gastritis (possibly secondary to *Helicobacter pylori*)
    d. Abnormal gastric motility (no definite association yet established)
    e. Psychosocial factors (no studies have identified a link between dyspepsia and personality)

B. Symptoms

Patients' description of symptoms usually includes some combination of

1. Nausea
2. Vomiting
3. Anorexia
4. Epigastric or substernal burning
5. Belching
6. Bloating
7. Food intolerance

C. Physical Examination

The physical examination may reveal *mild* epigastric or abdominal tenderness. However, it is generally benign in nonulcerative dyspepsia.

II. Diagnostic Approach

The diagnostic approach depends on whether a patient has a low or a high risk for PUD.

A. Low-Risk Group

1. Patients at low risk for PUD
   a. No evidence of organic disease by history or physical examination
   b. Age < 40 y
   c. No prior history of PUD
   d. No *regular* aspirin, nonsteroidal anti-inflammatory drug (NSAID), alcohol, or tobacco use
   e. Short duration of symptoms
2. For low-risk patients suggest
   a. Reassurance, explanation
   b. Discontinue any aspirin, NSAID, alcohol, and tobacco
   c. Treat symptoms of irritable bowel syndrome if present (see Chapter 47D)
   d. Empirical trial of antacids
   e. If no response in 7–10 d or lack of complete response in 6–8 wk, then upper endoscopy recommended

B. High-Risk Group

1. Patients at high risk for PUD
   a. Evidence of organic disease (eg, heme-positive stool, weight loss, early satiety)
   b. Age > 40 y
   c. Prior personal history or family history of PUD
   d. Severe, chronic symptoms
   e. Regular use of ulcerogenic substances such as aspirin, NSAID, alcohol, and tobacco
2. For high-risk patients suggest
   a. In the absence of apparent complications (bleeding, obstruction, etc.) can institute empirical therapy with H_2 blockers because endoscopy is unlikely to influence initial management
   b. Endoscopy indicated for patients who fail to respond to therapy within 7–10 d or for patients who relapse within 8 wk of completing therapy

III. Differential Diagnosis

A. Peptic Ulcer Disease (see Chapter 48A)

1. Must be excluded prior to the diagnosis of nonulcerative dyspepsia

B. Gastric Cancer

1. Diagnosed by esophagogastroduodenoscopy (EGD)

C. Gastroesophageal Reflux Disease (GERD, see Chapter 50)

1. History helps to differentiate

2. Patients with GERD will complain of heartburn, acid taste, excess salivation; symptoms exacerbated when reclining.

D. Biliary Tract Disease (see Chapter 51)

1. Patients with biliary tract disease will complain of episodic pain that can last hours.

2. Ultrasound or cholecystogram will help in diagnosis.

E. Chronic Pancreatitis

1. Typically constant, severe upper abdominal pain radiating to back

2. Patients at risk for pancreatitis (alcohol use or gallstones) should undergo x-ray/ultrasound

F. Irritable Bowel Syndrome (IBS, see Chapter 47D)

1. Patients with IBS will generally complain of more lower tract symptoms (loose stool, alternating diarrhea constipation, etc.) than will patients with nonulcerative dyspepsia.

2. Both IBS and nonulcerative dyspepsia are functional disorders.

3. Differentiating the two may be difficult and a trial of IBS therapy is warranted when the diagnosis is unclear.

IV. Treatment

A. H_2 blockers—at present, no evidence that H_2 blockers or sulcrafate are any better than placebo

B. Antacids—occasionally help and have the advantage of being inexpensive and relatively free of serious side effects

C. Eradication of *H. pylori*—has not yet been determined whether triple therapy against *H. pylori* (bismuth, amoxicillin or tetracycline, and metronidazole) benefits patients with nonulcerative dyspepsia, but may be worthwhile to treat infection if documented

D. Patient Education

1. Physician should explain that no serious pathology exists and that patients are not at increased risk for cancer or premature mortality.

2. Patients should be advised to avoid triggering factors (dietary, medications, stress).

3. The emphasis should be on symptom management rather than cure.

V. Indications for Referral to a Gastroenterologist

Two sorts of patients can benefit from referral to a gastroenterologist.

A. High-risk patients with history or physical findings supporting the presence of PUD should undergo EGD.

B. High-risk patients with no evidence of organic disease who have failed empirical therapy or relapsed after therapy completed should be referred for EGD.

VI. Indications for Hospitalization

Hospitalization is rarely indicated. Occasionally may be necessary to exclude other serious diagnoses when patients initially present complaining of severe symptoms.

VII. Annotated Bibliography

Health and Public Policy Committee, American College of Physicians. Endoscopy in the evaluation of dyspepsia. Ann Intern Med 1985;102:226–229. Recommends endoscopy only for patients who fail to respond to H_2 blockers or antacids.

Talley NS, Phillips SF. Non-ulcerative dyspepsia: potential causes and pathophysiology. Ann Intern Med 1988;108:865–879. Excellent review of potential causes and possible therapeutic strategies for nonulcerative dyspepsia.

Zell SC, Budhraja M. An approach to dyspepsia in the ambulatory care setting: evaluation based on risk stratification. J Gen Intern Med 1989;4:144–150. Describes a useful outpatient treatment algorithm for nonulcerative dyspepsia.

Chapter 49: Evaluation of Heme-Positive Stool

David S. Weinberg and Christine Laine

I. Clinical Presentation

A. General Information

The majority of fecal occult blood testing (FOBT) performed in the outpatient setting is done for cancer screening. Although patient and physician generally are fearful of malignancy, both must recall that, as listed below, there are many causes for occult blood from upper and lower GI sources. Systematic evaluation of a positive stool guaiac test based on the clinical situation is outlined below.

B. Important Facts about FOBT

1. 1–3% of adults older than 40 have positive FOBT; < 50% have a neoplasm. Of these, adenomas are 3 times more common than carcinomas.

2. Positive predictive values for adenoma and carcinoma range from 20–60%. The positive predictive value of a positive FOBT for cancer is about 10%.

3. Only 20–40% of patients with known adenomas have positive FOBT.

4. 2 mL of blood in the gut is necessary for a positive test.

5. Colorectal cancers and adenomas may bleed intermittently.

6. Polyps of < 1 cm rarely bleed.

7. FOBT more likely positive with more distal (and larger) polyps.

8. Most studies use Hemoccult cards. Several other testing cards are currently available or in trials. Their sensitivities and specificities remain to be determined.

C. Which stool samples should be used for FOBT?

1. A positive FOBT on random *digital* examination may result from

   a. True disease
   b. Trauma
   c. False positives stemming from food or medication

2. The best method for reliable testing is *home* testing.

   a. Give the patient 3 test cards. Use of 3 cards increases the sensitivity of FOBT. Each card has 2 windows, so a total of 6 stool smears is required.

b. Instruct the patient to avoid the following for 3 d prior to collecting stool specimens
   1) Red meat
   2) Foods high in peroxidase (broccoli, turnips, cantaloupe, radish, cauliflower), which can result in a false positive test
   3) Vitamin C (false negative), iron (no evidence that iron causes false positive, though stool color changes), aspirin and nonsteroidal anti-inflammatory drugs
c. After this preparation, the patient should smear samples of the next 3 stools (1 stool sample per card) onto the windows of the diagnostic cards. All cards should be returned to the physician.

3. For the most reliable results, the physician should

   a. Develop within 4–6 d of testing
   b. Whether or not samples should be rehydrated is controversial because rehydration will increase both the false positive and true positive rates.

D. Causes of false positives and negatives for stool hemoccult cards

1. False positive

   a. Red meat, uncooked fruits and vegetables
   b. Any source of non-GI bleeding into GI tract (epistaxis, gingival bleeding)
   c. Topical iodine

2. False negative

   a. Storage of slides > 7 d
   b. Vitamin C
   c. Lesion not bleeding at time of test
   d. Improper development or interpretation

II. Differential Diagnosis

Patients with acute GI bleeding typically present with clear evidence of active bleeding, eg, hematemesis or hematochezia. Chronic bleeding generally has a less impressive presentation; nonetheless the differential diagnosis for these two clinical situations is the same.

A. Upper GI Bleeding

1. Bleeding from nose or pharynx

2. Hemoptysis

3. Mallory-Weiss tear

4. Inflammation (esophagitis, gastritis, duodenitis)

5. Ulcer disease (esophageal or peptic)

6. Neoplasm

7. Arteriovenous malformation (AVM)
8. Hemobilia

B. Lower GI Bleeding

1. Hemorrhoids
2. Anal fissure
3. Inflammatory bowel disease
4. Neoplasm
5. Diverticulosis
6. AVM
7. Radiation colitis
8. Amyloidosis
9. Meckel's diverticulum
10. Vascular-enteric fistula

III. Diagnostic Studies

A. Lower GI Evaluation

1. Flexible sigmoidoscopy
    a. Usual first diagnostic test
    b. Detects polyps in 10–15% of asymptomatic persons over age 40
    c. Enemas for preparation, usually in conjunction with barium enema

2. Barium enema
    a. Air contrast study more sensitive than single contrast for detection of polyps
    b. Sensitivity 85–95% for colorectal polyps
    c. 5% false positive and 5% false negative rate

3. Colonoscopy
    a. Combines increased diagnostic accuracy with therapeutic capability
    b. 10% of time cecum not reached
    c. Requires sedation, more expensive than flexible sigmoidoscopy/barium enema, though may be more cost effective as positive flexible sigmoidoscopy/barium enema may require colonoscopy

B. Upper GI Evaluation

1. Upper Endoscopy (esophagogastroduodenoscopy [EGD])
    a. Most sensitive method to evaluate esophagus, stomach, and proximal duodenum
    b. Combines diagnostic and therapeutic capability
    c. Generally requires sedation

2. Upper GI and small bowel x-ray series
   a. Allows visualization of esophagus, stomach, and entire small bowel
   b. Single contrast, therefore detail often lost, particularly in small bowel
3. Small bowel enema (enteroclysis)
   a. Special barium study, with contrast instilled directly into duodenum via tube passed orally
   b. Double contrast so able to delineate subtle lesions not seen on conventional x-ray studies
   c. Not available in all settings, very dependent on expertise of radiologist

IV. Diagnostic Approach

In general practice, occult GI bleeding is discovered via FOBT. However, the clinical setting in which this testing is done—routine screening, screening for malignancy in high-risk patients, testing in the setting of iron deficiency etc.—will determine the subsequent work-up.

All patients with a positive FOBT, need to have a complete blood count, red blood cell indices, and iron studies (Fe, total iron-binding capacity, ferritin) checked.

A. FOBT positive in an asymptomatic patient *without* anemia

1. Usually in setting of screening for colorectal cancer
2. Colonoscopy versus flexible sigmoidoscopy/barium enema (depending on local availability and patient preference) should be initial test in any patient over 40. In patients < 40, especially with upper GI symptoms (nausea, vomiting, epigastric pain, etc.) upper endoscopy (or upper GI series) is more appropriate initial evaluation.
3. If evaluation is negative, and individual risk of cancer is low, can follow with regular blood testing and repeat FOBT in 3–6 mo

B. FOBT positive in the asymptomatic patient *with* anemia

1. Unless there is a clear non-GI bleeding source, an aggressive GI evaluation should be pursued.
2. GI lesions will be found in > 65% of all men and postmenopausal women with iron deficiency anemia.
3. Colonoscopy is the test of choice; if negative, upper endoscopy
4. X-ray studies in this setting are not suggested.
5. If evaluation to this point is negative, then small bowel enteroclysis should be obtained.
6. If bleeding source still not found, GI referral (if not already done) for further help with evaluation is mandated.

C. FOBT positive with GI symptoms

1. If symptoms are clearly upper GI, then EGD or upper GI with small bowel follow-through is recommended.
2. As a general rule, in elderly patients, or patients at high risk for colon cancer, even if a definitive lesion is found on upper GI evaluation, the lower tract should also be evaluated, because the chance of synchronous lesions is great enough to justify the effort.

D. Screening of patients at high risk for colon cancer (see Chapter 8)

V. Indications for Referral

A. Referral to a Gastroenterologist

1. For endoscopic evaluation (diagnostic and/or therapeutic)
2. Barium enema or upper GI study with positive findings
3. Any patient with previous colon cancer
4. Any patient with inflammatory bowel disease
5. Long-term screening for patients at high risk for colon cancer

B. Referral to a Surgeon

1. When surgery is indicated for resection of a neoplasm

VI. Indications for Hospitalization

A. Evidence of active bleeding

B. Elective surgical admission for removal of neoplasm

C. Flares of inflammatory bowel disease (may seek GI consultation first)

D. Rare instances where patient is unable to complete bowel preparation before diagnostic study

VII. Annotated Bibliography

Ahlquist D. Approach to the patient with occult gastrointestinal bleeding. In: Yamada T, ed. Textbook of Gastroenterology. Philadelphia: JB Lippincott; 1991:616–634. A comprehensive review of the subject, with a complete discussion of evaluation of occult bleeding in different clinical scenarios.

Ahlquist D, Wieand HS, Moertel CG. Accuracy of fecal occult blood screening for colorectal neoplasia. A prospective study using Hemoccult and HemoQuant tests. JAMA 1993;269(10):1262–1267. Recent prospective study of the predictive accuracy of several types of FOBT cards, as well as their generally poor ability to detect colorectal neoplasia.

Hsia PC, Al-Kawas FH. Upper endoscopy in the evaluation of asymptomatic patients with Hemoccult positive stool after negative colonoscopy. Am J Gastroenterol 1992;87(11):1571–1574. One of several similar studies that identifies the value of looking for upper sources of occult bleeding if colonoscopy is negative.

Chapter 50: Gastroesophageal Reflux Disease

David S. Weinberg and Christine Laine

I. Clinical Presentation

A. General Information

1. Epidemiology

   a. Gastroesophageal reflux disease (GERD) represents the effortless movement of gastric contents from stomach to esophagus. Manifested as "heartburn," it occurs in one third of the population monthly and 10% of the population daily. Up to 25% of pregnant women will experience symptomatic reflux daily.
   b. Conditions frequently associated with reflux
      1) Diabetes mellitus
      2) Pregnancy
      3) Zollinger-Ellison syndrome
      4) Scleroderma

2. Etiology

   a. Noxious substances in the stomach include HCl, bile salts, pancreatic enzymes, and pepsin.
   b. Etiology currently thought to be multifactorial, centering on interaction of hiatal hernia and decreased lower esophageal sphincter (LES) pressure. Neither hiatal hernia nor decreased LES pressure is synonymous with reflux.

B. Symptoms

1. Esophageal symptoms

   a. Heartburn
      1) Usually after meals, worse when reclining
      2) Frequency and severity not correlated with tissue damage
   b. Chest pain
      1) Sharp or dull
      2) Can radiate
   c. Waterbrash
      1) Excess salivation stimulated by refluxed materials
      2) Tastes bland or salty

d. Regurgitation
   1) Bitter or acid taste
e. Dysphagia/odynophagia
   1) Stricture or esophagitis can underlie complaints

2. Nonesophageal symptoms

   a. Oropharyngeal
      1) Sore throat
      2) Earache
   b. Laryngeal
      1) Hoarseness
   c. Pulmonary
      1) Wheezing
      2) Cough
      3) Bronchospasm
      4) Aspiration

C. Physical Examination

Physical exam is often nonspecific in GERD. The goal should be to look for evidence of other etiologies for the patient's symptoms.

II. Diagnostic Approach

Early diagnostic testing is warranted in any patient with symptoms or signs of esophageal damage such as odynophagia, dysphagia, heme-positive stool, or anemia.

A. General Tests

1. Upper GI series

   a. Very low sensitivity (20–30%) for reflux
   b. Dependent on radiologist noting reflux during the study

2. Continuous intraesophageal pH monitoring

   a. Accomplished with a nasally inserted pH probe placed 5 cm above the LES
   b. Sensitivity 85%, specificity 90%

B. Tests to Differentiate GERD pain from other causes of chest pain

1. Bernstein test

   a. Nasogastric tube is placed in mid esophagus and either acid or saline is infused.
   b. Occurrence of symptoms with acid infusion is a positive test for reflux.
   c. Sensitivity and specificity are approximately 80%.

2. Cardiac studies are sometimes necessary to rule out cardiac chest pain.

C. Tests to Assess Type and Degree of Esophageal Injury

Unless there is a complaint of dysphagia, or other concern about a stricture, endoscopic evaluation is the test of choice in GERD.

1. Esophagogastroduodenoscopy (EGD)
   a. Allows biopsy for tissue diagnosis
   b. Gold standard for documenting tissue injury (esophagitis and/or Barrett's esophagus)
2. Barium swallow can be helpful, and should be the first test for complaints of dysphagia.
   a. Single contrast
      1) Strictures
      2) Ulcers
      3) Hiatal hernia
   b. Double contrast
      1) Erosions
      2) Barrett's esophagus

III. Differential Diagnosis

A. Cholelithiasis (see Chapter 51B)

B. Peptic ulcer disease (see Chapter 48A)

C. Angina (see Chapter 21)

D. Esophageal motility disorders

E. Gastritis

F. Esophagitis secondary to infection, pills, or noxious ingestion

IV. Treatment

GERD is a slowly progressive disorder and is rarely life-threatening.

A. Medical Management is two-pronged.

1. Nonpharmacologic therapy should be the initial treatment in all patients with clinically apparent reflux.
   a. Elevate head of bed by 10 inches so that gravity will enhance acid clearance.
   b. Cease alcohol and tobacco use because these substances decrease LES pressure and alter epithelial function.
   c. Decrease meal size to decrease the number of times the LES spontaneously relaxes in response to gastric distention.

d. Decrease dietary substances that decrease LES pressure or stimulate acid secretion (fat, coffee, chocolate, cola beverages, spearmint, peppermint, tomato juice, citrus juice)
   e. Avoid drugs that decrease LES pressure
      1) Anticholinergics
      2) Theophylline
      3) Benzodiazapines
      4) Narcotics
      5) Calcium channel blockers
      6) β-Agonists
      7) α-Antagonists
      8) Progesterone
2. Pharmacologic therapy
   a. Liquid antacids
      1) Safe, effective, can be used PRN
      2) Problems with compliance due to frequency of dosing, taste, effect on bowel motility
      3) Magnesium- or aluminum-containing antacids (Maalox, Mylanta both 30 mL 4–6 times/d) can be problematic in patients with renal insufficiency.
      4) Patients requiring salt restriction should use Riopan (30 mL 4–6 times/d) because it is low in salt content opposed to other antacids.
   b. H_2 blockers are the pillars of continuous therapy; patients may need high doses.
      1) Cimetidine (Tagamet) 400–1600 mg qd in divided doses
      2) Ranitidine (Zantac) 300–600 mg qd in divided doses
      3) Famotidine (Pepcid) 20–40 mg qd in divided doses
   c. Omeprazole (Prilosec) 20 mg qd–b.i.d.
      1) Proton pump inhibitor that effectively turns off acid production
      2) Approved for use in erosive esophagitis or in GERD refractory to other therapy
      3) Not yet approved for long-term use because of concern regarding carcinoid production
   d. Sulcrafate (Carafate) 1 g PO t.i.d.–q.i.d.
      1) Topical agent that may be useful in protecting esophageal mucosa
      2) Patients with severe erosive esophagitis benefit the most.
      3) Constipation is the major side effect.
      4) Can interfere with the absorption of other medications
   e. Metoclopramide (Reglan) 10–20 mg PO t.i.d.–q.i.d.
      1) Dopamine antagonist that may increase gastric emptying and increase LES pressure
      2) No anti-inflammatory effect
      3) Significant CNS side effects particularly in the elderly (insomnia, drowsiness, agitation, dyskinesia)

B. Surgical therapy is rarely indicated, but when dedicated therapy for symptom relief fails or recurrent complications occur (stricture, malignancy, hemorrhage) surgery may be necessary.

C. Patient Education

The physician must advise the patient that the nonpharmacologic therapy is as important as the pharmacologic therapy.

V. Indications for Referral

A. When upper endoscopy is required because of high suspicion of tissue injury, gastroenterology referral is necessary.

B. Gastroenterology referral is often helpful for patients with symptoms refractory to the usual therapeutic modalities.

C. The management of complications stemming from GERD often requires referral to a gastroenterologist.

1. Barrett's esophagus—stratified squamous epithelium of the lower esophagus is replaced by metaplastic intestinal epithelium.

    a. Acquired lesion that develops as a result of reflux damage to the lower esophagus
    b. Seen in 10–15% of patients with esophagitis and 40% of patients with peptic strictures
    c. Barrett's esophagus is a premalignant lesion; approximately 10% of patients with Barrett's esophagus will develop adenocarcinoma.
    d. Average age of onset is 55 y.
    e. More common in men than in women
    f. Barrett's esophagus is asymptomatic and the diagnosis is made by endoscopy. Once it is known to be present, patient should have regular EGD with biopsy to detect significant dysplasia.

2. Stricture—bands of submucosal fibrous tissue that constrict the esophageal lumen and impede the passage of material from mouth to stomach

    a. Patients with stricture usually complain of dysphagia with solids more than liquids.
    b. Patients with stricture often report decreased heartburn because the fibrous tissue is less prone to acid injury than is normal tissue.
    c. Strictures are usually smooth walled and occur in the lower 1-4 cm.
    d. Whether a stricture is benign or malignant must be determined by endoscopy and biopsy.
    e. Bougie or balloon dilation is treatment of choice.

3. Hemorrhage—may occur secondary to esophageal ulcers

4. Perforation—due to severe tissue injury, rare

D. In cases refractory to medical therapy, referral to a surgeon may be necessary to have patient evaluated for surgical therapy to decrease reflux.

VI. Indications for Hospitalization

A. Hemorrhage

B. Perforation

VII. Annotated Bibliography

Cohen S. Pathogenesis of gastroesophageal reflux disease: a challenge in clinical physiology. Ann Intern Med 1992;117:1051–1052. An editorial addressing the role of LES competence, hiatal hernia, and other hypotheses about the determinants of GERD.

Gelfand MD. Gastroesophageal reflux disease. Med Clin North Am 1991;72:923–940. Extensively referenced article on all aspects of GERD with an emphasis on pathophysiology and diagnosis.

Spechler S, Goyal RK. Barrett's esophagus. N Engl J Med 1986;315:362–371. A complete review of Barrett's esophagus discussing pathogenesis, clinical features, and treatment options.

Chapter 51: Hepatic and Biliary Disease

51A Abnormal Liver Function Tests

Karen S. Scoles

I. Clinical Presentation

A. General Information

1. These are not actually tests of liver function, but elevations of certain liver enzyme levels reflecting hepatocyte injury.
2. They include alanine aminotransferase (ALT, formerly serum glutamic pyruvate transaminase), aspartate aminotransferase (AST, formerly serum glutamic oxaloacetic transaminase), alkaline phosphatase, and γ-glutamyl transpeptidase (GGTP).

   a. The aminotransferases, ALT and AST, are the most frequently measured tests in the evaluation of liver disease, especially in acute processes.
   b. AST is a mitochondrial enzyme present in large quantities in heart, liver, skeletal muscle, and kidney and thus may not be specific for liver disease.
   c. ALT is also present in the heart and skeletal muscle, but a greater proportion is present in the liver, making ALT more specific for liver damage than AST.
   d. Alkaline phosphatase is present in liver, bone, and intestine. The placenta is responsible for the elevation in alkaline phosphatase seen in the third trimester of pregnancy. An elevated alkaline phosphatase of liver origin is usually associated with cholestatic liver disease. It can be fractionated by electrophoresis to identify the origin of the enzyme elevation.
   e. γ-Glutamyl transpeptidase
      1) Found in many tissues including liver, kidney, pancreas, heart and brain
      2) An inducible microsomal enzyme
      3) Serum values are increased in cholestasis and hepatocellular disease.
      4) γ-Glutamyl transpeptidase (γ-GTP) can be used to confirm that increased levels of alkaline phosphatase are of hepatic origin because elevations of γ-GTP parallel alkaline phosphatase in cholestasis.
      5) γ-GTP can be elevated in ethanol abuse even without liver disease.
      6) May be elevated in other systemic disorders such as thyrotoxicosis, renal failure, myocardial infarction

B. Symptoms

1. Patients are most often asymptomatic and are found to have liver function abnormalities as a result of "screening" blood test panels.
2. These patients should be carefully questioned about medications, alcohol use, risks for hepatitis, IV drug use, and family history of liver disease.

II. Diagnostic Approach

A. Asymptomatic patients with under threefold elevation in liver function abnormalities should have follow-up testing in 1–3 mo.

B. Patients with persistent elevations or greater than threefold elevation on initial testing should be further evaluated.

C. If AST or ALT is mildly elevated (< 3 times) retest after 1–3 mo or after obesity is corrected, drugs discontinued, and the patient abstains from ethanol.

D. Abnormalities present > 6 mo are chronic.

E. The levels of enzyme elevation do not necessarily correlate with the severity of the disease.

F. The evaluation is guided by the patient's history and the pattern of enzyme elevation (Table 51A–1).

III. Differential Diagnosis

A. Hepatocellular Disease

1. May be secondary to hepatocellular injury due to ethanol, fatty infiltration, drugs, viral illnesses, autoimmune disease or inherited conditions
    a. Alcoholic liver disease
        1) Generally enzyme elevations < 300 units/L
        2) AST/ALT ratio > 2:1
        3) Need to rule out other causes of chronic hepatitis in alcoholics with transaminase levels > 300 units/L

Table 51A–1. Enzyme Elevation

Enzyme	Cholestatic	Hepatocellular
AST/ALT	N to +	+ + to + + +
ALK PHOS	+ + to + + +	N to +
γ-GTP	+ to + + +	+ to + +

b. Viral infections resulting in chronic hepatitis are diagnosed by serologic tests and persistent transaminase elevation (see Chapter 51C).
   1) Hepatitis B—positive hepatitis B surface antigen (HBsAg); negative hepatitis B core antibody IgM (anti-HBc-IgM)
   2) Hepatitis C—positive test for the antibody to hepatitis C virus (anti-HVC) is suggestive but the diagnosis should be confirmed with the more specific recombinant immunoblot assay.
   3) Identification of chronic hepatitis by liver biopsy is important because treatment may halt progression to cirrhosis.
c. Drugs responsible for hepatocellular disease
   1) Acetominophen
   2) Methyldopa
   3) General anesthetic agents
   4) Phenytoin
   5) Isoniazid
   6) Penicillins
   7) Niacin
   8) Procainamide
   9) Quinidine
d. Fatty liver (steatohepatitis)
   1) Can be confused with alcoholic liver disease
   2) Usually associated with AST/ALT < 3
   3) Never associated with hypoalbuminemia or prolongation of the prothrombin time
e. Autoimmune hepatitis
   1) Associated with significant (8 times) levels of transaminase elevation
   2) Hypergammaglobulinemia may also be present.
   3) Patients who have chronically elevated transaminases without obvious etiology should have antinuclear antibody and antismooth muscle antibody titers determined.
f. Other inherited diseases should be ruled out as well.
   1) Hemochromatosis
      i) Minimal enzyme elevations, AST and ALT < 3 times normal
      ii) Transferrin saturation > 62%
      iii) Confirmed by liver biopsy with iron staining
   2) Wilson's disease
      i) This diagnosis should be considered when patients younger than 40 present with chronically abnormal liver function abnormalities.
      ii) Diagnosed by liver biopsy with determination of hepatic copper content

B. Cholestatic Disease
1. May be secondary to biliary obstruction, infiltrating liver pathology, or nonobstructive cholestasis. Ultrasonography is used initially to detect gallbladder abnormalities, dilated bile ducts, or hepatic mass lesions. Further evaluation with liver biopsy, endoscopic retrograde cholangiopancreatography (ERCP), CT or MRI of the abdomen or transhepatic cholangiogram may be necessary.

2. Nonobstructive cholestasis may be due to
   a. Drugs—Patients may have fever, RUQ pain and tenderness secondary to drug-induced cholestasis.
      1) Oral contraceptives
      2) Anabolic steroids
      3) Oral hypoglycemics
      4) Phenothiazines
      5) Clavulanic acid
      6) Propoxyphene
   b. Primary biliary cirrhosis—mostly middle-aged women, greater than eightfold elevation in alkaline phosphatase, normal bilirubin, positive antimitochondrial antibody. Patients often present with generalized pruritus. Confirmed by liver biopsy.
   c. Primary sclerosing cholangitis—mostly younger men, associated with inflammatory bowel disease, diagnosed by ERCP
   d. Granulomatous liver disease such as sarcoidosis, tuberculosis or other infectious diseases

IV. Treatment

Abnormal liver function studies are a symptom of a specific process. Often the etiology of the abnormalities cannot be determined. When the etiology is determined, treatment depends on the disease process responsible for the elevation.

V. Indications for Referral

A. Patients should be referred for liver biopsy when liver enzymes are persistently elevated and results of other studies are not conclusive.

B. Patients should understand that liver biopsy may not reveal a treatable cause of chronic liver disease. When liver biopsy is not performed in asymptomatic patients with chronic liver disease, they should have repeat liver function studies q 4–6 mo. These patients should be reevaluated for biopsy if the clinical course deteriorates.

VI. Indications for Hospitalization

Patients undergoing liver biopsy are often admitted overnight for observation.

VII. Annotated Bibliography

Frank BB. Clinical evaluation of jaundice: a guideline of the Patient Care Committee of the American Gastroenterological Association. JAMA 1989;316(9):521–528. A clinical guideline for the effective evaluation of jaundice.

Gittlin N. Differential diagnosis of elevated liver enzymes. Contemp Intern Med January 1993;44–56. Two complete, well written reviews for the general internist or family practitioner.

Herrera J. Abnormal liver enzyme levels. Postgrad Med 1993;93(2):113–131.

Kaplan M. Laboratory tests. In: Schiff L, Schiff E, eds. Diseases of the Liver, 6th ed. Philadelphia: JB Lippincott;1988:219–252.

51B Cholelithiasis

Christine Laine and David S. Weinberg

I. Clinical Presentation

A. General Information

1. Epidemiology
   a. Approximately 20 million people in the United States have gallstones, making cholelithiasis the most prevalent biliary disorder in this country.
   b. More than 500,000 cholecystectomies are performed annually in the United States.
   c. The distribution of gallstones varies widely with ethnicity and geography, suggesting that both hereditary and life-style factors affect the development of gallstones.

2. Pathogenesis—Gallstones can be of two different types
   a. Cholesterol stones
      1) Develop as a consequence of
         a) Biliary cholesterol hypersecretion due to advancing age, obesity, hormonal fluxes, medications, or high-fat diet
         b) Bile salt hyposecretion due to excessive GI loss or underproduction
      2) Usually arise in the gallbladder
      3) The most common type of gallstone in the United States, especially prevalent in women, Pima Indians, and persons with ileal pathology
   b. Pigment stones
      1) Calcium bilirubinate stones arising from precipitation of indirect bilirubin
      2) Arise in gallbladder or in the cystic ducts
      3) Common in Asians, chronic parenteral nutrition, and patients with liver disease, hemolysis, or hemoglobinopathies
      4) Brown pigment stones are associated with the presence of bacteria (*Escherichia coli* and anaerobes); black pigment stones are not

B. Symptoms

1. One third of people with gallstones will develop symptoms or complications of cholelithiasis; two thirds will remain entirely asymptomatic.

2. Symptoms of biliary colic
   a. Pain secondary to spasm due to cystic duct obstruction by stones and inflammation of the gallbladder is not present.
   b. Pain tends to be episodic and severe, located in the RUQ or epigastrium, and usually lasts from 15 min to 3 h.
   c. Pain may radiate to precordium, scapulae, or right shoulder.
   d. Contrary to common belief, it is difficult to link symptom episodes with the consumption of fatty meals.

3. Symptoms of cholecystitis
    a. Cholecystitis is characterized by inflammation of the gallbladder.
    b. Can occur with stones or in the absence of stones
    c. Pain similar to biliary colic, but lasting for > 6 h should raise the suspicion of cholecystitis.
    d. Low-grade fever or emesis
    e. Symptoms may be absent in diabetic, immunosuppressed, or elderly patients.

C. Physical Examination
1. Biliary colic
    a. Abdominal tenderness, usually localized to the RUQ, without other findings
2. Cholecystitis
    a. Abdominal tenderness with positive Murphy's sign
    b. Gallbladder may be palpable.
    c. Low-grade fever may be present.
    d. Jaundice present in 15% of cases

II. Diagnostic Approach

Because cholelithiasis is prevalent, it often coexists with other pathology and the finding of gallstones does not always mean that you have uncovered the source of the patient's symptoms.

A. Many diagnostic tests are available. The challenge is to avoid unnecessary, costly studies.

1. Blood tests
    a. In uncomplicated biliary colic, there will be no hematologic or biochemical abnormalities.
    b. In cholecystitis
        1) Leukocytosis with left shift
        2) Elevated alkaline phosphatase
        3) Elevated transaminases (< 2.5 times normal)
        4) Bilirubin elevated to 2–10 mg/dL if choledocholithiasis is present; if > 15 mg/dL suspect malignant obstruction

2. Radiologic studies
    a. Plain films rarely helpful in the diagnosis of cholelithiasis because fewer than 20% of gallstones are radiopaque
    b. Ultrasound
        1) Highly sensitive and specific for gallstones and should be used to diagnose or exclude gallstones
        2) Thickened gallbladder wall, intramural gas, and pericholecystic fluid suggest infection.
        3) The significance of sludge in the gallbladder is unclear.

4) Inability to see a gallstone on ultrasound does not rule out choledocholithiasis.
  c. Hepatobiliary scintigraphy (HIDA)
    1) Failure to image the gallbladder by 90 min in the presence of adequate views of the liver, common bile duct, and small intestine strongly suggests acute obstructive disease.
    2) False positives can occur from nonfasting or prolonged fasting; repeat scanning in 4 h or giving morphine can help to decrease false positives.
  d. Oral cholecystography
    1) Rarely the initial diagnostic test
    2) Chief advantage over ultrasound is that oral cholecystography enables the assessment of gallbladder function and cystic duct patency.
  e. CT
    1) Test of choice when tumor is suspected
    2) Not as good as ultrasound in the diagnosis of common bile duct stones
  f. Endoscopic retrograde cholangiopancreatography (ERCP)
    1) Indicated when the biliary system must be visualized for diagnostic or therapeutic reasons
    2) A major advantage of ERCP is the ability to obtain tissue.
    3) Demonstrates the lower extent of an obstruction
    4) If ERCP not available, percutaneous transhepatic cholecystography can be considered; better than ERCP for proximal obstructions

III. Differential Diagnosis

A. Gastritis/duodenitis/ulcer disease

B. Irritable bowel syndrome

C. Acute pancreatitis

D. Appendicitis

IV. Treatment

A. Asymptomatic Cholelithiasis

When gallstones are an incidental finding in a patient with no symptoms referable to gallbladder disease, no treatment is indicated unless the patient has diabetes mellitus or if the stones are detected during laparoscopy.

B. Symptomatic Cholelithiasis

In the past, surgery was the only option. Several nonsurgical approaches now exist for appropriate patients. Cholecystectomy remains the only curative therapy for gallstones. Stones may recur after any therapy that removes the gallstones, but leaves the gallbladder in place.

1. Oral bile acids lead to the secretion of unsaturated bile and dissolution of gallstones.
   a. Ursodeoxycholic acid (UDCA)
      1) Patient selection criteria are similar to the criteria for CDCA, except that obesity or liver disease does not contraindicate UDCA.
      2) Higher efficacy and lower side effects make UDCA preferable to CDCA when oral bile acid therapy is the appropriate therapy.
      3) Dose range is 8–12 mg/kg/d generally for periods ≤ 2 y.
   b. Chenodeoxycholic acid (CDCA)
      1) Indications
         a) Cholesterol stones
         b) Stones < 1.5 cm in diameter
      2) Contraindications
         a) Pigment stones
         b) Stones > 1.5 cm in diameter
         c) Pregnancy
         d) Obesity
         e) Liver disease
         f) Hyperlipidemia
      3) Dose range is 12–15 mg/kg/d for 1–3 y.
      4) CDCA leads to 20–40% complete dissolution of gallstones.
2. Contact solvents
   a. When gallstones can be reached by catheter, solvents (eg, methyl tert butyl ether) can be applied directly to the stones.
   b. Works for cholesterol stones, little success with pigment stones
   c. None of the solvents have thus far proved to be easy, safe, and effective.
3. Extracorporeal shock wave lithotripsy (ESWL)
   a. Used in combination with UDCA
   b. Best results occur with single, small gallstones

V. Indications for Referral to a Gastroenterologist

A. Gastroenterology referral is indicated if
1. The diagnosis is unclear
2. ERCP is indicated

B. Surgical referral is necessary if cholecystectomy is indicated.

VI. Indications for Hospitalization

The patient should be hospitalized when acute cholecystitis is suspected.

VII. Annotated Bibliography

Bruckstein AH. Nonsurgical management of cholelithiasis. Arch Intern Med 1990;150:960-964. A comprehensive review of nonsurgical treatment options for cholelithiasis.

Gibney EJ. Asymptomatic gallstones. Br J Surg 1990;77:368-372. A review of the management of asymptomatic gallstones.

Lee SP, Sekijima J. Gallstones. In: Yamada T, ed. Textbook of Gastroenterology. Philadelphia: JB Lippincott; 1991:1966-1989. An overview of gallstones with an extensive discussion of pathogenesis.

Way LW, Sleisenger MH. Cholelithiasis; chronic and acute cholecystitis. In: Sleisenger MH, Fordtran JS, eds. Gastrointestinal Disease, 4th ed. Philadelphia: WB Saunders; 1989:1691-1714. This chapter contains a good discussion of the epidemiology and clinical management of gallstone disease.

51C Viral Hepatitis: A, B, and C
Carol M. Reife

I. Clinical Presentation

A. General Information

1. Acute viral hepatitis is a systemic infection affecting predominantly the liver. Clinical and epidemiologic features of the different types of hepatitis are variable and considerable overlap exists.

2. Incubation period

   a. Hepatitis A (HAV): 2–6 wk
   b. Hepatitis B (HBV): 4–26 wk
   c. Hepatitis C (HCV): 2–16 wk

3. Epidemiology

   a. HAV—Spread is almost entirely by the fecal-oral route. Spread is common from person to person in families and in institutions and in areas with poor hygiene and overcrowding. Large outbreaks as well as sporadic cases have been traced to contaminated food, water, milk and shellfish.
   b. HBV—The major route of transmission is by percutaneous exposure. HBV has been found in almost every body fluid. Prevalence is increased in:
      1) Sexual contacts of those with HBV
      2) Homosexuals
      3) Infants of mothers infected with HBV
      4) Those with occupational exposure to contaminated blood and body fluids (health care workers)
      5) Those receiving multiple transfusions
      6) IV drug users
      7) Some developing countries
   c. HCV—Spread may be by percutaneous as well as nonpercutaneous exposure. Prevalence is increased in those receiving multiple blood or blood product transfusions and in IV drug users. HCV also seems to be transmitted by intrafamily and intrainstitutional contact and by occupational exposures. Sexual transmission and vertical transmission appear uncommon. There is a high proportion of sporadic cases in patients with an entirely negative history.

B. Symptoms are variable.

1. Prodromal symptoms may precede the onset of jaundice by 1–2 wk and may include a variety of symptoms such as anorexia, nausea, vomiting, weight loss, fatigue, malaise, arthralgias, myalgias, headache, photophobia, pharyngitis, cough, coryza, fever, dark urine and clay-colored stools.

2. Many patients with viral hepatitis never become icteric but once jaundice appears, constitutional symptoms usually decrease.

3. Specific viruses

    a. HAV—Anorexia may be a prominent symptom. Children tend to be asymptomatic; older patients may have more severe symptoms.
    b. HBV—5–10% of patients with acute hepatitis B experience a prodromal serum sickness-like syndrome with rash, angioedema, fever, and arthritis and occasionally glomerulonephritis with the nephrotic syndrome.
    c. HCV—About 75% of cases are anicteric and relatively asymptomatic. Extrahepatic manifestations are rare compared to HBV infection although there has been a link with aplastic anemia.

C. Physical Examination

1. A low-grade fever is most often present in HAV but may also be present in HBV especially when there is a serum sickness-like syndrome.

2. After the onset of jaundice, there may then be RUQ pain and tenderness as the liver becomes enlarged. Splenomegaly and cervical adenopathy may be present in 10–20% of those with acute hepatitis.

D. Clinical Course

1. The prodromal symptoms of acute viral hepatitis may precede the onset of jaundice by 1–2 wk. Constitutional symptoms decrease as jaundice resolves but liver enlargement, RUQ pain, and liver function test abnormalities may persist. (Acute levels of transaminase elevation do not correlate with degree of hepatocellular damage.)

2. Patients with underlying medical illness or advanced age may have a more complicated course as do patients presenting with ascites, peripheral edema, or hepatic encephalopathy.

3. More severe disease and poorer prognosis are suggested by a prolonged prothrombin time, low serum albumin, hypoglycemia, or high serum bilirubin.

4. Specific viruses

    a. HAV—Almost all patients with hepatitis A recover completely within 1–2 mo with no sequelae. Occasionally, patients with hepatitis A develop "relapsing hepatitis" weeks to months after apparent resolution of infection with recurrence of symptoms and transaminase elevations. Hepatitis with protracted cholestatic jaundice may also occur. Fulminant hepatitis is extremely rare. There is no HAV carrier state (Figure 51C-1).
    b. HBV—90% or more of patients with hepatitis B have a favorable course and recover completely usually 3–4 mo after the onset of jaundice. Fulminant hepatitis with massive hepatic necrosis and extremely high mortality may be seen occasionally. Approximately 5–10% of patients with hepatitis B develop chronic disease. These patients may continue as asymptomatic carriers or may develop either chronic persistent or chronic active hepatitis. These latter entities are characterized by a combination of hepatocyte necrosis and inflammation of varying severity persisting for > 6 mo

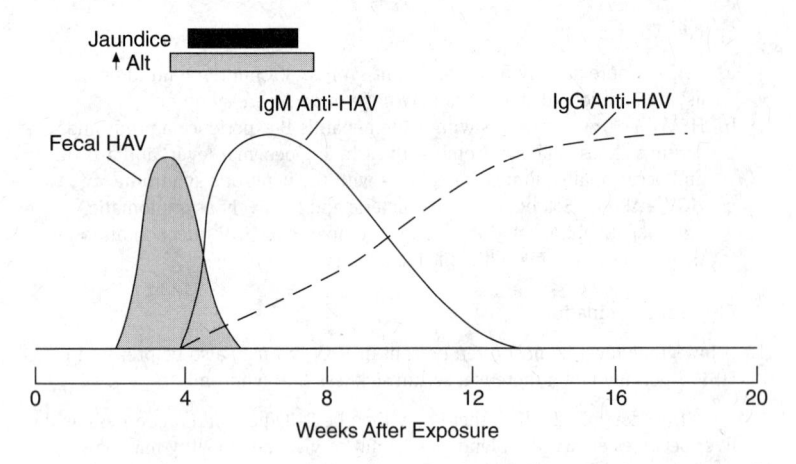

Figure 51C–1. Scheme of Typical Clinical and Laboratory Features of Viral Hepatitis Type A.

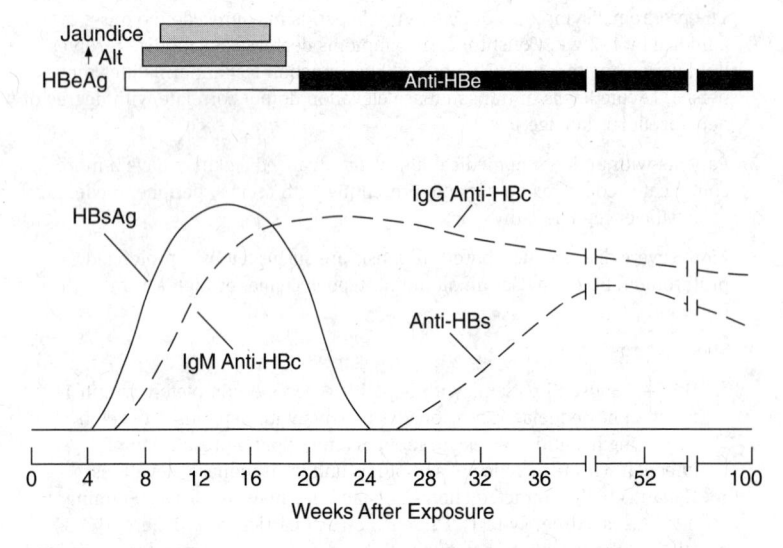

Figure 51C–2. Scheme of Typical Clinical and Laboratory Features of Acute Viral Hepatitis Type B.

(above). Carriers of HBsAg have an increased risk of developing hepatocellular carcinoma (Figure 51C-2).
c. HCV—50% of infected patients will develop clinical and biochemical evidence of chronic infection regardless of the route of infection. 20% of

these patients will develop cirrhosis, often with few clinical manifestations of liver disease, suggesting a more indolent form of cirrhosis. There is also an increased risk of hepatoma in these patients.

5. Chronic hepatitis—both HBV and HCV infection may progress to chronic hepatitis, defined as ongoing inflammation of the liver persisting for at least 6 mo.
   a. Chronic persistent hepatitis
      1) Inflammation is limited to the portal tracts. Disease is nonprogressive and hepatic failure does not occur. Fibrosis may be seen but development of cirrhosis is very rare.
      2) Most patients are asymptomatic although anorexia, fatigue, nausea and vomiting may occur.
      3) Physical examination is usually normal although the liver may be slightly enlarged and tender.
      4) During active phases, aminotransferase levels may resemble those seen in acute hepatitis but more frequently only mild liver function test abnormalities are seen.
   b. Chronic active hepatitis
      1) Inflammation involves the portal tracts as well as periportal parenchyma. There is ongoing inflammation, hepatic necrosis, and fibrosis.
      2) About one third of patients have disease that begins abruptly; most often, however, onset of disease is insidious and diagnosis may be incidental.
      3) Fatigue is common as are recurrent symptoms of jaundice, malaise, anorexia, and low-grade fever. Extrahepatic features may be prominent and symptoms due to complications of cirrhosis may occur. There may be long periods of time without overt disease although ongoing hepatic necrosis persists.
      4) Liver function tests are invariably abnormal but may not correlate with clinical severity. Laboratory abnormalities may be mild despite severe biopsy findings.
      5) Liver failure, cirrhosis, and ultimately death may occur.

II. Diagnostic Approach

A. Laboratory Values

1. Liver function tests—Serum aspartate aminotransferase (AST) and alanine aminotransferase (ALT) increase variably during the prodromal phase with peak levels of 400–4000 IU. When jaundice appears, serum bilirubin levels continue to rise (to ranges of 5–20 mg/dL) although serum aminotransferase levels may start to fall. Increased serum alkaline phosphatase levels may be seen.

2. Neutropenia and lymphopenia may be seen, followed by a relative lympocytosis. Atypical lymphocytes are common during the acute phase of illness.

3. The prothrombin time may be prolonged indicating extensive hepatocellular necrosis.

4. Hypoglycemia may be present due to inadequate PO intake and poor hepatic glycogen reserves.
5. A diffuse mild elevation in γ globulins may be present and antibodies including antinuclear antibody, heterophil antibody, and rheumatoid factor may be seen.

B. Serology

1. HAV—anti-HAV (antibody to hepatitis A virus)
   a. IgM anti-HAV appears early on in disease when aminotransferase levels are high and persists for several months. Diagnosis of acute hepatitis A is made by finding IgM anti-HAV during acute illness.
   b. IgG anti-HAV develops during convalescence and remains indefinitely, conferring protection against reinfection.
2. HBV
   a. HBsAg (hepatitis B surface antigen) appears first, before symptoms or liver function test elevations. It usually lasts 1–2 mo after the onset of jaundice and is rarely detectable after 6 mo.
   b. Anti-HBs (antibody to hepatitis B surface antigen) appears in the serum after HBsAg disappears and may remain indefinitely. It is a protective antibody. There may be a "window" period of several weeks or longer after HBsAg disappears before anti-HBs appears. 10–20% patients with chronic HBV infection may have low levels of anti-HBs despite the persistence of HBsAg.
   c. HBcAg (hepatitis B core antigen) is associated with the core of the hepatitis B virion but is not detectable in serum.
   d. Anti-HBc (antibody to hepatitis B core antigen) may indicate infection during the window period before anti-HBs appears. It may persist for years after HBV infection, at times longer than anti-HBs. IgM class antibody usually predominates during the first 6 mo of infection and IgG antibody beyond 6 mo.
   e. HBeAg (hepatitis B e antigen) is found only in HBsAg-positive serum. It appears transiently early in the course of illness and usually disappears in the first several months. Persistent HbeAg coincides with ongoing replication and correlates with infectivity.
3. HCV—Anti-HCV (antibody to hepatitis C virus) is detectable by a commercially available enzyme-linked immunosorbent assay (ELISA) test. It may take 6–12 mo for the antibody to appear and therefore assays for anti-HCV are of limited value in the diagnosis of acute hepatitis C. This antibody is not neutralizing and does not indicate immunity to the virus, only exposure. The false positivity rate of the ELISA test is high. A second test, using the recombinant immunoblot assay (RIBA) is much more specific.

C. Liver Biopsy

1. Definitive diagnosis can only be made by liver biopsy.
2. Liver biopsy is rarely indicated in acute viral hepatitis except when the diagnosis is in question.

3. Liver biopsy may be considered in some patients with chronic hepatitis. Because there is no consistent clinical or laboratory pattern to distinguish among different types of hepatitis, liver biopsy may be considered in patients with abnormal liver function tests, in the range of 1.5–2 times normal, persisting for at least 6 mo. Biopsy will provide more accurate information regarding diagnosis and will also give prognostic information.

III. Differential Diagnosis

A. Extrahepatic manifestations including arthritis, pleuritis, rash, abdominal pain, anemia, and azotemia may cause confusion with connective tissue disorders.

B. Other viral illnesses such as infectious mononucleosis or infection with cytomegalovirus, herpes simplex, coxsackie virus, and toxoplasmosis may present as acute hepatitis. Tests such as heterophile antibodies and serologic tests for the various agents may help in differentiating the cause of infection.

C. Various drugs, anesthetic agents and toxins (eg, isoniazid, halothane, carbon tetrachloride) can produce a picture like that of acute viral hepatitis or cholestasis.

D. Alcoholic liver disease may present as acute hepatitis (usually serum aminotransferase levels are not as high and other stigmata of chronic alcohol use are present).

E. Acute cholecystitis, common duct stone, or ascending cholangitis may present with RUQ pain, nausea, vomiting, fever, and jaundice. Malignancies metastatic to the liver may also have some similar symptoms. Radiographic studies may allow differentiation from hepatitis.

F. Right ventricular failure with passive hepatic congestion or hypoperfusion syndromes such as in shock, severe hypotension, or severe left ventricular failure may mimic acute hepatitis.

G. Occasionally genetic or metabolic disorders of the liver (Wilson's disease, α_1-antitrypsin deficiency) have features similar to those of viral hepatitis and can be differentiated by appropriate blood tests.

IV. Treatment

A. There is no specific treatment for most cases of acute viral hepatitis. Most patients require no dietary restrictions. IV fluids may be necessary if adequate PO intake cannot be maintained. Activity need not be restricted but patients should try to get adequate rest.

B. Drugs metabolized by the liver and those that may cause cholestasis should be avoided.

C. Isolation

1. HAV—Patients rarely need to be isolated except in cases of fecal incontinence. Gloves should be worn when bedpans or fecal material from patients with hepatitis A are handled.
2. HBV and HCV—Blood precautions should be advised, with strict handwashing and avoidance of contact with blood or body fluids (see patient education section).

D. Liver function tests and coagulation profiles should be monitored during the acute phase of hepatitis.

E. Prophylaxis (see also Appendix A)

1. HAV
   a. Immune globulin can prevent infection or attenuate symptoms of hepatitis A if given before or during the early incubation period. Preexposure prophylaxis is recommended for travelers to areas where hepatitis A is endemic. A dose of 0.02 mL/kg is recommended for travel periods of ≤ 3 mo as well as for household and intimate contacts of patients with hepatitis A. A dose of 0.06 mL/kg is recommended for travel abroad lasting > 3 mo.
   b. Vaccine against hepatitis A is currently available in other countries but has not yet been licensed in the United States.
2. HBV
   a. A plasma-derived hepatitis B vaccine as well as a recombinant vaccine prepared from yeast is available for active immunization against hepatitis B.
   b. Vaccine is given in 3 doses (1 mL IM each dose) at 0, 1 and 6 mo.
3. HCV
   a. Whether immune globulin prophylaxis is effective for prevention of HCV transmission is still uncertain.
   b. The Centers for Disease Control and Prevention currently recommends a dose of 0.06 mL/kg IM of immune globulin as prophylaxis after occupational exposure.

F. Treatment of Fulminant Hepatic Failure

1. Supportive therapy with fluid replacement and respiratory and circulatory support as needed should be initiated.
2. IV solutions should be given to maintain nutritional support.
3. IV H_2-receptor blockers may prevent GI bleeding.
4. Protein should be restricted.
5. Therapy for hepatic encephalopathy such as lactulose should be administered as indicated.
6. Liver transplantation may be considered in patients with stage III or IV hepatic coma.

G. Treatment of Chronic Hepatitis

1. Corticosteroids

   a. Administration of steroids to patients with chronic hepatitis B or C infection has not been shown to improve outcome. In some cases, its use has been deleterious.

2. Liver transplantation

   a. Liver transplantation for patients with liver failure from chronic hepatitis B or C infection has been associated with a very high rate of graft reinfection.
   b. Long-term survival after liver transplantation in patients with hepatitis B is only about 40–50%.
   c. Graft reinfection in patients with hepatitis C does not result in a high mortality rate.

3. Interferon

   a. HBV—Interferon alfa 2b has been shown to reduce HBV replication and liver inflammation in some patients. It is recommended for patients with abnormal liver function tests 1.5–2 times normal for at least 6 mo who are HBeAg positive and who also have a biopsy consistent with chronic active hepatitis.
   b. HCV—Interferon alfa 2b is recommended for chronic hepatitis C in patients without decompensated cirrhosis. Doses used are low and side effects are mild. 40–50% of patients achieve rapid normalization of their transaminase levels and improvement in hepatic function but there is a high relapse rate after cessation of treatment.

4. Other antiviral agents

   a. Studies using β and γ interferon, ribavirin, and ursodeoxycholic acid are currently ongoing.

V. Patient Education

A. Patients should be advised to maintain adequate oral intake and to rest when necessary.

B. Alcohol as well as drugs metabolized by the liver should be avoided.

C. Specific viruses

1. HAV—Strict handwashing should be observed. Isolation is unnecessary except in cases of fecal incontinence. Prophylaxis with immune globulin is advised for close personal contacts and should be given within 2 wk of exposure.

2. HBV—Infection may be spread by sexual contact or by contact with blood or body fluids. Barrier protection (condoms) should be used during sexual contact. To reduce risk of transmission, sexual contacts may be advised to

obtain vaccination against hepatitis B. Patients with hepatitis B should not donate blood or blood products, semen, or organs and should not share objects that may be contaminated with blood such as toothbrushes or razors.

3. HCV—Patients should be aware of the uncertainty regarding modes of transmission. Condoms should be used during sexual contact. Patients should not donate blood or blood products, semen, or organs and should avoid blood or body fluid exposure to others.

VI. Long-term Management

A. In patients with hepatitis B or C, transaminase levels and serologies should be followed to identify patients who may progress to chronic hepatitis. Disappearance of HBsAg must be documented even after patients appear clinically well and liver function tests have normalized.

B. Patients with chronic hepatitis (from either hepatitis B or C) have an increased risk of primary hepatocellular cancer. α-Fetoprotein levels should be obtained and ultrasound examination of the liver should be performed every 6 mo.

VII. Indications for Referral

A. Indications for Referral to a Gastroenterologist

1. Liver biopsy should be considered for patients in whom the diagnosis is in question or when there is a question of chronic active hepatitis. Biopsy may be used to determine stage of disease, and whether or not cirrhosis is present.

B. Indications for Hospitalization

1. IV fluid replacement may be necessary in dehydrated patients unable to replace fluids orally.

2. Patients with advanced age or severe underlying disease may have a poorer prognosis and may need to be hospitalized. Patients found to have prothrombin time prolongation, marked elevations of bilirubin, low serum albumin, or hypoglycemia or those presenting with ascites, peripheral edema, or hepatic encephalopathy may have a prolonged and complicated course and may require hospitalization.

VIII. Annotated Bibliography

Dienstag J, Wands J, Isselbacher K. Acute hepatitis. In: Wilson JD, Braunwald E, Isselbacher KJ, eds. Harrison's Principles of Internal Medicine, 12th ed. New York: McGraw-Hill; 1991:1322–1337.
Tang E. Hepatitis C virus. A review. West J Med 1991;155(2):164–168. Excellent review of much of what is currently known about hepatitis C.

Part X:
Geriatrics

Chapter 52: Dementia

Karen G. Kelly

I. Clinical Presentation

A. **Definition**

1. Acquired loss of intellectual abilities of sufficient severity to interfere with social or occupational functioning
2. No decline in level of consciousness
3. Cognitive deficit involves memory and some impairment of visual spatial ability, abstract thinking, judgment, personality, language or praxis.
4. Should be distinguished from delirium, which may also be superimposed.
5. Should be distinguished from mild memory loss of aging (see below)

B. **Epidemiology**

1. Incidence of dementing illnesses increases with age.
2. Due to increase in older age groups in the United States, predictions are that the prevalence of dementia will increase in the next 40 y.
3. Figure 52–1 presents prevalence estimate by age.
4. Incidence is higher in women than men.

C. **Causes**

1. Alzheimer's disease represents at least 60% of all cases.
2. Multi-infarct dementia—approximately 20%
3. A combination of Alzheimer's and multi-infarct dementia—approximately 10–20%
4. Parkinsonism with dementia
5. Multiple other diseases, which are all much less common (Table 52–1)
6. A small proportion with so-called reversible dementia (Table 52–2)

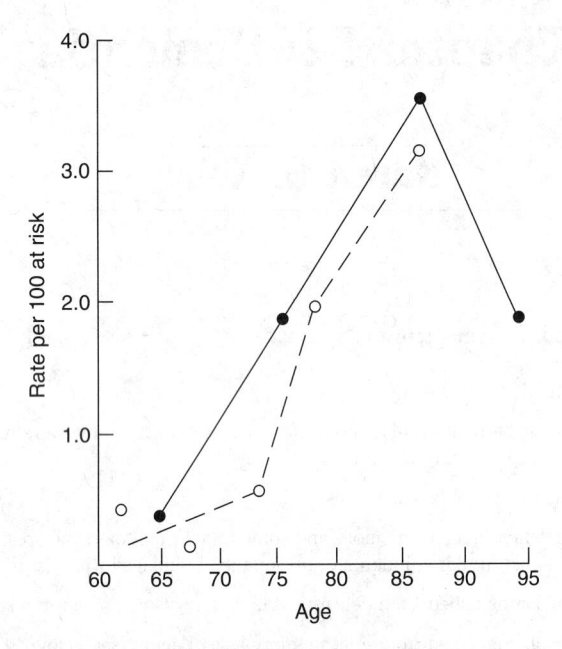

Figure 52-1. The Incidence of Development of Dementia per 100 Individuals at Risk per Year. ●, Data for women ○, Data for men.

SOURCE: Reprinted by permission from Katzman R, Row DW. Principles of Geriatric Neurology. Philadelphia: F.A. Davis, 1992.

Table 52-1. Partial List of Other Causes of Dementia
Degenerative dementias, eg, Pick's disease, Huntington's disease
Post-head trauma
Post-anoxia
Infections
AIDS, both primary and as a result of secondary infections
Creutzfeldt-Jakob
Herpes encephalitis
Neurosyphilis
Normal pressure hydrocephalus
Space-occupying lesions
Subdural hematomas
Brain tumors (primary or metastatic)
Heavy metal poisons (lead, mercury, arsenic)

Table 52-2. Possibly Reversible Causes of Dementia

Depression
Drugs, particularly sedative, hypnotics, and anticholinergics
Vitamin deficiencies
Metabolic problems—thyroid, hypercalcemia, kidney or liver failure
Remote effect of carcinoma (especially oat cell)

D. History

1. It is important to obtain a history from the patient *and* from the family or caregivers because the patient may deny or minimize problems.

2. Ask about loss of memory, decline in functioning, and changes in personality.

3. Common early symptoms might include

    a. Decrease in ability to handle finances correctly
    b. Repetitiveness of speech and difficulty finding words
    c. Loss of interest in usual activities
    d. Personality changes

4. Dementia of the Alzheimer's type—Ask about onset and progression. Should have gradual onset and insidious progression, but may be recognized acutely, eg, following the death of a spouse or during a hospitalization

5. Ask about medical problems, particularly those things that increase the risk for stroke or other diseases that might cause dementia.

6. Ask about medications, particularly psychotropic medications and anticholinergic agents, which may cause delerium.

7. Ask about symptoms of depression (sadness, sense of hopelessness, worthlessness, loss of appetite, trouble sleeping).

8. Ask about the inability to handle activities of daily living and instrumental activities of daily living (see Chapter 53).

E. Physical Examination

1. Complete physical examination essential

2. Neurologic examination particularly looking for signs of stroke and parkinsonism

3. Evaluate gait

4. Mental status examination in some standardized form, eg, Folstein mini mental status examination (Table 52-3).

Table 52–3. Mini Mental State Examination

Maximum Score	Patient Score	
		Orientation
5	_____	What is the (year) (season) (date) (day) (month)?
5	_____	Where are we (state) (county) (town) (hospital) (floor)?
		Registration
3	_____	Name three objects—one second to say each—then ask the patient all three after you have said them. Give one point for each correct answer. Then repeat them until patient learns all three. Count trials and record. Number of trials _____
		Attention and Calculation
5	_____	Serial sevens. One point for each correct answer. Stop after five answers. If subject refuses, ask to spell "World" backwards.
		Recall
3	_____	Ask for three objects repeated above. Give one point for each correct.
		Language
9	_____	Name a pencil and watch (2 points). Repeat the following : "No ifs, ands, or buts" (1 point). Follow a three-stage command: "Take a paper in your right hand, fold it in half, and put it on the floor" (3 points). Read and obey the following: "Close your eyes" (1 point). Write a sentence (1 point). Copy design (1 point).
30 (Maximum Score)	_____ (Patient Total)	
		Assess Level of Consciousness Along a Continuum
		Alert Drowsy Stupor Coma

A score of less than 24 is considered abnormal.

source: Reprinted with permission from Folstein MF: Mini-mental state. J Psychiatric Res 12:189. Copyright 1975, Pergamon Press PLC.

II. Diagnostic Approach

A. Goals

1. Establish cause (see below).
2. Identify aggravating factors.
   a. Medical conditions
   b. Environmental
   c. Medications

B. Establish Cause

1. Alzheimer's disease—see diagnostic criteria (Table 52-4)
2. Usual baseline studies would include complete blood count, electrolytes, calcium, liver function tests, thyroid function tests, urinalysis, creatinine, vitamin B_{12}, folate, test for syphilis, erythrocyte sedimentation rate, glucose
3. A neuroimaging study, CT, or MRI, would be indicated in most cases.
4. In selected cases, other testing should be based on previous evaluation or clinical suspicions—HIV testing, lumbar puncture, EEG, heavy metal screen

C. Identify Aggravating Factors

1. Medical problems and painful conditions
2. Anticholinergic and sedative medications

Table 52-4. Criteria for the Clinical Diagnosis of Alzheimer's Disease

Criteria for the Clinical Diagnosis of *Probable* Alzheimer's Disease

- Dementia established by clinical examination and documented by mental status test and confirmed by neuropsychologic tests
- Deficits in two or more areas of cognition
- Progressive worsening of memory and other cognitive functions
- No disturbance of consciousness
- Absence of systemic disorders or other brain diseases that in and of themselves could account for the progressive deficits in memory and cognition

Criteria for the Clinical Diagnosis of *Possible* Alzheimer's Disease

- May be made on the basis of the dementia syndrome, in the absence of other neurologic, psychiatric, or systemic disorders sufficent to cause dementia, and in the presence of variations in the onset, in the presentation, or in the clinical course
- May be made in the presence of a second systemic or brain disorder sufficient to produce dementia, which is not considered to be the cause of the dementia

SOURCE: Reprinted by permission from Katzman R, Rowe JW. Principles of Geriatric Neurology. Philadelphia: F.A. Davis, 1992.

3. Vision loss and hearing loss

4. Environmental problems (see below)

5. Depression (often coexists with dementia)

6. Delirium (may coexist with dementia)

III. Differential Diagnosis

A. Depression

1. May coexist with dementia

2. May show some fluctuating cognitive loss

3. May see apathy, slow responses, difficulty concentrating

4. Often have feelings of guilt, worthlessness, and preoccupation with somatic symptoms

5. Sleep disturbances and weight loss common

6. Treatable!

B. Delirium

1. Major difference is with level of consciousness, which is depressed in delirium but not in dementia. Onset is acute and hallucinations may be pronounced.

2. Delirium is commonly seen as a result of coexisting medical illness or medications

3. May coexist with dementia

4. Delirium needs to be identified so it can be managed appropriately.

C. Memory Loss of Aging

1. Short-term memory loss with no other cognitive dysfunction

2. May be difficult to distinguish from early dementia

3. Follow-up with sensory cognitive testing or send for more elaborate neuropsychological testing

4. Suggest compensating strategies

IV. Treatment

A. Will depend on cause

B. Most causes are not reversible. Control of risk factors for vascular disease may limit progression.

C. Alzheimer's disease

1. Tacrine has been approved for use in Alzheimer's disease, but is of limited use.

    a. If a therapeutic trial is desired, an initial dose of 10 mg q.i.d. is used.
    b. Hepatic function should be monitored weekly.
    c. The dose is increased at six week intervals to a maximum does of 40 mg q.i.d.
    d. If there is no measurable improvement in cognition or behavior at this dose, then it should be tapered and stopped.
    e. If cholinergic side effects (eg, nausea, vomiting) are a problem, the dose my be given after meals, but otherwise it should be given on an empty stomach.
    f. Tacrine does not stop the progression of the disease.

2. Other drugs are in clinical trials at present.

D. Education of the patient, if appropriate, and of caregivers

1. Safety issues

    a. Cooking
    b. Driving—No clear criteria for assessing ability to drive but all demented patients should be encouraged not to drive and if the patient is moderately demented caregiver support should be enlisted in preventing driving.
    c. Wandering—caregivers should be alerted to the fact that patients may begin to wander.
    d. Being alone—Would the patient be able to call for help in an emergency?

2. Education about common behavioral problems

    a. Need for regular structure and schedule
    b. Need to simplify tasks for the patient
    c. Need to avoid confrontation and redirect to distract the patient's attention when the patient starts to get agitated

3. Refer caregivers to

    a. Published material, eg, The 36 Hour Day (see bibliography)
    b. Local Alzheimer's associations or other support groups
    c. Social services

4. Discuss with the patient if possible, or with caregivers the need to

    a. Put financial affairs in the hands of a responsible person
    b. Think about end-of-life issues

5. Education is an ongoing process because caregivers are often overwhelmed when the diagnosis is initially presented.

V. Indications for Referral

A. Uncertainty with or about the diagnosis may require referral to an experienced neurologist or geriatrician or to a geriatric assessment program.

B. Care of these difficult patients often requires many types of health care professionals, eg, social service, home health nurses, geropsychiatry, occupational therapy.

C. The primary care physician should not desert the patient and family at this difficult time, even if consultation is required.

VI. Indications for Hospitalization

A. Psychiatric hospitalization if the dementia is severe and there are endangering behavioral problems

B. Medical hospitalization for usual medical problems

VII. Annotated Bibliography

Clarfeld AM. Reversible dementias: do they reverse? Ann Intern Med 1988; 109:467–486. Argues that few cases of dementia are truly reversible.

Consensus Conference on Differential Diagnosis of Dementing Disease. JAMA 1987; 258:3411–3416. Recommendations for evaluation.

Mace NL, Rabins PV. The 36 Hour Day. Baltimore: Johns Hopkins University Press; 1991. A guide for families caring for demented people. Very useful for physicians as well.

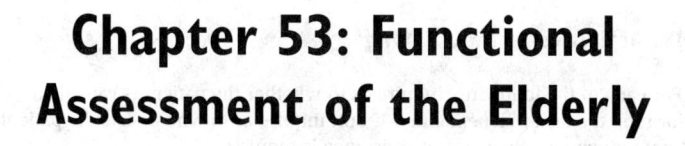

Chapter 53: Functional Assessment of the Elderly

Karen G. Kelly

I. Definition

Assessment of an elderly patient's functioning in physical, cognitive, and psychosocial realms

II. Epidemiology

Loss of function becomes increasingly common with age. The number of patients unable to perform common tasks of daily living roughly doubles each decade past age 60.

III. Importance of Functional Assessment

A. Assessment of function is a critical first step in helping the patient to have optimal quality of life, by identifying patients who need help and by focusing on ways to improve functioning.

B. Identification of a loss of function does not tell you why the function has been lost. Further work-up may be required to identify the cause. Dementia (see Chapter 52), depression (see Chapter 83), deconditioning, and a large number of medical problems may hinder function.

C. If the loss of function cannot be restored, the physician must help the patient find assistance. For example, if a patient can no longer prepare meals, Meals on Wheels may be arranged or family members may be enlisted to deliver food. Obviously identifying this problem before the patient has lost a significant amount of weight will be most useful.

D. Loss of previous function may indicate new physical or psychological problems, which may need to be evaluated and treated. Serial assessments of function are useful.

E. Serial functional assessments should be part of the ongoing care of the elderly. Information should be sought from the patient *and* caregiver or close relations or friends.

IV. Activities of Daily Living

A. For each of the following, inquire as to whether the patient is capable of performing the task independently. If not, inquire as to who assists the patient and how much and what sort of assistance is required.

1. Dressing
2. Bathing
3. Feeding
4. Transfers
5. Use of toilet
6. Continence

B. Goals are to identify care needs that are not being met and to identify areas of decreased function that may respond to therapy (eg, therapy for incontinence or rehabilitation therapy).

V. Instrumental Activities of Daily Living

A. Inquire from the patient and reliable observers whether the patient is able to independently manage the following tasks. If not, is assistance available?

1. Use of telephone
2. Shopping
3. Food preparation
4. Housekeeping
5. Laundry
6. Use of available transportation (car or public transportation)
7. Responsibility for medication
8. Responsibility for finances

B. Goals are to identify areas of limitation and unmet needs. Decline of function in these areas may be due to a variety of physical, psychological, or social factors that may require evaluation and treatment.

VI. Psychiatric

A. Some sort of cognitive assessment should be done periodically on all elderly patients because the frequency of dementia increases markedly with age.

B. In a patient with good functioning and no apparent cognitive decline, a reasonable screening test would be to ask the person to recall three objects after

1 min and to spell the word WORLD backwards. Failure to do either of these tasks would indicate the need for further testing.

C. The Folstein mini mental status examination is widely used (see Chapter 52).

VII. Gait

A. Particularly important and often abnormal

B. Gait abnormalities may identify patients who are likely to fall.

C. Observe the patient

1. Getting up from a chair without the use of his or her arms

2. Walking

3. Turning

4. Standing with feet together

5. Standing with eyes closed

D. No assessment of function is complete without *observing* the patient's gait.

E. Goal is to identify patients who

1. May benefit from strengthening

2. Should use assistive devices

3. Are not safe to walk alone

VIII. Sensory

A. Loss of vision may underlie or contribute to the loss of function. Visual acuity should be checked on all elderly patients.

B. Loss of hearing likewise may impair function. Screening for hearing loss should be done either with an audiogram or hand-held instrument. Refer to an audiologist if there is a > 40 db hearing loss.

IX. Social

A. The isolated elderly patient is particularly at risk when functional decline occurs.

B. The physician should inquire as to who could help the patient should the need arise.

C. Ask about social activities, friends, and interests.

D. Be familiar with local senior centers and services for aging in the area.

X. Formulating a Care Plan

A. At the end of the assessment the physician should have information to answer the following questions

1. Is the current living situation a safe one (ie, if the patient is cognitively impaired, is supervision adequate)?

2. Is additional assistance or equipment needed?

3. Is rehabilitation needed (eg, for strengthening to improve gait)?

4. Should friends or caregivers be enlisted to help the patient (eg, with shopping)?

5. Should elderly protective services or other social work agencies be contacted?

B. The physician cannot meet all these needs alone and should be familiar with other professionals in the area, such as rehabilitation physicians and therapists, home health agencies, audiologists, social workers, etc.

XI. Patient Education

A. Patients and families need to be informed if the physician feels the living situation is not safe.

B. Recommendations for equipment, rehabilitation, and assistance in the home should be made to the patient and family members.

XII. Indications for Hospitalization

A. Functioning rarely improves during a hospitalization. Thus hospitalization in an acute care facility is only indicated if

1. Loss of function is felt to be secondary to serious physical illness that requires hospitalization

2. In rare situations where safety is a major concern and there are no other options

B. Hospitalization in a rehabilitation or psychiatric facility may be indicated.

XIII. Annotated Bibliography

Lachs MS, Feinstein AR, Cooney LM, et al. A simple procedure for general screening for functional disability in elderly patients. Ann Intern Med 1990;112:699–706. A short simple approach to functioning screening. Includes the mini mental state examination.

Chapter 54: Prevention in the Elderly

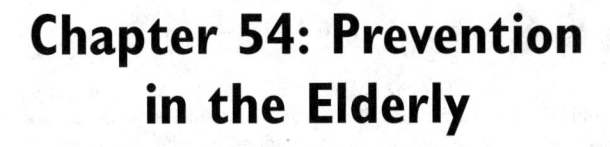

Karen G. Kelly

I. Definitions

A. Primary prevention—interventions in asymptomatic people to prevent condition, eg, immunizations, counseling regarding behavioral risk factors such as smoking

B. Secondary prevention—screening, early detection, therapy of modifiable risk

II. Consider Expense and Risk of Intervention versus Anticipated Gain in Life Expectancy or Quality of Life

A. Consider epidemiology of disease or condition you are trying to prevent.

B. Individualize the program based on the patient's risk and current condition. Remember that the average person at age 65 has approximately 16 more years of life ahead and an 85 year-old can expect an average of approximately 6 more years of life.

C. Use a flow sheet in the patient's chart or reminders to the patients.

III. U.S. Preventive Task Force Recommendations for Prevention in the Elderly

A. Primary Prevention

1. Smoking cessation counseling with scheduled follow-up for all smokers (see Chapter 15)

2. Exercise counseling regarding the importance of regular safe exercise (see Chapter 23)

3. Nutrition

   a. Counsel on the need to eat a healthy diet consisting of fat not > 30% of total calories, saturated fat < 10%, cholesterol < 300 mg, with an increase in fruits, vegetables, and fiber. Diet should be calorie limited if patient is obese (body mass index > $27/kg/m_2$)

b. The elderly should not be advised to lose excessive weight, but rather to improve the quality of their diet and increase their activity levels.
c. Screen for factors that are likely to increase the risk of poor nutrition (Table 54–1).

4. Alcohol and drug use
   a. Use of CAGE questionnaire to screen for alcohol use (2/4 positive answers suspicious for alcoholism)
   b. Routine inquiries about drug use

5. Injuries, particularly falls and motor vehicle accidents
   a. Counsel regarding safety in the home (fire alarms; adequate lighting, especially at night; removal of loose rugs, electrical cords, and other obstacles).
   b. Counsel on seat belt use and drinking and driving.
   c. Measure visual acuity and refer to ophthalmology if it is diminished.
   d. Monitor the use of drugs associated with an increase in the risk of falls (antihypertensive agents and long-acting sedatives).
   e. Encourage exercise programs to improve strength, mobility, and flexibility.

6. Dental
   a. Urge dental visit at least q 1–2 y.

7. Immunizations
   a. Pneumococcal vaccine should be given once to all persons over 65.
   b. Influenza vaccine annually to all persons over 65
   c. Diphtheria tetanus booster q 10 y

8. Chemoprophylaxis
   a. Low-dose aspirin (325 mg every other day) especially if the patient is at increased risk for myocardial infarctions and if there are not contraindications (Table 54–2)
   b. Estrogen replacement therapy (see Chapter 55)

Table 54–1. Risk Factors for Poor Nutrition in the Elderly
Advanced age (> 85)
Poverty
Social
Multiple medications
Alcoholism
Limited food intake (fewer than 3 meals/d restricted diets)
Dental problems
Functional disability

Table 54-2. Contraindications to Aspirin Therapy

Uncontrolled hypertension
Liver or kidney disease
Peptic ulcer disease
History of GI or other bleeding problems
Other risk factors for bleeding or cerebral hemorrhage

B. Secondary Prevention

1. Coronary artery disease (see above for smoking, diet, and exercise)

   a. Hypertension—check blood pressure q 2 y if < 140/85, annually if diastolic between 85–89; treat both systolic and diastolic hypertension.
   b. Elevated cholesterol—diet therapy for those with cholesterol > 240 or 200–239 with two or more risk factors for coronary artery disease. The effectiveness of drug therapy of hypercholesterolemia in the elderly is not established (see Chapter 39).
   c. Obesity—Counsel appropriately those who are 20% above ideal body weight especially if at increased risk for vascular disease.

2. Cancer

   a. Breast cancer—annual mammograms. The age at which to discontinue annual mammography is not entirely clear and should be individualized. The risk of breast cancer increases with age (see Chapter 7).
   b. Colorectal cancer—consider annual fecal occult blood testing and periodic sigmoidoscopy especially in those at increased risk. Age at which to discontinue screening is not clear and should be individualized. The risk of colon cancer increases with age (see Chapter 8).
   c. Cervical cancer—Pap tests should be done q 1–3 y on patients who are under age 65. May consider discontinuing screening after age 65 if at low risk and previous specimens were consistently normal (see Chapter 10).
   d. Prostate cancer—The role of prostate-specific antigen is not clear at this time in screening elderly men (see Chapter 9).
   e. Lung cancer—Chest x-ray is not recommended as screening.
   f. Skin cancer—Screen those at increased risk.
   g. Oral cancer—Screen those at increased risk (smokers and drinkers).
   h. Other, particularly screening for ovarian and pancreatic cancer currently not recommended

3. Miscellaneous

   a. Glucose measurements in those at high risk for diabetes mellitus (overweight, family history of diabetes)
   b. Thyrotropin or T_4 in women
   c. Purified protein derivative yearly especially in nursing home residents or other high-risk groups

d. Visual acuity
e. Screening for hearing loss either by audiometric test or questionnaire
f. Periodic inquiry regarding functioning of elderly patients (see Chapter 53)

IV. Annotated Bibliography

The Periodic Health Examination of Older Adults. The Recommendations of the U.S. Preventive Services Task Force Part I: Counseling, Immunizations and Chemoprophylaxis. J Am Geriatr Soc 1990;38:817–823. Part II. Screening Tests. J Am Geriatr Soc 1990;38:933–942. A consensus statement.

Part XI:
Gynecology

Chapter 55: Estrogen Replacement Therapy

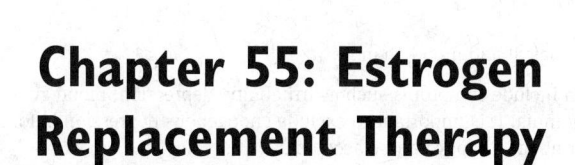

Kenneth R. Epstein

I. General Perspectives on Menopause

A. Current life expectancy of women in the United States is 78–80 y.

B. Mean age at menopause is 51–52 y.

C. Therefore, many women will spend over one half of their adult lives in the postmenopausal years.

D. See Chapter 56 for additional discussion of menopause management.

II. Benefits of Therapy

A. Perimenopausal Symptoms

Are the most common reason for the prescription of postmenopausal estrogen replacement therapy (ERT)

1. Vasomotor instability (hot flashes/flushes)
   a. Mechanism—thought to be due to effect of increased gonadotropin-releasing hormone levels on the hypothalamic thermoregulatory center.
   b. Estrogens clearly relieve the "hot flashes."
   c. In many cases the therapy can be stopped within several years without return of the symptoms.

2. Atrophic vaginal and urethral changes
   a. Some atrophic changes of the vagina occur in virtually all women within 4–5 y after menopause.
   b. Vaginal symptoms include vaginal itching, dyspareunia, and recurrent vaginitis.
   c. Urethral symptoms include dysuria, urgency, and stress incontinence. It is important to consider atrophic urethritis in older women with symptoms of urinary tract infection (UTI) and negative urinalysis.
   d. Vaginal estrogen cream or systemic estrogens are effective in reversal of symptoms. However, cream is well absorbed systemically, so may not be advantageous over oral therapy.

3. Psychological and mood changes
   a. Can include symptoms such as irritability, depression, mood swings, and insomnia. It is important to exclude endogenous depression before a hormonal etiology can be accepted.
   b. Some of the symptoms may be secondary to sleep disturbances from the hot flashes.
   c. Estrogen therapy can improve these symptoms.

B. Prevention of Osteoporosis

1. Magnitude of the problem
   a. Affects > 20 million persons in United States, mostly postmenopausal women.
   b. > 250,000 hip fractures occur in United States annually.
   c. 1.3 million total osteoporotic fractures annually
   d. In 1986, the public health cost was $7–10 billion.

2. Effect of ERT on osteoporosis
   a. Multiple studies have confirmed protective effect of postmenopausal estrogens on bone mineral density (BMD). Calcium slows down the rate of cortical, but not trabecular, bone loss. ERT prevents both types of bone loss but does not restore lost mass.
   b. More importantly, postmenopausal ERT decreases fracture rates, especially vertebral and hip fractures. Relative risk is 0.75 for hip fractures for ever-users compared with nonusers.
   c. No studies have yet been done on the differential effect of combined therapy with estrogen plus progestins on the risk of hip fracture.

C. Cardiovascular Disease

1. Incidence of cardiovascular disease (CVD) markedly increases postmenopausally. By 5–10 y after menopause, CVD is a disease of both sexes.

2. Reason for this change seems to be, at least in part, due to changes in lipid status.
   a. Before menopause—high-density lipoproteins (HDL) higher in women, low-density lipoprotein (LDL) lower, total cholesterol lower
   b. After menopause—HDL decreases, LDL increases, total cholesterol increases

3. ERT reverses these lipid changes—HDL cholesterol increases and LDL cholesterol decreases. Triglycerides are also moderately increased by ERT.

4. Numerous case-control and prospective cohort studies have documented a protective effect of estrogens on both incidence and mortality of CVD.

5. The relative risk for CVD in women who have ever used estrogen compared with never-users is 0.65. The protective effect of estrogen may even be stronger in women with preexisting CVD than in healthy women.

6. Only 25–50% of the risk reduction conferred by estrogens may be due to the favorable changes in lipids. Estrogens also directly affect the vasculature and may have antithrombotic effects. This may explain why current use is more protective than past use.

7. Recent studies have reported an equally significant improvement in metabolic status in women who use combination estrogen and progestin therapy. Likewise, a reduction in risk for CVD has been shown. The degree of protection for women on combination hormonal replacement therefore appears to be as great as that observed for women taking estrogen alone.

III. Risks of Therapy

A. Endometrial Carcinoma

1. *Unopposed* ERT has been clearly shown to increase the incidence of endometrial carcinoma. Case-control studies in the 1970s demonstrated a relative risk of 4–8, but more recent studies have demonstrated the risk to be more in the range of 2–3. The risk is elevated for all doses, and the risk increases with increasing dose.

2. At diagnosis, endometrial cancers in women who have used estrogens are generally of earlier stage, lower grade, and show less myometrial invasion than do tumors in women who have not used estrogens.

3. The increased risk is due to unopposed stimulation of the endometrium. Addition of progestational agents counteracts this effect.

4. Adding progestins for at least 10 d/mo totally eliminates the increased risk of endometrial cancer (relative risk = 1.0).

5. Therefore, almost all women with intact uteri should receive either sequential or continuous progestogens in addition to ERT. (See below for dosing.)

6. Endometrial screening

    a. Women who plan on taking unopposed estrogens should undergo a baseline endometrial evaluation (biopsy or transvaginal ultrasound) to detect latent endometrial cancer or hyperplasia.
    b. The woman should then report any signs of vaginal bleeding. If bleeding occurs and no recent endometrial evaluation has been done, a diagnostic endometrial evaluation should be performed.
    c. If bleeding does not occur, then screening endometrial evaluation should be done yearly.
    d. Women taking combination estrogen and progestin therapy do not require baseline or routine endometrial evaluation because the risk of cancer is not increased.
    e. If the progestin is given cyclically days 1–12 of the month, then if bleeding is going to occur, it occurs days 5–15. Endometrial evaluation should be performed if bleeding occurs at other times or if it persists for > 10 d.

B. Breast Cancer

1. Another potential adverse effect of ERT on women has been a reported increased incidence of breast cancer in estrogen users.
2. Some studies have shown an increased risk, whereas others have not demonstrated any change in incidence. Results of several recent meta-analyses have indicated only a minimally increased risk. The relative risk is 1.0 for all users, but the relative risk is 1.25 for women who have used estrogens for > 8 y.
3. It may be that the type of estrogen is important. Estradiol may be associated with increased risk of breast cancer, whereas conjugated estrogens may not be associated with an increased risk.
4. There seems to be no increased risk for women with fibrocystic breast disease.
5. The effect of adding a progestin to the estrogen is not known. Data are limited, but there may be an increased risk after long-term use.

C. Side Effects

1. Differ from risks in that side effects may be uncomfortable, but present no risk of long-term morbidity or mortality
2. Nausea and breast tenderness—due to initial sensitivity to estrogen. Advise patient to take with food. Can start with low dose, and increase to normal dose after several weeks.
3. Premenstrual symptoms—due to progestin. Symptoms may include bloating, headache, irritability, and fluid retention. Can decrease progestin dose or change to different progestin.
4. Endometrial bleeding—see indications for endometrial biopsy above. If heavy bleeding, decrease the estrogen dose. If resumption of withdrawal bleeding is a major concern to the woman, consider continuous progestin therapy.

IV. Contraindications

A. Absolute Contraindications

1. Breast cancer, current or in past
2. Endometrial cancer
3. Active liver disease
4. Active or recurrent thromboembolic disorders
5. Recent myocardial infarction, cerebrovascular accident, or transient ischemic attack—This contraindication may change if further studies demonstrate antithrombotic effects of postmenopausal estrogen.

B. Relative Contraindications

1. Can still prescribe, but involves clear consideration of risks versus benefits
2. Family history of first-degree relative with breast cancer
3. Uterine leiomyomata
4. History of disabling migraine headaches

V. Dosing and Regimens

A. Estrogen

1. Oral estrogen—Most commonly used in United States is conjugated equine estrogens. The usual dose is 0.625 mg.
   a. There is no advantage to higher dose in prevention of osteoporosis or CVD.
   b. Indication for higher dose (1.25 mg)—if no relief of perimenopausal symptoms (hot flashes) with 0.625 mg
   c. Indication for lower dose (0.3 mg)—side effects from estrogen
2. Transdermal preparation
   a. Starting dosage—0.5-mg patch twice/wk
   b. Advantage is convenience for some patients.
   c. *Theoretical* advantage—since no first-pass effect through liver, avoid estrogen's effect on hepatic protein synthesis. No clinical evidence of any advantage.
   d. *Theoretical* disadvantage—since no first-pass effect through liver, may not have as favorable an effect on lipoprotein synthesis. Evidence is mixed.
3. Estrogen vaginal cream
   a. Dosage—2–4 g (1/2–1 applicatorful) daily, intravaginally.
   b. Indication—treatment of atrophic vaginitis or urethritis
   c. Is absorbed systemically, but dose absorbed is not predictable; therefore, does not eliminate risks if there is a contraindication to oral estrogens
   d. Is useful for short-term therapy; if using long term, then consider oral or transdermal

B. Combination Therapy

1. Combination therapy of estrogen with progestins is indicated in almost all women with intact uteri to prevent endometrial cancer.
2. The most commonly prescribed progestin in the United States is medroxyprogesterone acetate (MPA). The usual dosage is 2.5–10 mg.
3. Regimens are still somewhat controversial.
   a. Traditional—estrogen for 25 d, MPA 5–10 mg days 11–25
   b. Alternative #1—estrogen continuously, MPA 5–10 mg days 1–14
   c. Alternative #2—estrogen continuously, MPA 2.5 mg continuously

4. There appears to be no advantage to having an estrogen-free period. It increases the risk of resumption of perimenopausal symptoms without any benefit. Therefore, most experts now recommend alternatives #1 or #2.
5. There may not be an advantage to cyclic progestins. Endometrial biopsies of persons receiving continuous progestins reveal endometrial atrophy, which is protective against cancer, and continuous therapy avoids resumption of menstrual bleeding. However, long-term studies are not yet available to assess the safety of this regimen.

VI. Conclusions

A. *Epidemiologically*, the benefits of prevention of osteoporotic fractures and CVD clearly outweigh the risks of endometrial and breast cancer (Table 55-1).

B. Based on an individual woman's risk factors, health status, and personal concerns, the woman and her health care provider need to determine the best course for her.

Table 55-1. Net Change in Life Expectancy for a 50-Year-Old White Woman Treated with Long-term Hormone Replacement

Variable	Life Expectancy	Estrogen	E + P*	E + P†
White woman, 50y				
No risk factors	82.8	+0.9	+1.0	+0.1
With hysterectomy	82.8	+1.1		
With history of coronary heart disease	76.0	+2.1	+2.2	+0.9
At risk for coronary heart disease	79.6	+1.5	+1.6	+0.6
At risk for breast cancer	82.3	+0.7	+0.8	-0.5
At risk for hip fracture	82.4	+1.0	+1.1	+0.2

(Net Change in Life Expectancy measured in y)

* Assuming that the addition of a progestin to the estrogen regimen does not alter any of the relative risks for disease seen with estrogen therapy, except to prevent the increased risk due to endometrial cancer (relative risk for endometrial cancer estimated to be 1.0). E + P = estrogen plus progestin.
† Assuming that the addition of a progestin to the estrogen regimen provides only two thirds of the coronary heart disease risk reduction afforded by estrogen therapy (relative risk for coronary heart disease).

SOURCE: Reproduced by permission from Grady D, Rubin SM, Pettiti DB, et al. Hormone therapy to prevent disease and prolong life in postmenopausal woman. Ann Intern Med 1992;117:1016–1037.

VII. Annotated Bibliography

Dupont WD, Page DL. Menopausal estrogen replacement therapy and breast cancer. Arch Intern Med 1991;151:67–72. A good meta-analysis of the controversial relationship between estrogens and breast cancer.

Ettinger BE, Genent HK, Cann CT. Long-term estrogen replacement therapy prevents bone loss and fractures. Ann Intern Med 1985;102:319–324. An example of the data demonstrating a decrease in osteoporotic fracture risk with estrogens.

Grady D, Rubin SM, Pettiti DB, et al. Hormone therapy to prevent disease and prolong life in postmenopausal women. Ann Intern Med 1992;117:1016–1037. An excellent review of the epidemiologic risks and benefits of postmenopausal hormonal therapy.

Nabulsi AA, Folsom AA, White A, et al. Association of hormone replacement therapy with various cardiovascular risk factors in postmenopausal women. N Engl J Med 1993;328:1069–1075. One of the first studies to clearly demonstrate that adding progestins to hormonal replacement does not adversely affect the beneficial effects on lipids and CVD incidence.

Stampfer MJ, Coldite GA, Willett WC, et al. Postmenopausal estrogen therapy and cardiovascular disease. N Engl J Med 1991;325:756–762. An example of the data demonstrating a decrease in cardiovascular morbidity and mortality with estrogens.

Walsh BW, Schiff I, Rosner B, Greenberg L, Ravnicker V, Seeks FM. Effects of postmenopausal estrogen replacement on the concentrations and metabolism of plasma lipoproteins. N Engl J Med 1991;325:1196–1204. Data demonstrating the effects of postmenopausal estrogen lipids.

Chapter 56: Menstrual Abnormalities

Rosemarie A. Leuzzi

I. Abnormal Vaginal Bleeding

A. General Information

1. The length of the menstrual cycle varies from 21–35 d with a duration of flow that varies from 2–9 d with approximately 30–60 mL of blood loss.

2. Abnormal menstruation may differ in duration, amount, or timing.
   a. *Menorrhagia* is excessive menstrual bleeding lasting > 7 d or menstrual blood loss exceeding 80 mL.
   b. *Metrorrhagia* is irregular uterine bleeding.
   c. *Menometrorrhagia* is vaginal bleeding that is excessive in amount and irregular in frequency.
   d. *Polymenorrhea* describes episodes of bleeding occurring with < 21-d intervals.
   e. *Oligomenorrhea* describes episodes of bleeding occurring with > 35-d intervals.
   f. *Hypomenorrhea* describes diminished menstrual flow.

3. All women may have occasional variations in bleeding pattern especially in the teenage years and during the premenopausal period.

B. History

1. Determine how the abnormal bleeding differs from the regular menstrual cycle.

2. Obtain a thorough gynecologic history including the regularity of menses, the usual amount of flow, and the date of the last normal cycle.

3. Determine if there is any chance of pregnancy and ask about symptoms of morning sickness or breast tenderness.

4. A thorough history should also include if the patient is using or has used a form of contraceptive. Breakthrough bleeding is common in women using oral contraceptives especially in the first year and anovulatory cycles may follow the discontinuation of the oral contraceptive agent. Women taking the mini-pill (progestin-only contraceptives) and those receiving long-acting progestin injections or implants (Norplant) may also experience this problem.

5. Question the patient regarding the presence of a vaginal discharge and the possibility of sexually transmitted diseases.
6. The presence of psychosocial stressors may commonly cause a change in hormonal balance that affects the interval between menstrual cycles either prolonged or shortened.
7. A thorough past medical history should include a history of liver disease, bleeding diasthesis, and coagulation problems.
8. Check the patient's other medications. Medications associated with disrupting the menstrual cycle include antipsychotic medications, tranquilizers, corticosteroids, seizure medications, antineoplastic drugs, and some antibiotics.
9. Risk factors for endometrial cancer should be assessed including estrogen therapy, nulliparity, and obesity, especially in patients older than 40 y.

C. Physical Examination

1. Vital signs should be obtained with particular attention to orthostatic changes in blood pressure and pulse.
2. The patient's conjunctiva, oropharyngeal mucosa, and lips should be checked for pallor.
3. A pelvic examination needs to be done to look for the site of the abnormal bleeding. The external genitalia should be carefully examined for evidence of infection or ulceration as well as evidence of injury. The vulvovaginal walls and cervix should be carefully inspected especially in women with postcoital bleeding. The uterus should be palpated to assess for size as well as the presence of fibroids. The rectal area should also be checked for hemorrhoids.

D. Diagnostic Approach

1. Laboratory studies that should be considered include
    a. Pregnancy test—Pregnancy must first be excluded in all women of reproductive age because reports of sexual abstinence and contraceptive use may not always be reliable.
    b. Complete blood count and platelet count
    c. Coagulation studies—prothrombin time/partial thromboplastin time (PT/PTT)
    d. Pap smear
    e. Gonorrhea and chlamydia cultures
    f. Thyroid function tests
2. A pelvic ultrasound may be considered to evaluate any abnormalities of the uterus or ovaries noted on physical examination.
3. Cervical and vaginal biopsy should be performed for any lesions of the lower genital tract. Pap smears may be insufficient to rule out cervical cancer.
4. Diagnostic algorithm (Figure 56-1)

```
Abnormal Vaginal Bleeding
```

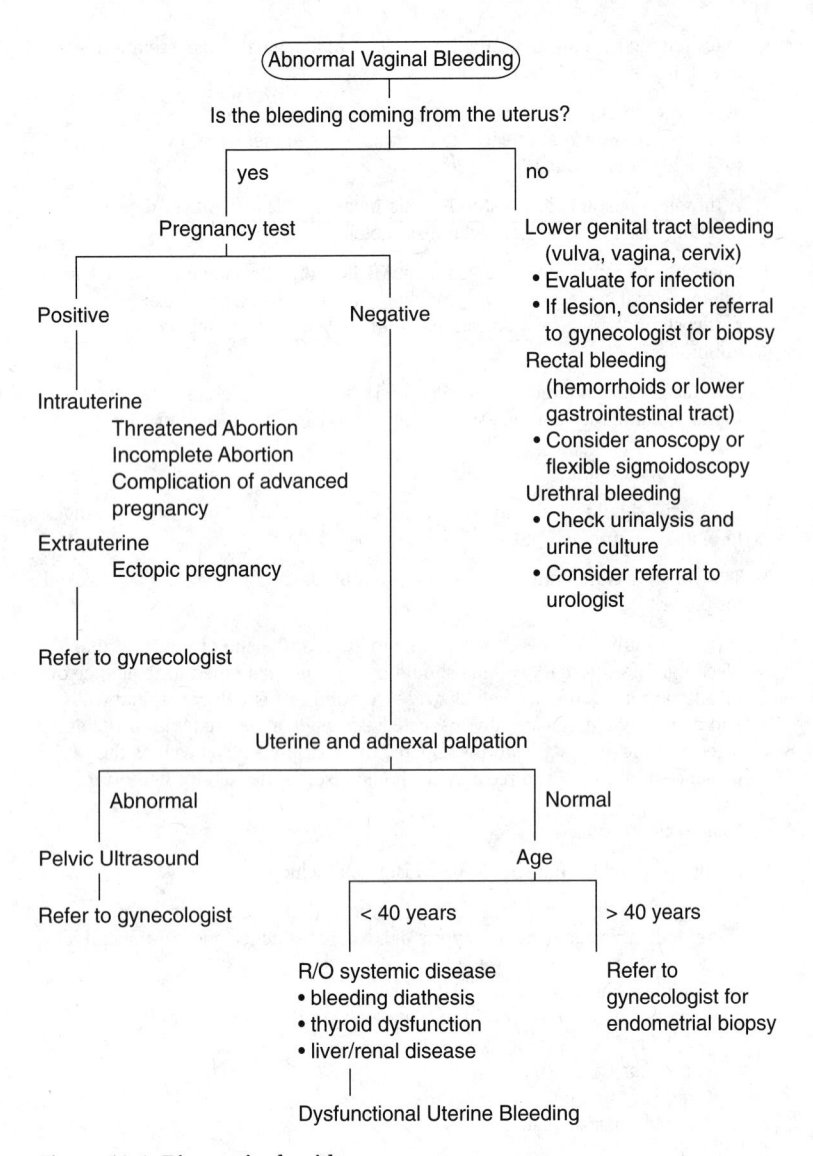

Is the bleeding coming from the uterus?

yes → Pregnancy test

- **Positive**
  - Intrauterine
    - Threatened Abortion
    - Incomplete Abortion
    - Complication of advanced pregnancy
  - Extrauterine
    - Ectopic pregnancy

  Refer to gynecologist

- **Negative** → Uterine and adnexal palpation
  - **Abnormal**
    - Pelvic Ultrasound
    - Refer to gynecologist
  - **Normal** → Age
    - **< 40 years**
      - R/O systemic disease
        - bleeding diathesis
        - thyroid dysfunction
        - liver/renal disease
      - Dysfunctional Uterine Bleeding
    - **> 40 years**
      - Refer to gynecologist for endometrial biopsy

no → Lower genital tract bleeding (vulva, vagina, cervix)
- Evaluate for infection
- If lesion, consider referral to gynecologist for biopsy

Rectal bleeding (hemorrhoids or lower gastrointestinal tract)
- Consider anoscopy or flexible sigmoidoscopy

Urethral bleeding
- Check urinalysis and urine culture
- Consider referral to urologist

Figure 56–1. Diagnostic algorithm.

E. Differential Diagnosis

1. Anovulatory or dysfunctional uterine bleeding is responsible for the majority of cases of abnormal uterine bleeding and is a diagnosis of exclusion.
   a. Dysfunctional uterine bleeding (DUB) occurs when the normal cyclic pattern of ovarian hormone production is interrupted. This imbalance of the hypothalamic-pituitary-ovarian axis results in bleeding unrelated to anatomic causes.
   b. Approximately 80% of cases are due to anovulation and may be caused by a recent stressor or illness.
   c. Treatment involves correcting the anemia, stopping the acute bleeding, and reversing the effects of unopposed estrogen on the endometrium. The general physician may elect to manage the problem or refer to a gynecologist.
      1) In young women, oral contraceptives containing estrogen are commonly used to promote endometrial maturation. Any preparation is acceptable and the usual dose is 1 tablet q.i.d. for 5–7 d. At the end of this treatment, withdrawal bleeding will occur. After bleeding has been controlled, cyclic birth control pills may be continued.
      2) In the perimenopausal woman, estrogen should not be given until endometrial hyperplasia or adenocarcinoma have been excluded.
   d. If hemodynamic instability is present and transfusion is necessary, hospitalization is indicated for treatment with IV estrogen (equine estrogen 25 mg IV q 4 h for a total of 4–6 doses). Consultation with a gynecologist is recommended because possible endometrial curettage may be necessary.

2. Estrogen withdrawal bleeding occurs when estrogen stimulation of the proliferating endometrium is reduced in cases following discontinuation of previously administered estrogen or bilateral oophorectomy.

3. Leiomyomas may present with abnormal uterine bleeding in approximately 30% of women and occur most commonly in the fourth and fifth decade of life. Severe iron deficiency may occur and referral to a gynecologist may be indicated for either removal of the fibroid or hysterectomy if fertility is no longer desired.

4. Cancer of the uterine corpus is the most frequent genital cancer that produces bleeding. Late menopause, nulliparity, obesity, hypertension, and cancer are frequently associated. The usual presenting symptom of endometrial cancer is uterine bleeding. All women with postmenopausal bleeding must be screened for endometrial cancer, even though only 20% will have carcinoma.

5. Cervical cancer causes abnormal bleeding when it becomes invasive. The typical appearance of cervical cancer is a red, raised, solid, friable tumor.

6. Vulvar or vaginal cancers may infrequently present with bleeding and the usual presentation is a vaginal or perineal mass. Any solid tumor at these sites should be evaluated for potential malignancy.

7. Systemic disease may rarely cause abnormal vaginal bleeding.

a. Thyroid dysfunction is the systemic disease most commonly associated with abnormal bleeding.
b. Women with renal failure who are undergoing dialysis may have abnormal bleeding due to abnormal platelet function and hypothalamic-pituitary dysfunction.
c. Bleeding secondary to a bleeding diathesis is usually caused by abnormalities in platelet function. Women on anticoagulants do not usually have excessive menstrual bleeding unless the degree of anticoagulation is excessive.
d. Women with severe liver disease may also experience abnormal bleeding due to changes in the metabolism of estrogen.

II. Dysmenorrhea

A. General Information

1. Defined as painful menstruation, dysmenorrhea is the most common gynecologic complaint of young women.
2. Dysmenorrhea occurs in > 50% of menstruating women and severe symptoms occur in 10% of women.

B. Types of Dysmenorrhea

1. Primary dysmenorrhea
    a. The onset of primary dysmenorrhea usually occurs within 1-2 y following menarche. Many young women do not ovulate at menarche and initially have irregular cycles. As a young girl matures and ovulation occurs, the menstrual cycle becomes more regular and dysmenorrhea develops.
    b. The pain is characterized by lower mid abdominal, crampy abdominal discomfort, which radiates to the back and upper thighs beginning within 1-2 d of the onset of menstruation. The abdominal cramps may also be associated with nausea, vomiting, abdominal bloating, and irritability.
    c. The discomfort is most severe during the initial several hours of menstrual flow and gradually fades over 2-3 d. The episodes usually become less severe with increasing age and may spontaneously fade after the first pregnancy.
    d. There is no identifiable pelvic pathology and the theory is that excessive production of uterine prostaglandins causes increased or abnormal myometrial contractions.

2. Secondary dysmenorrhea
    a. Dysmenorrhea that appears for the first time after the age of 25 or suddenly intensifies in a mature woman is more likely to be secondary rather than primary dysmenorrhea.
    b. Secondary dysmenorrhea is caused by pelvic pathology such as endometriosis, adenomyosis, or infection associated with an intrauterine contraceptive device.

c. The abdominal pain often begins a few days before the start of menstrual flow and in some cases may be present throughout most of the menstrual cycle. The pain from endometriosis is typically described as bilateral deep pain radiating to the rectum and the perineum.

C. Treatment

1. Mild symptoms
   a. Analgesics such as aspirin or acetaminophen are recommended beginning at the onset of menses and continued regularly q 4–6 h.
   b. Many OTC preparations are available but none have been proven more effective than aspirin or acetaminophen.
2. Severe symptoms
   a. Nonsteroidal anti-inflammatory drugs (NSAIDs) approved by the Food and Drug Administration for the treatment of dysmenorrhea include ibuprofen 400 mg q 6 h, naproxen 500 mg b.i.d., or mefenamic acid (Ponstel) 250 mg q 6 h. An agent should be given a 3-mo trial. If no response, switching to a different agent may prove helpful.
   b. Oral contraceptive agents may be necessary to suppress ovulation if symptoms are very severe.

D. Indications for Referral to a Gynecologist

1. If a patient with presumed primary dysmenorrhea does not respond to the above therapies, the diagnosis should be reconsidered and the patient evaluated for secondary causes of dysmenorrhea.
2. Any patient with secondary dysmenorrhea should be referred for further gynecologic evaluation. The possible causes of secondary dysmenorrhea can have serious implications for fertility and potentially serious complications for the woman's health.

III. Premenstrual Syndrome

A. General Information

1. This ill-defined complex of symptoms occurs in approximately 30–40% of women during the reproductive years.
2. By definition, premenstrual syndrome (PMS) significantly alters the ability of an afflicted patient to lead a normal life-style and interferes with interpersonal relationships. If the symptoms do not affect the patient's daily life in an adverse manner and cause great difficulty in her ability to function at work or at home, then these patients should be excluded from the strict diagnosis of PMS.

B. Symptoms

1. The hallmark of PMS is that symptoms occur during the luteal phase of the menstrual cycle, resolve within a day or two of the onset of menstrual flow, and are absent during the first part of the follicular phase of the menstrual cycle.

2. The American Psychiatric Association has set forth criteria for the *Late Luteal Phase Dysphoric Disorder* in the DSM-III to further classify the symptoms of PMS, which include
   a. Marked affective lability
   b. Persistent and marked anger or irritability
   c. Marked anxiety or tension
   d. Markedly depressed mood, feelings of hopelessness, or self-deprecating thoughts
   e. Decreased interest in usual activities
   f. Easy fatigability or marked lack of energy
   g. Subjective sense of difficulty in concentrating
   h. Marked change in appetite, overeating, or specific food cravings
   i. Hypersomnia or insomnia
   j. Other physical symptoms such as breast tenderness or swelling, headaches, joint or muscle pain, a sensation of "bloating," weight gain

3. A woman should not be diagnosed with PMS unless underlying medical problems related to rheumatic disease or thyroid dysfunction or an exacerbation of another mental disorder have been excluded. Migraine headaches, asthma, seizures, and psychiatric disturbances such as depression can become more severe in the luteal phase, but do not constitute PMS.

C. Diagnosis

1. The diagnosis is based on the prospective recording of signs and symptoms on a daily basis during at least two symptomatic cycles. Having patients keep a diary of menstrual history and symptoms as well as recording their basal body temperature can be helpful to demonstrate the cyclic nature of the symptoms.

2. There is no typical pattern of hormone or electrolyte abnormalities.

D. Treatment

1. Physician reassurance is important and information regarding availability of PMS support groups should be given.

2. Although there is no accepted treatment, the following recommendations may be given.
   a. Dietary changes to limit simple sugars, alcohol, and caffeine
   b. Life-style changes to increase regular exercise and use stress reduction techniques
   c. Vitamin therapy using pyridoxine—the dose should be limited to < 100 mg/d due to potential neurotoxicity with paresthesias and symmetric distal sensory loss.
   d. Diuretics—spironolactone is most commonly used if symptoms of bloating and weight gain are present.
   e. Bromocriptine (Parlodel) 2.5 mg qd–b.i.d. for breast discomfort symptoms
   f. Benzodiazepines—usually Alprazolam 0.25–0.50 mg PO t.i.d.
   g. Oral contraceptives

IV. Menopause

A. General Information

1. Menopause is the irreversible cessation of the menstrual cycle due to the permanent loss of ovarian response to gonadotrophins.

    a. Menopause is a single point in time describing the last menstrual period.
    b. The female *climacteric* describes the transitional period between the reproductive years to and beyond the last episode of menstrual bleeding.
    c. *Premenopause* refers to that time during the climacteric when the menstrual cycle becomes irregular.
    d. *Postmenopause* is the period starting 1 y following the last menstrual period.

2. Types of menopause

    a. *Physiologic menopause* occurs as the number of oocytes decreases and the remaining follicles fail to respond to the gonadotrophins. Menopause usually occurs in women between ages 45–55.
    b. *Premature menopause* or premature ovarian failure is defined as cessation of ovarian function prior to age 40, which may be the result of surgical removal of the ovaries, surgical disruption of the blood supply to the ovaries, or destruction of the ovaries due to infection, tumor, or radiation. Hysterectomy does not cause premature menopause unless both ovaries are removed with the uterus.

3. Pathophysiology

    a. As women approach age 35, there is a decrease in the serum estadiol level due to a decrease in the number of functioning oocytes in the ovary. Few oocytes remain and these appear to be nonfunctioning. The decrease in serum estradiol results in decreased negative inhibition of follicle-stimulating hormone (FSH) secretion; therefore, the FSH level increases and this results in a shortened follicular phase. This shortened follicular phase, along with a shorter luteal phase due to decreased progesterone levels, results in a shorter menstrual cycle. Anovulatory cycles and "missed cycles" also start to occur. The FSH and luteinizing hormone (LH) levels increase as the estradiol level becomes extremely low. The FSH level will rise earlier and to a greater extent than the LH level.
    b. Menses may remain irregular over a 1–2-y period and will eventually cease. The duration of the irregular menstrual cycles varies greatly among women.

B. Clinical Presentation

1. Hot flashes

    a. Hot flashes describe the sudden flushing and extreme warmth followed by profuse sweating that is caused by the estrogen deficient state.
    b. These occur in approximately 75% of women, but only 15% of women experience severe enough symptoms to warrant medical therapy.

c. The frequency of the episodes may vary from 1–2 episodes per hour to 1–2 episodes per week. The average duration of an episode usually is 2–5 min and is associated with an average temperature rise of 2.5°C, which may last up to 30 min.
d. Onset of episodes may begin in the premenopausal period due to the decreasing estrogen levels and may continue for 1–5 y following cessation of the menstrual cycle.
e. Patients frequently complain of "night sweats" and insomnia. There is a temporal relationship between the hot flashes and waking episodes, thereby resulting in a disruption of the sleep cycle.
f. The mechanism appears to be an exaggerated response of the neurosecretory nuclei which spread to the adjacent thermoregulatory centers of the hypothalamus and set off the hot flash.

2. Psychological changes
   a. The psychological changes range from severe emotional lability, irritability, depression, and withdrawal from usual activities. There may be a marked change in personality.
   b. These changes appear to be the most pronounced in the period just preceding menopause.
   c. Depression is commonly seen in patients with a history of depressive illness and may be aggravated by other factors such as a perceived change in femininity, divorce or marital difficulties, and the empty nest syndrome.
   d. There may be an increase in libido due to no further worries about pregnancy or a decreased interest in sexual activity due to a perceived loss of attractiveness or possibly associated with dyspareunia as a result of decreased lubrication.

3. Breast atrophy
   a. With loss of adipose tissue, the breast tissue may decrease in size and lose elasticity.

4. Atrophy of the urogenital system
   a. Relaxation of the pelvic ligaments and muscles along with changes in the distal urethra result in uterine and bladder prolapse, which may cause stress incontinence as well as urinary frequency and urgency.
   b. Atrophic vaginitis, which results in a patchy or diffuse reddening of the vagina, can cause symptoms of itching, local tenderness, and complaints of dyspareunia due to the decrease in lubrication. Minimal trauma during intercourse can cause slight vaginal bleeding.
   c. Pubic hair may become sparse.

5. Osteoporosis
   a. With the decrease in estrogen levels, there is an accelerated loss of bone mass.
   b. The vertebral body is the most common site of fracture.

c. 25% of aging women sustain a vertebral or hip fracture between the ages of 60 and 90 with the highest incidence in elderly white women.

C. Diagnosis

1. Clinical symptoms consistent with menopause
2. Elevated serum FSH level (menopausal range) is useful to confirm the diagnosis of menopause in a woman younger than expected or if similar symptoms could be related to an underlying medical or psychological problem.

D. Treatment

1. Patient education and reassurance by the physician are the most helpful because most women have minor, self-limited symptoms.
2. Estrogen replacement therapy is controversial. (Refer to Chapter 55 for further explanation of the risks and benefits of estrogen replacement therapy.)
3. Genital atrophy with vaginitis, dyspareunia, or urinary symptoms may respond to systemic estrogen or an estrogen-containing cream. (Refer to Chapter 55 for recommended preparations and dosages.)
4. Patients with depression or other psychiatric symptoms should be evaluated for evidence of a psychiatric diagnosis especially if there is a past history of psychiatric problems.

V. Annotated Bibliography

Avant R. Dysmenorrhea. Prim Care 1988;15(3):549–559. Good review of primary and secondary causes of dysmenorrhea.

Chihal H. Premenstrual syndrome: an update for the clinician. Obstet Gynecol Clin North Am 1990;17(2):457–479. Good review of treatment options for premenstrual syndrome.

Cowan B, Morrison J. Management of abnormal genital bleeding in girls and women. N Engl J Med 1991;324(25):1710–1714. Good overall view of abnormal vaginal bleeding and treatment for dysfunctional uterine bleeding.

Harman S, Blackman M. Common problems in reproductive endocrinology. In: Barker L, Burton J, Zieve PD, eds. Principles of Ambulatory Medicine. Baltimore: Williams & Wilkins;1991:1044–1066. Concise review of issues in ambulatory gynecology for the internist.

Chapter 57: Genital Infections

Rosemarie A. Leuzzi

57A Vaginitis

I. Clinical Presentation

A. General Information

1. Normal vaginal secretions consist mostly of cervical mucus along with upper tract secretions and glandular secretions. Normal secretions are odorless, clear or white, viscous, and homogenous, without pooling of secretions noted on pelvic examination.

2. The normal acidic pH of the vagina (usually 3.8–4.2) is the result of lactic acid production by the breakdown of glycogen in the vaginal secretions and the predominant organism is the acidophilic, anaerobic lactobacillus.

3. 90% of vaginal infections are due to bacterial vaginosis (caused by an overgrowth of anaerobic microorganisms and *Gardnerella vaginalis*), candidiasis (usually caused by *Candida albicans*), or trichomoniasis (caused by *Trichomonas vaginalis*).

B. Symptoms

1. Vaginal discharge
   a. A thin, white or yellow, homogenous discharge is usually suggestive of bacterial vaginosis.
   b. A thick, white vaginal discharge is noted in vulvovaginal candidiasis.
   c. Copious amounts of a diffuse, frothy, yellow-green discharge is typical of trichomoniasis.

2. Vulvar itching/irritation
   a. Women with vulvovaginal candidiasis usually complain of intense pruritis and vaginal burning/soreness usually worse during the week before menses; furthermore, dyspareunia and dysuria may be significant problems.
   b. Women with trichomoniasis usually present with vaginal irritation and pruritis; in addition, dyspareunia and dysuria may be present due to periurethral inflammation.

    c. Vulvar irritation occurs in only 15% with bacterial vaginosis and usually women do not complain of pruritis.

    d. Women with atrophic vaginitis may complain of vaginal dryness and irritation as well as dyspareunia and urinary incontinence.

3. Vaginal odor

    a. The most prevalent cause of a malodorous discharge is bacterial vaginosis with which most women note a "fishy" or "musty" odor. The odor may be more noticeable after sexual intercourse due to the interaction with alkaline seminal fluid causing the release of polyamines.

    b. A foul odor is noted in only 10% of women with trichomoniasis.

    c. Women with vulvovaginal candidiasis usually deny any abnormal odor to the discharge.

C. Physical Examination

1. Vaginal discharge with pooling of secretions is noted during pelvic examination.

2. Inflammatory changes of the vulvar and vaginal mucosa

    a. Vulvar and vaginal inflammation with white clumps of vaginal discharge adherent to inflamed mucosa is typical of vulvovaginal candidiasis. Vulvar erosions with satellite pustules may also be seen.

    b. Evidence of vaginal inflammation, vulvitis, and cervicitis with a characteristic "strawberry cervix" (petechial lesions noted on the cervix) is typical of trichomoniasis.

    c. The vaginal walls and cervix are usually not inflamed in bacterial vaginosis; however, a thin white-yellow discharge may be noted coating the walls of the vagina.

3. Pale vaginal mucosa with a loss of rugal folds, decreased subcutaneous tissue, and a loss of pubic hair may be seen in atrophic vaginitis.

II. Diagnostic Approach

A. Microscopic Examination of the Vaginal Discharge

1. Wet preparation

    a. The sample is diluted with 1–2 drops of 0.9% normal saline on one slide and covered with a cover slip.

    b. The motile trichomonads (intermediate in size between polymorphonuclear cells [PMNs] and epithelial cells) have a characteristic jerking motility pattern from its four flagellae and are visualized on the saline slide usually with many PMNs. The saline solution should be at room temperature because trichomonads may be immobilized with the use of cold saline.

    c. The "clue cells" of bacterial vaginosis (epithelial cells with a granulated surface and blurred margins due to the adherence of bacteria) may be identified on the saline slide.

2. Potassium hydroxide preparation
   a. The sample is diluted with 1–2 drops of 10% KOH on another slide and covered with a coverslip (warming over a flame is not usually necessary).
   b. Yeast with pseudohyphae is usually best identified using KOH because the KOH causes lysis of the epithelial cells and leukocytes that may obscure visualization of the budding filaments and pseudohyphae.

B. Vaginal Discharge pH

1. The pH of the vagina is normal with a pH < 4.5 in women with vulvovaginal candidiasis.
2. An elevated pH (> 4.5) is typical of trichomoniasis and the bacterial vaginosis infections.

C. Positive Whiff Test

1. Signifies the fishy odor of the vaginal discharge due to the production of polyamines by the anaerobic bacteria before or after the addition of KOH.
2. A positive whiff test is usually noted in bacterial vaginosis infection and trichomoniasis.
3. The whiff test is negative in women with vulvovaginal candidiasis.

D. Vaginal Culture

1. Culture for *T. vaginalis* or *Candida* species is usually more sensitive than microscopic examination.
   a. Vaginal culture is 90% sensitive in detecting *Trichomonas* organisms; however, cultures are not routinely used because fresh media is required although the processing of the culture is not difficult.
   b. Culture is the most sensitive method for detecting yeast; however, up to 25% of asymptomatic women without vaginitis will have positive yeast cultures, raising doubts about the specificity of the culture.
2. Culture of *G. vaginalis* is not recommended as a diagnostic tool because it is not specific and can be isolated from vaginal cultures in half of normal women.

III. Differential Diagnosis

A. Bacterial Vaginosis

1. Bacterial vaginosis, previously known as nonspecific vaginitis, is caused by a shift in the normal vaginal flora with replacement of the normal *Lactobacillus* species with high concentrations of anaerobic bacteria, *G. vaginalis*, and *Mycoplasma hominis*.
2. The cause of this alteration is poorly understood; however *Gardnerella* may play a part in the pathogenesis by disturbing the normal flora.

3. Bacterial vaginosis is not exclusively considered a sexually transmitted disease (STD); however, it is usually associated with multiple sexual partners and the presence of other STDs.
4. Clinical diagnosis requires three of the following criteria—a homogenous, thin, white, noninflammatory discharge that adheres to the vaginal walls; the presence of "clue" cells on microscopic evaluation; pH of the vaginal fluid > 4.5; and a positive whiff test.

B. Trichomoniasis

1. Trichomoniasis is caused by the protozoan *T. vaginalis*.
2. *T. vaginalis* is not an invasive type of organism; however, it attaches to epithelial cells causing superficial irritation and inflammation.
3. The prevalence of this infection correlates with sexual activity, number of sexual partners, and the presence of other STDs. Transmission may also occur nonvenereally via moist cloths because trichomonads may survive up to 3 h outside the vagina.
4. The majority of men are usually asymptomatic and tend to eliminate the organism quickly with infections remitting spontaneously (possibly due to clearing of the organism during urination or poor attachment of the organism to the urethral mucosal cells).

C. Vulvovaginal Candidiasis

1. Caused by *C. albicans*, vulvovaginal candidiasis is usually not sexually acquired or transmitted.
2. Identifying candida in the absence of symptoms should not lead to treatment because approximately 10–20% of women normally harbor Candida and other yeasts.

D. Atrophic Vaginitis

1. Atrophic vaginitis is commonly seen in postmenopausal women.
2. The lack of estrogen results in thinning of the vaginal and vulvar mucosa, decreased normal vaginal secretions, and increased susceptibility to traumatic irritation and perhaps infection.

E. Gonorrhea and chlamydial infections may initially present with an abnormal vaginal discharge and be misinterpreted as vulvovaginitis.

IV. Treatment

A. Treatment for Bacterial Vaginosis

1. Recommended regimen

   a. Metronidazole 500 mg b.i.d. for 7 d

b. Patients need to be asked about the potential possibility of pregnancy because metronidazole is contraindicated during the first trimester of pregnancy and advised to avoid alcohol during treatment due to the potential disulfiram-like reaction from the metronidazole blocking the metabolism of alcohol.

2. Alternative regimens

   a. Metronidazole 2 g PO in a single dose *OR*
   b. Clindamycin cream 2% 5-g applicator intravaginally qhs for 7 d *OR*
   c. Metronidazole gel 0.75% 5-g applicator intravaginally b.i.d. for 5 d *OR*
   d. Clindamycin 300 mg b.i.d. for 7 d

3. Asymptomatic infection does not require treatment because the goal of therapy is to relieve vaginal signs and symptoms; therefore, only symptomatic women require treatment.

4. Follow-up is not necessary if symptoms resolve; however, recurrence is common.

5. Management of sexual partners

   a. Routine treatment of sexual partners is not recommended.
   b. Male sexual partners are usually asymptomatic and treatment of male partners has not been shown to alter the clinical course of the infection or prevent recurrence.

B. Treatment for Trichomoniasis

1. Recommended regimen

   a. Metronidazole 2 g PO in a single dose

2. Alternative regimen

   a. Metronidazole 500 mg b.i.d. for 7 d
   b. Metronidazole gel has not been studied for the treatment of trichomoniasis and is only approved for the treatment of bacterial vaginosis.

3. Follow-up

   a. Not necessary if symptoms resolve
   b. If symptoms persist, consider reinfection and retreatment with metronidazole 500 mg b.i.d. for 7 d is recommended.

4. Sexual partners should be treated and patients should be advised to avoid sexual contact until the patient and partner are cured.

C. Treatment of Vulvovaginal Candidiasis

1. Recommended regimens

All of the following regimens are equivalent for treatment; however, single-dose treatments should be reserved for uncomplicated mild candidiasis and multiday regimens are preferred for moderate to severe infections.

a. Butoconazole (Femstat) 2% cream 5 g intravaginally for 3 d
  b. Clotrimazole (Mycelex or Gyne-Lotrimin)
     1) 1% cream 5 g intravaginally for 7–14 d OR
     2) 100-mg vaginal tablet for 7 d (or 2 tablets for 3 d) OR
     3) 500-mg vaginal tablet in single dose
  c. Miconazole (Monistat)
     1) 2% cream 5 g intravaginally for 7 d OR
     2) 200 mg vaginal suppository for 3 d OR
     3) 100 mg vaginal suppository for 7 d
  d. Terconazole (Terazol)
     1) 0.4% cream 5 g intravaginally for 7 d OR
     2) 0.8% cream 5 g intravaginally for 3 d OR
     3) 80 mg suppository for 3 d
  e. During pregnancy, candida infection can be more resistant; therefore, a 7-d regimen is recommended
  f. Topical formulations provide effective treatment; furthermore, no oral agent is approved by the Food and Drug Administration for treatment of acute vulvovaginal candidiasis.

2. Skin conditions that predispose to candida infection generally involve persistent moisture and development of maceration of the skin due to occlusive synthetic clothing.

3. Follow-up
   a. Patients with persistent symptoms should be instructed to return; retreatment with a longer course of antifungal therapy may be required and switching to a different imidazole topical agent should be considered.
   b. Recurrent vulvovaginal candidiasis
      1) Risk factors for recurrent yeast infections include diabetes mellitus, immunosuppression, pregnancy, broad-spectrum antibiotic use, corticosteroid use, and HIV infection.
      2) Women who experience three or more episodes per year should be evaluated for predisposing conditions, although the majority of women with recurrent vulvovaginal candidiasis will have no apparent risk factors.
      3) Ketoconazole 100 mg PO daily for up to 6 mo or routine prophylaxis with ketoconazole 400 mg PO daily for 5 d at the beginning of menses reduces the frequency of episodes of recurrent vulvovaginal candidiasis; however, the optimal treatment has not been established.

4. Management of sexual partners
   a. Treatment of sexual partners is not recommended and has not been shown to decrease recurrences.
   b. Men with balanitis may benefit from treatment with topical antifungal drugs to relieve symptoms.

D. Treatment of Atrophic Vaginitis

1. Refer to Chapter 55.

V. Indications for Referral to a Specialist

A. Women with frequent, recurrent episodes of vaginitis may be referred to either a gynecologist or infectious disease consultant for confirmation of the diagnosis with cultures and sensitivities as well as consideration of alternative antibiotic therapy.

B. The presence of a nonhealing ulcer or lesion on the vulva, vagina, or cervix should be referred for further evaluation and possible biopsy.

VI. Annotated Bibliography

Centers for Disease Control and Prevention. 1993 sexually transmitted diseases treatment guidelines. MMWR 1993;42:No. RR-14. Excellent handbook covering diagnosis and recommended therapy for vaginitis.

Cullins V, Huggins GR. Nonmalignant vulvovaginal disorders. In: Barker LR, Burton JR, Zieve PD, eds. Principles of Ambulatory Medicine. Baltimore: Williams & Wilkins; 1991. Concise review of types of vaginitis with good chart reviewing types of vaginal discharge and good illustrations of microscopic findings.

McCue JD. Evaluation and management of vaginitis: an update for primary care practitioners. Arch Intern Med 1989;149:565–568. Good review article covering three forms of vaginitis and diagnostic approach.

57B Cervicitis

I. Clinical Presentation

A. General Information

1. Cervicitis can be caused by *Neisseria gonorrhoeae* or *Chlamydia trachomatis*; although in many cases, neither organism can be isolated.
2. Transmission of gonorrhea from infected men to uninfected women or men is efficient and occurs in 90% of exposures.
3. *C. trachomatis* is isolated from the cervix of 30–60% of women with gonorrhea infection.
4. Some women with apparently uncomplicated cervical infection already have subclinical upper reproductive tract infections and complications of *N. gonorrhoeae* and *C. trachomatis* infection include pelvic inflammatory disease, ectopic pregnancy, and infertility.

B. Symptoms

1. Many women are asymptomatic.
2. Abnormal vaginal bleeding, usually following intercourse
3. Vaginal discharge, vaginal itching, dyspareunia, and dysuria (the result of the cervicitis, not vaginitis)
4. Lower abdominal discomfort
5. Anorectal symptoms with rectal fullness, painful defecation
6. Petechial or pustular acral lesions, asymmetric arthralgias, tenosynovitis, or septic arthritis may result from gonococcal bacteremia and disseminated gonococcal infection; these strains of *N. gonorrhoeae* tend to cause little genital inflammation.

C. Physical Examination

1. Cervicitis is characterized by a mucopurulent discharge from the cervical os or yellow endocervical exudate visible in the endocervical canal or in an endocervical swab specimen.
2. The cervix may appear inflamed, edematous, and friable.

II. Diagnostic Approach

A. Because many women are asymptomatic, routine screening for gonorrhea and chlamydia are important in women with a history of other sexually transmitted diseases or multiple sexual partners.

B. Gram Stain of the Cervical Discharge

1. Diagnostic when intracellular gram-negative diplococci are identified (insensitive but highly specific test)
2. Increased number of polymorphonuclear leukocytes may also be noted

C. Microbiologic Culture

1. Patients should have cervical specimens cultured for *N. gonorrhoeae* on chocolate agar media (sensitivity 80–90%)
2. *C. trachomatis* culture media is expensive and growth is slow; therefore, fluorescent antibody staining technique (Microtrak) and enzyme immunoassay (Chlamydiazyme) are inexpensive and reliable methods to detect *C. trachomatis*, using a cotton swab impregnated with calcium gluconate to obtain the sample.

D. Syphilis Serology

1. Persons treated for either gonorrhea or chlamydia should also be screened for syphilis.

III. Differential Diagnosis

A. Vaginitis (see Chapter 57A)

B. Primary syphilis chancre (see Chapter 71)

C. Herpes simplex virus

IV. Treatment

A. General Information

1. Treatment of infected patients prevents transmission to sexual partners and reduces the likelihood of subsequent ascending infections and decreases the incidence of long-term complications of tubal infertility and ectopic pregnancy.
2. Because of the high prevalence of coinfection with *C. trachomatis* among patients with gonococcal infection, presumptive treatment for chlamydia in patients being treated for gonorrhea is appropriate.
3. Treatment should be initiated while the results of the cultures are pending.
4. Treatment for gonorrhea and chlamydia is indicated in patient populations with a high prevalence of both infections.
5. If the prevalence of both infections is low and the patient is likely to return for a follow-up visit, waiting for test results to decide on treatment is appropriate.
6. For infected pregnant women, antibiotic therapy may prevent transmission of *C. trachomatis* to the infant during birth.

B. Treatment for Chlamydial Infections

1. Recommended regimen

    a. Doxycycline 100 mg PO b.i.d. for 7 d *OR*
    b. Azithromycin 1 g PO in a single dose

2. Alternative regimen

    a. Ofloxacin 300 mg PO b.i.d. for 7 d *OR*
    b. Erythromycin base 500 mg PO q.i.d. for 7 d

3. Recommended regimen in pregnancy

    a. Erythromycin base 500 mg PO q.i.d. for 7 d
    b. Doxycycline and ofloxacin are contraindicated in pregnancy and the safety of azithromycin has not been established.

4. Follow-up

    a. Patients do not need to be retested for chlamydia after completing treatment unless symptoms persist or reinfection is suspected.
    b. Patients should be instructed to avoid sexual intercourse until they and their partners are cured.

5. Management of sexual partners

    a. Patients should be instructed to refer their sex partners for evaluation and treatment.
    b. All sexual partners of *symptomatic* patients should be treated if their last sexual contact with the patient was within 30 d of onset of the patient's symptoms
    c. All sexual partners of *asymptomatic* patients should be treated if their last sexual contact with the patient was within 60 d of the patient's index diagnosis.
    d. If the patient's last sexual intercourse preceded these time intervals, the most recent sexual partner should be treated.

C. Treatment for Gonococcal Infections

1. Recommended regimens

    a. Ceftriaxone 125 mg IM in single dose *OR*
    b. Cefixime 400 mg PO in single dose *OR*
    c. Ciprofloxacin 500 mg PO in single dose *OR*
    d. Ofloxacin 400 mg PO in single dose
    e. *PLUS* a regimen effective against possible coinfection with *C. trachomatis*, such as doxycycline 100 mg b.i.d. for 7 d

2. Alternative regimens

    a. Spectinomycin 2 g IM in a single dose
    b. Many other antimicrobial regimens are effective in treating gonococcal infections including other injectable/oral cephalosporins and other quinolones.

3. Recommended regimen in pregnancy
   a. Cephalosporin treatment should be used because quinolone therapy is contraindicated.
   b. If the patient cannot tolerate a cephalosporin, a single dose of spectinomycin should be used.
4. If pharyngeal infection is a concern, either the ceftriaxone or ciprofloxacin regimen is recommended.
5. Follow-up
   a. Persons who have uncomplicated gonorrhea and who are treated with any of the above regimens need not return for a test of cure.
   b. For patients with persistent symptoms, repeat culture for *N. gonorrhoeae* should be done with antimicrobial sensitivity testing.
   c. Persistent infection is usually due to reinfection rather than treatment failure and patients should be instructed to avoid sexual intercourse until their sexual partner is also treated.
6. Management of sexual partners
   a. Sexual partners should be notified, evaluated, and treated.
   b. Partners of patients who are treated presumptively should receive the same treatment as the index patient.
   c. Same as above for treatment of Chlamydia—management of sexual partners

D. Treatment for Disseminated Gonococcal Infection

1. Hospitalization is recommended for initial therapy and patients should be examined carefully for evidence of meningitis or endocarditis.
2. All patients treated for disseminated gonorrhea should also be treated for concurrent *C. trachomatis* infection.
3. Recommended regimen:
   a. Ceftriaxone 1 g IM or IV q 24 h
4. Alternative regimens
   a. Cefotaxime 1 g IV q 8 h *OR*
   b. Ceftizoxime 1 g IV q 8 h *OR*
   c. Spectinomycin 2 g IM q 12 h
5. All regimens should be continued for 24–48 h after improvement begins, then therapy can be switched to either cefixime 400 mg PO b.i.d. or ciprofloxacin 500 mg PO b.i.d. to complete 1 wk of therapy.

V. Indications for Referral to a Specialist

A. Patients with persistent cervical inflammation and friable cervical tissue after antibiotic therapy should be referred to a gynecologist for further evaluation.

B. Once reinfection has been excluded, patients with persistent gonorrhea/chlamydia infection may need referral to an infectious disease specialist for further cultures and sensitivity testing.

VI. Annotated Bibliography

Centers for Disease Control and Prevention. 1993 sexually transmitted diseases treatment guidelines. MMWR 1993;42:No. RR-14. Excellent handbook covering all STDs including diagnosis, testing, recommended therapy as well as special consideration of pregnancy, children/adolescents, and HIV-infected patients. An essential guide to have available in ambulatory practice settings.

Cullins V, Huggins GR. Nonmalignant vulvovaginal disorders. In: Barker LR, Burton JR, Zieve PD, eds. Principles of Ambulatory Medicine. Baltimore: Williams & Wilkins; 1991. More generalized review for ambulatory setting.

Drugs for sexually transmitted diseases. Med Lett (36) January 7, 1994. Good, brief review of current treatments for STDs including new antibiotic regimens. Concise table covers drug of choice for each infection, dosage, and alternative therapy.

Hacker NF, Moore JG. Essentials of Obstetrics and Gynecology. Philadelphia: WB Saunders; 1986. Basic review of pelvic inflammatory disease and cervicitis.

Holmes KK. Pelvic inflammatory disease. In: Wilson JD, Braunwald E, Isselbacher KJ, et al eds. Harrison's Principles of Internal Medicine. New York: McGraw-Hill; 1991. For more in-depth review of infectious organisms and details regarding epidemiology and diagnostic testing.

57C Pelvic Inflammatory Disease

I. Clinical Presentation

A. General Information

1. Pelvic inflammatory disease (PID) involves the proximal spread of pathogens from the endocervix to the upper reproductive tract and includes a spectrum of inflammatory disorders including any combination of endometritis, salpingitis, tubo-ovarian abscess, and pelvic peritonitis.
2. Sexually transmitted organisms, especially *Neisseria gonorrhoeae* and *Chlamydia trachomatis* are implicated in the majority of cases; *Mycoplasma hominis* and *Ureaplasma urealyticum* have also been considered potential pathogens.
3. The presentation of PID may be acute, subacute, or chronic with a wide variation of presenting signs and symptoms; consequently, a delay in diagnosis and effective treatment may contribute to the inflammatory sequelae in the upper reproductive tract.
4. Complications of PID include bilateral tubal occlusion, ectopic pregnancy due to tubal damage without occlusion, chronic pelvic pain, and recurrent PID.
5. A single, mild episode of acute salpingitis will cause infertility in 13% of patients and this figure rises to 75% after three or more bouts of PID.

B. Symptoms

1. Lower abdominal pain, often bilateral, usually described as dull or aching
2. Purulent vaginal discharge
3. Dysuria and urinary frequency (due to urethritis)
4. Anorectal pain and tenesmus
5. Fever
6. Nausea and vomiting
7. Pleuritic right upper quadrant pain (caused by perihepatitis) may be present
8. The onset is frequently related to menses in women with gonorrhea or chlamydial infections.
9. Acute PID may be exacerbated by menses, sexual intercourse, strenuous physical activity, and even a pelvic examination.
10. Important risk factors for PID include a history of gonorrhea or salpingitis, use of an intrauterine contraceptive device, and exposure to a male sexual partner with urethritis.

C. Physical Examination

1. Fever (present in one third of patients with acute salpingitis)
2. Generalized lower abdominal tenderness without palpable masses
3. Cervical motion tenderness on bimanual examination
4. Uterine fundal tenderness may be due to endometritis and abnormal adnexal tenderness may be due to salpingitis, which is often bilateral.
5. On pelvic examination, a mucopurulent cervical discharge may be present.
6. Right upper quadrant tenderness may be present with perihepatitis (also known as Fitz-Hugh-Curtis syndrome), which occurs in 3–10% of women with acute PID.

II. Diagnostic Approach

A. No single historical, physical, or laboratory finding is both sensitive and specific for the diagnosis of PID; therefore, a clinical diagnosis of PID is difficult and many cases of PID go unrecognized.

B. Because of the difficulty of diagnosis and the potential damage to a woman's reproductive tract, maintaining a low threshold for the diagnosis is important.

C. As per the Centers for Disease Control and Prevention guidelines, the following clinical criteria are suggested to diagnose PID.

1. Minimum clinical criteria for pelvic inflammation (if all three are present and there is no other established cause other than PID, empirical treatment is recommended).

    a. Lower abdominal tenderness
    b. Adnexal tenderness
    c. Cervical motion tenderness

2. Additional *routine criteria* to increase the specificity of the diagnosis include

    a. Oral temperature > 38.3°C
    b. Abnormal cervical or vaginal discharge
    c. Elevated erythrocyte sedimentation rate
    d. Elevated C-reactive protein
    e. Laboratory documentation of cervical infection with gonorrhea or chlamydia

3. The *elaborate criteria* for diagnosing PID include

    a. Histopathologic evidence of endometritis on endometrial biopsy
    b. Tubo-ovarian abscess on sonography or other radiologic tests
    c. Laparoscopic abnormalities consistent with PID

D. Laboratory Testing

1. Complete blood count—Leukocytosis indicates acute infection.
2. Endocervical culture
   a. Gram stain for the presence of gram-negative diplococci (*N. gonorrhoeae*) and neutrophils
   b. Culture for *N. gonorrhoeae* on chocolate agar
   c. Chlamydia testing with culture or Chlamydiazyme
3. Pregnancy test—important to rule out the possibility of ectopic pregnancy
4. Urinalysis—rule out urinary tract infection
5. Erythrocyte sedimentation rate may be elevated (75% of cases).

E. Diagnostic Imaging

1. Pelvic ultrasound study may reveal a tubo-ovarian abscess, ectopic pregnancy
2. CT scan of the abdomen and pelvis may be needed to further evaluate abnormal ultrasound findings.

F. Following referral to a specialist, laparoscopy is the most specific method for diagnosis of acute salpingitis and can be used to obtain a more accurate bacteriologic diagnosis; however, endometritis and subtle inflammation of the fallopian tubes may not be detected.

III. Differential Diagnosis

A. Acute appendicitis

B. Urinary tract infection

C. Adnexal torsion

D. Endometriosis

E. Diverticular abscess

F. Ectopic pregnancy

G. Functional pain

IV. Treatment

A. Outpatient Therapy for PID

1. Recommended regimens
   a. Cefoxitin 2 g IM *PLUS* probenecid 1 g PO in a single dose concurrently or ceftriaxone 250 mg IM *PLUS* doxycycline 100 mg PO b.i.d. for 14 d *OR*

    b. Ofloxacin 400 mg PO b.i.d. for 14 d *PLUS* either clindamycin 450 mg PO q.i.d. or metronidazole 500 mg PO b.i.d. for 14 d

2. Follow-up

    a. Patients need to be clinically reevaluated in 48–72 h after the initial visit.

    b. Patients who do not respond to outpatient therapy within 72 h should be hospitalized to confirm the diagnosis and receive parenteral antibiotics.

B. Inpatient Therapy for PID

1. Recommended regimens

    a. Cefoxitin 2 g IV q 6 h or cefotetan 2 g IV q 12 h *PLUS* doxycycline 100 mg IV/PO q 12 h. Continue this regimen for at least 48 h after the patient begins to show clinical improvement, then switch to doxycycline 100 mg PO b.i.d. for a total of 14 d of therapy.

    b. Clindamycin 900 mg IV q 8 h *PLUS* gentamycin IV q 8 h. Continue this regimen for at least 48 h after the patient begins to show clinical improvement, then switch to doxycycline 100 mg PO b.i.d. or clindamycin 450 mg PO q.i.d. to complete 14 d of therapy (when tubo-ovarian abscess is present, clindamycin is recommended as continued therapy for better anaerobic coverage).

2. Follow-up

    a. Hospitalized patients receiving IV antibiotics should show substantial improvement within 3–5 d.

    b. If no improvement, further diagnostic evaluation or surgical intervention may be necessary.

C. Management of Sexual Partners

1. Evaluation and treatment of sexual partners who have PID is essential due to the risk of reinfection and the high likelihood of urethral gonococcal or chlamydial infection of the partner.

2. Sexual partners should empirically be treated for *both N. gonorrhoeae* and *C. trachomatis* regardless of the apparent etiology of PID in the patient (due to the insensitivity of culture results in asymptomatic men).

V. Indications for Hospitalization

A. Hospitalization is recommended in the following settings

1. Uncertain diagnosis and surgical emergencies such as appendicitis and ectopic pregnancy cannot be excluded

2. Suspected pelvic abscess

3. Pregnant patient

4. Adolescent patient

5. HIV-infected patient
6. Severe illness or nausea and vomiting preclude outpatient management
7. The patient is unable to follow or tolerate an outpatient regimen.
8. The patient has failed to respond clinically to outpatient therapy.
9. Clinical follow-up within 72 h of starting antibiotic therapy cannot be arranged.

VI. Indications for Referral to a Specialist

A. With the complaint of atypical abdominal pain, consultation with either a general surgeon or gynecologist may be helpful; further diagnostic evaluation or surgical intervention may be required.

B. Laparoscopy may be required to confirm the diagnosis of PID and exclude other possibilities, eg, endometriosis.

VII. Annotated Bibliography

Please refer to entries listed in Chapter 57B.

57D Human Papillomavirus Infection

I. Clinical Presentation

A. General Information

1. Exophytic genital and anal warts are most commonly caused by human papillomavirus (HPV) types 6 or 11.
2. HPV is transmitted by direct contract, usually sexual.
3. HPV lesions are more profuse in patients who are pregnant, diabetic, on oral contraceptives, or on immunosuppressants.
4. HPV types 16, 18, 31, 33, and 35 have been strongly associated with cervical dysplasia and carcinoma.

B. Symptoms

1. Asymptomatic, benign growths on the genitalia, perineal, or perianal area (moist areas)
2. Minor or no symptoms aside from their cosmetic appearance
3. The lesions may be small and discrete or may have coalesced into large masses.
4. Vaginal itching and discharge may be present, possibly due to an associated vaginitis or infection within the crevices of the wart. (Venereal warts often occur in association with trichomoniasis or bacterial vaginosis.)

C. Physical Examination

1. A 1–2-cm lesion first appears on the labia but then spreads, with congruent or discrete lesions appearing on the perineum, anus, vagina, or cervix.
2. The verrucous warts then may coalesce into large cauliflower-like lesions.

II. Diagnostic Approach

A. Usually a clinical diagnosis; however, biopsy of the lesion can confirm the diagnosis.

B. Serology for syphilis should be checked to rule out condyloma latum.

C. Female patients should have a Pap smear performed to exclude cervical dysplasia.

III. Differential Diagnosis

A. Condyloma latum of secondary syphilis

B. Squamous cell carcinoma

C. Skin tags

IV. Treatment

A. Goal of treatment is removal of the warts not the eradication of HPV; if left untreated, genital warts may resolve on their own, remain unchanged, or grow.

B. A treatment regimen should be chosen with consideration of the anatomic location, size, and number of warts as well as the expense, convenience, and potential adverse effects.

C. Treatment for External Genital/Perianal Warts

1. Cryotherapy with liquid nitrogen or cryoprobe
2. Podofilox 0.5% solution applied to warts with cotton swab b.i.d. for 3 d followed by 4 d of no therapy. This cycle may be repeated for a total of 4 cycles.
3. Podophyllin 10–25% solution in tincture of benzoin applied to warts and washed off after 1–4 h and repeated weekly as necessary.
4. Trichloroacetic acid (TCA) 80–90%
5. Electrodesiccation or electrocautery

D. Follow-up

1. After warts have responded to therapy, follow-up is not necessary.
2. With a history of HPV, female patients should be encouraged to have careful follow-up with annual cytologic screening for cervical dysplasia and cervical carcinoma.

E. Management of Sexual Partners

1. Patients with exophytic anogenital warts should be made aware that they are contagious to uninfected sexual partners, although the majority of partners are probably already subclinically infected with HPV, even if they do not have visible warts.
2. Even after removal of warts, patients may harbor HPV in the surrounding normal tissues as may persons without exophytic warts.
3. The use of condoms may prevent the transmission of HPV to uninfected partners.

V. Indications for Referral to a Specialist

A. Extensive warts may require carbon dioxide laser therapy or conventional surgery; referral to a dermatologist, gynecologist, or surgeon is recommended.

B. For patients with cervical warts, dysplasia must be excluded and referral to a gynecologist is recommended.

VI. Annotated Bibliography

Please refer to entries listed in Chapter 57B.

Part XII:
Hematology

Chapter 58: Abnormal Coagulation Tests

Barry Ziring

I. Clinical Presentation

A. General Information

1. In an asymptomatic population, the risk of an unsuspected coagulation disorder is very low.
2. As a result, the literature does not support the routine use of screening coagulation tests either in the general public or in the preoperative setting.
3. Preoperative coagulation studies should be drawn for patients undergoing surgery only where there is a high risk of bleeding.
4. Preoperative or diagnostic studies should be obtained in patients who have had episodes of abnormal bleeding. In this population up to 40% will be found to have a coagulation disorder.
5. The three most commonly ordered tests of coagulation are the prothrombin time (PT), activated partial thromboplastin time (aPTT) and the platelet count (Table 58-1).

B. History

1. Platelet disorders—Patients with abnormal platelets or thrombocytopenia will report bleeding primarily into skin and mucous membranes. This bleeding often stops with local pressure or packing.
2. Coagulation protein disorder—Patients with these deficits will report bleeding into subcutaneous tissue, muscle, and joints. This bleeding does not respond to local pressure.
3. Certain patients will have a coagulation disorder that predisposes to hypercoagulable states.
4. Family history of bleeding is important.
5. A careful history of medication use is important.

C. Physical Examination

1. Petechiae (discrete hemorrhagic areas < 2 mm in diameter) may indicate a platelet abnormality but can also be seen in infectious disease and vasculitis.

Table 58–1. Profiles of Hemostasis Screening Tests in Patients with Bleeding Disorders

PT	PTT	Platelet Count		Differential Diagnoses
↑	—	—	Common	Factor VII deficiency (early liver disease, early vitamin K deficiency, early warfarin therapy)
			Rare	Factor VII inhibitor
—	↑	—		Deficiency or inhibitor of factors VIII, IX, or XI; vWD, heparin, lupus inhibitor with qualitative platelet defect
↑	↑	—	Common	Vitamin K deficiency, liver disease, warfarin, heparin
			Rare	Deficiency or inhibitor of factors X, V, prothrombin, or fibrinogen; lupus inhibitor with hypoprothrombinemia; DIC
↑	↑	↓		DIC, liver disease, heparin therapy with associated thrombocytopenia
—	—	↓		Increased platelet destruction, decreased platelet production, hypersplenism, hemodilution
—	—	↑		Myeloproliferative disorders
—	—	—	Common	Variant vWD, acquired qualitative platelet disorders (uremia)
			Rare	Inherited qualitative platelet disorders, vascular disorders, fibrinolytic disorders, factor XIII deficiency, autoerythrocyte sensitization, dysfibrinogenemia

The differential diagnosis of bleeding disorders suggested by results of the PT, PTT, and platelet count is listed for each profile. ↑, increased; ↓, decreased; —, normal; PT, prothrombin time; PTT, partial thromboplastin time; vWD, von Willebrand's disease; DIC, disseminated intravascular coagulation. This table includes the differential diagnosis of hemostasis screening test results in patients with a history of bleeding. Consideration of patients with abnormal coagulation tests and negative bleeding histories is not included in this table.

2. Purpura (groups of petechiae or ecchymoses) similarly may indicate a platelet abnormality but can be seen in Rocky Mountain spotted fever, scurvy, and trauma.
3. Splenomegaly may be helpful in evaluating the cause of thrombocytopenia.
4. Bleeding into joints and muscles after minor trauma is indicative of a coagulation disorder.

II. Diagnostic Approach to Thrombocytopenia

A. Thrombocytopenia is defined as a platelet count < 150 (cells × 10^9/L).

B. The three general mechanisms of thrombocytopenia are decreased production, increased destruction, and sequestration.

C. Certain clinical patterns will be obvious from the history and physical examination including sepsis, lymphoma, and liver disease.

D. If no diagnosis is obvious after a thorough history and physical, examination thrombocytopenia should be further evaluated on the basis of the presence or absence of splenomegaly followed by a bone marrow examination.

E. Thrombocytopenia and Splenomegaly

1. Normal marrow
    a. Congestive splenomegaly
    b. Liver disease
    c. Storage disorders
    d. Neoplasm

2. Abnormal marrow
    a. Chronic leukemia
    b. Lymphoma (usually accompanied by adenopathy)
    c. Myeloid metaplasia

F. Thrombocytopenia and Normal Spleen

1. Normal marrow
    a. Drug-induced thrombocytopenia
        1) Quinidine
        2) Phenytoin
        3) Sulfonamide
        4) Gold salts
        5) Cephalosporins
        6) Heparin
    b. Acute postinfection thrombocytopenia
    c. Chronic autoimmune thrombocytopenia
    d. Disseminated intravascular coagulation
    e. Thrombotic microangiopathies
        1) Thrombotic thrombocytopenia purpura
        2) Hemolytic uremic syndrome
        3) Disseminated intravascular coagulopathy
        4) Vasculitis

2. Abnormal marrow
    a. Aplasia
    b. Acute leukemia
    c. Metastatic carcinoma

III. Diagnostic Approach to Thrombocytosis

A. Defined as platelet count of > 400 (cells $\times 10^9$/L)

B. Thrombocytosis may be associated with either clinical bleeding <u>or</u> thrombosis.

C. Primary causes of chronic thrombocytosis include

1. Myeloproliferative disorder

2. Essential thrombocytosis

3. Polycythemia rubra vera—increased red blood cell mass

4. Chronic myelocytic leukemia—leukocytosis with a shift to the left on white blood cell count

5. Myelofibrosis—splenic enlargement and leukoerythroblastosis

D. Secondary causes include

1. Chronic inflammation

2. Rheumatoid arthritis

3. Inflammatory bowel disease

4. Sarcoidosis

5. Polyarteritis nodosa

6. Chronic infection

7. Tuberculosis

8. Malignancy

9. Iron deficiency anemia

E. Following a thorough history and physical examination, laboratory and radiographic studies should be done to evaluate any abnormalities.

F. If the diagnosis is not apparent, all patients should be screened for common malignancies with a chest x-ray, mammogram, pelvic examination and Pap smear, stool hemoccult, and urinalysis for hematuria.

G. If no secondary cause of thrombocytosis is found, essential thrombocytosis must be distinguished from other myeloproliferative disorders. Diagnostic features of essential thrombocytosis are:

1. Platelet count > 600 (cells $\times 10^9$/L).

2. Absence of increased red blood cell mass.

3. Bone marrow that demonstrates normal iron stores.

4. Absence of bone marrow fibrosis.

5. Absence of Philadelphia chromosome.

IV. Diagnostic Approach for Qualitative Disorders of Platelet Function

A. Platelet function defects should be considered for patients with a history of bleeding who have a normal platelet count and coagulation studies.

B. There are very few reliable tests for evaluating platelet function.

C. The bleeding time can be helpful in this setting. A prolonged bleeding time in a patient with a history of bleeding requires further evaluation of platelet function.

D. Congenital platelet function defects include

1. von Willebrand's disease

2. Glanzman's thrombasthenia

3. Storage pool deficiency

E. Acquired platelet function defects include

1. Uremia

2. Paraproteinemias

3. Myeloproliferative disorders

4. Cardiopulmonary bypass

5. Drugs—aspirin, nonsteroidal anti-inflammatory drugs (NSAIDs), β-lactam antibiotics

F. When indicated, tests of platelet function can be performed in specialized coagulation laboratories including.

1. von Willebrand's Factor (activity and antigen).

2. Response to Ristocetin aggregatory agent.

3. Platelet membrane glycoprotein assays.

V. Diagnostic Approach to Elevated aPTT

A. The risks of unsuspected coagulation disorders in an aysmptomatic patient is very low.

B. If the PTT is elevated in an asymptomatic person, suspect a spurious result secondary to

1. Incomplete filling of the specimen tube

2. Heparin effects
3. Crossover effect from warfarin.

C. Most patients with an isolated elevated PTT are not prone to bleeding.

D. If a history of bleeding is present, a bleeding time should be done to evaluate for a concomitant platelet defect.

E. Perform a mixing study (often ordered through coagulation laboratory) at 0 and 60-min incubations.

1. Correction of elevated PTT at 0 and 60 min
    a. Perform specific factor assays VIII, IX, and XI.
    b. Factor VIII and factor IX deficiency are hemophilia A and B, respectively.
    c. Factor XI deficiency has a high frequency in Eastern European Jews. There is rarely bleeding associated with this disorder except during major surgical stress.

2. Incomplete correction at 0 and 60 min
    a. Suspect lupus type inhibitor.
    b. Perform specific tests for lupus inhibitor including tissue thromboplastin inhibition (TTI) and Russell's viper venom time and anticardiolipin antibodies.
    c. Patients with lupus inhibitor may be at risk for hypercoagulable state.

3. Incomplete correction that is time dependent.
    a. Suspect antibodies to intrinsic pathway coagulation protein.
    b. Perform factor VIII, IX, XI level, and assay of antibody titer.

VI. Diagnostic Approach to Elevated PT

A. The same general principles regarding elevated value in asymptomatic patient as for aPTT apply.

B. The common causes of elevated PT are

1. Factor VII deficiency (rare)

2. Acquired factor VII deficiency secondary to
    a. Early liver disease
    b. Vitamin K deficiency
    c. Warfarin therapy

VII. Prethrombotic or Hypercoagulable Disorders

A. Approximately 1–2% of all patients with thrombosis and 10–20% of patients with recurrent thrombosis will have a hereditary defect of coagulation.

B. At the present time, this group of diseases include

1. Protein C deficiency
2. Protein S deficiency
3. Antithrombin III deficiency
4. Abnormal fibrinogen or abnormal release of tissue plasminogen activator
5. Lupus anticoagulant and anticardiolipin antibody syndromes.

VIII. Treatment

A. The treatment strategies for this heterogenous group of disorders is beyond the scope of this outpatient textbook. A general review of the therapies available follows.

1. Factor VIII deficiency—cryoprecipitate or factor VIII concentrate
2. Factor IX deficiency—prothrombin complex concentrate (PCC) or factor XI concentrate
3. Factor XI deficiency—fresh frozen plasma.
4. von Willebrand's disease—desmopressincetate (DDAVP) or cryoprecipitate
5. Dysproteinemia—plasmaphoresis
6. Thrombocytopenia—hydroxyurea

B. An effort should be made to identify secondary causes of abnormal coagulation tests and treat these diseases.

IX. Patient Education

A. Patients who are found to have abnormal coagulation studies are often extremely concerned.

B. This group can be divided into two categories

1. Patients with a history of bleeding frequently do have diseases identified that are often treatable.
2. Patients without a bleeding history require reassurance while work-up is being performed because clinically significant bleeding disorder is rarely found.

C. Sports are not contraindicated for patients with coagulopathies but contact sports should be avoided.

D. Aspirin and NSAIDs should be avoided in any coagulapathy.

E. Patients may require family counseling and genetic counseling.

X. Indications for Referral to a Hematologist

A. Long-term management of patients with a coagulopathy

B. Bone marrow aspiration or special coagulation studies

C. Family or genetic counseling

XI. Annotated Bibliography

Green JB. Hereditary and acquired coagulation factor abnormalities. Postgrad Med 1984;76:118–131.

Palmer RL. Laboratory diagnosis of bleeding disorders. Postgrad Med 1984;76:137–162. Two good reviews of abnormal coagulation tests designed for the primary care physician.

George JN. Excessive bleeding and clotting. Schafer AI. Thrombocytopenia and disorders of platelet function. White GC. Disorders of blood coagulation. In: Stein TH, ed. Internal Medicine, 3rd ed. Boston: Little, Brown; 1990. A more complete and more recent review of this topic with discussion of pathophysiology.

Chapter 59: Anemia

Barry Ziring

I. General Considerations

A. General Information

1. Anemia is a sign of a pathologic process and not a specific diagnosis.
2. Anemia is defined as a hemoglobin concentration below the lower limit of the 95% reference range for age, sex, and geographical altitude.
   a. In a male patient this is generally < 14 g/dL or a hematocrit < 40%
   b. In a female patient this is generally a hemoglobin < 12 g/dL or a hematocrit < 35%
   c. There is a possible effect of age on red cell parameters and coexistent diseases increase with age. However, most healthy patients above age 65 will maintain normal values.

B. History and Symptoms

1. Orthostasis
2. Weakness, fatigue
3. Exertional dyspnea
4. Decreased appetite secondary to decreased intestinal blood flow (when anemia is severe)
5. Patients with chronic anemias may not manifest the above symptoms until the anemia becomes severe (6–8 g/dL).
6. Patients with an acute loss of blood may manifest acute symptoms even if the hemoglobin remains within the normal range.
7. The physician should inquire about conditions that result in anemia.
   a. History of GI blood loss or abdominal pain, hematemesis, hematochezia, melena
   b. Menorrhagia
   c. History of use of drugs including alcohol, antineoplastic drugs, antibiotics, zidovudine, anticonvulsants, α-methyldopa, nonsteroidal anti-inflammatory drugs (NSAIDs)
   d. History of bowel resection or bypass resulting in malabsorption

e. History of splenomegaly or jaundice, which may be an indication of hereditary spherocytosis or hemoglobinopathies
  f. Patients of African American, Mediterranean or Asian ancestry are at higher risk for thallasemia or glucose-6-phosphate dehydrogenase (G6PD) deficiency
  g. Vegetarian diet, which can result in iron deficiency

C. Physical Examination

1. The following features of the physical examination have been shown to correlate with anemia.
   a. Conjunctival pallor
   b. Absence of nail bed blanching
   c. Nail bed pallor
   d. Palmar crease pallor

2. The physical examination of the patient with known anemia should include
   a. Evaluation for enlarged liver or spleen
   b. Check for evidence of jaundice
   c. Rectal examination for occult blood
   d. Check for evidence of glossitis or angular stomatitis, which are seen in iron deficiency
   e. Check for orthostasis especially when acute blood loss is suspected

II. Diagnostic Approach

A. Several schemes are used for classifying anemias. In part the approach depends on the physician's level of comfort reviewing peripheral smears. The major classification schemes depend either on categorization by automated red cell indices or by review of the peripheral smear.

B. In outpatient practice most physicians rely heavily on automated red cell indices in their initial evaluation. Red cell size measured by the mean corpuscular volume (MCV) and reticulocyte count may be used to categorize anemias.

C. The reticulocyte index (RI) is a mathematical correction for the fact that younger reticulocytes have an increased maturation time in the peripheral blood, which is inversely proportional to the hematocrit value (Table 59–1)

D. Hypochromic Microcytic Anemia (MCV < 80)

1. Iron deficiency
   a. Most common cause of microcytic anemia
   b. As frequent as 14% of women and 2% of men
   c. Very important to identify underlying cause
   d. Transferrin saturation (ratio of serum iron to total iron-binding capacity) below 16% is consistent with iron deficiency anemia.

Table 59-1. Calculation of Reticulocyte Index

Hematocrit (HCT)	Maturation Time
45%	1.0
35%	1.5
25%	2.0
15%	2.5

$$\text{Reticulocyte index} = \text{Reticulocyte count} \times \frac{\text{Patient's HCT}}{\text{Normal HCT}} \times \frac{1}{\text{Maturation time}}$$

  e. Serum ferritin of below 12 ng/mL is specific for iron deficiency.
  f. In patients without chronic disease either the transferrin saturation or the ferritin level may be used to confirm iron deficiency anemia. The tests are not complimentary and do not need to be used together or sequentially.
  g. In patients with chronic diseases the transferrin saturation may be a more sensitive test. Liver disease, acute leukemia, Hodgkin's disease, and chronic inflammatory processes can raise the ferritin level and cause false negative results.
  h. Examination of the bone marrow for stainable iron is highly sensitive and specific for iron deficiency but is rarely necessary.
  i. A therapeutic trial of iron offers a less invasive and inexpensive alternative to bone marrow examination.
     1) The usual dose is 300 mg (60 mg of elemental iron) t.i.d.
     2) Response should be a moderate reticulocytosis of 3–10% within 10–14 d.
  j. If the diagnosis of iron deficiency anemia is made either on the basis of blood tests, bone marrow, or therapeutic iron trial, a search must be made for a source of blood loss. This includes a detailed menstrual history and evaluation for epistaxis, hemoptysis, hematemesis, hematuria, or blood in stool.

2. Thalassemia
   a. The thalassemias are the second most common cause of microcytosis among healthy people.
   b. Most patients have minimal anemia.
   c. An elevated A_2-hemoglobin concentration confirms the diagnosis of thalassemia minor. Routine hemoglobin electrophoresis often does not show A_2 concentration.
   d. Differentiating thalassemia from iron deficiency is important to avoid unnecessary tests.

3. Disorders of heme synthesis

a. Exogenous causes
   1) Alcohol
   2) Lead—Check lead level and peripheral smear to look for basophilic stippling and ringed sideroblasts. Also, abdominal pain and neuropathy may be present.
   3) Isoniazid or chloramphenicol
   4) Above causes may be treated by removing the offending agents and sometimes with a trial of pyridoxine at doses of 50–200 mg/d.
b. Sideroblastic anemia of unknown cause
   1) Rare cause of anemia in which smear reveals ringed sideroblasts and no exogenous cause is found. The course is slow but the anemia may be severe.
   2) Patient's should be given a trial of pyridoxine as above.

4. Anemia of chronic disease
   a. Due to block in release of iron from cells in the reticuloendothelial system.
   b. Transferrin saturation is usually above 16%.
   c. Ferritin is often elevated due to inflammatory process and not a reliable diagnostic tool. If it is measured and is low, iron deficiency is present.
   d. Will not respond to trial of iron therapy

E. Normochromic Normocytic Anemias (MCV 80–100)
1. Elevated reticulocyte index
   a. Sickle cell disease (sickle cells can be seen on smear)
   b. Traumatic hemolytic anemias
      1) Microangiopathic—smear will include schistocytes or burr cells.
      2) Valvular heart disease
      3) Marching, jogging, or distance running
   c. Other causes of hemolysis
      1) Membrane abnormalities (eg, hereditary spherocytosis)
      2) Enzymopathy (G6PD deficiency)
      3) Paroxysmal nocturnal hemoglobinuria
      4) Drugs including penicillin, quinine, α-methyldopa, procainamide, antimalarials, sulfa drugs, nitrofurantoin
      5) Cold reactive antibodies secondary to mycoplasma, Epstein-Barr virus, syphilis (Rouleaux formation may be seen on smear)
   d. Recent blood loss
   e. Early iron deficiency

2. Normal or low reticulocyte index
   a. Anemia of chronic disease (discussed under microcytic anemias)
   b. Liver disease
   c. Renal disease
   d. Hypothyroidism
   e. HIV disease or zidovudine use
   f. Marrow disorders
      1) Aplasia (primary aplastic anemia or secondary to drugs)

2) Dysplasia
3) Fibrosis
4) Leukemia, lymphoma, myeloma, metastatic disease—In these diseases nucleated red blood cell, tear drops, and immature white cell forms may be seen; bone marrow examination is usually diagnostic.

F. Macrocytic Anemias (MCV > 100)
1. Megaloblastic—presence of hypersegmented neutrophils and oval macrocytes on peripheral blood smear
   a. Vitamin B_{12} deficiency
      1) Physical findings include pallor, vitiligo, glossitis, diminished vibratory and position sense, and dementia.
      2) Megaloblastic changes almost always appear on smear.
      3) Vitamin B_{12} levels can confirm diagnosis.
      4) B_{12} deficiency may result from pernicious anemia (lack of intrinsic factor), gastrectomy, resected or diseased ileum, transcobalamin deficiency (rare), blind loop syndrome, and extreme vegetarian diets.
      5) Schilling test may be ordered to confirm diagnosis of pernicious anemia.
      6) Because of the association of hypothyroidism with megaloblastic anemias, thyroid studies should be obtained.
   b. Folate deficiency
      1) Physical findings include pallor, glossitis, signs of malabsorption, signs of alcohol abuse, exfoliative dermatitis. Isolated folate deficiency does not result in neurologic signs.
      2) Because folic acid does not accumulate in the body, dietary lack can result in anemia within 4–6 wk.
      3) Usually caused by a diet lacking in leafy vegetables, meats, yeast, and diary products
      4) Drugs that interfere with folate absorption include phenobarbitol, diphenylhydantoin, oral contraceptives, and methotrexate.
      5) Malabsorption of folate may occur due to diseases of the jejunum.
      6) Folate deficiency can also result from hemolytic anemias, pregnancy, and malignancies.
      7) Serum folate levels may be measured to confirm diagnosis
2. Nonmegaloblastic
   a. Reticulocytosis—Increase in reticulocytes can result in automated red cell index with a high MCV. Review of the peripheral smear will confirm this. Presence of a high red cell distribution width (RDW) is also suggestive of reticulocytosis.
   b. Alcohol
   c. Liver disease
   d. Hypothyroidism
   e. Marrow disorders (see discussion under normocytic anemias)

III. Treatment

A. Iron Deficiency Anemia

1. Treat primary cause
2. Iron salts in doses of 100–200 mg elemental iron daily. Usual iron sulfate preparation contains 300 mg (60 mg elemental iron).
3. Side effects include nausea, diarrhea, constipation, and cramps (fewer side effects with more expensive ferrous gluconate).
4. Modest reticulocytosis expected (3–10%) within 10–14 d. Hemoglobin and hematocrit should then begin to rise.

B. Vitamin B_{12} Deficiency

1. Administer vitamin B_{12} SQ in dose of 100 mg daily for 2 wk followed by 100–1000 mg monthly to bimonthly.
2. Reticulocyte levels should rise within 3–5 d followed by a rise in hemoglobin and hematocrit.

C. Folate Deficiency

1. Recommended dose is 1 mg folate daily orally.
2. Treatment with folate will correct anemia but allow neurologic symptoms to worsen if there is coexistent B_{12} deficiency. Therefore B_{12} should be given as above until vitamin B_{12} levels are available.

D. Erythropoietin

1. Indicated in patients with chronic renal failure
2. Indicated in patients with HIV disease taking zidovudine. Endogenous serum epoetin alfa level should be measured. Patients with levels > 500 milliunits/mL are unlikely to respond.
3. Dosage is started at 50–100 units/kg SQ three times weekly and may be titrated to response. Therapy is expensive.

IV. Patient Education

A. Patients should be advised that anemia is not a disease but rather a sign of underlying disease.

B. Work-up sometimes takes time and several diagnostic studies; however, thorough work-up is critical to make correct diagnosis.

C. Empirical therapy is sometimes indicated for diagnosis, but close follow-up is necessary regardless of the results.

V. Indications for Referral to a Hematologist

A. The majority of diagnostic evaluations can be performed by the primary care provider.

B. Referral is usually made for bone marrow biopsy and less frequently for diagnostic dilemmas and specialized diagnostic testing.

VI. Annotated Bibliography

Beissner RS, Trowbridge AA. Clinical assessment of anemia. Postgrad Med 1986;80:83–95. A good review of evaluation of anemia based on morphologic classification.

Cook IJ, Pavli P, Riley JW, et al. Gastrointestinal investigation of iron deficiency anemia. Br Med J 1986;292:1380–1382. Discusses the need for colonic assessment in elderly patients with iron deficiency anemia.

Guyatt GH, Oxman AD, Ali MA, et al. Laboratory diagnosis of iron deficiency anemia: an overview. J Gen Intern Med 1992;7:145–153. Reviews the use of ferritin in the diagnosis of iron deficiency anemia.

Simmons JO, Noel GL, Diehl LF. Does review of peripheral smears help in the initial work-up of common anemias? J Gen Intern Med 1989;4:473–482. Presents evidence for the utility of relying on automated testing for work-up of anemia.

Chapter 60: Lymphadenopathy

Barry Ziring

I. Clinical Presentation

A. General Information

1. Lymphadenopathy may either be found in the setting of symptoms (which might make the diagnosis more obvious) or as part of the routine physical examination.
2. The work-up depends on the characteristics of the node, the history and age of the patient, and associated symptoms.

B. Symptoms

1. Lymphadenopathy itself usually causes no symptoms unless the nodes are large enough to cause vascular or lymphatic obstruction or the lymph node presses on a nerve, which may cause pain.
2. Symptoms usually relate to the primary disease; the most frequent include
   a. HIV-generalized lymphadenopathy
   b. Carcinoma
   c. Infection including Epstein Barr virus (EBV), cytomegalovirus (CMV), tuberculosis, bacterial infections and cat scratch disease, sexually transmitted diseases (STDs)
   d. Lymphoma
   e. Drug reaction, including phenytoin, carbemazipine
   f. Granulomatous disease, such as sarcoidosis

C. Physical Examination

1. General considerations—Lymph nodes should be characterized as to size, tenderness, consistency, and if matting is present.
   a. Size—As a general rule benign lymph nodes are < 1 cm, suspicious lymph nodes are 1-2 cm, and worrisome lymph nodes are > 2 cm.
   b. Consistency—Stone hard nodes are malignant. Rubbery nodes are frequently lymphomas. Infectious nodes are frequently tender. However, soft supple nodes may be benign or malignant.
   c. Tenderness—usually indicates inflammation and therefore is usually of clinical significance. Often nonmalignant in etiology.
   d. Matting—Nodes feel as if they are connected. Such nodes usually represent a malignant condition but can be seen in chronic inflammation or sarcoidosis.

2. Location
   a. Generalized lymphadenopathy is always abnormal.
   b. Epitrochlear nodes—In the absence of dermatitis, trauma or infection of the hands, epitrochlear nodes are usually a clue to systemic disease including sarcoidosis, syphilis, lymphoma, HIV, or IV injection of drugs.
   c. Axillary nodes—Typically lymph nodes cannot be palpated in the axilla. Trauma or infection of the distal upper extremity can result in benign axillary adenopathy. In the absence of a benign cause, malignancy should be considered (especially breast cancer).
   d. Supraclavicular nodes—The clinician should have a high index of suspicion for malignancy. The left supraclavicular node (Virchow's, "sentinel" node) may signal an intra-abdominal or testicular carcinoma. Cancer of the breast or bronchus may metastasize to the ipsilateral supraclavicular node.
   e. Cervical nodes—Upper respiratory or ear infections typically result in cervical adenopathy. A single hard node is of concern for head and neck carcinoma. Many clinicians prefer endoscopic examination of the nasopharynx, larynx, and esophagus prior to lymph node biopsy because there is some evidence that lymph node aspiration or partial excision may lead to seeding of metastatic cells. The age of the patient and the patient's surgical risks help determine the diagnostic approach.
   f. Inguinal nodes—Often reactive but inguinal adenopathy can signal cancer of the genitourinary or GI tract, lymphoma, or STDs.
   g. Paraumbilical nodes (Sister Mary Joseph's node)—a sign of intra-abdominal or pelvic malignancy

II. Diagnostic Approach

A. The history, coincident symptoms, characteristics, and location of the lymphadenopathy should determine the diagnostic approach.

B. Biopsy—Surgical biopsy of an entire node is the diagnostic procedure of choice for adenopathy that is suspicious for malignancy. There is no benefit to waiting when there is a hard fixed node in a suspicious location. In some locations, studies are indicated prior to biopsy.

1. Head and neck—consider panendoscopy especially in an older patient or a smoker

2. Axillary—mammogram and breast examination

C. Aspiration—generally reserved for nodes suspected to be infectious. This procedure is suboptimal for malignancy and is difficult to interpret for lymphoma. Many authorities recommend against aspiration for the head and neck region.

D. Serology—often more helpful in the evaluation of generalized adenopathy. May include screening for HIV, syphilis, mononucleosis, CMV, and collagen vascular disease

E. Complete blood count—sometimes useful in the evaluation of lymphoma or infection

F. Chest x-ray—sometimes indicated if lymphoma, lung malignancy, or tuberculosis is suspected

G. Other radiologic imaging—CT, MRI, and nuclear scanning are unlikely to be diagnostic as screening tests. Waiting for these tests often delays biopsy. More helpful in staging of disease.

H. Conservative follow-up—Serial examination of adenopathy is a rational approach for adenopathy, which is low risk by history and physical. Discussion with the patient and follow-up are essential.

III. Differential Diagnosis

A. Malignancy—discussed above by location

B. Staph and strep lymphadenitis result in inflamed and tender nodes. More common in children.

C. Cat scratch disease—unilateral axillary or epitrochlear nodes, which usually occurs in autumn and winter. Constitutional signs may be present.

D. EBV and CMV infection

E. STDs

1. Syphilis—usually firm nodes that are bilateral

2. Genital herpes—usually bilateral and tender

3. Chancroid—usually unilateral and tender; often drains

F. Other infectious causes

1. Histoplasmosis—Ohio and Mississippi Valley. Diffuse lymphadenopathy. Often involves the liver and spleen. Diagnosed by culture.

2. Brucella—contact with farm animals. Severe constitutional symptoms and nocturnal fever. Diagnosis via blood culture and serology.

3. Toxoplasmosis—acquired from feces of cats or by ingesting undercooked meat. More frequent in AIDS patients. Diagnosis made by rising antibody titer.

4. Tuberculosis—Diagnosis can be made by culturing aspirated material or from biopsy showing caseating granuloma.

5. HIV

G. Collagen vascular diseases including Stills disease, rheumatoid arthritis, systemic lupus erythematosus, dermatomyositis

H. Metabolic diseases including Gaucher's, Nieman-Pick, hyperthyroidism

I. Drug induced—phenytoin

J. Miscellaneous

1. Amyloid
2. Sarcoidosis
3. IV drug use
4. Serum sickness

IV. Patient Education

A. Lymphadenopathy often represents a benign disease, but malignancy is always a possibility if a specific cause is not obvious or found at the time of work-up.

B. Biopsy is diagnostic in approximately 65% of cases. A nondiagnostic biopsy does not rule out malignancy.

C. If a biopsy is nondiagnostic or if a conservative approach is taken, follow-up is essential.

V. Indications for Referral

A. Rarely is referral necessary for diagnosis. The key to diagnosis is a methodical history and physical with biopsy if necessary.

B. Referral is indicated to a surgeon for lymph node biopsy or to an otolaryngologist for possible endoscopy if a head and neck cancer is suspected.

VI. Annotated Bibliography

Doberneck RC. The diagnostic yield of lymph node biopsy. Arch Surg 1983;118:1203–1205. This article focuses on the use of the lymph node biopsy for diagnosis.

Fijten GH, Blijham GH. Unexplained lymphadenopathy in family practice: an evaluation of the probability of malignant causes and the effectiveness of physician work-up. J. Fam Pract 1988;27:373–376.

Greefield S, Jordan MC. The clinical investigation of lymphadenopathy in primary care practice. JAMA 1978;240:1388–1393. A good review article of lymphadenopathy.

Slap GB, Brooks JS, Schwartz JS. When to perform biopsies of enlarged peripheral lymph nodes in young patients. JAMA 1984;252:1321–1326. A good review of lymphadenopathy in young patients.

Part XIII:
HIV Disease

Chapter 61: Pretest and Posttest HIV Counseling

Carol M. Reife

I. Pretest Counseling

A. General Principles

1. Pretest counseling is mandatory for anyone obtaining a human immunodeficiency virus (HIV) test and should be given in person.
2. During the pretest interview, the physician should educate, obtain a sexual and drug history, and provide counseling and guidance.
3. Counseling should include at least the following topics, described in detail below.

    a. What the HIV test is, why it is being requested, and how it is performed
    b. What HIV and AIDS are
    c. Meaning of a negative HIV test result
    d. Meaning of a positive HIV test result
    e. Meaning of an indeterminant test result
    f. Confidentiality of HIV testing
    g. Risks and benefits of HIV testing
    h. How to prevent infection with HIV
    i. How to prevent transmission of HIV
    j. Specific recommendations for behavior change based on assessment of risk
    k. Assessment of support systems and referral as indicated

4. After counseling is completed, one should make sure that the individual has understood the information presented and has had the opportunity to ask questions. He or she should be told the time and place to return for posttest counseling.

B. Specifics of Counseling

1. What the HIV test is, why it is being requested, and how it is performed.

   This is a blood test to determine if one has been infected with HIV, the virus that causes AIDS. It tests for antibodies to HIV, which is the body's response to infection. Blood is drawn and placed in a test tube. First the enzyme-linked immunosorbent assay (ELISA) is done. This is a sensitive test for detecting the presence of antibodies to the HIV virus. Because the test is very sensitive but not very specific, it may cross react with other antibodies and yield a false positive test result. If the ELISA test is positive, the more specific Western blot test is done to confirm the presence of antibodies. If the Western blot test is positive, one is considered to be infected with HIV.

2. What HIV and what AIDS are.

HIV is the virus that causes AIDS. HIV infection may be present for many years before signs or symptoms of AIDS appear. 60–70% of people who test positive for HIV do not develop AIDS within 7 y of infection. The virus acts by attacking cells of the immune system, making it difficult for them to fight off infections. There currently is no known cure for AIDS and there is no vaccine to prevent its occurrence.

3. Meaning of a negative HIV test result.

A negative test result means that no antibodies to HIV were detected in the blood sample tested. This almost always means that HIV infection is not present. However, because it may take as long as 6 mo for the body to develop antibodies, it may also mean that infection is present but there has not been enough time for antibodies to develop. If the test result is negative and one has recently engaged in high-risk behaviors (unsafe sex, IV drug use), the test should be repeated in 3–6 mo. A negative test result may also mean that the test just failed to detect antibodies that were really there (false negative result). This is very rare.

4. Meaning of a positive HIV test result.

A positive test result means that antibodies to HIV have been detected. It is almost certain that infection with HIV is present. It does not tell when infection occurred. A positive result does not mean that one has AIDS and does not tell when signs or symptoms of infection will develop. It does mean that HIV can be transmitted to others through contact with blood or body fluids. In a child < 18 mo of age, a positive HIV test is usually the result of the presence of HIV antibodies from the mother. Most babies born to HIV-infected women (approximately 70%) lose their mother's antibodies by 18 mo of age and then test negative.

5. Meaning of an indeterminant test result.

Occasionally the laboratory cannot definitely tell whether an HIV test is negative or positive. Indeterminant results generally present as a nondiagnostic band pattern on the Western blot confirmatory test. This happens when antibodies to some antigens but not all are present. When this occurs, the test should be repeated in 3–6 mo.

6. Confidentiality of HIV testing.

Most HIV testing is done confidentially but not anonymously. HIV test results are not automatically reportable to any outside health department or agency (though once the diagnosis of AIDS is made, it must be reported to the Department of Health). Because HIV test results are often part of one's permanent medical record, absolute confidentiality of test results cannot be guaranteed. Information may be obtained by persons given specific written permission, through court order, by a funeral director in the case of death, or by an insurer, to the extent necessary to reimburse health care providers. Because absolute confidentiality cannot be guaranteed, referral to an anonymous testing center should be offered during pretest counseling. In many cities, anonymous centers exist where blood specimens are obtained and tracked by code word alone and the identity of the individual requesting testing is never known.

7. Risks and benefits of HIV testing
    a. Risks of HIV testing include bruising or very rarely, local bacterial skin infection, when a blood sample is obtained. Anxiety and stress may occur while waiting for test results as well as after test results are obtained. Obtaining an HIV test, regardless of the outcome, may result in prejudice or discrimination by others (with possible negative effects on employment, housing, insurance, and personal relationships).
    b. Benefits include reduction in needless anxiety regarding HIV status. Knowing test results will allow one to make decisions about behavior and about personal health issues. Baseline HIV test results will be important in following occupational exposures. Knowing that test results are positive will allow one to seek early intervention, which can increase length and quality of life. Knowing test results will allow one to inform others so that risk of transmission is reduced.

8. How to prevent HIV infection

    HIV is transmitted by infected blood and body fluids. HIV infection can occur through

    a. Sexual contact with an infected person—This may occur through heterosexual contact from men to women or women to men. It may also spread through homosexual contact from men to men or women to women. The only way to absolutely prevent infection through sexual contact is by abstinence. It is safest to have sex with only one person who is known to be HIV negative and who does not engage in high-risk behaviors. Risk of infection can be decreased by using a latex barrier such as a condom during any sexual contact (vaginal, anal, or oral).
    b. IV drug use—The best way to avoid transmission by this route is to avoid using IV drugs. If drugs are used, it is safest not to share needles or equipment with others.
    c. Occupational injury by percutaneous or mucous membrane contact with contaminated fluids
    d. Transfusion of contaminated blood or blood products—Since 1985, all blood has been screened for antibodies to HIV. The chance of becoming infected by blood transfusion is very small, about 1 in 150,000 from each unit of blood.
    e. Perinatal transmission from an infected mother to her infant— Transmission can also occur through breast-feeding.

9. How to prevent HIV transmission once you are known to be HIV positive.
    a. Sexual contact—The only way to absolutely prevent sexual transmission of HIV is total sexual abstinence or by sexual contact with only one person who is known to be HIV negative. Risk can be reduced by limiting the number of sexual contacts and by using a latex barrier such as a condom during any form of sexual contact (vaginal, anal, or oral).

b. IV drug use—The best way to avoid HIV transmission from IV drug use is to stop using IV drugs. If drugs are used, needles and other equipment should never be shared.
   c. Do not donate blood or plasma, body organs, or sperm.
   d. Avoid causing pregnancy or becoming pregnant. (Perinatal transmission occurs in approximately 30% of infants born from HIV-positive mothers.) HIV can also be transmitted by breast-feeding.
   e. Do not share objects that may be contaminated with blood, such as razors or toothbrushes.
   f. Clean body fluid spills with a 10% bleach solution.
   g. Inform health care providers (dentist, physician, or other health care provider of HIV status.
   h. Encourage sexual partners and needle contact to be evaluated and tested.
10. Specific recommendations for behavior change should be made based on assessment of risk.
11. Assess coping skills and existing support systems and make referrals as indicated.

II. Posttest Counseling

Posttest counseling should be mandatory for anyone obtaining an HIV test and should be given in person. It should include at least the following topics

A. For Negative HIV Test Results

1. Meaning of a negative test result (see above)

2. Confidentiality of HIV test results (see above)

3. How to prevent infection with HIV (see above)

4. Retesting may be advised if high-risk behaviors occurred in the past several months.

5. Provide information (refer to support groups, hotlines) that may assist the person in adapting behaviors that decrease risk of infection in the future.

6. Assess need for and make referral for emotional or psychological support when indicated.

7. Make sure that information presented is understood and questions have been answered.

B. For Positive HIV Test Results

1. Meaning of positive test result (see above)

2. Confidentiality of HIV test result (see above)

3. How to prevent transmission of HIV (see above)

4. Who should know about a positive test result—The physician caring for the individual should be informed of the test result as well as a social worker or counselor if support is needed. It is important to inform anyone who may have been the source of infection as well as anyone who may have been infected to decrease the risk of transmission and to facilitate early intervention.
5. Make referral to a physician—Early evaluation and prophylactic treatments may increase length and quality of life. It is important to establish a rapport with a physician that will provide care if and when medical problems arise.
6. Assess need for and make referral for emotional and/or psychological support when indicated.
7. Review health insurance coverage and make referral for assistance when needed.
8. Assess patient's understanding of test results and answer any questions.

III. Annotated Bibliography

Rinaldi RC. HIV blood test counseling: AMA physician guidelines. J Ky Med Assoc 1989;87(8):372–374. Good general approach to basic concepts in HIV counseling.

Chapter 62: Management of the Symptomatic Patient

James Witek

I. General Background

A. Symptoms may develop at any stage of HIV infection, but they generally occur later in the course of the disease as immune function deteriorates.

B. Early symptoms may more commonly be related to the psychological effects of the disease, ie, symptoms related to depression or anxiety.

C. Later symptoms are more commonly associated with an opportunistic infection.

D. The diagnosis of AIDS was revised by the Centers for Disease Control and Prevention (CDC) in January 1993. AIDS occurs when an individual demonstrates evidence of HIV infection on the enzyme-linked immunosorbent assay (ELISA), which is confirmed by a specific antibody test (Western blot) (see Chapter 61 for details) and has one of the following:

1. CD4 count < 200 cells/mm^3

2. CD4 % < 14%

3. Clinical AIDS—evidence of opportunistic disease (see Table 62-1)

II. Evaluation of Symptoms—Overview

A. Patients should be monitored with a careful review of symptoms at each visit including fever, weight loss, headache, visual changes, cough, shortness of breath, dyspnea on exertion, and diarrhea.

B. When evaluating symptoms, it is important to look at the stage of disease and the clinical status of the patient. The most recent CD4 count is very helpful because, although there are exceptions, most opportunistic disease does not occur until CD4 counts fall below 200–300.

C. Persistent generalized lymphadenopathy, pneumococcal pneumonia, candidal vaginitis, Kaposi's sarcoma, lymphoma, and idiopathic thrombocytopenic purpura may develop earlier.

Table 62-1. AIDS—Defining Conditions

The presence of one or more of the following plus confirmed HIV antibody or evidence of HIV antigen constitutes the diagnosis of AIDS.

- Candidiasis of bronchi, trachea or lungs
- Candidiasis, esophageal*
- Coccidiomycosis, disseminated or extrapulmonary
- Cryptococcosis, extrapulmonary
- Cryptosporidiosis, chronic intestinal (> 1 mo duration)
- Cytomegalovirus disease (other than liver, spleen, nodes)
- Cytomegalovirus retinitis (with visual loss)*
- Encephalopathy, HIV related
- Herpes simplex: chronic ulcers (> 1 mo duration) or bronchitis, pneumonitis, or esophagitis
- Histoplasmosis, disseminated or extrapulmonary
- Isosporiasis, chronic intestinal (> 1 mo duration)
- Kaposi's sarcoma*
- Lymphoma: Burkitt's, immunoblastic, primary brain
- *Mycobacterium avium* complex or *M. kansasii,* disseminated or extrapulmonary
- *Mycobacterium tuberculosis,* any site
- *Mycobacterium,* other species, disseminated or extrapulmonary*
- *Pneumocystis carinii* pneumonia*
- Progressive multifocal leukoencephalopathy
- Salmonella septicemia, recurrent
- Toxoplasmosis of brain*
- Wasting syndrome due to HIV

Conditions added in 1993 expanded case definition:
- Pulmonary tuberculosis*
- Invasive cervical cancer
- Recurrent pneumonia*

* May be diagnosed presumptively based on CDC guidelines; however, when possible it is preferable to have definitive diagnosis for initial AIDS—defining condition.

D. Patients should be hospitalized to evaluate symptoms if they appear toxic, are hemodynamically unstable, unable to take fluids orally, develop a new seizure or focal neurologic deficit, are hypoxic or in rare circumstances, cannot be thoroughly studied as an outpatient.

E. When assessing and evaluating symptoms, remember that some opportunistic conditions may be diagnosed presumptively, allowing earlier treatment and less patient discomfort from invasive testing.

III. Evaluation of Common Symptoms

A. Fever

1. Occurs frequently and should be pursued when it is persistent, increased compared to baseline, > 100.5° F, or accompanied by changes in clinical status or laboratory values.
2. Evaluation should include careful history, physical examination, and documentation of the fever.
3. Localizing symptoms or physical findings should be explored. Sinuses should be carefully assessed because sinusitis frequently complicates HIV disease.
4. Consider that etiology may be drug fever, opportunistic malignancy, or infection. Drugs that are not necessary should be stopped.
5. If no localizing features, studies should be undertaken to identify potentially treatable infections—blood cultures for bacteria, fungi, cytomegalovirus (CMV) and mycobacteria; urinalysis with culture; serum cryptococcal antigen (may disseminate prior to localizing to CNS); purified protein derivative (PPD) with anergy; chest x-ray (some patients with *Pneumocystis carinii* pneumonia [PCP] have few pulmonary symptoms)
6. Other studies that may be helpful include bone marrow biopsy and lumbar puncture.

B. Dysphagia

1. Occurs commonly and may be due to esophageal candidiasis, herpes simplex virus (HSV), CMV, aphthous ulcers, acute retroviral infection, histoplasmosis, or lymphomatoid granulomatosis.
2. The presence of oral thrush is a diagnostic clue in the evaluation.
    a. If present, candida is the likely etiology for dysphagia and can be treated with fluconazole 100–200 mg/d (up to 400 mg/d in some cases) or ketoconazole 200 mg b.i.d. for 2–3 wk.
    b. Refractory candida may need to be treated with amphotericin B (0.3–0.5 mg/kg/d) +/– flucytosine (100 mg/kg/d) for 5–7 d.
    c. Following acute treatment, maintenance therapy must be given with ketoconazole 200 mg/d, nystatin 100,000–200,000 units gargled 5 times daily, fluconazole 50–100 mg/d or clotrimazole troches 100 mg 5 times daily.
3. If thrush is not present or symptoms persist after treatment for candida, further evaluation with either barium swallow or endoscopy is recommended.
    a. Barium swallow may reveal diffuse irregular nodularity of mucosa seen in candidal infection or the single or multiple punctate ulcerations of HSV, CMV, or aphthous ulcers.
    b. If ulcers are present, endoscopy with biopsy for histology and fungal and viral cultures are needed.

1) Dysphagia due to HSV may be treated with acyclovir 400–1000 mg PO 5 times daily or 5 mg/kg IV t.i.d. for 7–10 d with lower doses then used as maintenance therapy.
2) CMV can be treated with ganciclovir 5 mg/kg IV b.i.d. or foscarnet 60 mg IV q 8 h for 14–21 d. Maintenance therapy is not usually needed with CMV esophagitis.
3) Aphthous ulcers are treated with prednisone 40 mg PO qd for 14 d with a slow taper thereafter.

C. Cough

1. Occurs frequently and may represent sinusitis with postnasal drip, bacterial bronchitis or pneumonia, tuberculosis, PCP, or other opportunistic disease.
2. CD4 count will be helpful in the evaluation because PCP and opportunistic infection will rarely occur with a CD4 count > 300 cells/mm^3 whereas TB or bacterial infections may occur at any time in the course of the disease.
3. Evaluation begins with a physical examination and chest x-ray.
   a. If the chest x-ray is normal, bronchitis, sinusitis, or early PCP should be considered.
   b. TB may present more atypically in patients with HIV disease with chest x-ray findings including focal infiltrates, cavitary lesions, reticulonodular patterns, or pleural effusions.
      1) If TB is suspected, respiratory isolation should be instituted immediately while sputum cultures are being obtained for acid-fast bacilli stain and culture.
   c. If a lobar infiltrate is present on chest x-ray, bacterial pneumonia should be considered as well as fungal or mycobacterial infection.
      1) Appropriate cultures of sputum and blood should be obtained so that treatment can be instituted.
      2) If a diagnosis is not established, bronchoscopy may be necessary.
   d. PCP may present with a normal chest x-ray, lobar infiltrates, or cavitary lesions but is usually characterized by bilateral interstitial infiltrates.
      1) Most patients with PCP have had progressive symptoms for several weeks, their cough is usually minimally productive and accompanied by fevers, night sweats, dyspnea on exertion, and weight loss.
      2) Supportive findings include hypoxia, oxygen desaturation with exercise, elevated lactic dehydrogenase (LDH) and diffuse uptake on gallium scan.
      3) Diagnosis may be made by silver stain of induced sputum or by bronchoscopy with bronchoalveolar lavage and/or biopsy.
      4) PCP may be treated orally on an outpatient basis in mild cases (Table 62–2).
      5) Corticosteroids reduce the morbidity and mortality of PCP when used in moderate to severe PCP (arterial oxygen < 70 mm Hg). They should be started as soon as possible, but especially within the first 72 h of treatment. A common regimen is prednisone 40 mg b.i.d. for 5 d, then 40 mg qd for 5 d, then 20 mg qd for 10 d followed by a tapering dose.

Table 62-2. Oral Treatment of Pneumocystic Pneumonia

PCP can be treated orally as an outpatient if symptoms are mild and the patient is compliant. The patient should not have GI symptoms (nausea, vomiting, or diarrhea) that would inhibit delivery of the drug.

Regimens: 1) Trimethoprim 15–20 mg/kg/d in 3 or 4 divided oral doses
Sulfamethoxazole 75–100 mg/kg/d PO
(generally 2 double-strength tablets t.i.d)

2) Atovaquone (Mepron) 750 mg PO t.i.d with food

3) Dapsone 100 mg PO qd
Trimethoprim 20 mg/kg/d in 3 divided oral doses

4) Clindamycin 600–900 mg PO t.i.d.
Primaquine 15–30 mg PO qd

Treatment duration for all above regimens is 21 d after which time secondary prophylaxis will need to be administered.

---

    e. If the chest x-ray reveals cavitary disease, sputum should be cultured for bacteria, fungi, acid-fast bacilli, and nocardia.
       1) If cultures are unrevealing, bronchoscopy should be performed to establish a diagnosis.

D. Headache

1. Headaches may be due to CNS infections such as bacterial meningitis, neurosyphilis, cryptococcosis, or toxoplasmosis, systemic infections, migraines, tension, or medications.

2. A recent CD4 count may be helpful in the evaluation.

    a. If no fever is present, neurologic examination is normal and CD4 count is > 200 cells/mm^3, consider tension headache, migraine headache, or sinusitis and treat appropriately.

    b. If fever is present, neurologic examination is normal and CD4 count is > 200 cells/mm^3, consider sinusitis, systemic infection, or headache due to fever.

3. If mental status is altered or focal signs or seizure are present, obtain CT scan with contrast or MRI.

    a. If the scan is normal, proceed with lumbar puncture to obtain CSF for analysis to include cryptococcal antigen, stain and culture, acid-fast bacillus stain, and culture and bacterial culture. Base treatment on results of analysis.

    b. Toxoplasmosis is likely if one or more focal lesions are found, which enhance with contrast, especially if they occur in the basal ganglia. Although such lesions could also represent lymphoma as well as fungal or tuberculous abscesses, presumptive antitoxoplasmosis treatment is often

begun with pyrimethamine 100–200 mg loading dose then 50–100 mg PO qd and sulfadiazine 1—1.5 g PO q 6 h.
  1) A repeat scan is generally performed several weeks after treatment is begun to evaluate response. If no response is seen, stereotactic biopsy may be considered.
  2) Length of initial treatment is based on clinical response but is generally 4–8 wk. The patient is then placed on a chronic suppressive regimen of pyrimethamine 25–50 mg PO qd with or without sulfadiazine 0.5—1.0 g PO q 6 h.
  3) Dexamethasone may be used if a mass effect is present.
4. If fever and meningismus accompany headache, a lumbar puncture with opening pressure should be performed to assess CSF by routine analysis plus India ink stain, cryptococcal antigen, acid fast bacilli stains and culture.
  a. Cryptococcosis may be treated with amphotericin B 0.7–1.0 mg/kg/d IV with oral flucytosine 150 mg/kg/d in 4 divided doses or less favorably with fluconazole 400–800 mg PO qd.

E. Weight Loss/Wasting

1. Weight loss in HIV infection is often associated with an underlying opportunistic illness. When weight loss is observed, a careful review of symptoms and physical examination should be performed to screen for opportunistic disease. If found, such disease should be treated.
2. Dietary intake should be evaluated with at 24–72-hour food record. Caloric needs and body composition should be determined.
3. The patient's diet should be liberalized with increased consumption of fats and sugars encouraged.
4. One or two multivitamins containing the B complex vitamins, selenium, and zinc should be taken each day as many patients with HIV disease have deficiencies of these vitamins and minerals.
4. Standard oral polymeric supplements may be added to the diet. If not tolerated, elemental formulas may be used.
6. Appetite may be stimulated with megesterol acetate 80 mg PO q.i.d.
7. If nausea is inhibiting intake, dronabinol 2.5 mg PO before lunch and dinner may be helpful.
8. Some patients may require nasoenteric or parenteral feeding.

F. Neuropathic Pain

1. Painful peripheral neuropathy is seen frequently in HIV disease and is disabling for many patients.
  a. Early in HIV infection, subacute and chronic demyelinating polyneuropathies may be seen, which respond to plasma exchange or glucocorticoids.

b. Late in HIV infection, sensory axonal polyneuropathy may occur causing severe peripheral burning pain or tingling.
      1) Treatment is usually attempted with tricyclic antidepressants including amitriptyline 10–25 mg PO qhs (titrating up to 100 mg qhs) or nortriptyline 10 mg PO qhs to start (titrating up to 50 mg qhs).
      2) Phenytoin or carbamazepine may also be tried.
      3) Capsaicin cream or lidocaine ointment may be helpful applied topically to the affected areas.
      4) Pain medications including narcotics may be needed by some patients.
   c. ddI, ddC and d4t are associated with peripheral neuropathy.
      1) If symptoms of neuropathy develop, they should be stopped immediately; the neuropathic symptoms will generally resolve slowly.
      2) If symptoms need to be treated, the modalities mentioned above to treat sensory axonal polyneuropathy may be used.

IV. Prophylaxis for Opportunistic Infections

A. Because we now have a general sense of when certain opportunistic diseases may appear in the course of HIV infection, it makes sense to try to prevent the occurrence of these infections.

B. Although some regimens have been proved effective, many more are currently undergoing evaluation in clinical trials.

C. Prophylaxis for PCP has been best studied and is indicated in all patients once the CD4 count approached 200 cells/mm^3 or a patient has had PCP (see Chapter 63).

D. Prophylaxis may be effected for toxoplasmosis in several ways and should be considered in patients with CD4 cell < than 200 cells/mm^3.

1. If trimethoprim-sulfamethoxazole is used for PCP prophylaxis, it also effectively decreases the incidence of toxoplasmosis, making it the preferred agent.

2. Pyrimethamine 50 mg PO q wk combined with dapsone 50 mg PO qd decreases the incidence of toxoplasmosis. In one study pyrimethamine use was associated with a higher mortality rate, but this has not been substantiated in other studies.

3. Atovaquone is currently being investigated for use as a prophylactic agent against toxoplasmosis.

E. Prophylaxis for *Mycobacterium avium* complex can be achieved with many agents, but all are hampered in their effectiveness by the development of resistance.

1. Rifabutin 300 mg PO qd has been approved for use in patients with CD4 counts < 200 cells/mm^3. Higher doses have been associated with uveitis.

2. Clarithromycin and azithromycin have been used as well, but data are currently pending regarding their effectiveness.

F. The use of fluconazole to provide prophylaxis for candidal and cryptococcal infections is controversial because of the low incidence of cryptococcal meningitis and the development of resistance which occurs with its use.

G. In summary, all patients should receive PCP prophylaxis when their CD4 count falls close to 200 cells/mm^3. Ideally, if trimethoprim-sulfamethoxazole is chosen, this will also protect against toxoplasmosis (as well as bacterial infections). Rifabutin may be used in patients with CD4 counts < 200 cells/mm^3 to delay the development of *Mycobacterium avium* complex.

V. End-of-Life Issues

A. It is important to discuss end-of-life treatment with patients early in the course of their disease because dementia may cloud their decision-making ability later in the disease process.

B. Patients should be asked about their desired aggressiveness of care close to the end of life. They should be encouraged to express their wishes in writing via a living will or advance directive.

C. Because many HIV-infected individuals would prefer to have someone other than their legal next-of-kin making decisions regarding their care, patients should be encouraged to designate a proxy or durable power of attorney.

VI. Annotated Bibliography

AIDS Clinical Care—published monthly by Massachusetts Medical Society. This periodical provides practical, useful information from HIV caregivers.

AIDS/HIV Treatment Directory—complied by AMFAR. This booklet contains complete information about drug trials, experimental agents, research and opportunistic infections.

Bartlett, JG. Medical management of HIV infection. Physician and Scientists Publishing Co, Inc: Glenview, IL, 1994. This is an excellent resource for the primary care physician providing an abundance of data in a well organized format.

Internal Medicine—the 3/93 issue is devoted to HIV disease and geared to generalists.

Treatment Issues—published monthly by Gay Men's Health Crisis in New York. Although this publication is geared for people with HIV, it is well written, informative, and of high quality.

Chapter 63: Management of Early HIV Infection

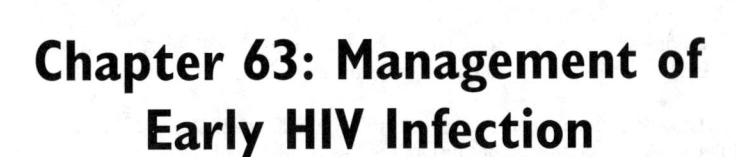

James Witek

I. General Background

A. Early HIV infection may be clinically quiescent but is a period of active viral replication. The time from actual infection to the appearance of clinical symptoms is variable, ranging from a few to as many as 12 to 15 y.

B. Early HIV infection may be accompanied by constitutional symptoms of weight loss, fever, night sweats, and lymphadenopathy.

C. Many early manifestations of HIV infection are psychosocial in nature.

II. Patient Presentation

A. Patients who know they are at risk for HIV infection may present for elective routine testing.

B. Patients may present for routine medical care not recognizing their risk for HIV infection.

C. 30–70% of patients may present with an acute retroviral syndrome marked by fevers, lymphadenopathy, malaise, sore throat, headaches, nausea, and weight loss. The duration of these symptoms is variable but approximates 2 wk.

D. Some patients will present with early evidence of immunocompromise, which the astute clinician will consider as possibly HIV associated. Examples include recurrent vaginal yeast infections or bacterial pneumonias.

E. Patients may present with opportunistic disease indicative of advanced HIV infection such as *Pneumocystis carinii* pneumonia (PCP).

III. Goals of Early Management

A. To provide the psychosocial supports the patient needs to continue a productive and meaningful life

B. To avoid or delay the complications of HIV infection

C. To maintain careful vigilance for signs of opportunistic disease so that treatment can be instituted early

D. To educate the patient about HIV disease and its transmission

IV. Initial Evaluation

A. Evaluate patient's risk factors.

B. Perform thorough history and physical examination.

C. Assess current life-style and habits.

D. Evaluate social supports

1. People of significance to the patient
   a. Family members and significant others
   b. Friends
   c. Coworkers and employers

2. Ask with whom the patient has shared their antibody status

E. Assess patient's psychological state.

1. Major depression occurs in up to 25% of patients and can often be readily treated.

2. Many patients experience anxiety related to their diagnosis.

F. Obtain baseline laboratory data

1. Complete blood count with differential

2. Quantitative platelet count

3. Liver function tests, blood urea nitrogen, serum creatinine

4. Rapid plasma reagin (RPR)

5. Hepatitis B surface antibody and antigen/hepatitis C antibody

6. CD4 cell count and percentage.

7. Toxoplasma, cryptococcal, herpes simplex virus, and cytomegalovirus (CMV) antibody titers (the need to obtain these is controversial)

G. Additional data

1. Purified protein derivative (PPD) with anergy controls

2. Pap smears
   a. It is important to perform Pap smears regularly in HIV-infected women because of the high incidence of invasive cervical cancer.

b. If CD4 count > 400 cells/mm^3, Pap smears should be performed q 6 mo initially. If first two consecutive smears are normal, then subsequent smears can be done annually.
c. If CD4 count < 400 cells/mm^3, Pap smears should be performed q 6 mo.
d. If a Pap smear reveals atypia, then colposcopy should be performed.

H. Immunizations

1. Influenza vaccine—given yearly

2. Pneumococcal vaccine—given once; may repeat q 6 y

3. Hepatitis B vaccine—given if hepatitis B surface antibody negative and patient is at risk for hepatitis B infection.

4. Diptheria/tetanus vaccines—q 10 y

V. Progression of Disease

A. The CD4 count is currently the most commonly used surrogate marker of the progression of HIV infection. The mean decrease in CD4 count appears to be 50–80 cells/mm^3/y but there is wide variability in the decline for an individual patient.

B. Although most opportunistic disease develops late in the course of HIV infection, patients may develop persistent generalized lymphadenopathy, tuberculosis, bacterial pneumonia, candidal vaginitis, Kaposi's sarcoma, lymphoma, and idiopathic thrombocytopenic purpura relatively early. Most other opportunistic illness associated with HIV does not occur until the CD4 count falls to < 200 cells/mm^3 and especially < 50 cells/mm^3.

VI. Monitoring of CD4 Counts and Interventions

A. The recommended frequency of obtaining CD4 counts and interventions at specific levels can be found in Table 63–1.

VII. Antiretroviral Agents

A. The antiretroviral agents are the only agents approved by the Food and Drug Administration (FDA) for use against the HIV virus. The recommendations regarding their use continually change as new knowledge is acquired through controlled studies. It is important for clinicians to keep abreast of these changes.

B. Clinical Use—Overview

1. AZT (zidovudine, Retrovir) appears better as initial therapy than ddI, ddC, or d4t.

2. AZT may delay progression of HIV infection and improve survival in asymptomatic patients.

3. AZT probably delays progression of HIV infection and improves survival in symptomatic patients.

Table 63–1. Frequency of Monitoring CD4 Counts and Recommended Initial Interventions

CD4 Count	Frequency of Repeat	Symptoms?	Intervention*
> 500	q 6 mo	yes or no	1) No therapy/observe or 2) early zidovudine 600 mg/d
300–500	q 6 mo	no	1) No therapy/observe or 2) zidovudine 600 mg/d
		yes	Zidovudine 600 mg/d
200–300	q 3 mo	no	1) No therapy/observe or 2) zidovudine 600 mg/d
		yes	Zidovudine 600 mg/d
< 200	????	yes or no	Zidovudine 600 mg/d[†] and PCP prophylaxis
< 100	?????	yes or no	Zidovudine 600 mg/d and consider anti-retroviral combinations and adding other prophylactic agents

See text for additional explanation regarding antiretroviral therapy and dosing.

* Consideration should always be given to possible enrollment in clinical trials.
† If clinical status is progressing, especially in these categories, consider a change from zidovudine to didanosine or zalcitabine or combinations.

4. The beneficial effects of AZT are of a limited duration due to the development of viral resistance.

5. Patients who take AZT may have some diminished quality of life related to side effects from the medication.

   a. Use of AZT perinatally in pregnant HIV infected women decreases the rate of fetal transmission.

C. Zidovudine (Retrovir, AZT)

1. Most widely studied agent with many studies providing conflicting results as to benefit and best time to initiate therapy.

2. It has been demonstrated to cause a mild increase in CD4 counts and seems to delay the progression of HIV infection to AIDS in symptomatic patients.

3. Current studies are evaluating the use of AZT early in HIV infection when it is best tolerated and when viral resistance to AZT occurs less. Preliminary results indicate that early AZT delays the decline in CD4 count but does not decrease AIDS defining diagnoses or deaths.

4. Generally given in total dose of 500–600 mg/d administered either 100 mg q 4 h or given 200 mg t.i.d.

5. In HIV dementia or idiopathic thrombocytopenic purpura a total of 1000 mg/d is recommended.
6. Nausea, headache, and fatigue may occur early in therapy but usually resolve after the first several weeks. Other side effects include rash, vomiting, confusion, and myopathy.
7. Bone marrow suppression may occur and a complete blood count should be initially obtained a few weeks after therapy is started and then at least q 3 mo.

D. Didanosine (Videx, ddI)
1. Terminates DNA synthesis similar to AZT and ddC.
2. Is considered an appropriate second-line agent in the treatment of HIV infection
3. Has more severe side effects of pancreatitis and peripheral neuropathy; may also cause diarrhea.
4. Dosage is based on weight; it is available as tablet or powder preparation and it must be taken on an empty stomach.

Wt > 75 kg	300 mg tablets b.i.d.
	375 mg powder b.i.d.
Wt 50–74 kg	200 mg tablets b.i.d.
	250 mg powder b.i.d.
Wt 35–50 kg	125 mg tablets b.i.d.
	167 mg powder b.i.d.

E. Zalcitabine (Hivid, dideoxycitidine, ddC)
1. Was initially approved for use only in combination with AZT but is now approved for use as monotherapy in patients who are intolerant of or had disease progression on AZT.
2. May be helpful in patients who are developing resistance to AZT monotherapy
3. Pancreatitis and peripheral neuropathy are limiting side effects. Stomatitis and oral ulcers can also be seen with ddC.
4. Most commonly used dosage range is 0.375 mg b.i.d. to 0.75 mg q8h.

F. Stavudine (Zerit, d4t)
1. Has FDA approval for use in adults with advanced HIV infection who are intolerant of AZT, ddI or ddC, or who have had disease progression while on these agents.
2. Peripheral neuropathy occurs in 15 to 21 percent of patients taking Stavudine. Pancreatitis, headache, and diarrhea are other common side effects.
3. Recommended dose is 20 mg PO b.i.d. Dose to 40 mg PO b.i.d. have been used but are associated with increased side effects.

VIII. Prophylaxis for Pneumocystis carinii Pneumonia (PCP)

A. PCP will occur in many patients with HIV infection and primary prophylaxis is indicated when CD4 count ≤ 200 cells/mm^3.

B. Secondary prophylaxis must be provided to patients who develop PCP because close to 70% will have a recurrence without prophylaxis.

C. Prophylactic Regimens
1. Trimethoprim-sulfamethoxazole is the most effective agent and it also provides protection from toxoplasmosis and some bacterial infections. The minimal effective dose studied is one double-strength tablet orally 3 times weekly but compliance is improved if given as one double-strength tablet each day. Adverse reactions to trimethoprim-sulfamethoxazole are common and include rash and fever.
2. Dapsone 50–100 mg orally each day is an alternate regimen, which may also provide protection from toxoplasmosis. Side effects include rash and nausea. It should not be given to patients with glucose-6-phosphate dehydrogenase deficiency.
3. Aerosolized pentamidine 300 mg/mo via Respigard II nebulizer may be used but is costlier and less effective. In addition it does not provide prophylaxis for toxoplasmosis. Common side effects include coughing and wheezing, which may be improved with pretreatment with a bronchodilator administered via metered-dose inhaler.
4. Atovaquone, pyrimethamine-sulfadoxine and clindamycin-primaquine are other agents that have not been well studied but that may be useful for prophylaxis.

IX. Management of the Positive Purified Protein Derivative

A. Patients with HIV disease should have a PPD (Mantoux method) with anergy panel controls (*Candida,* mumps, or tetanus toxoid) annually.

1. Any induration to the anergy controls 48–72 h indicates intact delayed-type hypersensitivity responses. Lack of a response to the controls indicates anergy.
2. The PPD is positive if there is ≥ 5 mm induration at 48–72 h.
   a. Active TB must be ruled out in these individuals with a thorough history and physical including a chest x-ray.
   b. Regardless of patient's age, prophylaxis is recommended with isoniazid 10 mg/kg (maximum 300 mg) PO qd for at least 1 y and some authorities advocate longer. If exposure to isoniazid-resistant strains is suspected, 12 mo of rifampin 600 mg/d can be used.
   c. Periodic liver transaminases should be monitored in patients on isoniazid who are > 35 y old and those with liver disease or alcoholism.

X. Management of the Positive Rapid Plasma Reagent

A. In HIV disease, syphilis (*Treponema pallidum*) may have atypical presentation, serology, and response to treatment.

B. An RPR should be obtained initially and on a yearly basis in the HIV infected.

C. If the RPR is positive, it is important to make attempts to appropriately "stage" the disease. Lumbar punctures have been advocated for all people with HIV disease and a positive RPR.

D. Treatment

1. Primary, secondary, or latent of < 1 y duration—benzathine pencillin G 2.4 million units IM once.

2. > 1 y duration (indeterminate duration, CNS, cardiovascular)—benzathine penicillin G 2.4 million units IM qwk for 3 wk. Lumbar puncture for CSF analysis should be considered in this group.

3. For neurosyphilis—aqueous penicillin G 12 million units IV qd for 10 d followed by benzathine penicillin G 2.4 million units IM qwk for 3 wk.

4. RPR should be repeated at 3, 6, 12, and 24 mo to demonstrate a gradual decline in titer; it is not uncommon for patients to get reinfected.

5. Retreat patient if clinical signs do not improve, a sustained fourfold increase in VDRL titer, an initial high titer fails to fall to < 1:8.

6. Some clinicians argue that more treatment may be needed than the recommended standards.

XI. Nutrition

A. Because wasting occurs frequently in patients with AIDS, it is important to maintain good nutrition.

1. Maintenance of a well-balanced diet should be emphasized. Early intervention from a nutritionist may be helpful.

2. Patients should be warned about safe eating habits.

   a. Raw eggs and seafood should be avoided.
   b. Poultry and seafood should be cooked thoroughly.

3. Weight should be monitored at each visit.

   a. Patients should be generally encouraged to avoid weight loss.
   b. Weight loss may be an early sign of opportunistic disease and when noted this possibility should be explored.
   c. If weight loss is observed, patients' diets should be liberalized to include larger portions and more high-caloric foods. An oral supplement may be added to the diet between meals and consideration given to having the patient eat six smaller meals per day.
   d. If weight loss does not respond to these initial efforts, megesterol acetate (Megace) 40–80 mg q.i.d. may be used as an appetite stimulant. Dronabinol (Marinol) 2.5 mg PO with lunch and dinner may improve nausea, which limits oral intake.

4. A multivitamin containing zinc, selenium, vitamin A, and the B complex vitamins should be taken daily because patients with HIV infection have been shown to be deficient in these substances.

XII. Exercise

A. Limited studies have demonstrated a beneficial effect of exercise on the course of HIV disease.

B. It should be encouraged for its physical and psychological benefits.

C. Exercise aids in maintaining lean body mass, which is important to prolong survival.

XIII. Psychological Support

A. Patients with HIV disease need psychological support as they deal with loss of function and employment, physical impairment, possible loss of significant others, and as they confront the dying process.

1. Supportive counseling on an individual or group basis may be helpful.
2. Many communities have support groups for HIV-infected and affected individuals.

B. Patients may express denial after learning of their HIV positivity.

C. Cognitive deficits due to HIV dementia or opportunistic disease may develop and contribute to depression and altered mental status.

D. Depression occurs frequently and responds well to treatment.

E. Many patients contemplate suicide and this should be explored with patients when assessing their psychological status.

XIV. Patient Education

A. Should include information about

1. How HIV is transmitted and appropriate precautions to avoid transmission
2. Basic disease pathophysiology/progression
3. Healthy living strategies: exercise, nutrition, safer sex, etc.
4. Antiretrovirals

XV. Annotated Bibliography

See entries in Chapter 62.

Part XIV:
Infectious Diseases

Chapter 64: Aphthous Stomatitis

Richard G. Paluzzi

I. Clinical Presentation

A. General Information

1. Painful noncontagious necrotizing ulcers that occur in 20–60% of the general population

2. Generally random, single, and recurrent, but may be multiple

3. Involve nonkeratinized mucosa, which is not bound to periosteum (buccal/labial mucosa, lateral border of tongue, lips, soft palate, pharynx)

4. Three forms

   a. Minor—generally single and < 1 cm in diameter but may be multiple. Generally occur in anterior portion of mouth.
   b. Major—multifocal, occurring throughout the mouth. Can range up to 2 cm in diameter. Very large, recurrent ulcers are termed periodontis mucosa necrotica recurrens.
   c. Herpetiform—very small and multiple. Very painful. Involve primarily lateral margin and tip of tongue. Can find intranuclear inclusion bodies within the ulcer but no other signs of viral etiology.

5. Etiology is unclear. May have autoimmune basis because autoantibodies and sensitized T lymphocytes against oral mucosa can often be isolated. See increased incidence associated with HLA-A$_2$ and B$_{12}$. Often seen in association with other autoimmune and inflammatory diseases (Behcet's, Reiters, inflammatory bowel disease, sprue, pernicious anemia) as well as nutritional deficiencies (B$_{12}$, folate, Fe).

6. Predisposing factors include stress, trauma, allergies, hormonal changes, menses, and acidic foods.

B. History

1. Generally present as spontaneous, painful lesions

2. May be a prodome of burning and tingling 2–3 d before ulceration.

3. Often recur in random patterns. Major and herpetiform types often have variable periods of quiescence with intense recurrences.

4. No associated fever, constitutional symptoms, or adenopathy unless ulcers are secondarily infected

C. Physical Findings

1. Usually involve the loose, nonkeratinized mucosa of the mouth, lips, cheeks, soft palate, ventral tongue, and pharynx.
2. Minor ulcers are usually single, shallow, and < 1 cm with raised red borders and a gray-white base.
3. Major ulcers can be single or multifocal, ranging up to 2 cm in size with ragged edges.
4. Herpetiform ulcers appear in crops and heal in 1–2 wk.

II. Diagnostic Approach

A. Diagnosis is primarily made by history of single or multiple painful ulcers that heal and recur in the face of an otherwise normal history and physical examination.

B. Location is often diagnostic.

III. Differential Diagnosis

A. Trauma—often see tissue tags along ulcer margins. Denture "sore spots" are common.

B. Herpes simplex—tends to occur on mucosal surfaces that are fixed to underlying periosteum; can perform a Tzank smear to confirm

C. Coxsackie virus—eroding oral ulcers with red areolae; associated with lesions on the hands and feet

D. Agranulocytosis with stomatitis

E. Behcet's syndrome—associated with genital ulcers and ocular lesions

F. Pemphigoid—immunofluorescence diagnostic

G. Angular chelitis—red, fissured lesion involving lateral commissure

H. Kaposi's sarcoma—red to purple macular lesion typically on hard palate, which ulcerates and erodes

I. Oral cancers—typically asymptomatic and chronic with an inflamed base

IV. Treatment

A. Primarily aimed at symptomatic relief. Aphthous ulcers typically heal spontaneously in 1–2 wk.

B. Good oral hygiene is of utmost importance.

C. Topical anesthetics or steroids (0.1% triamcinalone acetonide in paste—Orabase; 0.1% betamethasone valerate ointment—Valsone) provide pain relief and may aid healing.

D. Intralesional steroid injections may be required for pain control if ulcers are large and disabling.

E. Adjunctive therapies—None have been proven to speed healing or decrease recurrence rates.

1. Mouthwash containing alkaloid sanguinarine (Viadent) has bacteriocidal and bacteriostatic effects.

2. Antibiotics—tetracycline (250 mg q.i.d.) is preferred due to high gingival levels attained.

3. "Magic mouthwash"—equal parts of aluminum hydroxide gel, elixir of diphenhydramine HCl, and viscous lidocaine may provide pain relief.

V. Annotated Bibliography

Rogers RS 3d. Disorders of the mouth. In: Orkin M, Maibach JH, Duhl MV, eds. Dermatology. East Norwalk, CT: Appleton & Lange; 1991:572–584.

Shafer WG, Hine MK, Levy BM. A Textbook of Oral Pathology, 4th ed. Philadelphia: WB Saunders; 1983. Two excellent texts of diseases involving the mouth.

Chapter 65: Ear Infections

Richard G. Paluzzi

65A Otitis Externa

I. Clinical Presentation

A. General Information

1. Infection of the external auditory canal is similar to infections in other skin and soft tissue structures.
2. Trapping of fluid and debris leads to maceration and irritation, which allows entry of bacteria.
3. External auditory canal averages about 2.5 cm in length with numerous hair follicles in the lateral one third.
4. Lateral one half of the canal is cartilaginous with thick skin, dermis, and subcutaneous areas; the medial skin is thinner and attached directly to the periosteum where the canal tunnels through the temporal bone. The junction between these zones is narrow (isthmus), which protects the tympanic membrane but also leads to trapping of moisture.
5. Typical flora are similar to normal skin flora: *Staphylococcus epidermis*, *Staphylococcus aureus*, diphtheroids, and some anaerobes (*Proprionibacterium acnes*). *Pseudomonas* is also a frequent pathogen.

B. History

1. Classic symptoms are pain and itching, which can be severe due to limited room for expansion of inflamed tissues.

C. Physical

1. Findings vary based on site, extent, and etiology of the process (see differential diagnosis and treatment).

II. Differential Diagnosis

A. Acute Otitis Externa

1. Localized

- a. Basically represents a pustule or furuncle associated with a hair follicle
- b. Generally due to *S. aureus* but may see streptococcal erysipelas involving the chondra and the canal.
- c. Present typically with pain, may find blue-red hemorrhage bullae in the canal and on the tympanic membrane.
- d. Regional adenopathy may be present.

2. Diffuse
   - a. Also called swimmer's ear
   - b. Presents as moderate to intense itching and pain
   - c. Edematous, reddened skin in the canal
   - d. Usually due to gram-negative organisms, may see hemorrhagic otitis externa associated with hot tubs

B. Chronic Otitis Externa

1. Irritation and maceration of the skin of the external canal due to drainage from chronic suppurative otitis media
2. Presents with severe itching
3. Rare causes include TB, syphilis, yaws, leprosy, and sarcoid
4. May also be due to manifestations of primary dermatologic problems affecting the outer portion of the canal

C. Malignant Otitis Externa

1. Severe necrotizing infection, may spread to deep tissue cartilage and bone. May bypass tympanic membrane and enter mastoid air cells. Can be lethal with spread to the sigmoid sinus, jugular bulb, base of skull, meninges, and brain. *Pseudomonas* is frequent pathogen.
2. Presents with severe pain (otalgia), tenderness of surrounding tissues, and purulent drainage (otorrhea). May present with acute cranial nerve palsies (VII, also IX, X, XI, and XII).
3. Predisposing risk factors: elderly, debilitation, and diabetes mellitus
4. Death occurs in 15–20%. Prognosis is poor in the face of neurologic deficits.
5. Patient may appear systemically ill. Can see marked rises in erythrocyte sedimentation rate (ESR) with only minimal abnormalities in white blood cells and CSF. MRI is study of choice for defining the extent of the process.

D. Fungal Otitis Externa

1. Associated with local or systemic fungal infections
2. Primarily *Aspergillus* but may see *Candida* in children with chronic mucocutaneous candidiasis

E. Vibrio Otitis Externa

1. Occurs with exposure to seawater (swimmers, fishermen)
2. *Vibrio vulnificus* causes intense cellulitis, necrotizing vasculitis, and ulcers.
3. *Vibrio alginolyticus* can cause fatal bacteremia in immunocompromised patients.
4. Vibrio can lead to otitis media.

III. Diagnostic Approach

A. Because most cases are noninfectious, history and physical examination are usually diagnostic.

B. Localized cellulitis and pustules may be treated empirically based on typical pathogens.

C. Abscesses may be drained for culture.

IV. Treatment

A. Acute Otitis Externa

1. Localized infection often responds to local heat and topical antibiotics (polymyxin B/neomycin) such as Cortisporin otic 3-4 drops q.i.d. until clinically improved. If severe, may require incision and drainage and systemic antistaphylococcal antibiotics such as dicloxacillin 500 mg q.i.d., cephelexin 500 mg q.i.d., or clindamycin 150 mg for 7-10 d.
2. Diffuse infections require gentle cleansing of canal to remove debris.
3. Irrigation may be with hypertonic 3% saline or 70-95% alcohol with acetic acid to promote drying. (Mix 2/3 rubbing alcohol with 1/3 white vinegar.)
4. Hydrophilic solutions—otic Domoboros 3-4 drops q 3-4 h or Vosol (2% acetic acid) for 1-2 d may reduce inflammation.
5. Topical antibiotics may reduce infection. Topical steroids can be added if inflammation is intense but theoretically can worsen infection or allow fungal overgrowth. Should discontinue steroids as soon as clinical improvement begins.

B. Chronic

1. Mainstay of treatment is to treat underlying otitis media or primary skin disorder.
2. Symptoms may be controlled by treating inflammation as above.

C. Malignant Otitis Externa

1. Treatment requires extensive cleansing and debridement.

2. Topical antipseudomonal antibiotics with steroids may be adequate for minor cases.

3. More severe infection requires systemic antipseudomonal antibiotics (pipercillin, mezlocillin, or ticarcillin with aminoglycosides) for 4–6 wk. Quinolones, aztreonam, and imipenim may be adequate.

4. Relapse can occur 4–12 mo following treatment. Relapse rates increase if treatment is with single agents.

5. Severe cases require close follow-up (ESR, imaging).

D. Vibro

1. Response to tetracycline (or chloramphenicol or penicillin) is generally good.

2. Severe infection may require incision and drainage.

V. Indications for Referral

A. Refer to otolaryngology if localized otitis requires incision and drainage or extensive debridement.

B. Admit to hospital for systemic antibiotics and debridement if significant abscess occurs, if severe cellulitis is present, or if bone appears to be threatened.

VI. Annotated Bibliography

Hirsch BE. Infections of the external ear. Am J Otolaryngol 1992; 13(3):145–155. A thorough, well written review of the subject.

Klein JO. Otitis externa, otitis media, mastoiditis. In: Mandel GL, Douglas RG Jr, Bennet JE, eds. Principles and Practice of Infectious Diseases, 3rd ed. New York: Churchill Livingstone; 1990:505–506. An extremely short, superficial overview with an emphasis on risk factors.

Vernick DM, Branch WT Jr. The painful or discharging ear. In: Branch WT Jr, ed. Office Practice of Medicine, 2nd ed. Philadelphia: WB Saunders; 1987:285–295. A clear concise description of various clinical presentations and diagnostic approach to otitis.

65B Otitis Media

I. Clinical Presentation

A. General Information

1. Defined as fluid in the middle ear behind the tympanic membrane associated with signs and symptoms of illness

2. Peak incidence up to age 3 (most cases occur between 6–24 mo). Second small peak at age of school entry.

3. Eustachian tubes provide drainage and ventilation for the middle ear and protect the tympanic membrane from pharyngeal secretions. Obstruction of the tube increases the risk of infection.

B. Symptoms

1. Primarily otalgia and fever

2. Often see otorrhea, loss of hearing, lethargy and irritability

3. Can see vertigo, tinnitus, and nystagmus

C. Physical Examination

1. Diagnosis requires fluid in the middle ear. This leads to bulging of the tympanic membrane and decreased tympanic membrane mobility on pneumatic otoscopy. May see tympanic membrane retraction very early on.

2. May see erythema of the tympanic membrane and inner portion of the external canal or a dull yellow or gray discoloration at the tympanic membrane.

3. Buccal cellulitis may occur when *Haemophilus influenzae* is the pathogen.

II. Diagnostic Approach

A. Diagnosis generally made on physical examination

B. Transtympanic aspiration for culture may be necessary in patients who are critically ill, immunocompromised, or showing poor response to treatment.

C. Throat and nasal cultures are of little value.

III. Differential Diagnosis

A. Serous otitis media causes retraction of the tympanic membrane.

B. *Streptococcus pneumoniae, H. influenzae,* and *Branhemella catarrhalis* are primary pathogens.

C. Viral illness may be responsible for up to one fourth of all cases of otitis media via inflammatory obstruction of the eustachian tube. Generally due to influenza, enterovirus, rhinovirus, or respiratory syncytial virus.

D. Mycoplasma can rarely lead to otitis media but more commonly will cause hemorrhagic bullous myringitis if it affects the ear. On examination see multiple hemorrhagic blebs on the tympanic membrane.

E. Tuberculous otitis is rare but can lead to painless otorrhea with multiple tympanic perforations, early hearing loss, and mastoid bone necrosis. Occasionally causes facial nerve palsy. Up to 50% have no other signs of active TB.

F. Rare causes include *Vibrio* (seawater exposure), diphtheria, tetanus (can be associated with cephalic tetanus causing multiple cranial nerve palsies), and *Ascaris*.

IV. Treatment

A. Goals

1. Decrease sequelae—hearing loss, cholesteatoma, adhesive otitis media, chronic perforation, brain abscess
2. Decrease recurrence—increased risk of recurrence is associated with first episode of otitis media before age 1, male sex, exposure to group day care settings, and history of a sibling with otitis media. Risk for recurrence decreases in children who were breastfed.

B. Acute Management

1. Antibiotic choice is based primarily on epidemiology.
2. At all ages, primary pathogens are *S. pneumoniae, H. influenzae* (leads to toxicity with bacteremia and meningitis in up to 25%) and *B. catarrhalis*. Need to cover enterobacteriaciae in newborns, immunocompromised patients and when suppurative otitis media is present.
3. Trimethoprim/sulfamethoxazole 1 double-strength tablet b.i.d. or amoxicillin-clavolinate 250–500 mg t.i.d. (amoxicillin if little *Haemophilus* influenzae resistance is prevalent) for 7–10 d is treatment of choice. May substitute cefaclor, cefixime, or loracarbef.
4. May see spontaneous resolution due to drainage through the eustachian tubes or via tympanic perforation.
5. Most improve within 48–72 h. Lack of improvement should prompt reevaluation with consideration toward changing antibiotics and tympanocentesis.
6. Little additional benefit to using decongestants or antihistamines in most cases
7. Effusion may persist up to 3 mo after treatment.

C. Chronic Otitis Media

1. Indicates prolonged disease as well as frequent relapses
2. Prevention of frequent relapses may require prophylaxis.
   a. Chemoprophylaxis with single daily doses of 500 mg amoxicillin or sulfasoxazole, especially during peak upper respiratory infection seasons (winter/spring).
   b. Immunoprophylaxis with pneumococcal vaccine (minimally effective due to poor immunogenicity prior to age 2), and *Haemophilus* influenza vaccine.
3. Surgical management may be required.
   a. Myringotomy to speed drainage and relieve pain
   b. Adenoidectomy to decrease obstruction of eustachian tubes
   c. Tympanostomy tubes—provide ventilation and drainage—primarily indicated with persistent effusions despite treatment for > 3 mo.
4. Chronic suppurative otitis media requires treatment aimed at *pseudomonas* (responsible for over 70% of cases).

V. Indications for Referral to an Otolaryngologist

A. If transtympanic aspiration is required to speed diagnosis or because of suppuration

B. If patient fails to respond to treatment

C. If surgical intervention is required to alleviate chronic/recurrent otitis media

VI. Annotated Bibliography

Bahal N, Nahata NC. Recent advances on the treatment of otitis media. J Clin Pharm Therap 1992; 17(4):201–215. Review of treatment and prevention with an emphasis on nonantimicrobial modalities.

Brock I, Burke P. The management of acute, serous and chronic otitis media: the role of anaerobic bacteria. J Hosp Infect 1992; 22 (suppl A):75–87. Good guide for selection of empirical therapy based on anticipated pathogens.

Grebinh GS. Otitis media update: pathogenesis and treatment. Med Clin North Am 1991; 75(6):1277–1291. Addresses complications of otitis media as well as medical and surgical management.

Vernich DM, Branch WT Jr. The painful or discharging ear. In: Branch WT Jr, ed. Office Practice of Medicine, 2nd ed. Philadelphia: WB Saunders; 1987:285–295. A concise, clear description of clinical presentation, diagnosis, and management of otitis.

Chapter 66: Lyme Disease

Richard G. Paluzzi

I. Clinical Presentation

A. General Information

1. A spirochetal disease caused by *Borrelia burgdorferi*
2. First recognized in 1975 in Lyme, Connecticut
3. Transmitted by ticks—*Ixodes dammini* (Northeast and Midwest) and *Ixodes pacificus* (West) as well as other related ticks
4. Ixodes life cycle—nymphs (May–July), larva (August–September), adults (Fall–Spring). Immature forms are carried by small rodents (white-footed mouse) with adults generally found on larger mammals (deer) but various other vectors have been implicated.
5. The disease is primarily transmitted by nymphs. Transmission may require > 24 h of tick attachment.
6. There appear to be three distinct foci of disease in the United States—Northeast, Midwest, and West with sporadic cases reported elsewhere. Onset of disease is usually May 1 through November 30 (primarily June and July).
7. After infection, *Borrelia* organisms spread on the skin and lymphatics or may spread hematogenously

B. Symptoms

1. Generally the disease begins in summer with a flulike illness or meningitis symptoms.
2. Can see malaise, fatigue, fever and chills, headache, cough, sore throat, mild encephalopathy, orchitis, and migratory myalgias and arthralgias
3. Late stages
   a. Early dissemination—stage 2
      1) After several weeks to months some patients will develop cardiac, neurologic, and musculoskeletal symptoms associated with attacks of arthritis.
      2) Up to 80% of patients in the United States will develop some form of joint symptoms in stage 2.

3) Early on, migratory pain in joints, tendons, bursa, muscles, and bone can develop into frank arthritis with marked swelling, especially in large joints (knees).
4) Arthritis may occur in attacks lasting several months with more mild symptoms in between. Recurrences decrease by 10–20% per year but 10% of patients develop chronic arthritis, which may be erosive in stage 3.
5) Neurologic manifestations—Frank neurologic abnormalities occur in stage 2 and include fluctuating meningitis, cranial neuropathies (Lyme is one of the few causes of bilateral Bell's palsy), peripheral neuropathies, paresthesias, encephalomyelitis, organic brain syndrome, spastic paraparesis, transverse myelitis and dementia.
6) Cardiac involvement—chest pain, heart failure symptoms, and syncopal episodes; generally transient but may recur
7) Ocular involvement—Eye pain and visual changes may occur.

b. Chronic multisystem infection—stage 3
1) Generally characterized by persistence of stage 2 problems
2) Arthritis becomes chronic and in 10% of patients is erosive (increased risk in patients with HLA type DR4).
3) Neurologic manifestations become fixed and may be progressive; more common in Europe.
4) Cardiac involvement—Recurrent episodes of stage 2 problems are often associated with heart block and conduction abnormalities.

C. Physical Examination

1. Erythema chronicum migrans (ECM) occurs at site of tick bite within 1–5 wk in 70% of patients. Bites most commonly involve the thigh, groin, and axilla. Lesions expand with partial central clearing. 50% develop multiple annular satellite lesions. Rash may last 3–4 wk.

2. Years later, some patients will develop red violaceous plaques, which may atrophy (acrodermatitis chronica atrophicans).

3. ECM may be associated with malar rash, conjunctivitis, urticaria, and regional adenopathy.

4. Early on joints generally show little swelling, but swelling can be marked in later stages.

5. Neck stiffness and other meningeal signs may be present in the acute phase. In later stages any cranial or peripheral nerve may be involved but Bell's palsy may be most common.

6. Physical signs of myopericarditis and cardiomegaly may be seen.

7. Approximately 20% of patients will develop inflammatory hepatitis; some develop splenomegaly.

8. Various inflammatory eye problems may occur, including conjunctivitis, iritis, panophthalmitis, and optic neuritis.

II. Diagnostic Approach

A. Multiple constitutional symptoms during appropriate season should be suggestive, particularly if ECM is present or patient recalls a tick bite.

B. Laboratory Studies

1. Initially may see increase in sedimentation rate, total IgM and aspartate aminotransferase.
2. Complete blood count may reveal mild anemia and leukocytosis.
3. Microscopic hematuria may occur.

C. Serology

1. IgM peaks at 3–6 wk from disease onset. IgG rises slowly over months to years.
2. Indirect enzyme-linked immunosorbent assay (ELISA) is elevated in < 40% of patients early and in 50% during convalescence. IgM-capture ELISA is more sensitive.
3. Serology can cross react with other spirochetes but *Borrelia* organisms do not cause a false positive VDRL (should check VDRL in all patients who test positive for *Borrelia*).
4. Polyclonal B cell activation can lead to false positive serology in patients with autoimmune diseases (systemic lupus erythematosus and rheumatoid arthritis) and infectious mononucleosis.
5. Sensitivity and specificity vary widely within and between laboratories.
6. Immune blotting is the most specific test readily available; measures bands against various borrelial antigens.
7. Blood or any clinically affected body fluid can be tested.
8. Polymerase chain reaction may prove to be the most sensitive and specific diagnostic test but is still considered to be experimental.
9. Serologic tests can be negative early in disease or following early antibiotic usage and remain positive for months to years following treatment.

D. Cerebrospinal Fluid

1. In acute phase, CSF examination is negative.
2. During stages 2 and 3, may see a lymphocytic pleiocytosis with elevated protein
3. Serology on CSF may be positive in stages 2 and 3.

E. Culture

1. Low yield overall
2. Yield may be slightly higher in CSF

F. ECG

1. May show varying atrioventricular block or diffuse conduction abnormalities

G. Skin Biopsy

1. May show *Borrelia* organisms in ECM lesions stained with Warthim-Starry stain.

III. Differential Diagnosis

A. Broad and varied. Clinical suspicion of Lyme disease is extremely important.

IV. Treatment

A. Prophylactic treatment following tick bite has never been shown to be useful because not all Ixodes ticks harbor disease and transmission requires 24–48 h of tick attachment.

B. Acute Phase

1. Drug of choice is tetracycline 500 mg q.i.d. for 21 d (doxycycline 100 mg b.i.d. gives better CNS penetration).
2. 15% of patients may have Jarisch-Herxheimer-like reaction during the first day of treatment.
3. Alternatives include phenoxymethyl penicillin 500 mg q.i.d. or erythromycin 250 mg PO q.i.d. for at least 10 d.
4. Early treatment may blunt immune response and allow reinfection as well as give false negative serology.
5. About 50% of patients may still get *minor* late symptoms (headache, arthralgia, lethargy).

C. Disseminated and Chronic Phase Treatment

1. Neurologic symptoms, CSF abnormalities or heart block

   a. Penicillin G 20 million units IV daily in divided doses for 10 d. Ceftriaxone 2 g IV daily for 14–21 d, or cefotaxime 2 g IV q 8 h for 14–21 d.
   b. Symptoms generally respond by day 2 but can persist up to 2 months.
   c. Neurologic disease with normal CSF or first-degree heart block of < 0.4 sec may be amenable to oral therapy. (Careful neurologic follow-up is required after oral therapy.)
   d. Cardiac abnormalities may respond to steroids but their usage is questionable and has been inadequately studied.
   e. Other cephalosporins and macrolides may also be effective.

2. Arthritis
   a. Doxycycline 100 mg b.i.d. for 30 d
   b. Amoxicillin 500 mg q.i.d. with probenecid 500 mg q.i.d. for 30 d
   c. IV therapy as above for persistent symptoms
   d. Response is slow and retreatment may be required.

D. Lyme Disease in Pregnancy

1. Tetracycline and probenecid should be avoided.

2. Any appropriate regimen should be adequate but IV therapy is probably warranted due to several case reports of fetal morbidity and mortality.

E. Patient Education

1. Primarily aimed at avoidance of exposure

2. Persons in endemic areas should check themselves, their children, and pets for ticks daily.

3. Insect repellents containing diethyltoluamide are useful but are neurotoxic and should only be sprayed on clothing in children.

4. Long clothing tucked into shoes and gloves can prevent ticks from reaching skin.

V. Indications for Referral

A. Referral to specialists for the management of Lyme disease must be individualized. There are many practitioners from various fields who concentrate on the evaluation and care of patients with Lyme disease. Referral of patients to these physicians should generally be based on one's level of familiarity with Lyme disease as well as the level of expertise and comfort in managing its various manifestations and complications.

B. The care of patients with Lyme disease may require evaluation by a cardiologist both to investigate possible causation and in the event that temporary or permanent pacemaker insertion is required.

C. The various neurologic manifestations of Lyme disease may necessitate consultation with a neurologist to assist with the diagnosis as well as to perform various diagnostic tests (electromyography, lumbar puncture, etc).

D. Evaluation by a rheumatologist might be useful both to assist in the evaluation of joint symptoms as well as to possibly perform diagnostic and therapeutic procedures (arthrocentesis with or without infection).

VI. Annotated Bibliography

Kaslow RA. Current perspective on Lyme borreliosis. JAMA 1992; 267:1381–1383. A brief but thorough review of the clinical manifestations of Lyme disease.

Rahn DW, Malawister SE. Lyme disease: recommendations for diagnosis and treatment. Ann Intern Med 1991; 114:472–481. Guidelines for evaluation and treatment.

Sigal LH. Lyme disease testing and treatment. Who should be tested and treated for Lyme Disease and how? Rheum Dis Clin North Am 1993; 19:79–93. An excellent discussion of diagnostic modalities, use of serology, and selection of patients for treatment.

Steere AC. Lyme disease. N Engl J Med 1989; 321:586–596. The authoritative review of the disease.

Chapter 67: Genitourinary Tract Infections

67A Cystitis/Pyelonephritis

Richard G. Paluzzi

I. Clinical Presentation

A. General Information

1. Denotes infection of lower urinary tract (cystitis) and upper urinary tract (pyelonephritis)
2. Bacteria enter urinary tract through various means leading to colonization and infection (UTI).
    a. Ascending
        1) Massage pushes normal urethral flora into bladder.
        2) More common in women due to shorter urethra and proximity to vagina and rectum
        3) Can follow intercourse (female) and catheterization. A single catheterization is associated with UTI in 1% of ambulatory patients and 10% of hospitalized patients.
    b. Hematogenous
        1) Frequently follows staphylococcal bacteremia or endovascular infection
        2) Occasionally occurs with candidemia
        3) Rare with enteric gram-negative organisms
    c. Lymphatic—probably insignificant
3. Several factors protect against lower urinary tract colonization/infection
    a. Urine osmolality and pH (diminished in pregnancy)
    b. Flushing effect of urination
    c. Antiadherence properties of bladder mucosa
    d. Zinc-containing antibacterial substance from the prostate in males
4. Several factors increase risk of UTI
    a. Poor hygiene in women
    b. Urinary tract obstruction
    c. Urinary tract stones
        1) Lead to obstruction and irritation

2) May become colonized with bacteria leading to recurrent infection
3) May be caused by UTI with urea-splitting organisms (*Proteus, Klebsiella*)
d. Bladder dysfunction
e. Vesicoureteral reflux—can lead to upper tract infection; can also be due to infection

5. Epidemiology

    a. UTI in preschool age boys is often due to congenital abnormalities
    b. Prevalence of bacteriuria increases with age
        1) 1–3% of young, nonpregnant females
        2) 0.1% of adult men
        3) 10% of men and 20% of women after age 65 due to prostatic enlargement, diminished prostatic secretions, neurogenic changes in bladder function, fecal soiling of urethra, bladder instrumentation
    c. Approximately 10–20% of women experience a symptomatic UTI at some time. Risk is increased by pregnancy, intercourse, changes in vaginal flora, and usage of diaphragms.

6. Complications

    a. Hemorrhagic cystitis
    b. Abscess of bladder wall (pyocystitis)
    c. Papillary necrosis
        1) Can follow pyelonephritis or occur spontaneously. Usual risk factors are diabetes mellitus, obstructive uropathy, sickle cell disease, or analgesic abuse.
        2) Necrosing papilla can obstruct ureters.
    d. Chronic pyelonephritis
        1) Bilateral or unilateral with unequal scarring
        2) See inflammation in wall of renal pelvis with papillary atrophy and parenchymal fibrosis
        3) May follow noninfectious diseases (interstitial nephritis)
    e. Renal abscess
    f. Renal insufficiency or failure with vesicoureteral reflux, papillary necrosis, or recurrent/chronic pyelonephritis

7. Recurrent UTI can be due to relapse (same organism) or reinfection (different organism).

B. History

1. Lower tract infection (cystitis)

    a. Classically, complaints of dysuria, frequency, and urgency
    b. May note tenderness in suprapubic area
    c. Generally do not see fever in older children and adults
    d. May note turbid urine and hematuria
    e. In very young children, symptoms may be nonspecific—fever, vomiting, failure to thrive
    f. Elderly are often asymptomatic or present with nonspecific signs (change in mental status, malaise, decreased appetite).

2. Upper tract infection

   a. Lower tract symptoms and fever with or without chills
   b. May complain of lower back or abdominal pain

3. Need to obtain historical clues as to risk factors

   a. Previous UTIs
   b. Previous instrumentation of urinary tract
   c. Nephrolithiasis
   d. Sexually transmitted diseases (may lead to uretheral structure)
   e. Chronic urinary symptoms suggestive of bladder dysfunction or obstruction (benign prostatic hyperplasia [BPH])
   f. Temporal relationship of urinary symptoms to intercourse

C. Physical Examination

1. Generally normal with lower tract infection or may see mild to moderate tenderness in the suprapubic area

2. Bladder may be palpable if urinary obstruction precedes or follows infection.

3. Fever suggests upper tract infection and may be severe (103°F).

4. May find pain with flank percussion or occasionally with palpation of abdomen superior-lateral to the umbilicus

5. Need to examine thoroughly for anatomic abnormalities of the genitalia, evidence of bladder outlet obstruction (distended bladder, large prostate), or signs of other diseases associated with bladder dysfunction (multiple sclerosis, stroke, neuromuscular disease, spinal cord injury)

II. Differential Diagnosis

A. Inflammatory conditions of lower urinary tract

1. Urethritis

2. Radiation-induced or drug-induced cystitis (chemotherapeutics)

3. Diseases causing urinary symptoms without dysuria or fever—diabetes, BPH, uretheral stricture, neurogenic bladder

B. Upper tract diseases without infection—renal stones, renal infarction, spontaneous papillary necrosis

III. Diagnostic Approach

A. History and physical examination can be highly suggestive and prompt empirical therapy.

B. Urinalysis

1. Obtain midstream, clean-catch urine and centrifuge at 2000 rpm for 5 min.
2. Each white blood cell (WBC) seen per high power field (hpf) is equivalent to 5–10 WBC/mm^3 of urine
3. 10–50 WBC/mm^3 or 5–10 WBC/hpf is upper limit of normal. Pyuria is nonspecific (urethritis, prostatitis) and does not differentiate upper from lower tract infection. Absence of pyuria speaks against significant UTI but may occasionally be seen in patients with pyelonephritis and an obstructed ureter.
4. Leukocyte casts are suggestive but not diagnostic of pyelonephritis.
5. Hematuria (gross or microscopic) is a nonspecific finding.
6. Proteinuria (< 2 g/24 h) may occur with pyelonephritis.
7. Some bacteria can reduce nitrate to nitrite on the diazotization reaction/Griess test but false negative rate is high.
8. Threshold for bacteriuria changes depending on whether urine is spun and stained.
    a. > 1 bacteria/hpf in an unspun, stained (Gram, methylene blue) urine is equivalent to about 10^5 (100,000) bacteria/mL.
    b. > 10^5 bacteria/mL is a reliable indicator of active infection (upper or lower tract).
    c. Women may have active cystitis with only 10^3–10^5 organisms/mL.
    d. Urine obtained via bladder catheterization or suprapubic aspiration may have significant bacteriuria with < 10^5 organisms/mL.
9. In absence of microscopy can use dipstick analysis for leukocyte esterase (WBC), nitrite (bacteria), blood, and protein to suggest presence of UTI.
10. Pyuria with sterile bladder urine can occur with TB and *Chlamydia* (urethritis).

C. Bacteriology

1. Treatment is generally begun empirically with culture results used to adjust treatment. Culture is generally not necessary in young women with acute symptoms unless treatment fails.
2. Acute single episodes—generally *Escherichia coli*
3. Recurrent infections, patients with anatomic abnormalities or hospitalized patients—increased incidence of *Proteus, Pseudomonas, Klebsiella, Enterobacter,* enterococci, and staphylococci as well as polymicrobial infection
4. Increased risk of *Proteus* and *Klebsiella* with stones, especially struvite stones and staghorn calculi. 25–30% of preexisting stones become colonized with the causative organism following a UTI.
5. *Staphylococcus saprophyticus* in young sexually active women
6. *Candida albicans* in patients with indwelling bladder catheters, especially if on antibiotics or with diabetes

7. *Salmonella* frequently invades urinary tract in patients who are bacteremic.
8. *Mycobacteria tuberculosis* associated with renal/prostatic TB causes sterile pyuria.

D. Imaging Studies

1. Indicated in men with any form of UTI if underlying cause is not obvious
2. Indicated in women if response to treatment is poor or with frequent recurrences
3. Indicated following any UTI leading to bacteremia
4. Ultrasound has low morbidity and may suggest renal/perinephric abscess, ureteral obstruction (stones, necrosed papilla), or lower tract obstruction but cannot assess bladder function (other than postvoid residual urine volume), strictures or other various malformations
5. IV pyelogram is the procedure of choice due to its high sensitivity for the anatomic abnormalities. Risks include dye-induced allergy and renal failure.

E. Presence of staphylococci or *Salmonella* (or *Candida* if no bladder catheter is present) should prompt evaluation for a distant focus of hematogenous spread.

IV. Treatment

A. Asymptomatic Bacteriuria

1. Generally does not require treatment unless patient is at high risk of developing symptomatic UTI
2. Treatment is warranted in
    a. Pregnant women, particularly in the third trimester
    b. Patients with a predisposition to renal disease—diabetes, polycystic kidneys
    c. Patients with anatomic or urologic abnormalities of the urinary tract
    d. Immunocompromised patients
    e. Patients planning to undergo urologic manipulation
3. Treatment should be avoided in female patients with no underlying problems, elderly or nonambulatory patients, and patients with indwelling bladder catheters.
4. Treatment is frequently followed by reinfection.
5. Treatment should be based on culture.

B. Symptomatic UTI

1. Uncomplicated lower tract infection
    a. Can attempt single-dose therapy, particularly in women under age 25–40.

1) Amoxicillin/clavulanate 500 mg with amoxicillin 2.5 g (20–40% of *E. coli* are resistant to amoxicillin alone)
2) Trimethoprim/sulfamethoxazole (TMP/SMX)—2 double-strength tablets
3) Quinolines—ciprofloxacin 250 mg or norfloxacin 800 mg

b. Failure of single-dose therapy suggests upper tract infection or anatomic/neurologic abnormalities of the urinary tract.

c. Women over age 40 and inner city women tend to respond better to therapy given for 3 d.
1) TMP/SMX—1 double-strength tablet b.i.d.
2) Amoxicillin/clavulanate—250 mg t.i.d.
3) Ciprofloxacin 250 mg b.i.d. or norfloxacin 400 mg b.i.d.
4) Persistent infection or relapses should be treated for 14 d based on culture results.
5) Pyridium 200 mg t.i.d. before meals for 48 h may ease dysuria. Patients should be warned that urine will become discolored (red).

2. Upper tract infection

a. Uncomplicated pyelonephritis can be treated as per B-1-c above with therapy given for 14 d.
b. Adequate treatment of complicated infections generally requires removal of bladder catheters, relief of obstruction, or relief of urinary retention caused by neurologic abnormalities.
c. Persistent infections should be treated for at least 6 wk based on culture result.

3. Recurrent infections

a. Early recurrence is typically due to persistence of same infection, whereas late recurrence (more than a few weeks following acute treatment) typically represents reinfection.
b. Can manage each episode as an acute infection (may require reliance on culture results)
c. Frequent or severe recurrences may require prophylaxis.
1) Single bedtime doses of nitrofurantoin 100 mg, trimethoprim 400 mg, TMP/SMX 1 single-strength tablet, ciprofloxacin 250 mg or norfloxacin 400 mg
2) Acidification of urine with ascorbic acid 1000–1500 mg/d with or without a urinary antiseptic (mendelamine, hispurate)
3) Can attempt to discontinue prophylaxis after 3–6 mo but recurrence is frequent if structural abnormalities are present
4) Single postcoital dose of a prophylactic agent is usually effective to prevent UTI associated with intercourse.
5) Patients should be instructed to drink fluids generously and void frequently. Voiding after intercourse is helpful.

D. Follow-up

1. In all patients, bacteruria should clear within 24 h. Symptoms and pyuria may persist (occasionally more than 5–7 d with pyelonephritis).

2. Urine culture should be repeated at 72 h in men and in patients who had a pretreatment culture due to suspected pyelonephritis, structural abnormalities, or relapse.
3. Urine culture should be repeated 1–2 wk following completion of therapy in all but uncomplicated lower tract infections, which clinically responded to short course therapy.

V. Indications for Referral to Urology

A. Recurrent infection unresponsive to treatment

B. Significant complications of infection such as abscess requiring drainage

C. Structural or neurologic abnormalities of the urinary tract requiring intervention

VI. Indications for Hospitalization

A. Systemic toxicity necessitating hydration and support

B. Inability to take oral drugs or need for IV based on culture, immunocompromise, or complications

C. Management of suspected complications

D. Severely ill patients (fever, toxicity) may require therapy with IV antibiotic for several days until clinically improving. Therapy can then be completed with oral antibiotics.

VII. Annotated Bibliography

Andriole VT. Urinary tract infection and pyelonephritis. In: Wyngaarden JB, Smith LH Jr, Bennett JL, eds. Cecil Textbook of Medicine, 19th ed. Philadelphia: WB Saunders; 1991:593–598. A short, concise review of the topic with an excellent flowsheet to guide treatment duration.

Dolan JG, Bordey DR, Polito R. Initial management of serious urinary tract infection. J Gen Intern Med 1989;4:190–194. Subgroups patients providing epidemiologic guidelines for treatment.

Johnson JR, Stamm WE. Urinary tract infections in women: diagnoses and treatment. Ann Intern Med 1989;111(11):906–917. Excellent review of the most commonly presenting UTIs.

Sobel JD, Ky D. Urinary tract infections. In: Mandell GL, Douglas RG Jr. Bennett JE, eds. Principles and Practice of Infectious Diseases, 3rd ed. New York: Churchill Livingstone 1990:582–610. A long, very detailed review of diagnosis, presentation and management.

67B Urethritis

Kenneth R. Epstein

I. Clinical Presentation

A. General Information

1. Defined as an acute inflammation of the urethra
2. Usually occurs as a sexually transmitted disease (STD) in men and is divided into gonococcal and nongonococcal
3. Nongonococcal urethritis (NGU) is more common. Etiology of NGU is 30–50% *Chlamydia trachomatis*, 15–20% *Ureaplasma urealyticum*, and 2–5% *Trichomonas vaginalis*; in 20–30% no cause is found.
4. Gonococcal urethritis has coexistent *Chlamydia* in 20–30% of cases.
5. Between one third and one half of women with dysuria have negative urine cultures. Many of these cases are thought to be secondary to urethritis, either bacterial or chlamydial.

B. Symptoms

1. Men
    a. Urethral discharge—either mucoid or purulent
    b. Dysuria
    c. Itching sensation of distal penis
    d. 25% of men with NGU are asymptomatic. 10% of men with gonococcal urethritis are asymptomatic.
2. Women
    a. Dysuria
    b. Hematuria may or may not be present.
    c. Urinary frequency may be present.

C. Physical Examination

1. In men, the primary physical finding is a urethral discharge.
    a. In gonococcal urethritis, the discharge tends to be more copious and purulent.
    b. In NGU, discharge tends to be scantier and thinner.
2. In women, there may be no urethral physical findings. Findings are usually of an associated cervicitis or vaginitis.

II. Diagnostic Approach

A. Samples of the urethral discharge should be examined.

1. If the discharge is copious, sampling for Gram stain and gonococcal culture is easy.
2. If the discharge is not readily apparent, the urethra should be "milked" from the base of the penis to the meatus 3–4 times.

B. Endourethral sampling through use of a swab is indicated if there is no obtainable discharge and for chlamydial testing.

1. A calcium alginate swab should be used.
2. The swab should be inserted 2–4 cm into the male urethra and rotated to ensure an adequate specimen for chlamydial testing.
3. The patient should be informed that the test will be uncomfortable and that he may have increased pain with his first urination.

C. Gram Stain

1. For gonococcal urethritis, the Gram stain usually reveals many white blood cells and numerous intracellular diplococci.
2. For NGU, Gram stain reveals fewer leukocytes and no bacteria.
3. In a symptomatic man, urethral Gram stain has a sensitivity of 95–98% and a specificity of 95% in distinguishing gonococcal urethritis from NGU. In an asymptomatic man, the sensitivity is 70%.

D. Culturing

1. For chlamydia, an enzyme immunoassay test is usually used, although chlamydial culture remains the reference method.
2. For gonococcal urethritis, a sample from the swab should be plated immediately on a special isolation media, such as modified Thayer-Martin media, which has been warmed to room temperature.

E. In women, pelvic examination is important to assess for the presence of vaginitis and cervicitis.

III. Differential Diagnosis

A. Differentiating Gonococcal Urethritis from NGU in Men

1. Shorter incubation period for gonococcal urethritis
2. More abrupt onset of symptoms in gonococcal urethritis
3. Discharge more purulent in gonococcal urethritis

B. **Vulvovaginitis**

1. Vulvovaginitis may also cause burning on urination.
2. Women can often differentiate the external dysuria due to the passing of urine through the inflamed labia in vaginitis from the internal dysuria of urethritis.
3. Other symptoms of vaginitis include vaginal discharge, pruritis, and dyspareunia.
4. The diagnosis is made by pelvic examination.

C. **Atrophic Urethritis in Women**

1. Due to estrogen deficiency postmenopausally
2. Suspect in postmenopausal women with dysuria and a sterile urine
3. Pelvic examination will reveal evidence of atrophic vaginitis.
4. Responds to estrogen therapy

IV. Treatment

A. **Goals**

1. Cure the patient
    a. Avoid discomfort
    b. Avoid long-term sequelae
        1) Urethral stricture
        2) Prostatitis
        3) Epididymitis
2. Identify sexual partner to avoid symptoms and long-term sequelae in that individual
3. Avoid infection of other sexual partners

B. **Acute Management**

1. In almost all cases, should treat for both gonococcal and chlamydial infection because may coexist.
2. Gonorrhea
    a. Ceftriaxone 250 mg IM single dose—the treatment of choice
    b. Spectinomycin 2 g IM single dose—if the patient is allergic to penicillin
3. Chlamydia
    a. Doxycycline 100 mg PO b.i.d. for 7 d—standard treatment
    b. Erythromycin 500 mg PO q.i.d. for 7 d—alternative treatment
    c. Azithromycin 1 g PO, single dose—becoming treatment of choice due to avoidance of compliance concerns; is as effective as 7 d of doxycycline

4. The patient should avoid unprotected intercourse until the partner has been treated.

V. Patient Education

A. Necessity of Treating Sexual Partner

1. Even if the patient's sexual partner is asymptomatic, he or she must be treated.
2. It is essential that the patient understands that this is an STD. Person is at risk of reinfection unless the partner is treated.

B. Testing for Other STDs

1. The patient needs to understand that he or she is at high risk for other STDs.
2. The provider and patient should discuss the advisability of testing for syphilis and HIV. Additionally, vaccination for hepatitis B should be considered.

VI. Long-term Management

A. Persistent or Recurrent Infection

1. Patient should be instructed to return for evaluation if symptoms persist or recur.
2. Patients with persistent or recurrent infection should be retreated with the initial regimen if there is a question of compliance during initial therapy or if they were reexposed to an untreated sexual partner.
3. If symptoms persist, consider wet mount examination and culture for *T. vaginalis*. Also, consider herpetic infection.

B. Monitor for Long-term Sequelae

1. Urethral stricture
2. Epididymitis
3. Prostatitis—association with urethritis not proven
4. Reiter's syndrome—a reactive arthritis that may occur following NGU

VII. Indications for Referral

A. Routine referral is not necessary.

B. Refer to urologist for evidence of urethral stricture or other anatomic abnormality

VIII. Annotated Bibliography

Bowie WR. Effective treatment of urethritis. Drugs 1992;44:207–215. A good review on the diagnosis and management of patients with urethritis.

Stamm WE. Azithromycin in the treatment of uncomplicated genital chlamydial infections. Am J Med 1991;91(suppl 3A):19S–22S. Reviews the role of azithromycin in the treatment of urethritis.

Stamm WE, Hooton TM. Management of urinary tract infections in adults. N Engl J Med 1993;329:1328–1334. Has a good section on differentiating cystitis and vaginitis from urethritis in women.

67C Epididymitis
Richard G. Paluzzi

I. Clinical Presentation

A. General Information

1. Infection of the epididymal structures may be acute or chronic; usually unilateral
2. May be due to reflux of urine into the epididymis via the ejaculatory ducts and vas deferens
3. Can follow strenuous activity, vigorous sexual events, instrumentation of the urethra, or prostatic/bladder surgery or may be associated with prostatitis or other genitourinary pathology
4. Epididymitis is generally sexually transmitted under age 35–50. Typically due to *Chlamydia* but approximately 10% of cases are due to gonorrhea
5. Typically "nonspecific" past age 50 with enteric gram-negative organisms most commonly; occasionally caused by *Pseudomonas* and gram-positive cocci
6. More unusual causes include
   a. TB
   b. Colifirms and *Haemophilus influenzae* in homosexuals; often associated with urethritis
   c. Cytomegalovirus (CMV) in immunosuppressed patients
   d. Cryptococcus in patients with AIDS
   e. Rarely meningococcus following oral sex
   f. Inflammatory manifestation of lymphatic filariasis
   g. Recovery phase of typhoid
   h. Blastomycosis
7. Complications include
   a. Bacteremia—particularly when epididymitis is associated with bladder catheterization
   b. Testicular infarction
   c. Abscess formation
   d. Chronic draining sinuses
   e. Sterility—rare, can follow bilateral disease

B. History

1. Acute epididymitis
   a. Sudden onset of scrotal pain that can radiate along the path of the spermatic cord. Pain can be exquisite.

- b. Irritative voiding symptoms (frequency, urgency, dysuria) as well as uretheral discharge can occur.
- c. Can occasionally present as fever alone, particularly following instrumentation
- d. Sexual history including diseases in contacts is mandatory.

2. Chronic epididymitis
   - a. Chronic scrotal swelling, which may or may not be painful
   - b. Can occur gradually or result from recurrent episodes of acute epididymitis

C. Physical Examination

1. Acute epididymitis
   - a. Epididymis is extremely tender.
   - b. Swelling is variable.
   - c. Fever is variable but can be quite high (104°F).
   - d. Reactive swelling of the testicle (noninfectious) as well as hydroceles may be present.
   - e. Scrotal skin may be erythematous and indurated. Fixation of scrotal skin suggests epididymal abscess.
   - f. Pain eases with elevation of the scrotum (Prehn's sign).

2. Chronic epididymitis
   - a. Epididymis is swollen and indurated due to lymphocytic infiltration.
   - b. Pain is variable.
   - c. Chronic epididymitis with "beading" of the vas deferens may occur with TB. Usually associated with prostatitis. May develop draining cutaneous sinuses. 50% will have renal TB.

II. Diagnostic Approach

A. History and physical examination are generally diagnostic.

B. Leukocytosis is common in acute epididymitis.

C. Urinalysis

1. Pyuria and bacteruria are common in acute epididymitis but usually lacking in chronic epididymitis unless a concommitent prostatitis occurs.

2. Sterile pyuria may occur with TB.

D. Cultures

1. Cultures of urine and any urethral discharge should be performed, including swabs for *Chlamydia* antigen.

2. Cultures for mycobacteria are indicated in the face of chronic epididymitis with sterile pyuria.

E. Imaging Studies

1. Ultrasound
   a. Usually not necessary unless doubt exists about diagnosis (see Differential Diagnosis) or presence of abscess
   b. Doppler study of testicular blood flow can be used to rule out testicular torsion with diminished flow.
   c. Most useful in diagnosing presence of chronic epididymitis

III. Differential Diagnosis

A. Testicular or epididymal torsion or torsion of the testicular appendage (testicle may be rotated with the epididymis posterior and/or elevated in the scrotum)

B. Tumors of the testicle (pain generally due to stretching of the tunica albuginea due to mass effect or hemorrhage)

C. Tumors of the epididymis (rare)

D. Trauma

E. Mumps (unilateral epididymo-orchitis occurs in 20%)

IV. Management

A. Acute Epididymitis

1. Analgesics, antipyretics, ice, and scrotal elevation (athletic supporter) all provide symptomatic relief.
2. Empirical antibiotics pending culture
   a. Suspected sexual transmission (based on age and history)
      1) Ceftriaxone 250 mg IM then oral doxycycline 100 mg b.i.d. for 7 d
      2) If necessary, can substitute ciprofloxacin 500 mg for 1 dose or erythromycin 500 mg q.i.d. for 7 d for doxycycline and spectinomycin 1 g IM or amoxicillin 3 g with probenecid 1 g for ceftriaxone
   b. Suspected nonspecific cause (age over 50)
      1) Trimethoprim-sulfaxmethoxazole (TMP/SMX) 1 double-strength tablet b.i.d. for 7–10 d
      2) May substitute ampicillin 1 g q.i.d. or doxycycline 100 mg b.i.d. for 7–10 d

B. Chronic Epididymitis

1. Empirical antibiotics as above. Results are poor.
2. Anti-inflammatory agents (such as nonsteroidal anti-inflammatory drugs) to reduce swelling

3. Persistent cases may require local anesthetic injection or surgical excision.

C. Unusual Cases

1. Management of TB and other rare causes of epididymitis is directed at the underlying disease.

V. Indications for Referral to Urology

A. Suspected torsion or tumor

B. Abscess requiring drainage

C. Recurrent or nonresolving epididymitis

VI. Indications for Hospitalization

A. Clinical sepsis

B. Severe pain nonresponsive to oral analgesics

C. Need for surgical intervention

VII. Bibliography

Krieger JN. Epididymitis. In: Mandell GL, Douglas RG Jr, Bennet JE, eds. Principles and Practice of Infectious Diseases, 3rd ed. New York: Churchill Livingstone; 1990:973–974. A concise review of clinical presentation.

Loughlin KR, Whitmore WF III. Epididymitis in Branch WT Jr, ed. Office Practice of Medicine 2nd ed. Philadelphia: WB Saunders; 1987:561–562. A short but thorough overview of the disease with a good review of differential diagnoses and treatment.

Oriel JD. Male genital chlamydia trachomatis infections. Infect 1990;25(Supp 1):35–37. A thorough review of clinical manifestations of this sexually transmitted organism.

67D Prostatitis
Richard G. Paluzzi

I. Clinical Presentation

A. General Information

1. Most common prostate disease seen prior to age 45
2. Occurs in up to 50% of men
3. Prostate secretes immunoglobulins and a zinc-containing antibacterial factor that may be protective.

B. Symptoms

1. Most diagnoses are based on perineal, low back, lower abdominal, or pelvic pain associated with urinary discomfort or ejaculatory complaints.
2. Acute bacterial prostatitis may be associated with obstructive voiding symptoms due to prostatic edema. Fever and systemic toxicity are common.
3. Chronic bacterial prostatitis generally presents as recurrent urinary tract infections with the same organism.
4. Nonbacterial prostatitis (prostatodynia) generally leads to vague pelvic symptoms (spasm or dull ache) with urinary discomfort and ejaculatory changes.
5. Fever of unknown origin may occur in elderly or debilitated patients, particularly with prostatic abscess.

C. Physical Examination

1. Fever is common.
2. Digital rectal examination
   a. Tender, tense gland in acute bacterial disease
   b. Normal in chronic and nonbacterial disease
   c. Prostate firm and nodular but nontender in granulamatous prostatitis. This typically follows acute bacterial prostatitis but may be seen with TB, fungi, syphilis, and herpes zoster.
   d. May find palpable fluctuance if abscess has formed
   e. Cutaneous, rectal, and bladder fistulae may form with TB and fungi (primarily blastomycosis).

II. Diagnostic Approach

A. Culture may be diagnostic.

1. Collect first 5-10 mL urine (VB_1—urethral specimen) and a midstream sample (VB_2—bladder specimen); then do prostatic massage for expressed secretions (EPS) followed by another urine sample (VB_3).
2. In prostatitis, bacteria in VB_3 should be 10 times that in VB_1 or VB_2. Bacteria in EPS (or ejaculate) is diagnostic. EPS is inflammatory in nonbacterial prostatitis but not prostatodynia.
3. Urinalysis may show pyuria.
4. Transrectal ultrasound with needle aspiration may be diagnostic (and therapeutic in prostatic abscess).
5. Biopsy may be required to rule out prostate cancer, particularly in granulomatous prostatitis.

III. Differential Diagnosis

A. *Acute bacterial prostatitis*—enterobacteriaciae, *pseudomonas*, and entercocci

B. *Chronic bacterial prostatitis*—gram-negative bacilli (*Escherichia coli*, *pseudomonas*), and gram-positive cocci (entercocci and *Staphylococcus saprophyticus*)

C. Prostatic abscess is generally due to common urinary pathogens as well as gonorrhea and staphylcocci (suggests hematogenous spread). Predisposing factors include diabetes mellitus, immunocompromise, inadequate treatment of acute disease, and urethral obstruction.

D. Cryptococcus may be harbored in the prostates of patients with AIDS.

IV. Treatment

A. Many drugs penetrate inflamed prostatic tissues.

B. Minimize prostatic manipulation and give stool softeners.

C. Drugs of Choice

1. Trimethoprim (160 mg)/sulfamethoxazole (800 mg) b.i.d. for 3-6 wk
2. Ciprofloxacin 500 mg b.i.d. for 3-6 wk
3. Azithromycin 500 mg followed by 250 mg daily for 14 d
4. Severely ill patients should receive 5-7 d of parenteral therapy with ampicillin 2 g t.i.d. or ciprofloxacin 400 mg for 1 dose then 200 mg daily with an aminoglycoside. Treatment is then completed with an oral agent.
5. Abscesses must be drained.

D. Long-term Management

1. One third are cured with adequate treatment. One third improve but relapse.
2. Treatment failure may be due to inadequate treatment, poor drug penetration, drug inactivation by abnormal pH, or infected calculi.
3. Chronic prostatitis may require oral treatment for 3–6 mo.
4. Long-term suppressive therapy with low-dose antibiotics may be necessary if cure fails.

E. Granulomatous prostatitis generally resolves without treatment.

F. Nonbacterial prostatitis generally resolves without treatment. Doxycycline 100 mg b.i.d. for 10 d is generally given, however, to treat possible *Chlamydia* and *Ureaplasma*.

G. Anxiolytics, α agonists (prazosin, terazosin) and smooth muscle relaxants (propantheline) have all been suggested as adjunctive treatment for prostatodynia.

V. Indications for Referral to Urology (All Relative)

A. Inability to confirm diagnosis

B. Treatment failure

C. Severe symptoms/toxicity

D. Prostatic abscess

VI. Indications for Hospitalization

A. Need for systemic antibiotics in severely ill

B. Dehydration

C. Abscess requiring drainage

VII. Annotated Bibliography

Aaguard J, Madsen PO. Bacterial prostatitis: new methods of treatment. Urology 1991; 37 (3 suppl):4–8. Good discussion of factors involved in treatment success and failure.

Berger RE, Hanno PM. The fine points of prostatitis care. Patient Care. September 15, 1992:91–107. An easily read review of presentation and management.

Leigh DA. Prostatitis—an increasing clinical problem for diagnosis and management. J Antimicrob Chemother 1993;32(suppl A):1–9. Excellent overall review of presentation, diagnosis, and management.

67E Genital Ulcers

Rosemarie A. Leuzzi

I. Clinical Presentation

A. General Information

1. In the United States, most patients with genital ulcers have either genital herpes (most common), syphilis, or chancroid. Each of these infections is associated with an increased risk of HIV infection.
2. Other potential causes of genital ulceration, lymphogranuloma venereum (endemic in Asia and South America) and granuloma inguinale (endemic in the tropics) are both rare in the United States.

B. Symptoms

1. Genital ulcer
   a. Painful vesicles or pustules are usually suggestive of herpes infection and a prodrome of tingling, numbness, or paresthesias may precede the outbreak of the genital ulcer. The incubation period is usually 24–48 h after exposure.
   b. A tender papule that progresses to a pustule, then to a painful, nonindurated genital ulcer is strongly suggestive of the diagnosis of chancroid.
   c. A painless papule that progresses to a painless ulcer (chancre) is typical of primary syphilis. This occurs at the site of intimate sexual contact appearing 10–90 d after infection (mean 21 d).
   d. A small, painless genital vesicle or papule that progresses to an ulcer is characteristic of lymphogranuloma venereum infection; in most cases, the lesion heals quickly and goes unnoticed. The primary genital lesion occurs 3 d to 3 wk following exposure.

2. Inguinal lymphadenopathy
   a. Tender suppurative inguinal lymphadenopathy is the most common clinical manifestation of lymphogranuloma venereum and is frequently the presenting symptom (since the ulcer usually goes unnoticed); the adenopathy is unilateral in two thirds of cases.
   b. Tender inguinal lymphadenopathy occurs in only one third of patients with chancroid.

C. Physical Examination

1. Genital ulceration
   a. A painless ulcer with a smooth base and raised firm borders is consistent with the chancre of primary syphilis. This is usually a solitary, indurated ulcer ranging in size from a few millimeters to a few centimeters in diameter; multiple lesions are seen in up to 30% of cases.
   b. Multiple, painful, grouped ulcerations that appear vesicular with an erythematous base suggest herpes infection.

- c. Ulcers of chancroid infections are typically painful, nonindurated (soft), multiple, and appear to be superficial erosions with ragged edges.
- d. The small, painless genital ulcer in lymphogranuloma venereum infections is usually not seen.
- e. The genital ulcer of granuloma inguinale is painless and heaped up with granulation tissue.

2. Inguinal lymphadenopathy
   - a. Regional, nontender, rubbery, nonsuppurative bilateral lymphadenopathy occurs 3–4 d after the appearance of the chancre in primary syphilis.
   - b. In primary herpes infection, tender bilateral inguinal adenopathy develops.
   - c. In chancroid, tender, regional, painful, suppurative nodes develop.
   - d. Painful, matted, necrotic, large nodes develop in lymphogranuloma venereum with fistula tracts. Inflammatory involvement of the perirectal and perianal lymphatic tissues may result in hypogastric/deep iliac lymphadenitis (this occurs most commonly in women and homosexually active men).
   - e. There is usually no significant lymphadenopathy in granuloma inguinale.

II. Diagnostic Approach

A. Diagnosis based on history and physical examination is often inaccurate and at least 3–10% of patients will have more than one infection.

B. All patients should have serologic testing for syphilis. HIV testing should be considered.

C. Depending on test availability and clinical or epidemiologic suspicion, consider the following

1. Culture or antigen test for herpes simplex virus (HSV)

2. Culture for *Haemophilus ducreyi*

3. Darkfield examination or direct immunofluorescence test for *Treponema pallidum*

D. If the above causes of genital ulcers with tender adenopathy have been ruled out, a biopsy of the lymph nodes or involved tissue may be indicated.

III. Differential Diagnosis

A. Chancroid

1. The definitive diagnosis of chancroid requires identification of *H. ducreyi* on special culture media that are not commercially available and, even using these media, sensitivity is usually < 80%.

2. A probable diagnosis of chancroid may be made if the person has one or more painful genital ulcers AND (a) no evidence of *T. pallidum* infection by

darkfield examination of ulcer exudate or by a serologic test for syphilis performed at least 7 d after the onset of the ulcer *AND* (b) either the clinical presentation of the ulcer is not typical of HSV or the HSV tests are negative.

3. The combination of a painful ulcer accompanied by tender inguinal adenopathy is suggestive of chancroid and when accompanied by suppurative inguinal adenopathy is almost pathognomonic.

B. **Herpes Simplex Virus**

1. Of the two serotypes of HSV, HSV-type 1 and HSV-type 2, HSV-type 2 causes most genital ulcers.

2. Most infected patients never recognize signs suggestive of genital herpes; some will have symptoms shortly after infection and then never again. Furthermore, many cases of genital herpes are acquired from persons who do not know that they have a genital HSV infection or who were asymptomatic at the time of sexual contact.

3. A minority of patients will have recurrent outbreaks of genital lesions.

C. **Granuloma Inguinale**

1. Granuloma inguinale is a chronic, indolent, mildly contagious ulcerative disease involving the skin and lymphatics of the genital or perianal areas.

2. The disease may be sexually transmitted and is associated with the presence in affected tissues of an intracellular microorganism, identified as the Donovan body (*Calymmato-bacterium granulomatis*).

3. This infection begins as a papule that ulcerates and develops into a painless elevated zone of beefy red friable granulation tissue; the chronicity of the disease is of diagnostic importance because several months may lapse before patients seek treatment.

4. This ulcer is easily mistaken for the primary chancre in primary syphilis or resembles carcinoma; the diagnosis is confirmed by the finding of Donovan bodies in biopsied tissue.

D. **Lymphogranuloma venereum**

1. Caused by serovars L1, L2, and L3 of *Chlamydia trachomatis*, lymphogranuloma venereum is a sexually transmitted infection.

2. The most common clinical manifestation among heterosexuals is tender inguinal lymphadenopathy, most commonly unilateral. Women and homosexually active men may present with proctocolitis or inflammatory involvement of perirectal lymphatic structures resulting in fistulas and strictures.

3. When patients seek care, most no longer have the self-limited genital ulcer that occurs at the site of inoculation; the diagnosis is usually made serologically or by isolation of the strain from a biopsied lymph node or rectal tissue biopsy.

E. **Syphilis (see Chapter 71)**

F. Other considerations in the differential diagnosis: trauma, carcinoma, lichen planus, psoriasis, scabies, fungal infection, folliculitis, and a fixed drug eruption.

IV. Treatment

A. Even after complete testing, 25% of patients will have no laboratory confirmed diagnosis; therefore, the physician must treat the patient empirically for the most likely diagnosis. Many experts recommend treatment for both chancroid and syphilis if the diagnosis is unclear.

B. Treatment of Chancroid

1. Recommended regimen

    a. Azithromycin 1 g PO in a single dose *OR*
    b. Ceftriaxone 250 mg IM in a single dose *OR*
    c. Erythromycin 500 mg PO q.i.d. for 7 d

2. Alternative regimen

    a. Amoxicillin 500 mg/clavulanic acid 125 mg PO t.i.d. for 7 d *OR*
    b. Ciprofloxacin 500 mg PO b.i.d. for 3 d—Contraindicated for pregnant/lactating women and children < 17 y

3. Follow-up

    a. Consider HIV and syphilis testing at the time of diagnosis and retesting in 3 mo for HIV and syphilis if the initial results are negative.
    b. Reexamine in 3–7 d following the initiation of treatment. If successful, symptoms should improve in 3 d and ulcers should improve objectively in 7 d; however, larger ulcers may take longer to heal.
    c. If no clinical improvement, consider the following: incorrect diagnosis, coinfection with another sexually transmitted disease, noncompliance with therapy, HIV infected, or resistance of the *H. ducreyi* strain.
    d. HIV-infected patients may require a longer course of antibiotics.

4. Management of sexual partners—Persons who had sexual contact with the patient who has chancroid within 10 d before the onset of the patient's symptoms should be examined and treated even if they are asymptomatic.

C. Treatment of Herpes Infection

1. Primary herpes infection

    a. Recommended regimen—acyclovir 400 mg PO t.i.d. for 7–10 d
    b. Alternative regimen—acyclovir 200 mg PO 5 times/d for 7–10 d
    c. Topical acyclovir provides little or no benefit.
    d. Acyclovir taken PO or IV for 7–10 d shortens the duration of pain, viral shedding, and systemic symptoms in primary herpes simplex infections.
    e. For patients with recurrent herpes infection, acyclovir may be helpful in some patients if started early during the prodrome or within 2 d of the onset of the lesions.

2. Frequent severe recurrences of herpes infection (> 6 episodes/y)
   a. Continuous suppressive therapy may benefit some patients by markedly decreasing the rate of recurrence without the development of resistance.
   b. Suppressive therapy does not eliminate symptomatic or asymptomatic viral shedding or the potential for transmission.
   c. Recommended regimen—acyclovir 200 mg PO 2–5 times/d
   d. Alternative regimen—acyclovir 400 mg PO b.i.d.
   e. After 1 y of continuous suppressive therapy, the acyclovir should be discontinued to allow assessment of the patient's rate of recurrent episodes.
3. Treatment of immunocompromised patients
   a. Immunocompromised patients may have prolonged episodes with extensive outbreaks and may require more aggressive treatment and hospitalization for IV acyclovir.
4. Follow-up
   a. Patients need to be educated about the natural history of the lesions, the potential for recurrent lesions, asymptomatic viral shedding, and sexual transmission.
   b. The use of condoms should be encouraged during all sexual encounters.
5. Management of sexual partners—Sexual partners of patients with genital herpes should be counseled regarding the risk of exposure and evaluated for evidence of herpes infection.

D. Treatment of Granuloma Inguinale

1. Recommended regimen—tetracycline 2 g daily for at least 3 wk, preferably continued until healing of the ulcer is complete
2. Follow-up—Lack of clinical response within 7 d should lead to reassessment of the diagnosis and therapy.

E. Treatment of Lymphogranuloma Venereum

1. Recommended regimen—doxycycline 100 mg PO b.i.d. for 21 d
2. Alternative regimens
   a. Erythromycin 500 mg PO q.i.d. for 21 d *OR*
   b. Sulfisoxazole 500 mg PO q.i.d. for 21 d
3. Treatment cures the infection and prevents further tissue damage, although tissue reaction can result in scarring and buboes may require aspiration.
4. Follow-up—Patients should be followed clinically until signs and symptoms have resolved.
5. Management of sexual partners—Persons who have had sexual contact with a patient who has lymphogranuloma venereum within the 30 d before the onset of the patient's symptoms should be examined and tested for evidence of chlamydial infection and offered therapy.

F. Treatment of Syphilis (see Chapter 71)

V. Indications for Referral to a Specialist

A patient with nonhealing ulcer should be referred to a specialist for possible biopsy of the lesion to confirm the diagnosis and evaluate therapy.

VI. Annotated Bibliography

Centers for Disease Control and Prevention. 1993 sexually transmitted diseases treatment guidelines. MMWR 1993;42 (No. RR-14). Excellent concise handbook reviewing diagnosis and therapy—an essential guide to have available in the ambulatory care setting.

Holmes KK. Donovanosis (granuloma inguinale). In: Wilson JD, Braunwald E, Isselbacher KJ, et al, eds. Harrison's Principles of Internal Medicine. New York: McGraw-Hill; 1991. In-depth review of granuloma inguinale covering etiology, clinical presentation, diagnosis, and therapy.

Peterson PK, Dahl MV. Dermatologic Manifestations of Infectious Disease. Kalamazoo, MI: The Upjohn Company; 1987. Brief chart covering symptoms and findings as well as good photos demonstrating the various types of genital ulcers.

Chapter 68: Management of Positive PPD

Richard G. Paluzzi

I. Clinical Presentation

A. General Information

1. Two tuberculin preparations are available
   a. Old Tuberculin (OT)—filtrate of sterile killed concentration of tubercle bacilli developed by Koch
   b. Purified protein derivative (PPD)—filtrate of OT available in three strengths
      1) Standard 5 TU (intermediate)
      2) 1 TU (first strength) rarely used
      3) 250 TU (2nd strength)

2. Two testing methods
   a. Multiple puncture (tine) test—OT or PPD introduced via coated applicators. Used to screen low-risk groups. Any vesiculation is considered positive and should be followed up with a Mantoux.
   b. Mantoux test—intradermal injection of 0.1 mL PPD containing 5 TU. Induration at injection site is measured at 48–72 h.

3. Booster reaction—delayed-type hypersensitivity due to previous mycobacterial infection or bacille Calmette-Guérin (BCG) exposure may wane over years leading to an initially negative skin test. A second test given within 1 y may be positive, thus appearing to be a new conversion due to a "boosted" reaction from the first test.

4. Two-step testing—useful in situations where skin testing will be repeated periodically. An initially negative Mantoux test is followed in 1 wk by a second test. A positive test represents a booster reaction and is considered positive and the patient should be managed accordingly.

5. A second negative test is likely to truly be negative and any subsequent positive test represents a new conversion.

B. Interpretation

1. Area of induration at site of injection is measured at its greatest diameter at 48–72 hours.

2. Interpretation as positive is based on associated risks.
    a. > 5 mm is positive in close contacts of persons with active TB, in those with fibrocystic changes on chest x-ray, and in those with HIV infection.
    b. > 10 mm is positive in immigrants from epidemic countries, in impoverished low socioeconomic groups, IV drug users, residents of long-term care facilities, prisons, and those with other risk factors known to increase the incidence of TB such as diabetes, silicosis, immunosuppressive therapy/steroids, end-stage renal disease, intestinal bypass, gastrectomy, carcinomas of oropharynx/upper GI tract, hematologic diseases, and in those > 10% below ideal body weight.
    c. > 15 mm is positive in all other groups.
    d. False positives occur in patients infected with atypical mycobacteria.
    e. False negatives occur in any disease that suppresses cell-mediated immunity and also in 20% patients with active TB. This can be confirmed by the use of anergy panels—intradermal injections of two to three common antigens (mumps, candida, trichophytin, tetanus) to which the majority of immunocompetent patients will make at least one response.
3. Following BCG vaccination, skin tests remain positive for varying lengths of time. Suspicion of true disease should increase as the size of the reaction and time lapse after BCG use increases, in persons who are in close contact with patients who have active disease, and in persons from countries of high TB prevalence.

II. Risk of Developing Active TB

A. Positive skin test of unknown duration with no other risk factors—0.1%/y.

B. Recent converters (within 2 y)—3–5% in first year

C. Positive skin tests in household contacts—2.5–5% in first year

D. Positive skin test with abnormal chest x-ray or inadequate previous treatment—1–4.5%/y

E. Positive skin test with chronic illness—risk variable

F. Positive skin test in HIV-positive patients—14% over 2 y

III. Management

A. Candidates for Preventive Therapy
1. High-risk group with positive skin tests regardless of age
    a. Patients with HIV infection (confirmed or suspected)
    b. Close contact of patients with active TB
    c. Recent skin test converters

d. Patients with abnormal chest x-rays who were previously untreated or inadequately treated
   e. IV drug users
   f. Those with illnesses that increase risk of TB (see above)
   g. Health care workers who have close contact with patients with active TB

2. High-risk groups with positive skin tests who are under age 35 y

   a. Immigrants from countries with high incidence of TB
   b. Low-income groups/high-risk minorities
   c. Residents of long-term care facilities and prisons

B. Prophylactic Regimens

1. Most regimens use isoniazid 10 mg/kg (up to 300 mg) daily. 12 mo of therapy decreases risk of active TB by 70–90%; 6 mo of therapy decreases risk by about 65%.

2. Patients with abnormal chest x-rays or who are HIV infected should receive 12 mo of therapy.

3. Isoniazid at 15 mg/kg (up to 900 mg) may be given twice weekly if needed to improve compliance.

4. Close contacts of patients with active, isoniazid-resistant TB should receive rifampin 600 mg daily for 1 y.

5. Major toxicity of INH is hepatitis. Risk is negligible before age 35 y, about 1–2% after age 35, and 2–3% after age 50.

6. Pyridoxine 50 mg/d can reduce the risk of isoniazid-related neuropathy and should at least be given to pregnant women, patients with seizure disorders, and those with diseases associated with neuropathies (diabetes/alcoholism).

C. Monitoring

1. Pretreatment

   a. Exclude active TB
   b. Exclude previously completed prophylactic therapy
   c. Exclude contraindications—prior isoniazid toxicity, active liver disease
   d. Identify patients at increased risk of toxicity—over age 35, use of other chronic medications, daily alcohol usage, previous isoniazid side effects, chronic liver disease, peripheral neuropathies, diabetes, pregnancy

2. Monthly monitoring during therapy

   a. Compliance (dispense 1 mo of medication only)
   b. Watch for symptoms of neurotoxicity (paresthesias).
   c. Watch for signs of acute hepatitis. Approximately 10–20% will develop elevated transaminases. These should only be routinely monitored in high-risk patients and all patients over age 35 y. Therapy should be stopped for any transaminase level > 3–5 times normal.

IV. Annotated Bibliography

Barnes PF, Barrows SA. Tuberculosis in the 1990s. Ann Intern Med 1993; 119(5):400–410.

Centers for Disease Control. Core Curriculum on Tuberculosis. U.S. Department of Health and Human Services. 00–5763, April 1991. Two thorough reviews of current management of TB.

Chapter 69: Respiratory Tract Infections

Richard G. Paluzzi

69A Pharyngitis

I. Clinical Presentation

A. General Information

1. Most cases are viral. Sore or scratchy throat occurs in 20–80% of colds.

2. Large number of mild cases are due to adenovirus or coronavirus.

3. Most cases occur during colder months.

4. Most important bacterial cause is group A β *Streptococcus pyogenes* (strep), which is responsible for 15% of cases and can result in rheumatic fever and glomerulonephritis.

5. Pathogenesis likely involves the local release of inflammatory mediators.

6. Examination alone often won't define etiology. Need to evaluate nonpharyngeal signs and symptoms as well as known epidemics, symptoms in contacts, and season of occurrence.

B. History

1. Season of occurrence provides clues to etiology: fall/spring—rhinovirus, winter—coronavirus, epidemics from December to April—influenza, summer—adenovirus.

2. Sore throat is generally mild. Severe pain is more common with strep and ulcerating lesions—herpes and coxsackie virus (herpangina).

3. Fever may occur.

4. Constitutional symptoms are common in viral illnesses but do occur frequently in strep and other nonviral causes.

C. Physical Examination

1. Should use a mirror to examine above and below the oropharynx.

2. Viral etiologies generally lead to edema and hyperemia of tonsillar and pharyngeal mucosa. Examination is generally normal with common colds.

3. Strep infections typically cause an intense inflammatory response with exudates and hemorrhages.

4. Exudates
   a. Occurrence inconsistent
   b. Rare with most viruses and influenza
   c. Presence is suggestive of strep, adenovirus, herpes, infectious mononucleosis, and bacteria (*Clostridia, Yersina,* anaerobes); occasionally seen in *Mycoplasma*
   d. Not reliable in diagnosing strep in children under age 3

5. Vesicles/ulcers
   a. Herpes—diffuse
   b. Herpangina—soft palate, uvula, anterior tonsils

6. Rash
   a. Strep, clostridia, acute HIV infection, infectious mononucleosis

7. Conjunctivitis
   a. Adenovirus—pharyngeal-conjunctival fever associated with swimming

8. Adenopathy—strep (tender, at angle of jaw), mycoplasma (tender, anterior cervical), *Yersenia*, viruses (nontender), herpes (tender), mononucleosis (tender, posterior cervical)

9. Pseudomembranes—light to dark gray adherent collection of necrotic epithelium and leukocytes seen in diphtheria

II. Diagnostic Approach

A. Key is to differentiate viral etiologies from strep and other more unusual etiologies.

B. History and physical examination should suggest etiology using epidemiologic clues and associated signs and symptoms.

C. Can swab tonsillar pillars and oropharynx for rapid strep screen

1. Latex agglutination, takes 10–70 min

2. 95–99% sensitive, 70–90% specific

3. Positive test confirms diagnosis, negative test warrants culture.

D. Can scrape ulcer base and do Tzank smear for herpes

E. If suspect gonorrhea, need to culture on chocolate agar

III. Differential Diagnosis

A. Strep (Group A β *S. pyogenes*)

1. Spreads person to person, increased by crowding
2. 2–4 d incubation followed by abrupt onset of malaise, fever and headache
3. See hyperemia of tonsils and pharynx with edema, posterior lymphoid hyperplasia and gray exudates
4. Tender nodes at angle of the jaw are suggestive.
5. May have leukocytosis
6. Can lead to acute rheumatic fever and poststreptococcal glomerulonephritis
7. Can be associated with otitis and sinusitis as well as septic shock, and peritonsillar abscess (Quincy)
8. Erythrogenic lesions can result in scarlet fever (can also occur with nonpharyngeal strep infections)

B. Common Cold

1. Rhinovirus (fall/spring), coronavirus (winter)
2. Symptoms are generally mild and examination is essentially benign.

C. Adenovirus

1. Summer months
2. More severe than common cold with malaise, myalgias, headache, dizziness and chills
3. Exudates are common and one third get follicular conjunctivitis

D. Influenza

1. Epidemics during winter months
2. Sore throat can be predominant complaint but usually see classic symptoms of myalgia, coryza, fever without exudates or tender nodes.

E. Infectious Mononucleosis

1. Typically due to Epstein-Barr virus
2. Approximately 50% get exudative pharyngitis/tonsillitis associated with fever, posterior cervical adenopathy, and headaches. About half get splenomegaly.
3. Cytomegalovirus can cause mononucleosis with sore throat and normal examination.
4. Can confirm diagnosis serologically; generally see atypical lymphocytosis on blood smear

F. Gonorrhea

1. Suspect with chronic or recurrent sore throat not responsive to antibiotic therapy or sore throat in context of a suspicious sexual history

G. Herpangina

1. Coxsackie virus
2. Small vesicles on soft palate, uvula, and anterior tonsils, which rupture to form small white ulcers
3. May be febrile illness in children and can cause abdominal pain

H. Acute Herpetic Pharyngitis

1. Mild cases look similar to other viruses
2. Severe cases can present with inflammatory exudates, vesicles, and shallow ulcers
3. May see tendor adenopathy, fever, and gingivostomatitis

I. Mycoplasma

1. Sore throat is uncommon and generally mild.
2. See posterior erythema and exudates with headache, cough, coryza, and tender anterior nodes

J. Acute HIV

1. 3–5 wk incubation period
2. Pharyngitis is part of primary infection.
3. See fever, myalgia, arthralgia, lethargy, and a nonspecific maculopapular rash
4. Adenopathy follows in about 1 wk.

K. Diphtheria

1. Rare in United States
2. Slow onset with minimal pain, low-grade fever and gray, adherent membranes
3. Two forms
    a. *Corynebacterium hemolyticum*—young patients with puritic scarlitina form, desquamating rash, chronic skin ulcers and pharyngeal membranes
    b. *Corynebacterium ulcerans*—mild pharyngitis associated with raw milk consumption in summer months

L. Yersinia

1. Exudative pharyngitis associated with enterocolitis, fever, prominent adenopathy, and abdominal pain
2. May be fullminant and fatal

M. Candida (Thrush)

1. Cheesy exudates throughout oropharynx and oral cavity associated with immunosuppressive illnesses and occasionally in patients using antibiotics

N. Noninfectious Causes

1. Pemphigoid
2. Systemic lupus erythematosus
3. Behcet's syndrome
4. Paraquat ingestion

O. Anaerobic pharyngitis (Vincents' angina)

1. Caused by fusobacterium and spirochetes
2. Can be associated with gingivitis (trench mouth)
3. Can lead to jugular septic phlebitis, septicemia, and metastatic infection to the lung (postanginal sepsis-Lemiere's disease).

IV. Treatment

A. Acute Management

1. Viral etiologies
   a. Symptomatic treatment with warm saline gargles, analgesics as needed, and fluids
2. Streptococcal pharyngitis
   a. If nonsuppurative, pharyngeal infection is generally self-limited and resolves in 3-5 d.
   b. Treatment is aimed at reducing incidence of rheumatic fever (ARF), otitis, and sinusitis. Treatment may not decrease incidence of glomerulonephritis. Treatment within 9 d of onset should prevent ARF.
   c. Can initiate treatment and discontinue if culture is negative
   d. Drug of choice is penicillin V 250 mg q.i.d. for 10 d. Alternatively erythromycin 250 mg q.i.d. for 10 d.
   e. 5-30% will continue to harbor the organism following treatment. No clear need for retreatment except in areas with reported ARF.
   f. Up to 25% disease occurrence in family contacts. Treat prophylactically in areas with known ARF.
3. Gonorrhea
   a. Ceftriaxone 250 mg IM as a single dose *OR*
   b. Erythromycin 500 mg q.i.d. for 10 d
4. Membranous pharyngitis
   a. Caused by diphtheria, mycoplasma.
   b. Erythromycin 500 mg q.i.d. for 10 d or penicillin G 1 g q.i.d. for 10 d

B. Chronic Management

1. Tonsillectomy may reduce incidence of recurrent pharyngitis in children.
2. Adenovirus vaccines have been used in the military.
3. Streptococcal vaccines are in development.

V. Indications for Referral to Otolaryngology

A. Multiple, recurrent or severe episodes of pharyngitis that might benefit from tonsillectomy

B. Presence or suspicion of abscess formation

VI. Indications for Hospitalization

A. Inability to maintain hydration

B. Need for IV antibiotics or surgical drainage (peritonsillar abscess, cellulitis)

VII. Annotated Bibliography

Goldstein MN. Office evaluation and management of the sore throat. Otolaryngol Clin North Am 1992; 25 (4): 837–842. Good description of differentiating between viral and bacterial etiologies.

Kind AC, Williams DN. Antibiotic treatment of pharyngitis. Sem Respir Infect 1991; 6 (2): 69–76. Discusses diagnosis and treatment of various bacterial pathogens.

Peter G. Streptococcal pharyngitis: current therapy and criteria for evaluation of new agents. Clin Infect Dis 1992; 14 (suppl 12): 5218–5223. Detailed but somewhat tedious overview of various treatment regimens for streptococcus.

Vukimer RB. Adult and pediatric pharyngitis: a review. J Emerg Med 1992; 10 (5): 607–616. Excellent review of differential diagnosis with an emphasis on treatment of streptococcal disease.

69B Acute Sinusitis

Kenneth R. Epstein

I. Clinical Presentation

A. General Information

1. Usually follows viral upper respiratory infection (URI) or allergic rhinitis
2. Maxillary sinusitis may follow dental abscess.
3. Suspect if URI persists beyond 10 d
4. Generally more than one sinus is involved (order of frequency is maxillary > frontal > ethmoid and sphenoid).

B. Symptoms

1. Pain (may be described as headache) over the area of the sinuses:
   a. Maxillary—over cheeks or upper teeth
   b. Frontal—over medial forehead
   c. Ethmoid—over bridge of nose or retro-orbital
   d. Sphenoid—over occiput or vertex of skull
2. Pain tends to be dull, persistent, worse on bending over, and may be referred to teeth (present as dental pain).
3. Nasal congestion
4. Purulent nasal discharge
5. Postnasal drip with persistent low-grade pharyngeal irritation and halitosis
6. May induce an asthma attack in adults with preexisting asthma

C. Physical Examination

1. Fever—usually low grade; only 50% of adults are febrile.
2. Nasal edema and erythema
3. Purulent exudate in ostia to sinusus
4. Occasionally can see facial edema or erythema, especially periorbital edema
5. Sinus tenderness over involved sinus

II. Diagnostic Approach

A. Suspect on history and physical—If the patient's symptoms clearly suggest the diagnosis, and obtaining a test would not alter therapy, then the test is probably unnecessary initially. If symptoms persist, then test may become necessary.

B. Transillumination

1. Method

   a. Requires a strong light source (eg, from otoscope head) in a completely darkened room
   b. Maxillary sinus—place over the patient's inferior rim of orbit and observe hard palate
   c. Frontal sinus—place at superior rim of the orbit and observe frontal area

2. Interpretation

   a. Complete opacity is reliable indication of active infection.
   b. Dullness correlates poorly with acute infection.

3. Problems

   a. Poor interobserver consistency
   b. Cannot visualize ethmoidal or sphenoidal sinuses
   c. Poor sensitivity and specificity—often have acute bacterial sinusitis without complete opacity, or dullness without sinusitis

C. Sinus X-rays

1. Views

   a. Caldwell (occipitofrontal)—for ethmoid and frontal sinuses
   b. Waters (occipitomental)—for maxillary or frontal sinuses
   c. Lateral—for sphenoidal sinuses

2. Interpretation

   a. Completely normal—usually rules out sinusitis
   b. Air-fluid levels and complete opacification of sinus—correlates well with active infection
   c. Mucosal thickening—can occur either with acute disease or in asymptomatic individuals, therefore correlates poorly with sinusitis

3. Problems

   a. Lack of usefulness—If completely normal, then rules out the disease (ie, few false negatives). However, there are many false positives due to presence of mucosal thickening in many asymptomatic individuals who perhaps had previous episodes of sinusitis.
   b. Therefore, sinusitis can usually be diagnosed on history and physical examination and x-rays are unnecessary in simple, uncomplicated cases.
   c. Indications for x-rays
      1) If diagnosis is in question
      2) If patient is much sicker than expected
      3) If there is no response to therapy

D. Nasal or nasopharyngeal cultures are not reliable and are not recommended.

III. Differential Diagnosis

A. Viral URI

B. Chronic sinusitis (see Chapter 69C)

C. Tension or migraine headache

IV. Treatment

A. Goals

1. Control of infection
2. Reduction of tissue edema
3. Facilitation of drainage
4. Maintenance of patency of the sinus ostia

B. Acute Management

1. Antibiotics
   a. Choice is based on suspected bacteriology—usually is *Streptococcus pneumoniae* or nontypeable *Haemophilus influenzae*, less common is *Brahmenella catarrhalis*, group A streptococci, various anaerobes.
   b. Treat for at least 2 wk with an additional 10 d if purulent discharge persists.
   c. First choice is amoxicillin 500 mg t.i.d. If allergic to penicillins or cephalosporins, alternate first choice is trimethoprim/sulfamethoxasole double strength, one tablet b.i.d.
   d. If failed amoxicillin, and concerned about resistant Haemophilus influenzae, then one of the following:
      1) Cefuroxime axetil 250 mg b.i.d.
      2) Cefaclor 500 mg t.i.d.
      3) Amoxicillin/clavulinic acid 500 mg t.i.d.

2. Topical nasal decongestants (eg, phenylephrine HCl 0.5% or oxymetazoline HCl 0.5%)—very useful in first several days to promote drainage, but only prescribe for first 3–4 d

3. Oral decongestants (eg, phenylpropanolamine or pseudoephredine)—can be prescribed for several weeks safely

4. Antihistamines—dry nasal secretions, not indicated

5. Nasal steroids—decrease edema, mucous membrane size, thereby improving drainage; consider only if allergic rhinitis is present concurrently

6. Nonpharmacologic measures include rest with head elevated, humidification (saline nasal sprays and steam humidification), adequate hydration, and analgesics (ASA, acetaminophen).

V. Patient Education

A. If patient smokes, encourage to quit

B. Educate patient on dangers of prolonged use of topical decongestants.

C. Encourage compliance with entire 2–3 wk of antibiotics to minimize chance of progression to chronic disease.

VI. Long-term Management

A. Inadequate treatment can lead to mucosal thickening and ostial scarring, resulting in poorly draining sinuses and chronic sinusitis. Therefore, if infection (tenderness, purulent drainage) has not cleared after initial 2 wk of treatment, continue for an additional 10–14 d.

B. Observe for evidence of chronic sinusitis (see Chapter 69C)

C. If sinusitis fails to clear and exudate is very thick, consider fungal sinusitis, often due to *Aspergillus fumigatus*. If diabetic, consider *Mucormycosis*. Refer to otolaryngologist for possible biopsy.

VII. Indications for Referral to Otolaryngologist

A. Indications for *immediate* referral to otolaryngologist for antral puncture or nasopharyngoscopy

1. If patient appears toxic

2. If patient is immunocompromised

3. If clinician suspects any serious or life-threatening complication of sinusitis, such as periorbital or orbital cellulitis, orbital abscess, cavernous sinus thrombosis, meningitis, brain abscess, subdural empyema, and frontal osteomyelitis.

B. If patient does not improve at all after 2–3 d of appropriate therapy

C. Chronic sinusitis

D. Persistent subacute disease

E. When to suspect fungal sinusitis—diabetics who fail to improve, immunocompromised persons

VIII. Annotated Bibliography

Kennedy DW, ed. First-line management of sinusitis: a national problem? Otolaryngol Head Neck Surg 1990; 103 (suppl):845-888. An entire supplement filled with useful articles on diagnosis and management of sinusitis from varied perspectives.

McMahon JT. Paranasal sinusitis, geriatric considerations. Otolaryngol Clin North Am 1990;23:1169-1177. Good review of sinusitis in the elderly.

White JA. Paranasal sinus infections. In: Ballenger JJ, ed. Diseases of the nose, throat, ear, head, and neck, 14th ed. Philadelphia: Lea & Febiger, 1991:184-202. A well-written chapter on sinus infections in a textbook on otolaryngology.

69C Chronic Sinusitis

I. Clinical Presentation

A. General Information

1. It is not clear that chronic sinusitis is primarily an infectious process.
2. Untreated, inadequately treated, or repeated episodes of acute sinusitis can lead to permanent and irreversible changes in the mucosal lining of the sinuses with disruption of normal mucociliary function.
3. Other causes include mucosal swelling due to allergies, pollutants, and dental infections as well as obstruction of drainage due to anatomic abnormalities.
4. All causes eventually lead to obstruction of drainage, stagnation of mucus, and potential secondary infection.
5. Diminished oxygen tension predisposes to secondary infections involving anaerobic organisms. 70% of positive cultures show anaerobes: α streptococci, *Bacteroides veillonella*, and Corynebacterium.

B. Symptoms

1. Patients complain primarily of slowly progressive postnasal drip associated with nasal congestion and facial pressure or headache.
2. Nasal discharge may be purulent and malodorous or thin and clear or mucoid.
3. Fever and frank pain are uncommon.
4. Taste and smell may be diminished.
5. If eustachian tube obstruction or middle ear infections occur, popping and clicking in the ears and diminished hearing may result.

C. Physical Examination

1. Findings are predominately similar to acute sinusitis.
2. May see anatomic abnormalities such as septal deviation or nasal polyps, which may predispose to obstruction

II. Diagnostic Approach

A. Cultures and Cytology

1. Examine spontaneously expressed secretions or secretions obtained from swabbing/scraping the inferior turbinate.
2. > 5 neutrophils/high power field (hpf) is significant (92% sensitive, 40% specific in adults). < 5 neutrophils or > 5 eosinophils/hpf makes sinusitis less likely.

3. Routine cultures are inaccurate and of low diagnostic yield unless obtained via antral puncture or via endoscopy.

B. Rhinopharyngoscopy (Fiberoptic)

1. More sensitive than radiographs in detecting chronic sinusitis
2. Purulent drainage from either meatus documents the presence of sinusitis.
3. Useful in evaluating other causes of chronic obstruction (polyps, septal deviation etc.)
4. Requires topical anesthetics/decongestants

C. Radiographs

1. Plain radiographs are fairly insensitive due to the inability to detect mucosal thickening.
2. CT scanning can elucidate the extent of the sinus disease as well as associated anatomic abnormalities and can guide surgery.
3. Increased density within the lumen of the sinus is suggestive of fungal sinus disease.

III. Differential Diagnosis

The main differentiation is between chronic sinusitis and recurrent acute sinusitis, which can usually be made on history.

IV. Treatment

A. Medical Management

1. Empirical trials of antibiotics are frequently used. Therapy should include anaerobic coverage and should be continued for at least 3 wk. Choices include amoxicillin/clavulinate 500 mg t.i.d., trimethoprim/sulfamethoxazole (TMP/SMX) 1 double-strength b.i.d., cefixime 400 mg daily, or penicillin G 1 g q.i.d.
2. Topical nasal steroids are useful to reduce chronic inflammation of the nose and paranasal sinuses. Systemic steroids may be useful if anterior nasal edema is so severe as to prevent penetration of the topical agent.
3. The most severe cases of chronic sinusitis often have associated allergic and lower respiratory diseases. Antihistamines, decongestants, and mucolytics are often useful as adjuvant therapy as discussed in Chapter 69.

B. Surgical Intervention

1. Indications

    a. Failure to respond to at least 3 wk of medical management

b. Chronic sinusitis resulting in worsening of underlying pulmonary disease or asthma
2. Procedures
   a. Caldwell-Luc procedure—complete removal of maxillary sinus mucosa through an incision above the upper incisors
   b. Functional endoscopic sinus surgery
      1) Has generally supplanted the Caldwell-Luc procedure; can usually be done in an outpatient setting under local anesthesia
      2) Directed removal of obstructive process
      3) Preservation of mucosa allows return of mucociliary function.
      4) Relatively contraindicated in the face of severe destruction or osteomyelitis or if osteomeatal abnormalities are not clearly defined
   c. External ethmoidectomy
      1) Often considered the gold standard for the management of chronic pansinusitis

V. Indications for Referral

A. Chronic sinusitis not responding to medical management

B. Chronic sinusitis with recurrent secondary infections

C. Severe infection threatening the orbit or surrounding bone

VI. Indications for Hospitalization

A. Severe secondary infection with clinical toxicity

B. Infection involving soft tissue, bone, skin

VII. Annotated Bibliography

Bolger WE, Kennedy DW. Guidelines for diagnosis, medical therapy and surgery: current perspectives on sinusitis in adults. J Respir Dis 1992;13:421-445. Good overview on presentation, evaluation and management.

English GM. Sinusitis. In: English GM, ed. Otolaryngology. Philadelphia: JB Lippincott, 1988:2:1-43.

Shaefer SD, Manning S, Close LG. Endoscopic paranasal sinus surgery: indications and considerations. Laryngoscope 1989;99:1-5. Patient selection and good overview of surgical techniques.

69D Acute Bronchitis

I. Clinical Presentation

A. General Information

1. Acute inflammatory condition of the tracheobronchial tree associated with generalized respiratory infections
2. Peak incidence in winter months with occurrence rate of approximately 40–50/100,000
3. Mucosal edema and hyperemia lead to increase in secretion production.
4. Incidence and severity may be increased by exposure to cigarette smoke and pollutants.
5. Can lead to prolonged abnormalities of airway resistance and reactivity

B. Symptoms

1. Cough is predominant symptom and can persist up to 2–3 wk (cough is dry with mucoid sputum, which may become purulent in late stages or if bacterial).
2. May be associated with nasal and pharyngeal symptoms (rhinorrhea, postnasal drip, sore throat)
3. May have chest tightness or burning substernal pain
4. Fever may occur with certain pathogens—influenza, adenovirus, *Mycoplasma*
5. Rarely see dyspnea and cyanosis in the absence of underlying lung disease

C. Physical Examination

Lungs are generally clear but may hear rhonchi, coarse rales, or expiratory wheezes.

II. Diagnostic Approach

A. Diagnosis of exclusion primarily suggested by history and physical

B. Chest x-ray is indicated only if lung examination is abnormal.

C. Gram stain is useful to guide therapy in patients producing purulent sputum.

D. Can obtain cultures for influenza and *Bordetella* as well as serology for *Mycoplasma* if confirmation of these diseases is desired. Bacterial cultures are generally contaminated by oral flora and should be reserved for nonresolving symptoms.

E. Prolonged cough should be evaluated by chest x-ray and possibly culture, sputum cytology, purified protein derivative (PPD), and in some cases, bronchoscopy.

III. Differential Diagnosis

A. Diagnosis of exclusion

B. Must consider pneumonia, cardiac disease, and thromboembolic disease

C. Vast majority of cases are viral.

1. Common colds—rhinovirus, coronavirus

2. Lower respiratory pathogens—influenza, adenovirus, respiratory syncytial virus

3. Occasionally Coxsackie virus, echovirus, parainfluenza, reovirus or herpes viruses (herpes simplex virus, cytomegalovirus)

4. Measles can lead to a severe bronchitis.

D. Nonviral cases

1. Mycoplasma

2. *Bordetella pertussis*

3. TWAR strain of *Chlamydia*—associated with severe laryngitis

4. Rarely pneumococcus and *haemophilius influenzae*

IV. Treatment

A. Generally symptomatic treatment

1. Cough suppressants

2. Fluids to prevent drying of secretions

3. Smoking cessation

4. Antihistamines and decongestants may help decrease cough and postnasal drip.

B. Antibiotics are generally useless for viral etiologies but are indicated if nonviral illness is suspected (constitutional syndrome of *Mycoplasma*, purulent sputum).

1. Erythromycin 500 mg q.i.d. for *Mycoplasma*

2. Ampicillin 500 mg q.i.d. or trimethyoprim/sulfamethoxazole 1 double-strength tablet b.i.d. for *H. influenzae, Streptococcus pneumoniae*

3. May substitute doxycycline 100 mg b.i.d. (also ampicillin/sulbactam, cefuroxime, cefixime, or quinolones), especially if TWAR suspected.
4. Doxycycline 100 mg b.i.d. for TWAR

C. Consider amantadine 100 mg b.i.d. to decrease severity of influenza if begun within 48 h of symptom onset (see chapter 69F).

D. Treatment should continue for 7–10 d.

E. Patients with severe, recurrent episodes of purulent bronchitis should receive pneumococcal and influenza vaccines.

V. Indications for Hospitalization

Usually not required unless the patient has significant underlying lung disease or other chronic illnesses that are being exacerbated by the acute infection.

VI. Annotated Bibliography

Dere WH. Acute bronchitis: results of US and European trials of antibiotic therapy. Am J Med 1992; 92(6A):53. Justification for antibiotic selection.
Gwaltney JM Jr. Acute bronchitis. In: Mandell GL, Douglas RG Jr. Bennett JE, eds. Principles and Practice of Infectious Diseases, 3rd ed. New York: Churchill Livingstone 1990:529–531. Thorough, easy to follow discussion of presentation and epidemiology.

69E Pneumonia

I. Clinical Presentation

A. General Information

1. Pneumonia is defined as inflammation in the lung parenchyma; synonymous with pneumonitis

2. Organisms can reach the lung via

    a. Inhalation
    b. Aspiration
    c. Hematogenous spread
    d. Direct spread from a contiguous site

3. Can be predisposed to pneumonia by

    a. Abnormal host defenses—immunocompromise, concomitant illnesses (diabetes, steroid usage), malnutrition, alcohol
    b. Altered consciousness—can lead to aspiration
    c. Ineffective cough—neuromuscular weakness, kyphoscoliosis, diaphragmatic dysfunction, following abdominal surgery
    d. Abnormal mucociliary transport—cigarette smoking, age, alcohol, chronic obstructive pulmonary diseases (COPD), bronchiectasis

4. Can be classified by type

    a. Typical (bacterial)
    b. Atypical pneumonia
    c. Aspiration pneumonia
    d. Aerobic gram-negative bacillary pneumonia
    e. Pneumonia with immunocompromise

5. Pneumonia has a mortality rate of approximately 13% in patients who require hospitalization.

B. History

1. Typical pneumonia generally presents with rapid onset of fever, chills, pleuritic chest pain, and productive cough.

2. Atypical pneumonia often presents with gradual onset of dry cough with prominent constitutional symptoms (headache, myalgia, nausea, diarrhea, fever).

3. Must obtain history of underlying diseases—diabetes, COPD, alcohol usage, HIV exposure/AIDS, heart failure, previous respiratory infection, smoking

4. Search for evidence of potential exposure to unusual organisms—travel, occupational/environmental exposures, hobbies, unusual activities, tuberculosis exposure

C. Physical Examination
1. Vital signs
    a. Temperature—should ideally be taken rectally because rapid mouth breathing may alter oral temperature
    b. Respiratory rate
    c. Pulse rate—generally rises by 10 beats/min for every degree of temperature elevation. Pulse temperature deficit (relative bradycardia) may suggest underlying cardiac conduction abnormality, viral disease, mycoplasma, psittacosis, tularemia, legionellosis, typhoid, hypothyroidism, specific drug therapy (β blockers)
    d. Blood pressure with orthostatic changes
2. Signs of cyanosis and accessory muscle use for breathing
3. Lung examination looking for signs of consolidation—bronchial breath sounds, rales, egophony, dullness to percussion
4. General physical examination to elicit clues to specific etiologies of pneumonia—adenopathy, hepatosplenomegaly, skin rashes

II. Diagnostic Approach

A. Although history and physical examination should suggest the diagnosis, other testing is useful not only to confirm the diagnosis but more importantly to guide treatment. (Table 69E-1)

B. Sputum should be obtained in all cases if possible.
1. Gross examination may suggest etiology (can also be misleading)
    a. Rust colored—*Pneumococcus*
    b. Currant jelly—*Klebsiella*
    c. Creamy yellow—*Staphylococcus*
    d. Green—*Pseudomonas*
    e. Bloody—*Klebsiella*, influenza, meningococcus, tuberculosis
    f. Foul smelling—anaerobes (aspiration)
2. Gram stain
    a. Adequate specimen shows < 10 epithelial cells and > 20 white blood cells per low-power (10x) field
    b. Gram stain can be more sensitive and specific for making diagnosis than culture, particularly with fastidious organisms (*Pneumococcus, Haemophilus influenzae, Moraxella*).
    c. Finding of polymorphonuclear leukocytes (PMN) *and* organisms suggests a bacterial pneumonia.
    d. Finding PMNs but no organisms suggests a nonbacterial process—viral, TB, mycoplasma, legionella, Q fever, psittacosis
    e. Presence of mononuclear cells may suggest legionella, mycoplasma
    f. Mixed microbial flora in an otherwise adequate specimen suggests aspiration pneumonia.

Part XIV: Infectious Diseases • 581

Table 69E-1. Characteristics of Various Pneumonias

Organism	Symptoms	Epidemiologic Clues	Chest X-Ray	Sputum	Labs	Diagnosis	Treatment Choice	Alternative
Streptococcus pneumoniae	Fever, cough Single rigor Rusty sputum Sinusitus	Recent URI COPD Alcoholism Diabetes Recent influenza	Lobar consolidation Bulging fissure	PMNs Lancet shape Gram ⊕ diplococci	Leukocytosis Leukopenia may occur Hypogammaglobulinemia	Gram stain Sputum culture (low yield) Blood culture (30%)	Pen V/C 500 mg PO q 6 h Pen G 1 million units IV q 4 h	Erythromycin 500 mg PO/IV q 6 h Cefazolin 1 g IV q 6-8 h
Staphylococci	Fever, rigors Pleuritic pain Purulent sputum	Recent influenza Nursing home resident IV drug abuser Nosocomial	Lobular to lobar consolidation Pneumatoceles Effusions	PMNs Gram ⊕ cocci in clumps Intracellular organisms	Leukocytosis	Gram stain Sputum culture Pleural fluid culture	Nafcillin 1-2 g IV q 4 h	Vancomycin Clindamycin 900 mg IV q 8 h
Streptococcus Group A/C	Fever Pleuritic pain Pharyngitis	Military recruits Recent influenza COPD	Bronchopneumonia Large effusion	PMNs Gram ⊕ cocci in long chains	Leukocytosis	Gram stain Sputum culture	Pen G 1 million units IV q 4 h	Erythromycin 500 mg PO/IV q 6 h
Klebsiella pneumoniae	Abrupt fever Rigors Dyspnea Currant jelly sputum	Nosocomial Alcoholism Diabetes UTI Nursing home resident	Lobar consolidation Bulging fissure Thick cavity	PMNs Gram ⊖ rods	Leukocytosis	Gram stain Sputum culture Blood culture (30%)	Cefazolin 2 g IV q 8 h or Cefotaxime 2 g IV q 8 h plus Aminoglycoside	Ampicillin/ Sulbactam 1.5-3 g IV q 6 h TMP/SMX 160 mg/800 mg b.i.d.
Haemophilus influenzae	Fever, chills Pleuritic pain Sinusitus	COPD Alcoholism Nursing home resident	Lobar consolidation Bulging fissure	PMNs Pleomorphic gram ⊖ coccobacilli	Leukocytosis Hypogammaglobulinemia	Gram stain Sputum culture Blood culture (75%)	Ampicillin/Clavulinate 500 mg PO q 8 h Cefaclor 500 mg q 8 h Cefotaxime 1-2g IV q 8 h	TMP/SMX 160 mg/800 mg b.i.d. Imipenem 0.5-1 g q 6 h Quinolones

582 • Manual of Office Medicine

Table 69E–1. Characteristics of Various Pneumonias (continued)

Organism	Symptoms	Epidemiologic Clues	Chest X-Ray	Sputum	Labs	Diagnosis	Treatment Choice	Alternative
Moraxella catarrhalis	Fever, cough Dyspnea	Recent URI or pneumonia COPD Immuno-compromise	Lobar pneumonia	PMNs Gram ⊖ cocci	Leukocytosis	Gram stain Sputum culture	Ampicillin/Clavulinate 500 mg q 8 h Erythromycin 500 mg q 6 h TMP/SMX 160 mg/ 800 mg b.i.d.	Cefazolin 1 g q 8 h Quinolones
Aspiration Gastric acid Inert matter Particulate matter Oropharyngeal secretions		Decreased gag Altered mental status or level of consciousness	ARDS Lobar obstruction Lobar consolidation in dependent segments Effusion and/or abcess form in 50%	PMNs Mixed flora	Leukocytosis	Clinical	Supportive if aspiration of gastric contents without signs of infection Suctioning of particulate matter Clindamycin 600–900 mg IV q 6 h Pen G 2 million units IV q 4 h	Cefoxitin 2 g IV q 6 h Ticarcillin/ Clavinulate 3.1 g IV q 4–8 h
Mycoplasma pneumoniae	Fever, cough Headache Chest pain Myalgias/ arthralgia Pharyngitis Bullous myringitis Diarrhea Erythema mutiforme Confusion Myocarditis	Children/young adults Summer/fall season Exposure to younger patients Group settings	Lower lobe reticular pattern progressing to patchy consolidation Effusion (20%) Bilateral hilar adenopathy	Neutrophils Monocytes No organism		Compliment fixation titer Cold agglutinins	Erythromycin 500 mg PO q 6 h (Self-limited disease; treatment may speed resolution)	Doxycycline 250 mg PO q 6 h

Table 69E-1. Characteristics of Various Pneumonias (continued)

Organism	Symptoms	Epidemiologic Clues	Chest X-Ray	Sputum	Labs	Diagnosis	Treatment Choice	Alternative
Legionnaires' Disease (*Legionella pneumophila*)	Fever, cough Chest/abdominal pain Myalgias Diarrhea Headache Confusion Ataxia Hemoptysis Relative bradycardia	Summer/fall months Elderly or immunocompromised Exposure to contaminated water source (air conditioning)	Lower lobe lobar consolidation Nodular consolidation Rapid progression	Few neutrophils Monocytes No organism	Hyponatremia Hypophosphatemia Elevated AST/ALT Microscopic hematuria Azotemia	Sputum Direct fluorescent antibody Compliment fixing antibody (4x rise or titer > 1:256)	Erythromycin 1 g IV q 6 h for 1 wk, then 500 mg PO q 6 h for 2 wk Add rifampin if severe	Clarithromycin 500 mg PO q 12 h Rifampin 600 mg IV/PO q 12 h
Chlamydia pneumoniae (TWAR)	Pretibial rash Fever, cough Mucoid sputum Laryngitis Pharyngitis Myalgias	College students Military recruits Young adults	Diffuse nonsegmental infiltrates or Single circumscribed infiltrates	Little sputum produced	Low-grade eosinophilia	IGM compliment fixation Immunofluorescent antibody	Erythromycin 500 mg PO q.i.d.	Doxycycline 100 mg PO b.i.d. Clarithromycin 500 mg PO q 12 h

Table 69E–1. Characteristics of Various Pneumonias (continued)

Organism	Symptoms	Epidemiologic Clues	Chest X-Ray	Sputum	Labs	Diagnosis	Treatment Choice	Alternative
Q Fever (*Coxiella brunetti*)	High fever Rigors Malaise Headache Vomiting Abdominal pain Hepatosplenomegaly Relative bradycardia Cardiac, ocular, neurologic involvement Thrombophlebitis	Exposure to milk or excrement of livestock (sheep, cattle, goats) Parturient cats	Patchy lower lobar infiltrates Linear atelectasis	Mononuclear cells No organism	Elevated AST/ALT	Antibody titer	Doxycycline 100 mg PO b.i.d.	Chloramphenicol 50 mg/kg/d in 4 divided doses Ciprofloxacin 500 mg PO b.i.d.
Psittacosis (*Chlamydia psittaci*)	Fever Nonproductive cough Headache, meningism Myalgias Splenomegaly Relative bradycardia Facial macules (Horder's spots)	Exposure to birds/bird droppings	Bronchopneumonia with patchy reticular infiltrates	Mononuclear cells No organisms	Increased AST/ALT Proteinuria Occasional DIC	Compliment fixing antibody Specific antibody (titer ≥1:32)	Tetracycline 2–3 g/d PO	Chloramphenicol 50 mg/kg/d in 4 divided doses Quinolones may be effective.

Table 69E-1. Characteristics of Various Pneumonias (continued)

Organism	Symptoms	Epidemiologic Clues	Chest X-Ray	Sputum	Labs	Diagnosis	Treatment Choice	Alternative
Tularemia (*Francisella tularensis*)	Fever, chills Malaise Adenopathy Nonproductive cough Maculopapular rash Cutaneous ulcers Hepatomegaly	Tick bite Exposure to infected animals (rabbits)	Patchy ovoid infiltrates Lobar infiltrates Bilateral hilar adenopathy Effusions		Elevated AST/ALT	Agglutination titers	Streptomycin 15–20 mg/kg/d IM	Tetracycline 1–2 g/d
Viral Pneumonia	URI Sore throat Rhinitis Low-grade fever Nonproductive cough Headache, myalgia Photophobia GI symptoms Relatively clear lungs Conjunctivitis (adenovirus)	Epidemics of influenza Exposure to infected children Military recruits (adenovirus)	Patchy or lobar disease Shifting infiltrates Perihilar infiltrates	PMNs No organisms		Throat swabs Rapid antigen screens	Ribavirin for life-threatening RSV Amantidine/Rimantidine for influenza Gancyclovir for HSV Acyclovir for HSV	Vaccines

Table 69E–1. Characteristics of Various Pneumonias (continued)

Organism	Symptoms	Epidemiologic Clues	Chest X-Ray	Sputum	Labs	Diagnosis	Treatment Choice	Alternative
Pneumocystis carinii	Dry cough Dyspnea on exertion Fever	AIDS Immunosuppression	Interstitial infiltrates Lobar consolidation Cavitation Effusion	Organism seen on silver stain	Leukopenia Elevated LDH	Methenamine silver stain	TMP/SMX 20 mg (TMP) kg d Pentamidine 4 mg/kg/d IV	Dapsone 100 mg/d with TMP 20 mg/kg/d Trimetrexate with leucovorin Clindamycin with primaquine Atovaquone 750 mg b.i.d.

ARDS, adult respiratory distress syndrome; AST/ALT, aspartate aminotransferase/alanine aminotransferase; COPD, chronic obstructive pulmonary disease; DIC, disseminated intravascular coagulation; GI, gastrointestinal; HSV, herpes simplex virus; LDH, lactate dehydrogenase; Pen, penicillin; RSV, respiratory syncytial virus; TWAR, ; URI, upper respiratory infection; UTI, urinary tract infection; TMP/SMX, trimethoprim/sulfamethoxazole

3. Culture
   a. Even a pure culture of a single organism can sometimes be due to contamination. Correlation to clinical setting and findings on Gram stain is useful.
   b. More fastidious organisms (*Pneumococcus, H. influenzae, Moraxella,* and *Legionella*) require proper technique and may not grow.
   c. A negative culture from an adequate sputum specimen should essentially exclude aerobic gram-negative organisms and staphylococci.
4. Blood culture
   a. 20–30% of patients with bacterial pneumonia will be bacteremic.
   b. A positive blood culture may be more specific for the infecting organism than a positive sputum culture.
5. Complete blood count with differential
   a. A normal white blood cell count does not exclude significant pulmonary infection.
   b. A predominant left shift in the differential may suggest serious illness.
   c. A predominance of lymphocytes or monocytes may suggest nonbacterial pneumonia.
   d. A predominance of eosinophils might suggest a noninfectious syndrome of pulmonary infiltrates with eosinophilia ("eosinophilic pneumonia") as well as chlamydial, coccidioidomycosis, and parasitic infiltration.
   e. Leukopenia may be seen in influenza, TB, and pneumocystis infection.
6. Chest x-ray
   a. *Cannot* define etiologic agent of infection but can help exclude noninfectious causes
   b. Several patterns may be seen.
      1) Lobar pneumonia—air bronchograms, "silhouette sign"
      2) Bronchopneumonia—segmental infiltrates without air bronchograms
      3) Interstitial pneumonia—linear or reticular pattern, often bilateral
      4) Aspiration pneumonia—involves lung segments that were most dependent at the time of the aspiration
         a) Patient upright—basilar segments of lower lobes
         b) Patient supine—posterior segments of the upper lobes or superior segments of the lower lobes, especially on the right
      5) Some suggestive findings of common infectious etiologies
         a) Bulging fissure—Klebsiella, Pneumococcus, Haemophilus organisms
         b) Shaggy heart border—pertussis
         c) Miliary pattern—TB, histoplasma, coccidioidomycosis
         d) Peripheral infiltrates—actimomycoses, Nocardia
         e) Perihilar infiltrates—viral pneumonias, Chlamydia, Pneumocystis carinii
         f) Rapidly progressing infiltrates—aspiration, Legionella, P. carinii, gram-negative pneumonia due to bacteremia
         g) Bilateral hilar adenopathy—histoplasma, tularemia, varicella, mycoplasma

h) Nodules—Legionella micdadei, *histoplasma, adenovirus, other fungi*
i) Cavitation
   i. Thick walled—staphylococci, *Klebsiella, Escherichia coli, Pseudomonas*, TB, fungi, anaerobes, septic emboli
   ii. Thin walled—TB, some fungi, *Pneumocystis*
j) Pleural effusions
   i. Small—pneumococcus, mycoplasma
   ii. Moderate—*Haemophilus influenzae*, tularemia
   iii. Large—group A streptococci

7. Arterial blood gas
   a. Hypoxemia suggests critical illness.
   b. Acidemia may suggest systemic sepsis or impending respiratory failure.

8. ECG
   a. Look for stress-induced arrhythmia or ischemia
   b. Underlying cardiac disease might suggest noninfectious etiologies

III. Differential Diagnosis

A. **Noninfectious**

1. Generally more insidious onset and afebrile—congestive heart failure, pulmonary malignancy

2. May be related to systemic illness—rheumatoid arthritis, systemic lupus erythematosus, sarcoidosis, vasculitis

3. May be part of a drug reaction—nitrofurantoin, methylsergide, chemotherapeutics, drug-induced lupus erythematosus

B. **Infectious (see Table 69E–1)**

1. Can be subdivided by findings on Gram stain

   a. Polymorphonuclear cells (PMNs) and gram-positive cocci
      1) Pneumococcus
         a) *10–50% of all community-acquired pneumonias*
         b) *Clinical picture generally includes abrupt fever, single shaking chill, and cough with rusty sputum; may see an associated outbreak of herpes simplex.*
         c) *Chest x-ray—lobar infiltrate*
         d) *Culture negative 45–50% of the time; Gram stain shows lancet-shaped diplococci (92% sensitive, 85% specific)*
      2) Staphylococci
         a) *About 10% of cases, tends to follow influenza or be seen as a nosocomial infection*
         b) *Clinical picture includes fever with rigors, pleuritic chest pain, and purulent sputum.*

c) Chest x-ray may show significant pulmonary necrosis with thin-walled cavities (pneumatocoeles).
    3) *Streptococcus pyogenes*
        a) Uncommon, tends to occur in children and among military recruits; may follow influenza
        b) Chest x-ray shows bronchopneumonia with large effusion.
  b. PMNs and gram-negative rods
    1) *Klebsiella pneumoniae*
        a) Most common gram-negative bacillary pneumonia (8–10% of all community-acquired cases)
        b) Often occurs in middle-aged or elderly patients with chronic underlying diseases—alcoholism, diabetes
        c) Clinical picture includes abrupt onset of fever with rigors, dyspnea, and productive cough with currant jelly sputum.
        d) Chest x-ray shows lobar consolidation, often of the upper lobes with bulging or sagging of the fissure.
    2) Other gram-negative rods
        a) Generally seen in hospitalized or immunocompromised patients
        b) 75% of patients become colonized with gram-negative rods within several days of hospitalization. Patients on respirators often develop Pseudomonas *infection.*
  c. Gram-negative cocci
    1) *H. influenzae*
        a) May be seen in younger, healthy patients, but most commonly seen in older patients with chronic obstructive pulmonary disease (COPD) or alcoholism; accounts for 5–15% of all nosocomial pneumonias.
        b) Clinical picture includes fever, chills, pleuritic chest pain, and productive cough.
        c) Sputum shows abundant white blood cells and pleomorphic coccobacilli.
    2) *Moraxella catarrhalis*
        a) Associated with COPD or immunocompromise, often follows a Haemophilus *influenzae or pneumococcal pneumonia*
        b) Clinical picture includes fever, dyspnea, productive cough, and an elevated leukocyte count.
        c) The usual presentation is bronchitis or a lobar pneumonia.
    3) *Neisseria meningitidis*
        a) Often occurs after a respiratory infection and in military recruits
        b) Generally not associated with meningitis or cutaneous signs of meningococcemia
  d. Mixed flora with PMNs
    1) May be seen in bronchitis or aspiration
    2) Aspiration may involve distinct syndromes
        a) *Aspiration of toxic fluids causing a chemical pneumonitis*
            i. Gastric acid, acid, bile, mineral oil, hydrocarbons, alcohol
            ii. Lung injury occurs within seconds with superinfection 48–72 h later.
            iii. Treatment generally not useful unless signs of true infection occur

- b) *Aspiration of inert substances*
  - i. Water, blood, buffered gastric fluid
  - ii. Generally does not lead to infection
- c) *Aspiration of particulate matter—obstruction can lead to pneumonia*
- d) *Aspiration of oropharyngeal secretions*
  - i. Bacterial-laden secretions
  - ii. Generally occurs in patients with altered mental status or decreased level of consciousness
  - iii. Symptoms develop over several days

e. PMNs with no organisms seen (treatable causes)
  1) *Mycoplasma pneumoniae*
     - a) *Predominantly young patients (age 15–30), occasionally older patients*
     - b) *Typically mild illness with myalgias, headache, diarrhea, fever, and nonproductive cough. Pleuritic pain, rigors, and hemoptysis infrequently occur.*
     - c) *5% get bullous myringitis.*
     - d) *Chest x-ray shows segmental bronchopneumonia, often bilateral.*
     - e) *Diagnosis is confirmed through serology and/or cold agglutinin levels.*
  2) Legionella
     - a) *Normal and immunocompromised hosts (renal transplants, elderly men); often follows exposure to contaminated aerosols (air conditioner, hospital water supplies)*
     - b) *Clinical picture includes myalgias, headache, fever, pleuritic pain, and nonproductive cough.*
     - c) *Extrapulmonary features include abdominal pain, diarrhea, renal failure, mental status changes, hyponatremia, hypophosphatemia, and increased creatine phosphokinase.*
     - d) *Diagnosis is via culture, direct fluorescence antibody, or use of antibody titer*
  3) Q fever—*Coxiella burnetii*
     - a) *Occupational exposure to livestock*
     - b) *Clinical picture includes headache, fever, chills, myalgias, chest pain, and nonproductive cough. Unlike other rickettsial illnesses, there is no rash.*
     - c) *Can lead to culture-negative endocarditis*
     - d) *Diagnosis is via an antibody compliment fixation test.*
  4) Psittacosis—*Chlamydia psittaci*
     - a) *Exposure to infected birds*
     - b) *Clinical picture includes severe headache, myalgias, nonproductive cough, and splenomegaly.*
     - c) *Diagnosis is via serologic testing.*
  5) Tularemia—*Francisella tularensis*
     - a) *Follows tick bite or exposure to infected animals (rabbits)*
     - b) *Clinical picture includes pneumonia and pleural effusion with a cutaneous ulcer and regional adenopathy.*

6) Nonbacterial pneumonias
   a) *Influenza*
      i. Rapid onset of fever, headache, and myalgias (can progress to encephalitis or myocarditis)
      ii. Pneumonia can be primary or secondary to bacterial superinfection (staphylococci, pneumococci).
   b) *Adenovirus*
      i. Common in military recruits
      ii. May be associated with conjunctivitis and perihilar infiltrates
   c) *Respiratory syncytial virus*
      i. Can cause upper and occasionally lower respiratory infections in adults
      ii. Often follows exposure to infants
      iii. Diagnosis is via isolation of virus from secretions.
7) Tuberculosis
   a) *Consider in any patient whose Gram stain shows no organism*
   b) *Often see insidious progressive illness with night sweats, weight loss, and cough*
   c) *Chest x-ray may show apical infiltrates or scarring, nodular densities, cavitation, or miliary spread.*
8) *P. carinii* pneumonia
   a) *Immunocompromised host, especially HIV infected*
   b) *See progressive dyspnea with exertional oxygen desaturation with fever and nonproductive cough*
   c) *Chest x-ray typically shows interstitial infiltrates, but may show lobar consolidation, cavitation, and effusions.*
   d) *Characteristically see elevated serum lactate dehydrogenase*
   e) *Diagnosis is via silver stain of secretions.*

IV. Treatment

A. Initial treatment is generally empirical based on historical and physical clues and Gram stain.

B. Generally, otherwise healthy patients who are not seriously ill and who have nondiagnostic sputum can be managed with

1. Erythromycin 500 mg PO q.i.d. for 10–14 d

2. Clarithromycin 500 mg PO b.i.d., which is generally better tolerated and may be more effective than erythromycin

3. Ofloxacin 400 mg PO b.i.d., which has better streptococcal coverage than ciprofloxacin

C. More seriously ill patients or patients requiring hospitalization

1. In all cases possible, therapy should be guided by the clinical scenario and sputum Gram stain (Table 69E-1).

2. Empiric therapy when unable to direct therapy or before laboratory data available.
   a. If bacterial etiology suspected, broad-spectrum therapy
      1) Ampicillin/sulbactam 1.5–3.0 mg IV q 6 h with an aminoglycoside
      2) Ticarcillin/clavulinate 300 mg/kg/d divided q 4 h with an aminoglycoside
      3) Ceftazidime 2 g IV q 8 h with an aminoglycoside
      4) Cefotaxime 2 g IV q 8 h with an aminoglycoside
      5) Ceftriaxone 1–2 g IV qd with an aminoglycoside
      6) Aztreonam 2 g IV q 8 h or imipenem 500 mg IV q 6 h with an aminoglycoside
   b. If an atypical pneumonia is suspected—erythromycin 0.5–1 g IV q 6 h

D. Repeated chest x-ray is generally not helpful because radiographic resolution generally lags behind clinical resolution (up to 3–6 weeks)

E. Treatment is generally continued for 10–14 d (21 d for *Legionella* and *Pneumocystis* pneumonia); generally can change IV therapy to PO as the patient improves.

F. All patients with significant predisposing illness (COPD, diabetes, alcoholism) or who are elderly or immunocompromised should be considered to receive polyvalent pneumococcal vaccine once and yearly influenza vaccine.

V. Indications for Hospitalization

A. Severe Illness

1. Hypotension
2. Significant tachycardia
3. Altered mental status
4. Respiratory distress, hypoxemia
5. Suppurative complications—empyema, metastatic infection
6. Severe hemotologic or metabolic abnormalities—neutropenia, hyponatremia, azotemia

B. High Risk for Significant Complications

1. Immunodeficiency
2. Airway obstruction
3. Suspicion of virulent organisms—staphylococci, gram-negative bacilli

C. Suspicion of opportunistic or unusual infection

D. Underlying diseases that may reduce host defenses or pulmonary reserve

E. Consider hospitalization for patients who may not comply with treatment or follow-up

VI. Indications for Referral to a Pulmonologist

A. Recurrent pulmonary infections

B. Pulmonary infections that fail to resolve

C. Suspected airway obstruction

D. Significant persistent symptoms (cough, dyspnea) following apparent resolution of infection

VII. Annotated Bibliography

Johnson DH, Cunha BA. Atypical pneumonias. Postgrad Med 1993;93:69–82.

Levison ME, Paukey GA. Pneumonia: choosing empiric therapy. Patient Care 1992;January:129–148. A quick but thorough review of differentiating the etiology of pneumonia and selecting treatment.

Montgomery JL. Pneumonia. Pearls for interpreting patients' radiographs. Postgrad Med 1991;90:58–73. A brief but useful overview of the various x-ray findings in pneumonia.

Pomilla PV, Brown RB. Outpatient treatment of community acquired pneumonia in adults. Arch Intern Med 1994;154:1793–1802. A concise, thorough review of the presentation, etiology, and treatment of community-acquired pneumonia.

Tuazon CU, Decker CF. 'Atypical' pneumonias: not so atypical anymore. J Respir Dis 1993;14:1279–1303. A good review of features that help differentiate among the atypical pneumonias.

69F Influenza

I. Clinical Presentation

A. General Information

1. Epidemic, self-limited febrile illness in winter months (October to April)
2. Etiology
    a. The A strain of influenza is responsible for most significant outbreaks. B strain generally causes sporadic, milder outbreaks, typically in group setting; C strain is widely isolated but may not be responsible for illness.
    b. Strains vary by internal proteins (M, NP, P) found in the envelope and nucleocapsid.
    c. Subtypes within each strain vary by surface glyoproteins possessing hemoglutinin (H) or neuramidase (N) activity (three hemaglutinins and two neuramidases have been isolated).
    d. Antigenic variation allows virus to remain infectious. Antigenic drift occurs almost seasonally and is due to point mutations in the RNA generally coding for H. Antigenic shift is less common and produces completely new H and/or N resulting from genetic rearrangement when two viruses coinfect a cell. More than one subtype may circulate together.
3. Epidemiology
    a. Epidemics are localized outbreaks of influenza that peak in 2–3 wk and generally last 5–6 wk. Overall disease rate is approximately 10–20% but rises to 40–50% in some settings.
    b. Pandemics are more widespread outbreaks typically caused by a new viral type to which there is no immunity.
    c. Transmission is via aerosal route. Virus attaches to respiratory epithelia and replicates for 4–6 h prior to viral release and subsequent cell death. Time to onset of illness is approximately 18–72 h.

B. Symptoms

1. Very abrupt onset
2. Primarily due to cell death with some contribution of interferon, which appears 2–3 d into illness
3. Predominate symptoms are headache and myalgias associated with arthralgias, fever, chills, malaise, photophobia, tearing, and painful eye movements. Respiratory symptoms (dry cough, nasal discharge and sore throat) are generally mild.
4. Early symptoms generally correlate with fever and decrease in 3–5 d at which time respiratory symptoms increase and persist 3–4 d.

C. Physical Examination

1. Early on, patient appears toxic and flushed.
2. Fever peaks within about 12 h from onset and gradually wanes.
3. Cervical adenopathy and mild mucosal hyperemia without exudates are common.
4. Complications
   a. Pulmonary
      1) Primary viral pneumonia—generally occurs in patients with underlying cardiac disease especially rheumatic mitral stenosis but has also been described in other chronic diseases and pregnancy
      2) See rapid development of significant fever, cough, dyspnea, and cyanosis with findings consistent with acute respiratory distress syndrome and hypoxemia
   b. Secondary bacterial pneumonia (superinfection)
      1) Usually occurs in the elderly or in the face of chronic diseases
      2) Patients recover from typical flu then represent in 1–4 d with symptoms/signs of bacterial pneumonia
      3) Typical pathogens are *Streptococcus pneumoniae*, *Staphylococcus aureus* and *Haemophilus influenzae*.
   c. Mixed pneumonias
      1) Milder or localized forms of either pulmonary or secondary bacterial pneumonia or features of both
      2) Localized viral pneumonia may be confused with *Mycoplasma*.
   d. Exacerbations of chronic obstructive pulmonary disease
5. Nonpulmonary complications
   a. Myositis, myoglobinuria—mostly children
   b. Myocarditis, pericarditis—rare
   c. Transverse myelitis, Guillan-Barre syndrome—unclear relationship to influenza
   d. Reyes syndrome
      1) More common with influenza B and in children under 16; questionably associated with aspirin use
      2) Normal influenzal illness followed in 1–2 d by nausea, vomiting, liver function abnormalities, and encephalopathy
      3) 10% mortality

II. Differential Diagnosis

Can present similar to and can be mimicked by many viral illnesses that produce headache, fever, myalgia and cough.

III. Diagnostic Approach

A. Classic symptoms presenting in context of epidemics should be diagnostic.

B. Other tests are useful in confirming the diagnosis early in the course of epidemics.
1. Virus may be isolated from throat washings, nasal specimens, and sputum in the first 2–3 d of illness.
2. Serologic testing (enzyme-linked immunosorbent assay [ELISA]) may be confirmatory but requires a convalescent titer 10–14 d following the acute illness.

IV. Treatment

A. Acute Management
1. Mainstay of care involves symptomatic treatment, with rest, fluids, antipyretics, analgesics, and cough suppressants. Aspirin should probably be avoided.
2. Amantadine 100–200 mg daily for 3–5 d may reduce the duration of symptoms of influenza A by 50% if begun within 48 h of onset. About 10% get CNS side effects (anxiety, insomnia, poor concentration). Dosage must be adjusted for renal failure.
3. Rimantadine 100 mg daily is similar to amantadine but has fewer side effects and does not require dosage adjustment.
4. Aerosolized ribavirin may be useful.
5. Primary viral pneumonias require intensive supportive care with supplemental oxygen.
6. Secondary bacterial and mixed pneumonias require treatment based on culture or directed empirically against typical pathogens.

B. Prophylaxis
1. Vaccine
   a. Inactivated influenza virus vaccine, usually trivalent, usually made up of most recently circulating subtypes of influenza A and B
   b. 80% effective in reducing the incidence of disease, 25% may have mild local reactions, 1–2% develop low-grade fever and systemic symptoms peaking at 8–12 h after injection.
   c. Priorities for vaccination
      1) Persons with chronic cardiopulmonary conditions and residents of chronic care facilities
      2) Health care workers, especially those with extensive contact with high-risk patients
      3) Patients over 65 and those with other chronic diseases
      4) Any person wishing vaccination
   d. Must be given annually and is contraindicated in persons allergic to eggs

e. Vaccine administration should begin in the fall and continue until epidemics have peaked.
f. Vaccine cannot cause influenza, is safe in pregnancy, and can be administered simultaneously with pneumococcal vaccine. False positive ELISA test for HIV has been reported to occur for up to 6 wk following vaccination.

2. Amantidine/rimantadine
   a. Equally effective in preventing influenza A; neither is effective against influenza B.
   b. Amantadine 200 mg daily or rimantadine 100 mg daily can be given
      1) For the season (or part thereof, eg, 5–7 wk) to patients in high-risk groups who have contraindications to vaccination, OR
      2) When vaccine is unavailable, OR
      3) In patients who are immunocompromised and may not have adequate response to vaccination
   c. May be administered for 2 wk following vaccination if local influenza outbreaks have begun
   d. Resistance can develop.

V. Indications for Hospitalization

Hospitalization is indicated in patients who require supportive care, hydration, antibiotics, or other measures.

VI. Annotated Bibliography

Belts RF, Douglas RF Jr. Orthomyxoviridae: influenza virus. In: Mandell GL, Douglas RF Jr, Bennet JE, eds. Principles and Practice of Infectious Disease, 3rd ed. New York: Churchill Livingstone; 1990:1306–1325. Somewhat difficult to follow but thorough review of virology and presentation.

Centers for Disease Control. Prevention and control of influenza. Part I. Vaccines. MMWR 1989; 38:297–298, 303–311. Detailed discussion of vaccine usage.

Douglas RF Jr. Prophylaxis and treatment of influenza. N Engl J Med 1990; 322(7):1993–1950. Excellent overview of usage of antiviral drugs and vaccine.

Chapter 70: Selected Skin Infections

Richard G. Paluzzi

70A Animal Bites

I. Clinical Presentation

A. General Information
1. Animal bites account for about 1% of all emergency room visits.
2. Most commonly due to dog bites, particularly large dogs.
3. Injuries can be crush type, lacerations, avulsions, punctures, and scratches. Cat wounds are generally small punctures and scratches.
4. Most bites are to extremities. Facial bites typically occur in young children.
5. Infection risk increases with age over 50, delayed treatment, puncture wounds, and wounds to the upper extremities. Even with treatment, 15–30% of wounds become infected.

B. Signs and Symptoms
1. Generally see localized cellulitis with pain and foul discharge.
2. Puncture wounds may become abscessed.
3. Less than 20% develop high fever, lymphangitis, and regional adenopathy.
4. Bites can penetrate to and cause infection in bones and joints.
5. Significant sequelae of bite infections are uncommon but include signs of sepsis (particularly if immunosuppressed), meningitis, endocarditis, and brain abscess.
6. *Pasturella multocida* is a common pathogen in dog and cat bites. This organism can cause significant wound swelling within hours, associated with serosanguinous drainage. One third of patients get regional adenopathy.

II. Bacteriology

A. Pathogens can come from skin flora, animal oral flora, and the environment.

B. Dog oral flora includes *P. multocida* (20% of all bites develop infections), *Staphylococcus aureus*, coagulase-negative staphylococci, and others.

C. Cat bites often lead to *P. multocida* infection.

D. Monkey bites can transmit B virus (herpes virus simiae).

E. Gram stain of wound is a specific but nonsensitive predictor of bacterial growth.

III. Management

A. All bites should be irrigated and debrided.

B. Tetanus toxoid (Td 0.5 mL IM) should be given.

C. Clinically clean wounds can be closed primarily. (See Appendix A)

D. Hand bites and all nontrivial bites should receive antibiotic prophylaxis.

1. Amoxicillin-clavulinate (Augmentin) 500 mg t.i.d. for 5 d is treatment of choice.

2. Doxycycline 100 mg b.i.d. may be substituted.

E. 15–30% of bites develop infection despite treatment.

IV. Rabies

A. In the United States, 40% of all cases of rabies are due to skunk bites. Other reservoirs include raccoons, foxes, coyotes, bobcats, and bats. Rodents and rabbits are uncommon sources and dogs are rare causes.

B. Should suspect rabies if the animal or the victim exhibits hydrophobia, aerophobia, agitated behavior, or unexplained myelitis/encephalitis in endemic areas.

C. 20% of cases have no known exposure.

D. Virus can be isolated from saliva by day 2 but antibody production requires 1–2 wk.

E. Risk is decreased by vigorous wound cleansing.

F. Rabies is uniformly fatal if untreated by day 3.

G. Postexposure prophylaxis is with human diploid cell rabies vaccine 1 mL IM on days 0, 3, 7, 14, 28 (day 0, 3 if previously vaccinated).

V. Human Bites

A. Generally lead to higher complication and infection rates than animal bites.

B. Most infections are due to self-inflicted bites leading to paronychia and infections of the lip.

C. Risk of infection is related to extent and depth of damage.

D. Most infections are polymicrobial; most common isolate is *Viridens* strep but also see *S. aureus*, Bacteroides fragilis, and gram-positive oral anaerobes.

E. All wounds should be Gram stained, cleansed, and debrided.

F. Antibiotic of choice is amoxicillin-clavulinate (Augmentin) 500 mg t.i.d. or a penicillinase-resistant penicillin combined with penicillin G or erythromycin q.i.d. or clindamycin 150 mg q.i.d.

VI. Indications for Referral

A. Large deep and contaminated wounds should be surgically debrided.

B. Hand wounds with any evidence of compartment compromise should be evaluated by a surgeon, preferably a hand surgeon.

C. Facial wounds may require closure by a plastic surgeon.

VII. Indications for Hospitalization

A. Patients presenting with significant cellulitis following a bite wound may require hospitalization. (The rapidly developing cellulitis of *P. multocida* often responds well to oral antibiotics.)

B. Patients with bite wounds causing threatened compartment syndrome or neurovascular compromise of an extremity should be hospitalized for observation.

C. Bite wounds to fingers must be observed closely for the development of osteomyelitis or tenosynovitis.

VIII. Annotated Bibliography

Dire DJ. Emergency Management of dog and cat bite wounds. Emerg Med Clin North Am 1992;10:719.
Goldstein EJ. Bite wounds and infections. Clin Infect Dis 1992;14(3):633–638. A thorough review of management of animal and human bite wounds.
Rest JG, Goldstein EJC. Management of human and animal bite wounds. Emerg Med Clin North Am 1985;3:117.
Weber DJ, Hansen AR. Infections resulting from animal bites. Infect Dis Clin North Am 1991;5(3):663–680. Detailed Review of the epidemiology, presentation, and treatment of animal bites with a detailed discussion of infections due to *P. multocida*.

70B Cellulitis and Erysipelas

I. Localized Infections and Pyodermas

A. Impetigo

1. Generally a Group A streptococcal infection of facial skin in children but may occur in adults. Occasionally results in poststreptococcal glumerulonephritis.
2. Begins as vesiculopustular lesion in area of minor trauma. Vesicles rupture resulting in a superficial erosion with a characteristic honey-gold crust. Regional adenopathy can occur.
3. Lesion is pruritic and can be spread by contact and scratching.
4. Treatment
    a. Soak off crusts with cool compresses.
    b. Penicillin is drug of choice—benzathine penicillin G 1–2 million units IM (300–600,000 units in children) as a single dose or penicillin VK 500 mg q.i.d.
    c. Alternatives—erythromycin 500 mg q.i.d. *OR* cephelexin 500 mg q.i.d. for 10 d
    d. Topical clindamycin or erythromycin may inhibit spread.
5. Staphylococcal impetigo forms flaccid bullae that rupture, resulting in varnish-like crust.
    a. Treatment consists of dicloxacillin 500 mg q.i.d. *OR* erythromycin 500 mg q.i.d. *OR* clindamycin 300 mg q.i.d. *OR* cephalexin 500 mg q.i.d. for 10 d

B. Folliculitis

1. Small pruritic papules with central pustules at base of hair follicles; common in bearded areas
2. Causes
    a. Vast majority are staphylococcal
    b. May be due to *Pseudomonas aeruginosa* following hot tub/whirlpool usage. See appearance of various stages of pruritic papulourticurial lesions, which form pustules. Often associated with otitis externa and mild constitutional symptoms
    c. *Candida* in intertriginous areas of patients on antibiotics or steroids; see primary lesions with pruritic satellites
3. Treatment
    a. Typical staphylococcal disease generally responds to warm compresses or frequent washings with chlorhexidine soaps or selenium sulfide shampoo. Severe cases may be treated as above for impetigo.
    b. Hot tub folliculitis is generally self-limited (5 d).
    c. *Candida* disease usually responds to topical 1% clotrimazole, miconazole, or ketoconazole. Severe areas may require oral ketoconazole 200 mg daily until resolved.

C. Furuncle

1. Extensive, deep infection of a hair follicle (carbuncle if involves multiple follicles with multiple septated sites of drainage); typically on buttocks, neck, back and thighs
2. Primarily staphylococcal; increased risk with obesity, diabetes
3. May lead to fever, cellulitis, occasionally bacteremia and cavernous sinus thrombosis if on the face
4. Treatment
    a. Warm compresses 3–4 times daily. Lesion may resolve spontaneously or form a central necrotic white area ("head"), which then requires drainage
    b. In patients with fever, cellulitis, facial/perineal lesions, or risk for endocarditis should add antibiotics as above for impetigo.
    c. Recurrent folliculitis or furunculosis may respond to frequent washing of hands and area of lesions, intranasal bacitracin to decrease staphylococcal carriage, frequent changes of towels/bed linens and/or prophylaxis with twice daily doses of antibiotics.

D. Hidradenitis Supprativa

1. Recurrent abscesses of sweat glands of the axilla and perineum following ductal plugging
2. Can lead to sinus tracts and scarring
3. Generally secondarily infected with staphylococci or streptococci and occasionally gram-negative bacilli or anaerobes
4. Treatment
    a. Hot compresses followed by incision and drainage (if persistent)
    b. Antibiotics as above for impetigo
    c. Frequent occurrences may respond to daily usage of topical clindamycin.

E. Erythrasma

1. Waxing and waning superficial red-brown macula patches in genitocrural area
2. Pruritic and slowly spreading
3. Increased risk in males, diabetics, and obese patients
4. Caused by *Corynebacterium minutissimum*, which fluoresces coral red under Wood's light
5. Treatment
    a. Erythromycin 250 mg q.i.d. for 14 d
    b. Topical treatment with erythromycin or 2% clindamycin applied b.i.d. for 14 d

II. Cellulitis and Erysipelas

A. Clinical Presentation
1. General information
   a. Acute spreading infection of the skin
      1) Cellulitis involves subcutaneous tissues.
      2) Erysipelas is superficial with prominent lymphatic involvement.
   b. Predisposing factors include trauma, wounds, or underlying skin diseases. Rarely due to hematogenous spread from elsewhere.
   c. Erysipelas commonly occurs in areas of venous stasis, lymphatic obstruction, or edema and tends to recur in same area. Risk is increased in diabetics and alcoholics.
   d. Most commonly caused by group A streptococci or staphylococci. Enteric organisms may infect perineal skin and anaerobes are often involved in infections of foot wounds in diabetics, traumatic wounds, and deep abscess.
   e. Occasionally leads to bacteremia and/or thrombophlebitis
2. History
   a. Rapidly developing local pain followed by malaise, fever and chills
   b. Need to question about even minor trauma, surgical incisions, and previous history of processes leading to abnormal venous/lymphatic drainage (vein harvest, lymphedema)
   c. Need to assess other medical conditions such as diabetes, systemic lupus erythematosus, immunocompromise, medications (steroids) and exposures (fresh water, salt water), which may predispose to unusual pathogens (see section II-B-4)
3. Physical examination
   a. Cellulitis
      1) Erythematous, hot swollen skin with no clear demarcation or raising of edges
      2) Lymphagitis (red streaking) is more common with streptococcal infection.
      3) Regional adenopathy and fever are common.
      4) May see local abscess and skin necrosis
   b. Erysipelas
      1) Skin is painful, bright red, edematous, and indurated (peau d'orange).
      2) Borders are very sharply demarcated.
      3) Lymphangitis is common.
   c. In all forms should look for portal of entry including macerated interdigital areas due to tinea pedis

B. Differential Diagnosis
1. Phlebitis and other inflammatory skin conditions—generally lack impressive fever, lymphangitis, adenopathy, and leukocytosis. Pain is much less localized with deep venous thrombosis.

2. Venous stasis—may be associated with lipodermatosclerosis, which is red and fairly well demarcated but not associated with warmth, fever, lymphangitis, adenopathy, or leukocytosis.
3. Inflammatory carcinomas and lymphatic cutaneous metastases
4. Specific types of cellulitis
   a. Postsaphenous vein harvest (coronary bypass)
      1) Cellulitis/lymphangitis in distribution of venectomy
      2) Prominent fever, chills, toxicity
      3) Often predisposed by tinea pedis
      4) Leads to further lymphatic obstruction and recurrences
   b. Postoperative
      1) Group A streptococcal infection spreads quickly (6–48 h postoperatively) with early bacteremia and toxicity. Staphylococcal infection spreads slowly (days).
   c. Salt water exposure
      1) *Vibro* species
      2) Leads to bullae, necrotic ulcers, and occasionally bacteremia and extensive necrosis
   d. Fresh water exposure
      1) *Aeromonas hydrophilia*
   e. Immunocompromise and diabetes
      1) Various gram-negative organisms and fungi
      2) Pneumococcal cellulitis is a rare occurrence, particularly in patients with systemic lupus erythematosus. Looks like erysipelas
      3) Peripheral vascular disease and diabetes predispose to infection of the feet. Staphylococci and streptococci are the most common pathogens but incidence of gram-negative organisms, enterococci, and anaerobes is increased.
   f. Workers with salt water fish, shell fish, poultry meat, and hides
      1) Erysipelothrix rhusiopathine
      2) Primarily occurs in summer months
      3) Painful violaceous areas with distinct raised borders, peripheral spread, and central clearing—erysipeloid

C. **Diagnostic Approach**
1. Leukocytosis is common.
2. Aspirate of leading edge of area with or without saline instillation yields organism in only 10%.
3. Skin biopsy is diagnostic in 25%.
4. Culture of obvious break in skin in area of cellulitis is helpful in about one third of cases (up to 88% in one series).
5. Blood cultures should be drawn in all patients who appear systemically ill/toxic.
6. Treatment is almost always empirical.

D. Treatment

1. Elevation and immobility of affected part may decrease swelling.
2. Cooling may initially decrease pain and should be followed in approximately 24 h by local heat.
3. Antibiotics
   a. Mild cases—oral treatment with dicloxacillin 500 mg q.i.d., cephalexin 500 mg q.i.d., erythromycin 500 mg q.i.d. *OR* ciprofloxacin 500 mg b.i.d. (may miss some streptococci) for 7–14 d based on clinical response
   b. Severe cases—IV therapy with cefazolin 1 g q 6–8 h, nafcillin 1–2 g q 4 h, clindamycin 600 mg q 8 h or vancomycin. Ciprofloxacin may be substituted but misses some streptococci. Treat until afebrile and cellulitis subsiding and then change to oral therapy for 7–14 d.
   c. In diabetic patients with peripheral vascular disease and immunocompromised patients, consideration should be given to broad-spectrum coverage with cefoxitin, clindamycin with ciprofloxacin, ticarcillin/calavulinate, or a penicillinase-resistant penicillin and an aminoglycoside (Aztreonam) and clindamycin (or vancomycin)
   d. Suspected *Vibrio*—tetracycline with an aminoglycoside
   e. *Aeromonas*—ciprofloxacin, norfloxacin, trimethoprim/sulfamethoxazole
4. Interdigital fungi should be treated with topical clotrimazole or miconazole.
5. Tetanus prophylaxis should be updated if not received within last 10 y.
6. Reduction of chronic edema with diuretics or compression stockings may reduce recurrences
7. Frequent recurrences, especially in patients with venectomies or lymphedema, may require prophylaxis with single or twice daily doses of the same antibiotics used for treatment.

E. Indications for Referral to Surgery or Dermatology

Pyodermas or abscesses requiring extensive incision and drainage

F. Indications for Hospitalization

1. More than trivial involvement of face or perineum
2. Systemic toxicity, high fevers, rigors
3. Uncontrolled diabetes
4. Significant debilitation or immunocompromise

III. Annotated Bibliography

Haynes H, Branch WT Jr. Dermatology in primary care. In: Branch WT Jr, ed. Office Practice of Medicine, 2nd ed. Philadelphia: WB Saunders; 1987: 1154–1181. A very short section regarding bacterial skin infections, which is surprisingly informative.

Swartz MN. Cellulitis and superficial infections. In: Mandel GL, Douglas RG Jr, Bennett JG, eds. Principles and Practice of Infectious Disease, 3rd ed. New York: Churchill Livingstone 1990;796–807. A somewhat difficult to follow overview of skin infections with good guides to treatment.

70C Herpes Simplex

I. Clinical Presentation

A. General Information

1. Approximately 90% of U.S. population is infected at some time with herpes simplex virus (HSV).
2. About 10–15% experience recurrent disease.
3. HSV is an icosohedral double-stranded DNA virus with lipid membrane and 40 antigenic types.
   a. HSV-1—causative agent of most herpetic infections of oral, ocular, and other facial structures (infections about the waist); can infect any skin site
   b. HSV-2—causative agent of most genital herpetic infections (infections below the waist).
4. Changing sexual practices may be altering the classic site specificity.
5. Spread is via skin to skin or secretion to skin contact with latency within sensory nerve ganglia. Recurrent infection is due to endogenous reactivation.

B. Symptoms

1. Can see infection at any skin site.
2. Primary oral infection
   a. Majority due to HSV-1.
   b. Generally a mild to asymptomatic infection in childhood with an incubation of 3–20 d.
   c. Can present with malaise, fever and sore throat
3. Recurrent oral infection (herpes labalis)
   a. Occurs in 20–40% of population
   b. Often triggered by sunlight, fever, trauma, menses, stress, or trigeminal nerve manipulation
   c. Often preceded by a short prodrome (usually < 6 h) of burning, tingling, or itching, followed by pain at the site of the outbreak
   d. Can cause photophobia and excessive tearing with ocular involvement
4. Primary genital infection
   a. 70–95% are due to HSV-2.
   b. Generally occurs during sexually active periods of life
   c. Typically presents with fever, anorexia, malaise, and pain at the site of the eruption with inguinal adenopathy. Incubation averages 2–7 d.
   d. Can see painful sacral radiculopathies
   e. Severity of symptoms varies, but they tend to be less severe in patients previously infected with HSV-1.

f. Anal/perianal HSV-2 infection can lead to pain, itching, and tenesmus-also associated with fever, chills, headache, sacral paresthesias, and urinary difficulty.

5. Recurrent genital infection

   a. Tends to be less severe than primary infection but tends to be more severe in women than men
   b. Prodrome may only last several hours.
   c. Healing occurs in 6–10 d but viral shedding resolves more slowly in women and may occur between attacks.

6. Primary finger (periungual) infection—Whitlow.

   a. Generally involves index finger with local pain, neuralgia, and regional adenopathy
   b. HSV-1 in health care workers, HSV-2 in the community

C. Physical Examination

1. Lesions

   a. Vesicular lesions on an erythematous base
   b. Recurrent eruptions are often stereotypical.
   c. Genital lesions
      1) Typically occur on the glans or shaft of the penis, on the vulva or cervix, in the vagina, on the skin of the perineum, perianal area, or buttocks
      2) 10–20% of patients get extragenital lesions.
      3) Genital lesions may persist for days in men or ulcerate in women, exuding a grayish exudate.
   d. Oral lesions
      1) Typically occur at vermillion border of the lip, in the anterior nares, or on the hard palate
      2) Oral lesions generally ulcerate and crust within 48 h. Healing generally occurs in 8–10 d but may take weeks.

2. Adenopathy

   a. Local and regional adenopathy are not uncommon.

3. Ocular disease

   a. Can involve any layer of the eye, leading to keratitis, blepharitis, conjunctivitis, and uveitis
   b. Can see dendritic ulceration and stromal invasion of the cornea
   c. Visual acuity may be compromised and excessive tearing and photophobia may occur.

D. Complications

1. Urethral stricture and labial fusion have been reported.
2. Recurrent disease can occur in the extremities, leading to several neuralgia, edema and lymphangitis.

3. Allergic, cutaneous, and mucous membrane disorders can occur. Up to 75% of cases of erythema multiforme follow HSV infections.
4. HSV-2 may be causally related to some cases of cervical cancer.
5. HSV infection of patients with AIDS can lead to progressive perianal ulcers, colitis, esophagitis, pneumonia, and neurologic disease.
6. Encephalitis
   a. Hemorrhagic necrotizing disease of temporal lobes usually caused by spread of HSV-1 infection.
   b. Influenza-like prodrome followed by headaches, fever, behavioral change, speech disturbance, focal seizures, and olfactory hallucinations.
   c. Can lead to death within days. Overall mortality range is 60–80% and < 10% escape some neurologic sequelae.
7. Pregnancy
   a. Primary infection can lead to abortion, premature labor, intrauterine growth, retardation as well as fetal skin lesions, choreoretinitis, and microcephaly.

II. Diagnostic Approach

A. Can unroof lesions and scrape base for Tzank smear. Multinucleated giant cells are pathologic findings.

B. Can do tissue culture looking for cytopathic effects

C. Serology—positive serology indicates exposure, but not acute infection.

D. In cases of encephalitis, CSF examination reveals a moderate sterile pleocytosis with a slight increase in protein. Brain biopsy guided by EEG or MRI is diagnostic.

III. Treatment

A. Acute Management

1. Acyclovir 400 mg t.i.d. or 200 mg 5 times daily given orally or IV may shorten the duration of pain, viral shedding, and symptoms during primary infections.
2. Treatment for primary infection should be for 10 days; for reoccurences, 5 days of treatment is recommended.
3. Topical acyclovir has little benefit.

B. Encephalitis requires hospitalization and aggressive IV therapy with acyclovir or vidarabine.

C. Long-term Management

1. There is probably little benefit to most patients treated for recurrent infection but acyclovir may help some patients if begun very early, preferably during the prodromal phase. Dose and duration are as above.

2. Patients who have more than six severe recurrences per year may benefit from suppressive therapy with oral acyclovir 400 mg b.i.d. or 200 mg 2–5 times daily. Viral shedding is not eliminated and transmission can still occur.

D. Patient Education

1. Patients need to be counseled on routes of transmission as well as potential for recurrent disease and viral shedding.

2. Condoms should be used for sexual contacts.

IV. Indications for Hospitalization

A. Need for IV acyclovir for the treatment of severe primary infection as well as management of encephalitis or herpetic infections in immunocompromised hosts

B. Need for supportive care in patients with severe systemic symptoms or massive cutaneous or visceral dissemination

V. Annotated Bibliography

Gurevich I. Varicella zoster and herpes simplex virus infections. Heart Lung 1992; 21(1):85–91. Discussion of manifestations, transmission and treatment with an emphasis on high-risk patients.

Hirsch MS. Herpes simplex virus. In: Mandell GL, Douglas RG Jr, Bennett JE, eds. Principles and Practice of Infectious Diseases, 3rd ed. New York: Churchill Livingstone; 1990:1144–1153. An excellent description of clinical presentation of all forms of HSV.

70D Herpes Zoster

I. Clinical Presentation

A. General Information

1. Latent varicella virus lies dormant in a dorsal root ganglion.
2. Reactivation leads to zoster (shingles).
3. Affects 10% of the population. About 40% of affected persons will have a second episode. Third occurrences are rare.
4. Severity and frequency increase with age.

B. Symptoms

1. Often predisposed by physical/emotional stress, debilitation, steroids, diabetes, or sunburn.
2. Generally presents as pain, intense burning, or pruritus followed in 48–72 h by a grouped vesicular eruption in a dermatomal distribution, which persists for 10–15 d.
3. Rarely, may see symptoms of pneumonia, hepatitis, or encephalitis.
4. Dermatomal pain lasting more than 1 mo (postherpetic neuralgia) occurs in 20–50%, particularly if over age 50.

C. Physical Examination

1. Unilateral vesicular eruption within one dermatome (usually thoracic or lumbar). Vesicles on erythematous base generally become pustular by day 3–4 and crust by day 7–10. Often heals with scarring. May see 10 or fewer lesions outside of the dermatone involved.
2. Involvement of the trigeminal nerve can lead to zoster ophthalmicus (V_1), or intraoral disease (V_2 or V_3). Ocular disease can involve any part of the eye (retinal infection leads to blindness in 64%).
3. Involvement of the geniculate ganglion can lead to ipsilateral facial palsy, loss of taste (anterior two thirds of tongue), lesions in the external auditory meatus and possibly hearing loss (Ramsey Hunt syndrome—herpes zoster oticus).
4. Anterior horn cell involvement can lead to painful paralysis or transverse myelitis.
5. Dissemination of lesions (> 30 lesions outside a single dermatome) can occur in immunocompromised patients and with advanced age (> 70) and is associated with a 30% incidence of visceral and brain involvement, which can be fatal if major organs become involved.
6. Occasionally see meningoencephalitis and granulomatous angiitis of the carotids.

II. Diagnostic Approach

A. Diagnosis is generally made by physical examination.

B. Can confirm diagnosis with Tzank smears or tissue cultures taken from lesion base or by serology (enzyme-linked immunosorbent assay).

III. Differential Diagnosis

A. Classic dermatomal zoster generally is definitive.

B. Disseminated disease can look similar to acute varicella or other vesicular viral exanthems including herpes simplex.

C. Zosteriform herpes simplex should be considered in patients with maxillary (V_2) or sacral root involvement or in patients with prior eruptions.

IV. Treatment

A. Acute Disease

1. Appears to be little true benefit to treatment in immunocompetent patients but acyclovir 800 mg 5 times daily may speed healing and lessen acute pain if begun within 72 h of rash onset.

2. Antiviral therapy appears to be warranted in significantly immunocompromised patients to improve healing, lessen acute pain, and perhaps decrease the risk of visceral dissemination but does not alter postherpetic neuralgia.

    a. Acyclovir 30 mg/kg/d divided q 8 h IV for 7 d. Monitor renal function and hydration.
    b. Vidaribine 10 mg/kg/d IV for 5–7 d may be substituted.

3. Therapy appears to decrease occular complications in ophthalmic zoster—acyclovir 800 mg PO 5 times daily for 10 d

4. Systemic steroid usage is controversial and probably should be avoided. Topical and intralesional steroids may decrease scarring.

B. Postherpetic Neuralgia

1. Pain management tends to be difficult.

2. Multiple therapies have been tried including tricyclic antidepressants, phenothiazine tranquilizers, phenytoin, carbamazepine, topical capsaicin, transcutaneous, electrical nerve stimulation, nerve blocks, or sympathetic blocks.

3. Little evidence that antibiotics or steroids prevent or lessen neuralgia.

4. Neuralgia resolves within 2 mo in 50% and within 1 y in 70-80%.

C. Prophylaxis

Consideration should be given to administering varicella-Zoster immune globulin (VZIG) within 96 h of exposure to person with close contact to infected patients and who are susceptible to varicella or have underlying immunosuppression or defective cellular immunity or who are pregnant. Transmission is thought to be via vesicular fluid contacting mucosal surfaces.

V. Indications for Referral

A. Patients with zoster ophthalmicus should immediately see an ophthalmologist.

B. Patients with zoster oticus may require the assistance of an otorhinolaryngologist.

VI. Indications for Hospitalization

Patients who are immunocompromised or those with significant cutaneous or visceral dissemination should be hospitalized for IV therapy.

VII. Annotated Bibliography

Huff JC, Drucher JL, Clemmer A, et al. Effect of oral acyclovir on pain resolution on herpes zoster: a reanalysis. J Med Virol 1993;(suppl 1):93-96. Single study showing effectiveness of antiviral therapy on acute symptoms of zoster.

Rowbotham NC. Treatment of post-herpatic neuralgia. Semin Dermatol 1992;11(3):218-225. Good overview of risk factors and treatment modalities.

Strauss SE, Ostrove JM, Inchauspe G, et al. Varicella-zoster virus infections: biology, natural history, treatment, and prevention. Ann Intern Med 1988;108:221-227.

Tyring SK. National history of varicella zoster virus. Semin Dermatol 1992;11(3):211-217. Two excellent reviews of pathophysiology, presentation, and management.

70E Pediculosis and Scabies

I. Pediculosis

A. Clinical Presentation
1. General information
    a. Pediculosis—three major species affecting human beings
        1) Pediculosis humanis var capitus (head lice)
        2) Pediculosis humanis var corporus (body lice)
        3) Phithirus pelvic (pubic or crab lice)
    b. Eggs are attached to hair shafts and hatch to form nits. Nymphs appear after 7–10 d and must feed within 24 h.
    c. Primary risks for contraction and spread are overcrowding and poor sanitation for body lice.
    d. Often spread via sharing of clothing and bed linens. Pubic lice often spread through sexual or other close body contact.
2. Symptoms
    a. Most common complaint with all forms is pruritis, which may be intense.
    b. Patient may actually see nits and eggs, particularly after combing.
3. Physical examination
    a. In most forms, may see nits/eggs on close inspection of hair.
    b. Head lice
        1) See excoriations due to scratching, primarily at occipital and temporal regions
        2) Nits at base of hair shafts
        3) Most common in young males, unusual in blacks
        4) Occasionally see a mobiliform pruritic eruption on the upper back due to a hypersensitivity reaction
    c. Body lice
        1) Pruritic maculopapular eruption
        2) Eggs are laid in seams of clothing with lice leaving the clothes to feed. Lice are generally not found on the body.
        3) Hypersensitivity reaction can occur.
        4) Can transmit disease (typhus, trench fever, relapsing fever)
        5) Can lead to chronic hyperpigmentation with numerous healed excoriations—Vagabond's disease
    d. Pubic lice
        1) Pruritis with occasional erythematous macules/papules
        2) Can infest pubic hair, eyebrows, eyelashes, axillary, back, and chest hair
        3) Find nits and adults attached to hair shaft
        4) Anticoagulant in the insect saliva can leave small gray-blue macules, particularly on the trunk and proximal extremities (maculae cerulae)
    e. Secondary infection of excoriations can occur, usually due to staphylococci

B. Diagnostic Approach

1. Suspicion is raised by clinical picture, particularly if close contacts are affected.
2. Close inspection (combing of involved areas) may reveal nits/eggs attached to hair shafts.

C. Differential Diagnosis

1. Common
    a. Other infestations (scabies, fleas, etc.)
    b. Atopic dermatitis
    c. Dermatitis herpetiformis
    d. Seborrheic dermatitis
    e. Folliculitis
    f. Syphilis

2. Less common—herpes gestationalis, linear IgA dermatosis, bullous pemphigoid, papular urticarial, and plaques of pregnancy, lichen planus, nodular prurigo, pityriasis rosea

D. Treatment

1. Three available agents
    a. Nix—0.5% permethrin (head lice only)
    b. Rid—piporonyl butoxide with pyrethrins
    c. Kwell (lindane)—1% γ benzene hexachloride. Available by prescription only because absorption through skin can lead to neurotoxicity. Avoid in infants and pregnant women.

2. Head lice
    a. Wash hair
    b. Rub on Rid or Nix for 10 min or Kwell for 4 min then rinse and comb hair with a fine comb.
    c. Repeat Rid or Kwell in 7 d.
    d. Boil combs/brushes or soak in 2% Lysol. Heat sterilize bedding and clothing (or disinfect with 1% malathion or 10% DDT).

3. Body lice
    a. Apply Rid for 10 min or Kwell for 4 min then rinse, repeat in 7 d.
    b. Clothing/bedding as above

4. Pubic lice
    a. Apply Rid or Kwell to affected areas for 24 h. May repeat in 1 wk.
    b. Remove lice and nits with combs and cotton-tipped applicators.
    c. Infestation of eyelashes should be treated with 0.25% physostigmine ophthalmic ointment b.i.d. for 10 d.

5. Pruritis can be managed with antihistamines or medium-potency topical steroids.

II. Scabies

A. **Clinical Presentation**

1. General information
   a. *Sarcopteus scabiei* var *hominis*—endoparasite that burrows into the skin
   b. Females burrow into skin and lay 2–3 eggs/day. Larva emerge in 72–84 h and form adults in about 17 d.
   c. Spread is enhanced by crowding, poor hygiene/sanitation, and probably by sexual promiscuity although transmission through casual contact may occur.
   d. Not a known vector of disease
   e. Probable cause of "7-year itch"

2. Symptoms
   a. Generally causes intense pruritus, which worsens at night and following hot baths

3. Physical examination
   a. Erythematous papules with excoriations
   b. Primary sites—interdigital webs, wrists, elbows, anterior axilla, pelvis, periumbilical area, buttocks, penis, knees, soles of feet
   c. May see small linear burrows (can add ink to enhance visualization)
   d. Hypersensitivity reaction can lead to eczematous eruption or nodular hyperpigmentation.
   e. In debilitated, immunosuppressed, or institutionalized hosts can see widespread infestation with varying degrees of pruritus (Norwegian scabies), which may lead to thickened nails, alopecia, hyperpigmentation, eosinophilia, and pyoderma.

B. **Diagnostic Approach**

1. Diagnosis is suggested by clinical presentation.
2. Mites can be seen under a microscope in skin scrapings.
3. May see thousands of mites in Norwegian scabies.

C. **Differential Diagnosis**

1. Similar to pediculosis
2. Norwegian scabies can mimic psoriasis.

D. **Management**

1. Single application of permethrin 5% cream (Elimite) is treatment of choice. Applied to all cutaneous surfaces (especially fingernails, waist, and genitalia) at bedtime and washed off in morning.

2. 0.5% permethrin (Nix) and piporonyl butoxide (Rid) are ineffective and lindane (Kwell) is neurotoxic in children.
3. All family members and regular guests should be treated and bedding and undergarments changed.

III. Annotated Bibliography

Elpart ML. Scabies. Dermatol Clin 1990;8(2):253–263.

Elpart ML. Pediculosis. Dermatol Clin 1990;8(2):219–228. Two thorough reviews of epidemiology, transmission, and treatment.

Hogan DJ, Schachner L, Tanglersampan C. Diagnosis and treatment of childhood scabies and pediculosis. Pediatr Clin North Am 1991;38(4):941–957. Excellent overview of various clinical presentations.

Chapter 71: Syphilis

Rosemarie A. Leuzzi

I. Clinical Presentation

A. General Information

1. Syphilis is a sexually transmitted infection caused by the spirochete, *Treponema pallidum*.
2. Stages of infection
   a. Primary syphilis—The primary lesion, a painless chancre, appears at the site of infection and often is associated with regional lymphadenopathy; this follows an incubation period of 10–90 d with an average incubation of 20 d.
   b. Secondary syphilis—A secondary bacteremic stage occurs in patients with untreated primary syphilis 6 wk to 6 mo after the initial contact. Involvement of the skin and mucous membranes predominates; however, the liver, bones, lymph nodes, kidneys, and CNS may be affected. Untreated, secondary syphilis lasts 2–6 wk and may relapse in 20% of cases during the first year.
   c. Latent syphilis—a latent period of subclinical infection when there are no clinical manifestations and usually diagnosed by routine serologic testing
      1) Early latent syphilis—patients with latent syphilis who are known to have been infected within the preceding year
      2) Late latent syphilis—syphilis of unknown duration
   d. Tertiary syphilis—occurs in approximately one third of untreated cases and is characterized by gummatous, cardiac, or neurologic problems
      1) Late benign syphilis—granulomatous involvement (gummas) of the skin, bone, cartilage, soft tissue, and viscera
      2) Cardiovascular syphilis—ascending aorta is involved resulting in aortic insufficiency and heart failure
      3) Neurosyphilis—either asymptomatic or symptomatic with a broad range of neurologic and psychiatric manifestations, eg, meningovascular syphilis, tabes dorsalis, or general paresis

B. Symptoms

1. In primary syphilis, skin ulceration is usually a *painless* genital ulcer (usually overlooked in women because painless and located inside the labia or on the cervix)

2. Painless regional and generalized lymphadenopathy
3. Nonpruritic rash
4. Oral and genitorectal lesions
5. Systemic symptoms such as malaise, fever, headache, anorexia, myalgias, and sore throat may occur in the secondary stage of syphilis.
6. Systemic manifestations, occurring in 1–2% of patients with secondary syphilis, may include hepatitis (presenting with jaundice and abdominal pain) and frank meningitis (possibly presenting with headache, neck stiffness, and tinnitus).

C. Physical Examination

1. The chance of primary syphilis starts as a painless papule ranging in size from a few millimeters to a few centimeters in diameter and progresses to a painless ulcer with indurated edges; this occurs at the site of intimate contact. If superinfected, the ulcer may become painful and multiple lesions occur in 30% of patients.
2. Nontender, regional or generalized lymphadenopathy may be noted.
3. A generalized maculopapular rash can involve all areas of the body, especially the trunk, palms, and soles in secondary syphilis.
4. Scalp and eyelash involvement can lead to characteristic "moth-eaten alopecia" with patchy, diffuse hair loss.
5. Mucosal lesions (gray oral patches on an erythematous base) as well as lesions found in moist areas such as the axillary or genital regions are highly infectious.
6. Condyloma latum (flat, wartlike lesions usually found in the genital or anal area) are also highly infectious.
7. Syphilitic meningitis is characterized by papilledema and involvement of the cranial nerves III, VI, VII, and VIII.
8. Anterior uveitis and iritis may also occur.
9. An enlarged, tender liver may be present with syphilitic hepatitis with mild elevation of transaminases.

II. Diagnostic Approach

A. Evaluation should include a careful history of previous rashes or lesions, history of previous sexually transmitted diseases and previous tests for syphilis, as well as inquiry into a patient's sexual practices and recent sexual partners.

B. Physical examination should include a careful skin examination with attention to the genital and perianal regions and palpation for lymphadenopathy.

C. Direct microscopic examination of the exudate of any suspicious lesions

1. Examination of the exudate from a suspicious lesion using darkfield microscopy or direct fluorescent antibody tests for *T. pallidum* (DFA-TP) is the definitive method for diagnosing early syphilis. This examination is positive in most chancres; however, the diagnosis in secondary lesions is less likely.

2. Method—Abrade the skin lesion gently with gauze to produce a nonbloody serous exudate; after wiping the surface, squeeze the lesion between gloved fingers; collect the exudate in either a capillary tube or a microscope slide.

3. For oral lesions, the DFA-TP test is more specific.

D. Serologic Testing

1. Nontreponemal tests
   VDRL (Venereal Disease Research Laboratory)
   RPR (rapid plasma reagin)

   a. Nontreponemal tests that detect reagin, a nonspecific antibody to cardiolipin, are used as the initial screening tests for syphilis. Any patient who presents with a genital ulcer should have nontreponemal serologic testing for syphilis.
   b. The nontreponemal tests usually correlate with disease activity and results are reported quantitatively as a titer.
   c. A fourfold change in titer (a twofold dilution) is necessary to demonstrate a substantial difference between two subsequent nontreponemal test results using the same serologic test.
   d. The VDRL and the RPR are equally valid, but quantitative results cannot be directly compared because RPR titers are usually slightly higher than VDRL titers.
   e. False positive nontreponemal serologic tests may occur in patients with disordered immunity such as rheumatoid arthritis, systemic lupus erythematosus, chronic liver disease, and in IV drug abusers.
   f. 15–25% of patients treated with primary syphilis may revert to being serologically nonreactive after 2–3 y.

2. Treponemal tests
   FTA-ABS (fluorescent treponemal antibody absorbed)
   MHA-TP (microhemagglutination assay for antibody to *T. pallidum*)

   a. Treponemal tests will usually remain reactive for a lifetime regardless of treatment or disease activity.
   b. The treponemal tests should be used selectively only when the nontreponemal tests are reactive or when primary or tertiary syphilis is highly suspect (due to the increased sensitivity of the treponemal tests compared to nontreponemal tests in patients with primary and tertiary syphilis).
   c. Because they correlate poorly with disease activity, treponemal tests should not be used to assess response to treatment.

E. CSF Analysis

1. Indications for lumbar puncture—As per the 1993 Centers for Disease Control and Prevention (CDC) guidelines, patients with any of the below criteria should have a CSF examination before treatment.

   a. Neurologic or ophthalmic signs or symptoms
   b. Other evidence of active syphilis (aortitis, gumma, iritis)
   c. Treatment failure
   d. HIV infection
   e. Serum nontreponemal titer > 1:32, unless duration of infection is known to be < 1 y
   f. Nonpenicillin therapy planned, unless duration of infection is known to be < 1 y

2. For neurosyphilis, the diagnosis can be based on various combinations of reactive serologic test results, abnormalities of CSF cell count or protein, or a reactive CSF-VDRL with or without clinical manifestations/abnormalities of CSF.

3. CSF leukocyte count is usually elevated with active neurosyphilis (> 5 cells/mm^3) and is a sensitive measure of therapy.

4. CSF-protein measurement may be elevated with a decreased CSF-glucose value.

5. A reactive CSF-VDRL result, in the absence of significant contamination of the CSF sample with blood, is considered diagnostic for neurosyphilis (positive in 90% of cases of active meningitis).

6. Some experts recommend performing an FTA-ABS test on CSF. This test is highly sensitive although less specific (yields more false positives).

III. Differential Diagnosis

A. The primary chancre of primary syphilis can be easily mistaken for lesions due to other infections, eg, chancroid, herpes (see Chapter 67E).

B. Secondary syphilis of the skin can be confused with diseases that produce widespread, symmetrical skin lesions including viral exanthems and drug reactions. The associated diffuse lymphadenopathy and hepatosplenomegaly may raise the possibility of lymphoma or infectious mononucleosis.

C. Late, tertiary lesions of the skin need to be differentiated from other chronic infections such as tuberculosis or fungal infections, rashes found in autoimmune diseases such as systemic lupus erythematosus, or sarcoidosis. Late syphilis of the bone may be confused with osteomyelitis or osteogenic sarcoma.

IV. Treatment

A. General Information

1. Parenteral penicillin G is the preferred drug for all stages of syphilis. The preparation used, dosage, and length of treatment depend on the stage of the infection.

2. All patients with syphilis should be tested for HIV and consider retesting in 3 mo.
3. Jarisch-Herxheimer reaction
   a. An acute febrile reaction with headache, myalgias, tachycardia, and hypotension due to vasodilatation may occur within the first 24 h of starting any therapy for syphilis, most commonly among patients with primary and secondary syphilis.
   b. Patients should be advised of the potential adverse reaction and treated with antipyretics.
4. Penicillin-allergic patients
   a. Patients with neurosyphilis and pregnant women who report a previous allergic reaction to penicillin should almost always be treated with penicillin and undergo desensitization if necessary.

B. **Treatment of Primary and Secondary Syphilis**
1. Recommended regimen—benzathine penicillin 2.4 million units IM in a single dose
2. Recommended regimen for nonpregnant penicillin-allergic patients—doxycycline 100 mg orally b.i.d. for 2 wk *OR* tetracycline 500 mg PO q.i.d. for 2 wk
3. Unless clinical signs or symptoms of neurologic involvement are present with auditory, cranial nerve, meningeal, or ophthalmic manifestations, lumbar puncture is not recommended for routine evaluation of patients with primary or secondary syphilis.
4. Follow-up—assessing treatment response is difficult; therefore, patients should be evaluated clinically and serologically at 3 mo and then again at 6 mo following treatment.
5. Treatment failure
   a. If signs or symptoms persist or recur or if there is a sustained fourfold increase in nontreponemal test titer (compared with either the baseline titer or to a subsequent result), or failure of the nontreponemal test titer to decline by fourfold by 3 mo after therapy, the patient should be considered a treatment failure or reinfected.
   b. These patients should be retreated after evaluation of their HIV status and unless reinfection is likely, a lumbar puncture should be performed.
   c. Recommended regimen for retreatment—benzathine penicillin G 2.4 million units IM weekly for 3 wk (unless CSF results suggest neurosyphilis)

C. **Treatment of Latent Syphilis**
1. Treatment of latent syphilis is intended to prevent occurrence or progression of late complications; all patients with latent syphilis should be evaluated carefully for evidence of tertiary disease (aortitis, neurosyphilis, gumma, and iritis).

2. Recommended regimen for early latent syphilis—benzathine penicillin G 2.4 million units IM in a single dose
3. Recommended regimen for latent syphilis of unknown duration—benzathine penicillin G 3 doses of 2.4 million units IM weekly
4. Recommended regimen for nonpregnant penicillin-allergic patients—doxycycline 100 mg b.i.d. for 2 wk *OR* tetracycline 500 mg q.i.d. for 2 wk if duration of infection is known to have been < 1 y; otherwise, for 4 wk (Nonpenicillin regimens should be used only after CSF examination has excluded neurosyphilis.)
5. Follow-up
   a. Quantitative nontreponemal serologic tests should be repeated at 6 mo and again at 12 mo.
   b. If titers increase fourfold, or if an initially high titer (> 1:32) fails to decline at least fourfold within 12–24 mo, or if the patient develops signs or symptoms attributable to syphilis, the patient should be evaluated for neurosyphilis and retreated appropriately.

D. **Treatment of Tertiary Syphilis**

1. The following regimen refers to patients with gummatous disease and patients with cardiovascular syphilis, but not with neurosyphilis.
2. All patients should undergo CSF examination to rule out neurosyphilis.
3. Recommended regimen—benzathine penicillin G 2.4 million units IM weekly for 3 doses.

E. **Treatment of Neurosyphilis**

1. CNS disease can occur during any stage of syphilis; therefore, any patient with clinical evidence of neurologic involvement warrants CSF examination.
2. Recommended regimen—Aqueous crystalline penicillin G 12–24 million units daily administered as 2–4 million units IV q 4 h for 10–14 d
3. Alternative regimen—procaine penicillin 2.4 million units IM daily plus probenecid 500 mg PO q.i.d., both for 10–14 d
4. Some experts recommend administering benzathine penicillin 2.4 million units IM after completion of the neurosyphilis regimen to increase total duration of therapy.
5. Patients who report a penicillin allergy should undergo desensitization.
6. Follow-up
   a. If CSF pleocytosis was present initially, CSF examination should be repeated q 6 mo until the cell count is normal and to evaluate changes in the CSF-VDRL or CSF-protein in response to therapy.
   b. If the cell count has not decreased at 6 mo or if the CSF is not entirely normal by 2 y, retreatment should be considered.

7. Management of sexual partners
   a. Sexual transmission of *T. pallidum* occurs only when mucocutaneous lesions are present.
   b. As per the 1993 CDC guidelines:
      1) Persons exposed to a patient with primary, secondary, or early latent syphilis within the preceding 90 d might be infected even if seronegative and should be treated presumptively.
      2) Persons who were sexually exposed to a patient with primary, secondary, or early latent syphilis > 90 d before examination should be treated presumptively if the serologic test results are not immediately available and the opportunity for follow-up is uncertain.
      3) The time periods before treatment used for identifying at-risk sexual partners are 3 mo plus duration of symptoms for primary syphilis, 6 mo plus duration of symptoms for secondary syphilis, and 1 y for early latent syphilis. Patients who have syphilis of unknown duration and have high nonteponemal test titers (> 1:32) may be considered to be infected with early latent syphilis for purposes of partner notification.
      4) Long-term sex partners of patients with late syphilis should be evaluated clinically and serologically for syphilis.

F. Syphilis in HIV-Infected Patients

1. Both nontreponemal and treponemal serologic tests are accurate for the majority of HIV-infected patients with syphilis; however, there have been reports of false negative serologic results or delayed appearance of seroreactivity.

2. If serologic tests are nonreactive or confusing, alternative tests such as biopsy or fluorescent antibody staining of a lesion may be helpful.

3. Some case reports have suggested the HIV-infected patients with early syphilis are at increased risk for neurologic complications and have higher rates of treatment failure with currently recommended regimens; therefore, careful follow-up after therapy is essential.

4. Patients should be evaluated clinically and serologically at 1 mo and at 2, 3, 6, 9, and 12 mo after therapy.

5. Although of unproven benefit, some experts recommend performing CSF examination before and at 6 mo after completion of therapy.

G. Syphilis During Pregnancy

1. All women should be screened serologically for syphilis during the early stages of pregnancy.

2. For patients at high risk, serologic testing should be repeated during the third trimester and again at delivery.

3. Seropositive women should be considered infected unless there is clear documentation of treatment and sequential serologic antibody titers have declined.

4. Treatment during pregnancy should be the penicillin regimen appropriate for the woman's stage of syphilis. There are no proven alternatives to penicillin to adequately treat a pregnant woman; therefore, desensitization is indicated if necessary.

5. Women who are treated for syphilis during the second half of pregnancy are at risk for premature labor and/or fetal distress if the therapy precipitates the Jarisch-Herxheimer reaction. Women should be warned of the potential symptoms and told to seek medical attention immediately if they begin having contractions or note any change in fetal movements.

V. Indications for Referral to a Specialist

A. Consultation with an allergist may be indicated to confirm the penicillin allergy with skin testing and to arrange for desensitization in patients with either neurosyphilis or pregnant women with diagnosed syphilis.

B. A persistent skin lesion may warrant referral to a dermatologist or gynecologist for biopsy.

VI. Annotated Bibliography

Centers for Disease Control and Prevention. 1993 sexually transmitted diseases treatment guidelines. MMWR 1993;42 (No. RR-14). Excellent concise handbook reviewing diagnosis and therapy with special consideration of HIV-infected patients, pregnancy, and children/adolescents—an essential guide to have available in the ambulatory care setting.

Dans PE, Griffin DE. Selected spirochetal infections: syphilis and lyme disease. In: Barker LR, Burton JR, Zieve PD, eds. Principles of Ambulatory Medicine. Baltimore: Williams & Wilkins; 1991. Good review of management of syphilis in the outpatient setting with a thorough review of the sensitivity and specificity of serologic testing methods.

Lukehart SA, Holmes KK. Syphilis. In: Wilson JD, Braunwald E, Isselbacher KJ, et al, eds. Harrison's Principles of Internal Medicine. New York: McGraw-Hill; 1991. In-depth review of syphilis covering etiology, natural course, clinical presentation, diagnosis, and therapy.

Peterson PK, Dahl MV. Dermatologic Manifestations of Infectious Disease. Kalamazoo, MI: The Upjohn Company 1987. Brief chart covering the differential diagnosis of genital ulcers as well as good photographs demonstrating the various types of genital ulcers.

Part XV:
Neurology/ENT

Chapter 72: Carpal Tunnel Syndrome

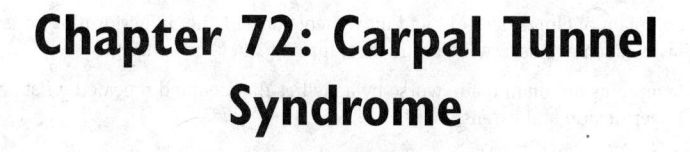

Carol M. Reife

I. Clinical Presentation

A. General Information

1. Carpal tunnel syndrome is one of the most common entrapment syndromes. It results from compression of the median nerve as it passes across the wrist in the "tunnel" between the carpal bones and the transverse carpal ligament on the palmar side of the wrist.

2. The incidence of carpal tunnel syndrome is highest in the fifth and sixth decades, affecting women more than men.

3. The syndrome appears as an isolated entity in the majority of patients but a generalized polyneuropathy or systemic illness (amyloidosis, multiple myeloma, acromegaly, hypothyroidism) may predispose to nerve entrapment. Symptoms may appear during pregnancy and resolve after delivery.

4. Signs and symptoms of carpal tunnel syndrome may result from or be exacerbated by extensive use of one's hands especially when repetitive motion involving flexion and extension is involved. Thus, carpal tunnel syndrome is often an occupational injury.

B. Symptoms

1. Painful paresthesias in the distribution of the median nerve (the palmar surface of the thumb, index and middle fingers, and radial half of the fourth finger) are the most common symptoms. Complaints of pain and numbness outside the median nerve distribution are not unusual and symptoms involving the entire hand may occur. Pain is often referred to the more proximal parts of the arm including the wrist, elbow and at times, the shoulder.

2. Symptoms are frequently most severe at night and are often relieved by shaking or rubbing the affected hand or letting it hang over the bedside.

3. Because of compression of peripheral vasomotor fibers, the affected limb may appear swollen, cold, or erythematous.

4. Weakness of median nerve-innervated hand muscles may cause decreased strength of abduction, opposition, and flexion of the thumb. Patients may

complain of clumsiness of hand movements or difficulty in performing certain tasks (such as unscrewing bottle tops, turning a key, or knitting).

5. Symptoms are often made worse by activities that demand repeated wrist and finger flexion and extension.
6. Although entrapment frequently occurs bilaterally, the dominant hand is usually more severely involved.

C. Physical Examination

1. Decreased touch or hypesthesia to pinprick may be demonstrated over the fingers supplied by the median nerve. Often the earliest objective sign is failure to appreciate textures. Sensory signs are best found in the fingertips where impairment is usually more pronounced.
2. Symptoms may be reproduced or exacerbated by applying pressure over the flexor aspect of the wrist, by prolonged passive flexion at the wrist, or by hyperextension of the wrist.
3. Tinel's sign—Paresthesia induced by percussion over the median nerve on the flexor surface of the wrist, (this is not specific to carpal tunnel syndrome).
4. Phalen's maneuver—Paresthesia or pain in the fingers reproduced by full flexion of the wrist for 1 min.
5. Weakness and atrophy of the thenar muscles may appear later and can occur without significant sensory symptoms. Advanced cases of carpal tunnel syndrome may show weakness and wasting of the abductor pollicis brevis, the opponens pollicis muscle, and other medianinnervated thenar muscles. Thenar muscle weakness is manifested by decreased strength of abduction, opposition, and flexion of the thumb.
6. Physical examination may be normal and all clinical tests (percussion of the nerve in the wrist, flexion, or hyperextension of the hand) may be within normal limits.

II. Diagnostic Approach

A. Symptoms compatible with carpal tunnel syndrome or physical examination showing sensory and/or motor deficits in the distribution of the median nerve warrant evaluation for carpal tunnel syndrome.

B. Blood tests—Sedimentation rate, rheumatoid factor, thyroid function tests, fasting or 2-h postprandial blood sugar may reveal causative factors for carpal tunnel syndrome or other causes of neuropathy.

C. Electrophysiologic Studies (see also Chapter 76E)

1. Indications

    a. Referral for electrodiagnostic studies should be made if history or physical examination is suggestive of carpal tunnel syndrome.

2. Diagnostic findings
   a. Median nerve conduction studies generally show increased motor latency and decreased sensory nerve conduction across the wrist. In some cases the amplitude of the sensory response is reduced early in the course of the disease. The amplitude of the motor response is diminished in more advanced cases, as motor fibers are lost.
   b. Advanced cases may show electromyographic signs of denervation, ie, fibrillation potentials and positive sharp waves in the medianinnervated intrinsic hand muscles.
   c. Electrophysiologic studies may occasionally be entirely normal.

III. Differential Diagnosis

A. Nerve root disease may mimic carpal tunnel syndrome. The distribution of distal sensory symptoms and proximal radiation of pain may suggest the diagnosis of a C-6 or C-7 root compression. Median nerve lesions cause predominantly palmar location of symptoms, whereas sensory impairment in isolated root compression is over the dorsal and palmar aspects of the thumb in C-6 lesions and of the first two fingers in C-7 lesions. Also, in C-6 and C-7 lesions, there is often weakness of muscles in the arm and forearm and brachioradialis or triceps reflexes may be impaired.

B. Cervical rib or compression of the brachial plexus from any type of anatomic derangement may cause wasting of the muscles of the hand.

C. Thoracic outlet syndrome may cause loss of bulk or strength in the hand muscles other than the thenar eminence.

D. Diffuse diabetic or amyloid neuropathy involving the distal parts of the upper limbs may cause paresthesias, which mimic carpal tunnel syndrome.

IV. Treatment

A. In cases when only mild sensory symptoms exist or when the condition is self-limited (pregnancy) or medically treatable (hypothyroidism), conservative measures may be indicated.

1. Anti-inflammatory medications
2. Splinting of the wrist in the neutral position
3. Steroid injections into the transverse carpal ligament

B. Injection of corticosteroids into the transverse carpal ligament may relieve symptoms for only a short period of time but in some cases, may cause remission of symptoms that will last for several years. If needed, injections may be given multiple times.

C. If symptoms persist or motor abnormalities are present, surgical decompression of the carpal tunnel with release of the transverse carpal ligament and debridement is indicated. Surgery is accompanied by relief of symptoms in the majority of cases.

V. Patient Education

A. Avoid work that requires repeated flexion, pronation, and supination of the wrist (eg, sewing, driving, typing) because these may exacerbate symptoms.

B. Follow-up if prescribed measures do not relieve symptoms or if worsening, especially motor symptoms, occurs

VI. Long-term Management

A. If symptoms are controlled and there is no evidence of motor deficit, conservative measures such as anti-inflammatory medication, wrist splints, and steroid injections should be continued.

B. If symptoms progress or repeated examination reveals evidence of muscle damage, surgical release should be considered.

VII. Indications for Referral

A. Referral for electrodiagnostic studies should be made if history or physical examination is suggestive of carpal tunnel syndrome.

B. Surgical consultation should be sought if there is objective evidence of slowing of nerve conduction or evidence of motor dysfunction.

VIII. Annotated Bibliography

Dyck P, Thomas P, Lanmbert E. Peripheral Neuropathy. Philadelphia: WB Saunders; 1975:695–697. Comprehensive text covering all aspects of peripheral neuropathy from basic science to clinical features, diagnosis, and treatment.

Kimura J. Electrodiagnosis in Diseases of Nerve and Muscle: Principles and Practice. Philadelphia: F A Davis; 1983:494–496. Detailed text intended for clinicians performing electrodiagnostic procedures; very thorough.

Chapter 73: Cerebrovascular Disease

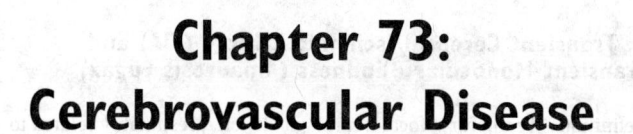

Robert D. Aiken

I. Asymptomatic Cervical Bruits

A. Prevalence

1. 3–4% of normal adult population
2. Increases with advancing age
   a. 8% of normal persons > 75 y
   b. 10% of persons > 85
   c. 13% of persons > 95

B. Significance

1. In general, it signifies underlying pathology in the cartoid artery, implying carotid stenosis, although not necessarily on the same side.
2. Using carotid Doppler correlation, there is 64% incidence of underlying carotid stenosis ipsilateral to the neck bruit, 33% incidence on the contralateral side.

C. Stroke Risk

1. About 1%/y in community studies, but not necessarily related to the side of the stroke, and includes all types of cerebrovascular disease(ischemia, hemorrhage, subarachnoid hemorrhage)
2. Using carotid Doppler studies, once stenosis has reached 75%, annual risk is closer to 5%.
3. Prospective studies ongoing to define role of carotid endarterectomy in patients with asymptomatic carotid disease
4. Other vascular risks
   a. Carotid bruits and carotid stenosis directly correlate to higher risk of fatal cardiac disease.
   b. Severity of carotid stenosis is related to risk of cardiac death.

II. Transient Cerebral Ischemic Attacks (TIA) and Transient Monocular Blindness (Amaurosis Fugax)

A. Definition—Temporary, focal neurologic deficit, presumably related to ischemia, lasting < 24 h. Typical TIAs are brief, lasting minutes or less.

B. Natural History

1. Patients who suffer stroke from extracranial carotid disease have known prior TIA incidence of 50–75%
2. Low incidence (about 10%) of TIA in association with all types of stroke
3. Prevalence varies widely 1.1–77/1000
4. Incidence 2.2–8/1000
5. Stroke risk after TIA varies widely, ranging from 2–50%, 35% over 5 y or 5–6%/y

C. Treatment (see III-D.)

III. Stroke

A. Clinical Presentation—depends on vessel affected

1. Internal carotid artery

    a. Contralateral hemiplegia
    b. Contralateral hemiparesthesias
    c. Aphasia (with dominant hemisphere involvement)
    d. Stupor/semicoma common

2. Anterior cerebral artery

    a. Weakness and sensory loss of contralateral leg > proximal arm
    b. Cortical sensory abnormalities
    c. Apraxia, agraphia, and tactile anomia due to callosal disconnection
    d. Akinetic mutism, abulia
    e. Language disturbance in dominant hemisphere involvement

3. Middle cerebral artery

    a. Paralysis of contralateral face, arm, leg
    b. sensory loss (primary and cortical sensations)
    c. Fluent or nonfluent aphasia (dominant hemisphere involvement)
    d. Homonomous hemianopsia
    e. Paralysis of gaze to the opposite side

B. Diagnostic Approach

1. Brain imaging: MRI generally preferrable to CT, if possible

a. CT
     1) Advantages
        a) *simple and quick to perform*
        b) *largely noninvasive*
        c) *able to accurately distinguish infarction from hemmorhage*
     2) Disadvantages
        a) *Does not define the full extent of the infarction for several days. Subtle changes may not be seen for up to 4 h.*
        b) *Brain stem and cerebellar structures are poorly displayed because of bony artifacts.*
  b. MRI
     1) Advantages
        a) *Clearly displays hemispheric, brain stem, and cerebellar pathology*
        b) *Displays ischemic change as early as 45 min after onset of ischemia*
        c) *Displays sequential changes during evolution of cerebral hemorrhage that enables distinction from infarction days or weeks after the event*
        d) *More reliable detection of venous infarction than CT*
     2) Disadvantages
        a) *Longer imaging time (45 min) may introduce motion artifact*
        b) *May cause anxiety in patients with claustrophobia*
        c) *If there are magnetic metallic objects in the body or brain, study cannot be performed*
  c. Carotid Doppler ultrasonography—noninvasive evaluation of extracranial carotid/vertebral arteries
  d. Transcranial Doppler—noninvasive evaluation of intracranial basilar artery and middle cerebral artery
  e. Cerebral angiography—remains the "gold standard" for evaluation of cerebrovascular disease
  f. Single photon emission computed tomography with Tc-HMPAO
  g. Positron-emission tomography—mainly a research tool
2. Cardiac imaging—useful in suspected cardioembolic situations
  a. Transthoracic echocardiography
  b. Transesophageal ecocardiography
3. Laboratory studies—complete blood count, differential, platelets, prothrombin time (PT) activated partial thromboplastin time, collagen vascular studies, tests of "hypercoagulability," if applicable (lupus anticoagulant, phospholipid antibodies, protein S, protein C)

C. Differential Diagnosis

1. Cardioembolic
  a. Atrial arrhythmia—fibrillation/flutter
  b. Valvular disease
  c. Dyskinetic cardiac segment or cardiomyopathy
  d. Myxoma

2. Hematologic
   a. Polycythemia
   b. Platelet disorders
   c. Bleeding disorders
   d. Hemoglobinopathies, ie, sickle cell disease
   e. Phospholipid antibody syndromes

3. Intracranial
   a. Brain tumor or abscess
   b. Subdural hematoma
   c. Subarachnoid hemorrhage (SAH)
   d. Intracerebral hemorrhage
   e. Migraine

4. Infections and inflammatory conditions
   a. Arteritis—giant cell and Takayesu's arteritis
   b. Endocarditis
   c. Rheumatologic—lupus erythematosus, polyarteritis nodosa
   d. Syphilitic, fungal infections

5. Cartoid artery disease
   a. Atheroembolic
   b. Carotid ulceration
   c. Arterial dissection
   d. Fibromuscular dysplasia
   e. Carotid aneurysm

D. Treatment

1. Atherothrombotic infarction (cerebral ischemic infarction)
   a. Acute phase management
      1) Medical therapy
         a) Bed rest
         b) Manage severe hypertension, if present
         c) Avoid orthostasis
         d) Hypervolemic hemodilution—maintain hematocrit 33–35 mg/dL with dextran, albumin, or plasmanate
         e) Thrombolytic therapy–streptokinase, tissue plasminogen activator (experimental)
      2) Anticoagulant drugs—may halt progression in some
         a) Valuable in observed progressive stroke, also in some lacunar syndromes
         b) Useful in patients with atrial fibrillation, acute myocardial infarction, cardiomyopathy, ventricular aneurysm, and valvular prostheses
         c) Initial therapy is IV heparin to aPTT 1.5 times control for up to 1 w, followed by oral warfarin, usually to an INR of 3.0–4.5.

3) Antiplatelet drugs
   a) *Aspirin*—*optimum dose not established, recommended doses vary from 30 mg to 1300 mg/day*
   b) *Dipyridamole - no advantage over aspirin*
   c) *Ticlopidine—role in therapy unclear—possibly more effective than aspirin*
4) Therapy for cerebral edema
   a) *Dexamethasone 4–6 mg q 4–6 h*
   b) *Mannitol 50 grams IV bolus or infusion*

b. Long-term management
   1) Anticoagulant drugs
   2) Antiplatelet drugs
   3) Carotid surgery—thromboendartectomy
      a) *Clear benefit established for TIA or mild nondisabling stroke with ipsilateral high-grade (70–99%) stenosis of the internal carotid artery*
      b) *Potentially beneficial in TIA or nondisabling stroke with at least 50% stenosis or large ulcerated plaque*
      c) *Not indicated in vertebral-basilar TIA/stroke, multiinfarct dementia, patients with severe neurologic deficits, and cerebral hemorrhage*
      d) *Relative contraindications include heart failure, myocardial infarction, active angina, and advanced malignancy*

2. Nontraumatic brain hemorrhage
   a. Acute phase management; principles include
      1) Identify site and extent of hemorrhage.
      2) Prevent subsequent damage from rebleeding, edema, hypertension.
      3) Correct electrolyte and coagulation parameters.
      4) Administer anticonvulsants in loading dose to prevent seizures.
      5) Intubate and ventilate patient, if necessary, maintaining PCO_2 30–35 mm Hq.
      6) Give mannitol if stuporous or comatose.
      7) Antihypertensive management
      8) Intracranial pressure (ICP) monitoring in selected patients
      9) Surgical management
         a) *Small hemorrhages with mild to moderate deficits require observation.*
         b) *Drainage of clot is helpful if ICP increased or neurologic deficits worsen despite optimum therapy.*
         c) *Cerebellar hemorrhage—hematomas > 3 cm should be removed emergently. Hematomas < 2 cm can be managed medically in the ICU/NICU.*
   b. Long-term management—search for underlying cause, such as ruptured arteriovenous malformation, hypertension, amyloid angiopathy, and treat if possible.

IV. Vertebral-Basilar Insufficiency

A. Clinical Presentation

1. Symptoms—site specific

   a. Vertigo, usually accompanied by staggering or diplopia
   b. Headache
   c. Facial pain
   d. Vestibular dysfunction
      1) Feeling of dysequilibrium
      2) Nausea and vomiting
   e. Ataxia, due to cerebellar dysfunction
   f. hiccups

2. Signs—site specific

   a. diminished sensation on ipsilateral face
   b. diminished sensation on contralateral body
   c. Horner's syndrome
   d. Ataxia
   e. Nystagmus
   f. Oculomotor disturbances
   g. Hoarseness, due to vocal cord paralysis or palatal weakness
   h. Ipsilateral facial weakness

B. Differential Diagnosis

1. Cervical spondylosis, compression of vertebral arteries by osteophytes
2. Neck rotation or trauma
3. Vertebral dissection
4. Fibromuscular dysplasia
5. Arteritis
6. Chronic basilar meningitis (fungal and tuberculous meningitis)
7. Subclavian steal syndrome
8. Lacunes
9. Also see differential diagnosis for cerebral infarctions

C. Treatment (see under cerebral infarction)

V. Indications for Referral

A. Most patients with brain hemorrhages require referral to a neurologist or neurosurgeon.

B. Patients with cerebral infarction or TIA need thorough evaluation for cause and planning of proper therapy.

VI. Indications for Hospitalization

All patients with TIA, acute cerebral infarction, SAH, and brain hemorrhage should be hospitalized.

VII. Annotated Bibliography

Barnett H, Mohr JP, Stein BM, Yatsu, FM. Stroke: Pathophysiology, Diagnosis, and Management, 2nd ed. New York: Churchill Livingstone, 1992.
   Comprehensive review of all aspects of cerebrovascular disease
Donnen G. Investigation of patients with stroke and TIA. Lancet 1992;339:473–477.
Hart R. Cardiogenic embolism to the brain. Lancet 1992;339:589–594.
Pulsinelli W. Pathophysiology of acute ischemic stroke. Lancet 1992:339:533–539.
Ropper AH. Neurological and Neurosurgical Intensive Care, 3rd ed. New York: Raven Press, 1993. Excellent review of all aspects of critical care neurology.
Wade D. Stroke: rehabilitation and long-term care. Lancet 1992:330:791–793.
   These reviews in *Lancet* are topical cogent articles that are accurate and up to date.

Chapter 74: Headache

Barry Ziring

I. Clinical Presentation

A. General Information

1. There are several headache patterns. The diagnosis is frequently made on the basis of the history and physical examination. As a general rule, acute severe headaches require more intensive investigation than chronic relapsing headache.

2. Common headache patterns include

    a. Acute headache
        1) Intracranial or subarachnoid hemorrhage
        2) Meningitis
    b. Chronic relapsing headache
        1) Migraine
        2) Cluster headache
        3) Muscle contraction headache
        4) Psychogenic headache
    c. Headaches associated with trauma
        1) Postconcussion syndrome
        2) Subdural hematoma
    d. Headache with atypical symptoms
        1) Trigeminal neuralgia
        2) Acute sinusitis
        3) Acute closed angle glaucoma
        4) Cranial (giant cell) arteritis/polymyalgia rheumatica
        5) Occipital headaches secondary to cervical arthritis
        6) Temporomandibular joint dysfunction
    e. Headaches associated with brain tumors
    f. Headaches in the immunosuppressed population
    g. Headaches associated with food or medication

B. Symptoms and History

1. General concerns regarding headaches include

    a. Symptoms suggesting increased intracranial pressure (ICP), such as vomiting or altered consciousness

b. Change in the headache pattern or a "typical" headache which fails to resolve.
c. Symptoms that are atypical for age group (eg, trigeminal neuralgia in a young person)
d. Unusual severity of headache (eg, description of worst headache of patient's life)

2. History of immunosuppression significantly expands the differential diagnosis of headache.

C. Physical Examination

1. Evaluation of most headache syndrome requires a general physical examination and complete neurologic examination.

2. In addition, certain features may help to indicate the etiology of a particular headache syndrome.

   a. Lacrimation and partial Horner's syndrome—suggestive of cluster headache
   b. Tender temporal artery—temporal arteritis
   c. Signs of meningeal irritation—seen in meningitis and subarachnoid hemorrhage
   d. Fever—seen in meningitis, temporal arteritis, and headaches in immunosuppressed patients

3. Focal neurologic deficits are always a concern in the setting of a headache.

II. Differential Diagnosis and Diagnostic Approach

A. Acute Headaches

1. Intracranial or subarachnoid hemorrhage

   a. The onset of headache is almost always sudden and severe from the moment of onset.
   b. Often accompanied by syncope
   c. Usually described as worst headache of patient's life
   d. Usually over age 35
   e. Headache may last for several days.
   f. 30–40% are fatal.
   g. Physical signs include
      1) Altered consciousness
      2) Vomiting may be present.
      3) Focal signs may be present.
      4) Stiff neck
   h. If signs of increased ICP are present, CT scan should be performed as soon as possible.
   i. Because subarachnoid hemorrhage can present with signs that are similar to meningitis, lumbar puncture should be performed if CT scan is negative.

j. If there are no signs of increased ICP, lumbar puncture may be considered as initial diagnostic procedure for acute headache.
2. Meningitis
   a. The headache of viral meningitis may be accompanied by other symptoms of viral illness.
      1) Neck stiffness is mild or absent.
      2) Consciousness is usually not altered.
      3) Lumbar puncture does not always need to be done. If performed, often shows mild increased leukocyte count.
   b. Bacterial meningitis
      1) The headache is severe, diffuse, and develops rapidly.
      2) Vomiting is common.
      3) There is usually a high fever although the elderly and immunosuppressed patients do not always have a fever.
      4) Most patients are confused or have altered consciousness. The presence of altered consciousness mandates further evaluation.
      5) If there are no signs of increased ICP, the patient with clinical suspicion of bacterial meningitis should have a lumbar puncture performed.
      6) If there are signs of increased ICP, the diagnosis is unclear or CT screening is immediately available, a CT scan may be performed before lumbar puncture.

B. Chronic Relapsing Headache
1. Migraine
   a. Classic type
      1) Has frequent incidence
      2) Often begins during childhood to young adulthood
      3) Unilateral, throbbing
      4) Often associated with aura
      5) Last 2–6 h
      6) Often associated with vomiting and pallor
      7) Female predominance
      8) Family history of headache
   b. Common type
      1) Common incidence
      2) Often begins during childhood to young adulthood
      3) Frontal, unilateral, or bilateral
      4) No significant aura
      5) Can last 1–3 d
      6) Can have an aura and vomiting
      7) Female predominance
      8) Migraines may be worse during the menstrual period.
   c. Complicated type
      1) May present without headache
      2) Usually a neurologic aura

3) Patients with this syndrome can have mild neurologic signs including speech disorder, hemiparesis, unsteadiness, cranial nerve III palsy.
4) Ophthalmologic migraine can present with cranial nerve III palsy, visual loss, ptosis, and pupillary dilatation.
5) Basilar migraine can present as syncope (often in adolescents).
6) The differential diagnosis in the above group of patients includes aneurysm and arteriovenous malformation.

2. Cluster headaches (Horton's headache, histamine headache)
   a. Uncommon
   b. Usually young to middle age men
   c. Male predominence
   d. Repetitive nature of pain, each pain lasts approximately 1 h but episodes may last a week or more.
   e. Pain is around eye, temple, and cheek.
   f. Lacrimation, nasal stiffness, scleral injection, and partial Horner's syndrome can confirm diagnosis.

3. Muscle contraction or tension headache
   a. Probably the most common headache syndrome
   b. Usually young adult to middle age
   c. No sex bias
   d. Often a family history of headache
   e. The location and quality is variable but often described as bandlike, squeezing, or localized to neck muscles.
   f. Often worse with stress.

4. Psychogenic headaches
   a. Headaches associated with psychiatric illness are often a diagnosis of exclusion.
   b. Headaches may be secondary to depression and may be accompanied by changes in sleep and eating patterns.
   c. Headaches can represent a conversion reaction.
   d. Great care should be taken before ascribing headache to psychiatric disease because headaches can cause depression and other mood changes.

5. Hypertension
   a. High blood pressure is an infrequent cause of headache.
   b. Moderately severe (diastolic blood pressure > 120 mm Hg) hypertension may produce dull, throbbing, diffuse, or occipital headaches.
   c. The physician must be aware that although hypertension rarely causes headache, it may predispose to intracranial bleeding discussed under acute headache.
   d. Paroxysmal headache associated with hypertension is suggestive of pheochromocytoma.

e. Abrupt onset of severe headache, mental confusion, seizure, and visual loss can be seen with hypertensive encephalopathy without hemorrhage.

C. Headache Associated with Trauma

1. Postconcussion syndrome

    a. Occurs a few hours after injury
    b. Cause unknown
    c. Patients should be examined for focal neurologic signs that may indicate more serious injury.

2. Subdural hematoma

    a. Patients with subdural hematomas usually have headaches.
    b. Headaches gradually worsen with time after injury.
    c. In advanced stages, focal neurologic signs and stupor may develop.

D. Headaches with Atypical Symptoms

1. Trigeminal neuralgia (tic douloureux)

    a. Can usually be distinguished from a true headache on basis of symptoms alone.
    b. Presents as lancinating, burning, or needle-like pain in cheek or jaw
    c. A less common syndrome of glossopharyngeal neuralgia can cause pain in the throat, tongue, or ear.
    d. The pain almost always occurs in spasms that can be extremely severe but resolve between episodes.

2. Acute sinusitis

    a. Usually presents with facial pain, purulent nasal discharge and is often accompanied by a headache
    b. Temperature elevation occurs in < 50% of patients.
    c. Erythema, swelling, and tenderness may be found over the involved sinus but usually are not present.
    d. Transillumination of the maxillary and frontal sinuses can be helpful if there is complete opacity or normal illumination of the sinuses.

3. Acute closed angle glaucoma

    a. Usually asymptomatic; patients can experience eye pain and headache when intraoclular pressures are suddenly high.
    b. The diagnosis is usually obvious at this point due to red eye, dilated pupils that do not respond to light, watery secretions, and decreased vision.

4. Cranial (giant cell) arteritis (GCA) and polymyalgia rheumatica (PMR)

    a. Characteristically over age 50.
    b. The pain of GCA is often localized to the scalp or to tender aching temporal arteries.
    c. PMR may present with shoulder and neck pain and stiffness, which can be confused with true headache. GCA may accompany PMR.

d. Due to the risk of irreversible vision loss in GCA or PMR with associated GCA, early diagnosis is imperative. Temporal artery biopsy should be considered whenever there is strong clinical suspicion for GCA or when PMR is accompanied by evidence of systemic involvement including fever, anemia, elevated liver enzymes, or neurologic signs.

5. Headaches associated with cervical arthritis
   a. Head pain is a common characteristic of cervical spine disorder.
   b. It results from root compression, vertebral artery pressure, compression of sympathetic nerves, and posterior occipital muscle spasm.
   c. The diagnosis is suspected based on the cervical or occipital distribution of the pain and decreased range of motion of the neck or findings of a cervical radiculopathy.

6. Temporomandibular joint (TMJ) dysfunction
   a. May account for as many as 10–15% of patients with chronic headache
   b. Pain is usually unilateral, located around the temple, above or behind the eye, or in and around the ear.

7. Headaches associated with brain tumors or intracranial space-occupying lesion
   a. Frequent features of this type of headache include worsening with motion, exercise, cough, or strain.
   b. Headaches may be worse in morning and may awaken patient from sleep.
   c. Headache secondary to brain tumors are rare.
   d. This diagnosis should be considered when
      1) Patient presents with an atypical pattern such as trigeminal neuralgia in a young person
      2) Symptoms progress or headache does not remit
      3) Any finding of focal neurologic deficit or subtle change of mental status
      4) New onset of symptoms or change in symptoms complex especially in middle age
   e. MRI or CT scan can be used if there is clinical suspicion for a brain tumor.

8. Headaches associated with food or drugs
   a. Caffeine or alcohol withdrawal
   b. Nitrates
   c. Chocolate
   d. Hunger

9. Headache in the immunosuppressed patient
   a. In a patient with AIDS or immunosuppression secondary to drug therapy, headache can be a signal of serious illness.
   b. Chronic or progressive headache in this population is the most prevalent symptom suggesting CNS involvement.
   c. *Toxoplasma gondii* is the most frequent cause of encephalitis in AIDS patients.
      1) Headache, focal neurologic signs, and occasionally, seizures are typical.

2) Fever is often not present.
3) Diagnosis is made by CT scan showing a ring enhancing lesion.
  d. *Cryptococcus neoformans* is the most frequent form of meningitis in AIDS patients.
    1) Headache is the most frequent complaint.
    2) Fever is common.
    3) Meningeal signs are usually absent.
    4) CT should be done to exclude increased ICP or mass lesion.
    5) Diagnosis is made by lumbar puncture.

III. Treatment

A. Migraines

1. Avoid contributing factors (eg, oral contraceptive, anxiety, precipitating foods, monosodium glutamate).

2. Abortive therapy
    a. Nonsteroidal anti-inflammatory drugs (NSAIDs)
        1) May be the first choice for mild to moderately severe migraine attacks
        2) No particular drug has been shown to be superior.
        3) These drugs do not always relieve nausea and vomiting.
        4) Metoclopramide (Reglan) may speed absorption and reduce nausea and vomiting.
    b. Ergotamine preparations
        1) Oral dose is 2 mg sublingually then 1–2 mg sublingual q 30 min to maximum 6 mg daily (also IM, rectally or by inhalation).
        2) Contraindicated in patients with peripheral vascular disease, impaired hepatic or renal function, or pregnancy
    c. Sumatriptin—a serotonin (5-hydroxytryptamine) agonist
        1) Available in SQ injection or tablet
        2) Results in transient increase in blood pressure
        3) Angina has been reported.
        4) Nausea and vomiting reported with the tablet.
        5) The dose is 10 mg orally or 6 mg injection. This may be repeated.
    d. Combination drugs
        1) Midrin (isometheptene, dichloralphenazone and acetaminophen)
        2) Fiorinal (butalbital, caffeine, aspirin)
        3) No strong evidence that either combination is more effective than other analgesics.
        4) Both combinations have addictive potential.
        5) Both combinations can cause withdrawal headache.

3. Prophylactic therapy
    a. First-line
        1) Cyproheptadine (Periactin) 8–16 mg/d in divided doses; may cause weight gain

2) β Blockers—propanolol (only β blocker with a Food and Drug Administration indication) at 40–160 mg/d in divided doses. Nadolol is also effective at 40–240 mg/d.
3) Tricyclic antidepressants (eg, amitriptyline) 10–150 mg PO, particularly beneficial in depressed patients but also has independent effects against migraine.
  b. Second-line
    1) Methysergide (Sansert) 2–8 mg/d in divided doses, may precipitate or worsen angina or symptoms of peripheral vascular disease. Contraindicated in patients with severe arteriosclerosis, renal or hepatic disease, serious infections, or pregnancy.
    2) Verapamil 240 mg/d
    3) Anticonvulsants—phenytoin, phenobarbitol, or carbamazepine
  c. Third-line
    1) Lithium
    2) NSAIDs
    3) Steroid—short course
4. Other techniques for migraine
  a. Biofeedback
  b. Relaxation techniques (yoga, hypnosis)
  c. Antiemetics for accompanying nausea
  d. Avoid narcotics and combination drugs

B. Chronic Tension Headache

1. Analgesics

   a. Acetaminophen
   b. Aspirin
   c. NSAIDs

2. Antidepressants

   a. The choice of antidepressants depends on the unique characteristics of each agent.
      1) Desipramine, protriptyline, buproprion, and fluoxetine are non-sedating and preferred for patients without a sleep disorder. May be able to use a lower dose for headache than for depression.
      2) Patients with symptoms of serotonin deficiency (myalgias, arthralgias, fatigue, carbohydrate craving, irritability, disturbed memory, and concentration) respond better to fluoxetene.

3. Adjunctive therapy

   a. Angiotensin-converting enzyme (ACE) inhibitors
   b. Lithium

C. Cluster Headaches

1. Abortive therapy is preferable to treatment.

a. Methysergide 4–12 mg/d
b. Lithium carbonate 600–1200 mg/d
c. Prednisone 15–60 mg/d
d. Verapamil 240 mg/d

2. Headaches can also be treated with indomethacin.

IV. Patient Education

A. Avoidance of precipitating foods, stressors, or drugs (as described previously) is very important.

B. Prophylactic drug therapy and early abortive therapy are more effective than treatment of headache when severe.

C. A change in pattern of headaches from chronic pattern may signal a new medical problem.

D. Brain tumors are often a concern of patients. Patients should be reassured that brain tumors are extremely rare. If the patient's symptoms fit a typical headache pattern, imaging studies are rarely necessary or helpful.

E. A major complication of chronic headaches is analgesic or narcotic overuse. Patients should be warned of the side effects of these medications.

V. Long-term Management

A. Nonpharmacologic therapy can play a role in treatment of vascular, mixed, and muscle contraction headaches. This includes

1. Reassurance and supportive care
2. Physical therapy and exercise
3. Biofeedback
4. Nutritional counseling
5. Changes in life-style

B. Minor analgesics are the mainstay of therapy for muscle contraction headaches. However, chronic use of narcotics should be avoided.

VI. Indications for Referral

A. Acute headaches where there is suspicion for a subarachnoid hemorrhage or meningitis require very rapid diagnosis and treatment. In general, this group of patients should be seen or sent directly to any emergency room.

B. Chronic headaches of most types can be treated by the primary care physician. Patients with headaches that do not respond to therapy or present with atypical features may be referred to a neurologist or headache clinic.

C. The wide availability of CT scanning and MRI has decreased the necessity of referring patients with suspected brain tumors to subspecialists for diagnosis. These patients are usually referred to qualified centers for treatment.

D. If patients fail to respond to standard therapy or if there is obvious psychiatric disease, referral to a psychiatrist may be indicated.

VII. Annotated Bibliography

Edmeods J. Headache and facial pain. In: Stein JM, ed. Internal Medicine. Boston: Little, Brown;1990. Thorough, practical discussion of headache.

Headache Classification Committee of the International Headache Society, Classification and Diagnostic Criteria for Headache Disorders, Cranial Neuralgias, and Facial Pain. Cephalalgia 1988; 8:(suppl 7):1–96. The current complete guide to headache and facial pain classification.

Solomon GD. Pharmacology and use of headache medications. Cleve Clin J Med 57:627–635, 1990; An excellent review of headache treatment.

Weiner SL. Acute head pain. In: Differential Diagnosis of Acute Pain by Body Region. New York: 1993. McGraw-Hill; Provides thorough, practical discussion of headache.

Chapter 75: Hoarseness

David Zwillenberg

I. Clinical Presentation

A. Symptoms and Signs

1. Acute change in voice

   a. With upper respiratory infection—generally viral laryngitis
   b. With vocal abuse; eg, cheering at a ball game, a family argument, etc—generally due to laryngeal edema

2. Chronic hoarseness

   a. Defined as hoarseness for 3 wk or more. All such patients should undergo laryngoscopic examination.

3. Associated signs and symptoms

   a. Pain—The presence of pain in the throat or the ears in the presence of chronic hoarseness suggests grave pathology such as carcinoma.
   b. Dysphagia—may also indicate severe pathology when associated with hoarseness
   c. Aspiration—The presence of aspiration generally indicates vocal cord paralysis.
   d. Dyspnea or stridor—Obstruction may be imminent.
   e. Neck mass—suggestive of malignancy

B. Physical Examination

1. Indirect laryngoscopy should be performed in the outpatient setting. If inadequate:

2. Fiberoptic direct laryngoscopy should be performed. If a suspicious lesion is seen or if fiberoptic exam is inadequate:

3. Direct operative laryngoscopy should be carried out.

II. Diagnostic Approach

A. Acute Change in Voice

1. After extubation—If either intubation or extubation were traumatic, laryngoscopy is imperative.
2. After a cerebrovascular accident—Laryngoscopy is important to rule out vocal cord paralysis and aspiration.
3. After neck trauma—Laryngoscopy is imperative.
4. After thoracic or neck surgery (eg, coronary artery bypass graft, thyroidectomy, anterior cervical fusion, etc.)—Laryngoscopy is indicated.

B. Who Should be Examined by Laryngoscopy

1. All patients with chronic hoarseness
2. All patients with acute hoarseness and any of the above signs or clinical scenarios

III. Differential Diagnosis

A. Viral Laryngitis

1. Probably most common cause of hoarseness
2. Generally self-limited without treatment

B. Vocal Nodules or Polyps

1. Very common
2. Generally follows persistent vocal abuse
3. Often seen in singers (singer's nodules), preachers (preacher's nodules), teachers, mothers of young children, etc.
4. Generally hoarseness is fluctuating—better after rest, worse after abuse

C. Vocal Cord Hemorrhage

1. Generally follows a particularly stressful period of voice use
2. In miduse the voice suddenly becomes hoarse.

D. Laryngocele

1. Cystic dilation of the laryngeal saccule. Can be
    a. Internal—within the cartilagenous larynx
    b. External—outside the cartilagenous larynx and palpable in the neck
    c. Mixed—internal and external

E. Mucous Retention Cyst

1. Can occur anywhere in the larynx
2. Those causing hoarseness generally occur on the true cords.

F. Neurogenic—Vocal Cord Paralysis or Paresis

1. Subdural hematoma
2. Meningocele
3. Arnold-Chiari malformation
3. Polio
5. Guillain-Barré syndrome
6. Mononucleosis
7. Myasthenia gravis
8. Tumors of the neck or mediastinum
    a. If the examination of the larynx shows a paralyzed cord without a lesion, a CT or MRI scan of the neck and superior mediastinum should be done.
9. Postsurgical
    a. Thyroidectomy
    b. Cardiac surgery
    c. Anterior cervical fusion
    d. Tracheoesophageal fistula repair
    e. Intubations
10. Cerebrovascular accident

G. Laryngeal Papilloma

1. Most common laryngeal tumor of childhood
2. Caused by human papillomavirus 6 and 11
3. Pediatric papillomas associated with vaginal birth and maternal condylomata
4. Also occurs in adults who generally have a more indolent course
5. Pediatric papillomata have a tendency to spread and recur and require surgical interventions.
6. In both children and adults malignant transformation may occur.

H. Malignancy

1. Squamous cell carcinoma accounts for >95% in most series.
2. Signs suggestive of malignancy include
    a. Otalgia
    b. Dysphagia
    c. Neck mass
3. Diagnostic work-up includes laryngoscopy with biopsy and bronchoscopy and esophagoscopy as well as chest x-ray due to the high incidence of synchronous and metachronous second primaries.

4. Generally associated with tobacco and ethanol use. Continued smoking and/or drinking has a significant negative effect on prognosis after treatment.

I. Trauma

1. Arytenoid dislocation
   a. Generally after traumatic intubation or extubation or severe coughing

J. Rheumatoid Disease

1. Cricoarytenoid arthritis can produce fixation of one or both cords.

K. Candidiasis

1. Laryngeal candidiasis can be seen in association with oral and/or esophageal candidiasis in the immunocompromised host.

L. Angioneurotic edema

1. Acute onset
2. Abnormal C4 levels

M. Reflux Laryngitis

1. Other reflux symptoms may or may not be present.
2. Usually worse in the morning
3. Usually worse under stress
4. Barium swallow with water siphonage or 24h pH monitoring may be indicated.

IV. Treatment

A. Viral Laryngitis

1. Voice rest will help hasten complete resolution.

B. Vocal Nodules or Polyps

1. Voice rest and speech therapy are the mainstays of treatment.
2. Excision may be necessary if unresponsive to the above.

C. Vocal Cord Hemorrhage

1. Voice rest is appropriate. In professional singers and the like, immediate drainage may be indicated.

D. Laryngocele

1. Excision of laryngocele

E. Mucous Retention Cyst

1. Marsupialization or excision are the treatments of choice.

F. Neurogenic—Vocal Cord Paralysis or Paresis

1. Hydrocephalus—treatment shunt
2. Generally treating the primary disease is adequate. Teflon injection or phonosurgery may be needed.

G. Laryngeal Papilloma

1. Repeated laser excision
2. Other therapies including interferon are controversial.

H. Malignancy

1. Treatment of early lesions consists of either radiation or surgery. More advanced lesions will require both surgery and radiation.
2. Chemotherapy may also prove useful in advanced lesions.

I. Trauma

1. If comminuted, perform tracheotomy immediately for airway protection and reduce.

J. Candidiasis

1. Topical and systemic treatments are indicated.

K. Angioneurotic Edema

1. Treat with epinephrine and steroids. Tracheotomy may be needed.

L. Reflux Laryngitis

1. H_2 Blockers or antacids may be indicated.

M. Acute Change in Voice

1. With upper respiratory infection—no treatment necessary
2. With vocal abuse—Voice rest is the best treatment.

V. Indications for Referral

A. All patients with hoarseness of > 3 or 4 wk duration

B. All patients with associated otalgia, neck mass, or dysphagia

C. All patients with hoarseness of new onset and a history of malignancy elsewhere

D. Hoarseness combined with shortness of breath may indicate an emergency situation.

VI. Indications for Hospitalization

A. Hoarseness with dyspnea

B. Treatment of any of the conditions listed in differential diagnosis may require hospitalization for airway support, treatment of malignancy, etc.

VII. Annotated Bibliography

Spofford B. History and Physical Exam in Otolaryngology-Head and Neck Surgery, Vol 3. St. Louis: CV Mosby; 1986:1792–1793. A very good overview of this area.

Weynuller E. Airway Management. In: Cummings CW, Fredrickson JM, Harker LA, Krause CJ, Schulle DE, eds. Otolaryngology-Head and Neck Surgery, Vol 3. St. Louis: CV Mosby; 1986:2417–2418.

Chapter 76: Peripheral Neuropathy

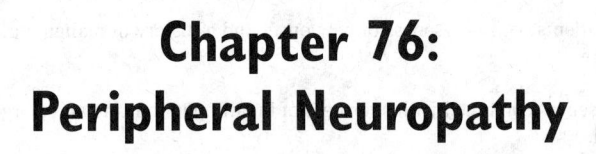

Kenneth R. Epstein

I. Clinical Presentation

A. General Information

1. Peripheral nerves consist of a bundle of axons. Large and medium-sized axons are usually covered by myelin sheaths, whereas small nerve fibers are usually not myelinated.

2. Peripheral nerves are usually mixed nerves that carry afferent (sensory) fibers, efferent (motor) fibers, and autonomic fibers. Most peripheral neuropathies affect both sensory and motor nerves, and some affect the peripheral autonomic nerves.

3. Large diameter afferent fibers are involved in position and vibration sense. Large diameter efferent fibers are involved in muscle innervation. Small diameter unmyelinated fibers carry pain and temperature sense as well as autonomic information.

4. Peripheral neuropathies may affect predominantly the axons (axonal neuropathy) or the myelin sheaths (demyelinating neuropathy). Secondary demyelination can occur with advanced axonal neuropathies, but axonal loss is rare in demyelinating disorders. Many of the common neuropathies involve both axonal degeneration and demyelination.

5. In both axonal and demyelinating neuropathies, the longer and larger nerves are affected earlier and more severely than are the shorter ones. This explains the frequent involvement of the feet and hands in peripheral neuropathies.

6. Peripheral neuropathies are usually classified into three predominant categories.
    a. Mononeuropathy—a lesion of an individual nerve root or peripheral nerve; usually due to a local cause, such as trauma or entrapment
    b. Multifocal neuropathy (also called mononeuropathy multiplex)—lesions of at least two discrete nerves, usually asymmetrically and noncontiguously; usually due to ischemic damage to nerves from a systemic process
    c. Polyneuropathy—a generalized disease process involving diffuse injury to the peripheral nervous system; affects peripheral nerves in a symmetrical, usually distal, distribution

B. Symptoms

1. A detailed history is essential to screen for the presence of symptoms suggestive of systemic diseases.
2. The specific neurologic symptoms depend on the type of neuropathy (mononeuropathy, multifocal neuropathy, or polyneuropathy), as well as the type of nerves affected (sensory, motor, autonomic).
3. Sensory symptoms (symptoms may precede physical signs) include
   a. Loss of sensation (anesthesia)
   b. Pain
   c. Paresthesias (pins and needle sensation)—polyneuropathies usually initially present with parethesias or anesthesia of the distal extremities, especially the feet.
   d. Hypersensitivity to nonnoxious stimuli (eg, light touch perceived as burning)
4. Motor symptoms include
   a. Weakness or clumsiness—ask about difficulty with specific functional activities
   b. Muscle cramps
   c. Fasciculations (muscle twitching)
5. Autonomic symptoms include
   a. Loss of ability to perspire or hyperhydrosis
   b. Impotence
   c. Urinary retention or overflow incontinence
   d. Constipation or diarrhea

C. Physical Examination

1. A complete physical examination is essential to look for the presence of systemic disease.
2. In addition to peripheral nerve examination, an examination for mental status and cranial nerve dysfunction is important.
3. Sensory examination includes
   a. Pin prick
   b. Light touch
   c. Deep pressure
   d. Paresthesia or anesthesia
   e. Vibration sense
   f. Temperature sense
   g. Position sense
4. Motor examination includes
   a. Strength—The patient may have objective evidence of muscle weakness before he/she is aware of it (ie, signs may precede symptoms, the opposite

of situation for sensory deficits). Examine distal extremity musculature in particular.
   b. Muscle atrophy
   c. Diminished deep tendon reflexes—are often decreased in peripheral neuropathies out of proportion to the motor weakness
5. Autonomic examination includes
   a. Trophic skin changes
   b. Rectal tone
   c. Postural changes in blood pressure and heart rate (> 20 mm Hg fall in systolic blood pressure going from lying to standing, with an inadequate compensatory increase in heart rate)
6. In polyneuropathies, the sensory loss is often initially a distal loss of pain and vibration, in a stocking-glove distribution.
7. In polyneuropathies, the motor weakness is also often initially distal, affecting the intrinsic muscles of the hands and feet. The patient may have difficulty with dorsiflexion of the feet and toes. The patient may eventually develop high arched feet, hammer toes, and muscle wasting of the small muscles of the hands and feet.

II. Diagnostic Approach

A. The key to diagnosis is a detailed history and physical examination. In particular, investigate for evidence of

1. Trauma
2. Alcohol consumption
3. Nutritional deficiencies
4. Occupational or environmental toxic exposures
5. Recent introduction of new medications
6. Endocrinopathies
7. Malignancies
8. Infections, such as recent viral illness
9. Metabolic abnormalities
10. Family history of neuropathy—is important to ask even in older adults

B. In polyneuropathies, the sensory and motor findings are usually symmetrical. If there is a unifocality or asymmetry, consider the multifocal neuropathies.

C. There are many ways to divide polyneuropathies. One method is to divide them based on three axes: time course, selective functional involvement, and distribution (Table 76–1).

Table 76–1. Differential Diagnosis of Polyneuropathies (with selected examples)

I. Course
   A. Acute (days), eg, Guillain-Barré syndrome
   B. Subacute (weeks), eg, many toxins, nutritional neuropathies
   C. Relapsing
   D. Chronic (many months or years), eg, diabetic or alcoholic neuropathies
   E. Very chronic (childhood onset), eg, inherited motor-sensory neuropathies

II. Selective Functional Involvement
   A. Predominantly motor, eg, Guillain-Barré syndrome
   B. Predominantly sensory
      1. Global sensory loss, eg, diabetic or carcinomatous sensory neuropathy
      2. Dissociated loss of pain and temperature sensation, eg, amyloidosis
      3. Dissociated loss of joint position and vibration sense, eg, subacute combined degeneration
   C. Autonomic neuropathy, eg, diabetes, amyloidosis

III. Distribution
   A. Proximal weakness, eg, Guillain-Barré
   B. Proximal sensory loss, eg, porphyria
   C. Temperature-related distribution, eg, lepromatous leprosy

SOURCE: Adapted by permission from Griffen JW, Cornblath DR. Peripheral neuropathies. In: Harvey AM, Johns RJ, McKusick VA, et al. The Principles and Practice of Medicine, 22nd ed. Norwalk, CT: Appleton & Lange; 1988:1092–1096.

D. If the cause of the peripheral neuropathy is not obvious by history and physical examination, then certain selected screening tests are indicated.

1. Complete blood count
2. Erythrocyte sedimentation rate
3. Fasting blood glucose
4. Creatinine
5. Thyroid function tests
6. Serum protein electrophoresis
7. Chest x-ray
8. Other laboratory or radiologic tests based on clinical suspicion by history and physical examination

E. Nerve Conduction Studies (NCS) and Electromyography (EMG)

1. Are indicated in almost all patients with suspected peripheral neuropathy
2. NCS involve stimulating a nerve at one point and recording the conduction velocity along the path of the nerve. For a motor nerve, this would be distally at the muscle, and for a sensory nerve, at a proximal point along the nerve.

3. EMG studies involve the percutaneous insertion of an electrode directly into the muscle, to record the action potential within the muscle. The action potentials are measured both at rest (looking for spontaneous activity) and with contraction of the muscle (looking for voluntary activity).

4. In primarily axonal neuropathies, one may see normal NCS, but denervation by EMG.

5. In primarily demyelinating neuropathies, one may see a normal EMG with slowed conduction by NCS.

6. The limitation of these tests is that they only measure nerve function between the two sites that are being measured. A more proximal or distal lesion may be missed. They are, therefore, not very useful for suspected nerve root lesions.

F. Nerve Biopsy

1. Occasionally indicated for diagnosis in asymmetric multifocal neuropathies if etiology after noninvasive work-up remains unclear. It may be helpful in diagnosis of specific diseases, such as amyloid, vasculitis, or sarcoid. Also indicted if a nerve is palpably enlarged

2. Is almost never necessary in symmetric distal polyneuropathies

3. The sural nerve of the ankle is the preferred site.

III. Differential Diagnosis

A. Mononeuropathy

1. Trauma

2. Entrapment or compression, eg, carpal tunnel syndrome (see Chapter 72)

3. Vasculitis

4. Neoplasia—either compression or direct invasion

5. Toxic, eg, accidental injection in a nerve

6. Infectious, eg, herpes zoster

B. Multifocal Neuropathy

1. Diabetes mellitus (see below)

2. Vasculitis

C. Polyneuropathy

See Table 76–1 for list of common causes. For rarer causes, refer to a neurology textbook.

D. Diabetic Neuropathies

1. Mononeuropathies or multifocal neuropathies

a. Etiology is often ischemic, ie, nerve infarction
  b. Diabetic patients have an increased incidence of compression and entrapment neuropathies such as carpal tunnel syndrome or peroneal palsy.
2. Diabetic amyopathy
  a. A specific form of multifocal neuropathy involving the proximal muscles
  b. Presents with the gradual or subacute onset of weakness of the proximal musculature, particularly the quadriceps and iliopsoas muscles
3. Diabetic Polyneuropathy
  a. Is a symmetric distal sensorimotor neuropathy. The sensory symptoms usually predominate over the motor symptoms.
  b. The patient's primary complaint usually involves pain and temperature sensation. The pain is often described as a burning dysesthesia or hypersensitivity.
  c. The distal upper limbs usually become involved when the lower extremity symptoms have extended to the upper one third of the foreleg.
  d. The patient may develop sensory ataxia with loss of position sense. This may lead to gait disturbances and Charcot joints, which is a type of osteoarthritic joint damage due to the loss of both proprioception and pain sensation.

IV. Treatment

A. The treatment of peripheral neuropathies is specific to the etiology of the neuropathy. Because the differential diagnosis is long, as shown in Table 76-1, therapy for specific disorders will not be addressed.

B. General Principles of Treatment for All Neuropathies

1. Identify and treat the underlying disorder.
2. Prevent further damage
   a. For sensory neuropathies, prevent trauma due to lack of sensation of affected extremities. Keep skin well hydrated and nails well groomed.
   b. For motor neuropathies, prevent contractures and minimize atrophy with splints as necessary and physical therapy.
3. In sensory neuropathies, treat pain, which is often chronic and disabling.
   a. Analgesics—Start with aspirin or acetaminophen. Avoid narcotics due to risk of addiction.
   b. Tricyclic antidepressants—can have significant effect for chronic pain. Start with low dose, eg, amitriptyline or nortriptyline 25–50 mg qhs, and increase slowly until achieve therapeutic effect. If dose exceeds 100 mg, monitor serum levels to avoid toxicity.
   c. Anticonvulsants—Phenytoin and carbemazepine have variable effects on chronic neuropathic pain. As with antidepressants, start at low dose

(phenytoin 200–300 mg/d or carbamazepine 100 mg b.i.d.) and increase until achieve therapeutic effect.

d. If above medications do not improve symptoms at maximum dose or with therapeutic blood levels, then there is no value in continuing the medication.

V. Patient Education

A. Patient education is specific to the etiology of the peripheral neuropathy.

B. Patients with sensory neuropathies of the lower extremities should be educated to inspect their feet daily, keep their feet clean and dry, always wear shoes, and report any lesions immediately.

VI. Indications for Referral

A. Indications for Referral to Neurologist

1. If unclear of the indications for or interpretation of NCS or EMG studies

2. Any patient with unexplained neuropathy after history, physical examination, and screening blood tests above

B. Indications for Referral to Physical Therapist or Occupational Therapist. Most patients with chronic motor neuropathies will benefit from evaluation by a physical and occupational therapist.

VII. Annotated Bibliography

Cohen JA, Gross KF. Peripheral neuropathy: causes and management in the elderly. Geriatrics 1990;45(2):21–34. Reviews the evaluation of peripheral neuropathies in the elderly.

Griffin JW, Cornblath DR. Peripheral neuropathies. In: Harvey AM, Johns RJ, McKusick VA, et al. The Principles and Practice of Medicine, 22nd ed. Norwalk, CT: Appleton & Lange; 1988:1092–1096. A concise review of peripheral neuropathies, with helpful table on the differential diagnosis of polyneuropathies.

Harati Y. Frequently asked questions about diabetic peripheral neuropathies. Neurol Clin 1992;10:783–806. A thorough review of many details of diabetic neuropathies.

Josifek LF, Bleker ML. Peripheral neuropathy. In: Barker LR, Burton JR, Zieve PD, eds. Principles of Ambulatory Medicine, 3rd ed. Baltomore: Williams & Wilkins; 1991:1155–1170. Well written chapter on the evaluation and treatment of peripheral neuropathies.

Chapter 77: Seizures

Robert D. Aiken

I. Clinical Presentation

A. See Chapter 6 for discussion of acute management of seizures.

B. History

1. General history

   a. Initial interview should include an eyewitness who has observed the phenomenon, if possible.
   b. Family history of seizures, blackouts
   c. Birth, perinatal history, growth and development
   d. Other factors that might bear on diagnosis—diabetes, concussive head injury, drug/alcohol/substance abuse
   e. Psychosocial development

2. Seizure history

   a. Aura or prodome, if present
   b. The clinical seizure, most reliably given by an eyewitness
   c. Postictal symptoms
   d. Precipitating factors, if any
   e. Frequency
   f. Age of onset
   g. Evolution of symptoms over time
   h. Antiepileptic drug history including doses, duration of treatment, and response, if known

C. Physical Examination

1. General physical examination is directed toward finding a specific disease process or malformation that is the cause of seizures. Particular attention is to craniofacial appearance, skin for birthmarks, liver and spleen for storage diseases, and musculoskeletal development and symmetry.

2. Neurologic physical examination

   a. Higher cerebral function
      1) Impairment common in patients with generalized convulsions and complex partial seizures

2) Retardation may be a sign of static encephalopathy.
   b. Motor and sensory testing—Focal or lateralized features help to distinguish partial from generalized epilepsy and may provide localization information.
   c. Coordination—clumsiness, abnormal postures
   d. Deep tendon reflexes and pathologic reflexes
3. Observation of the epileptic seizure—"One picture is worth a thousand words."
   a. Aura, if any, and description if possible
   b. Ictal period
      1) Mental status
         a) *Alert or dulled*
         b) *Amnesic*
      2) Sensory—sometimes helpful (visual field examination and pin prick if cooperative)
      3) Motor—observe initial site of seizure including nature of initial motions (clonic, tonic, positioning)
   c. Postical period
      1) Abnormal behavior and responsiveness
      2) Focal, lateralizing, or cognitive defects (Todd's paralysis)
      3) Tests of recall
      4) Description of the aura, preictal event if recalled

II. Diagnostic Approach

Individualize testing to the patient's problem.

A. Laboratory Tests

1. Complete blood count, differential, platelets, electrolytes, liver and hepatic function, coagulation studies, Ca, mg—routine
2. CSF by lumbar puncture—not routine unless history and physical examination suggest a specific problem associated with known CSF abnormalities
3. Prolactin—elevated after complex partial and generalized convulsions. May help to distinguish between epileptic and nonepileptic episodes. Draw within 20 min of the event and compare with another drawn remote from an event or on another day.

B. Electroencephalogram (EEG)

1. Most informative test in diagnosis of epilepsy
2. Routine—Standard 10–20 system of lead placement, awake and asleep recording
3. Nasopharyngeal electrodes—helpful to evaluate for mesial temporal region seizures
4. Sphenoidal electrodes—rarely used because application of leads is painful.

5. Ambulatory EEG recording—occasionally helpful for infrequent seizures
6. Video/EEG monitoring—helps to correlate EEG and behavioral manifestations

C. Tests of Cerebral Morphology

1. CT scan
2. MRI

D. Other Tests of Cerebral Function (Occasionally Valuable)

1. Neuropsychological testing
2. Single photon emission CT/position-emission tomography scanning to map the epileptic focus—especially useful for candidates considering seizure surgery

III. Differential Diagnosis

A. Syncope due to cardiac, vasomotor causes

B. Hyperventilation

C. Breath holding (infants only)

D. Toxins

1. Alcoholic blackouts
2. Encephalopathy due to hepatic, renal failure
3. Confusion and hallucinations (eg, porphyria, psychotomimetic drugs)

E. Narcolepsy/sleep disturbances

F. Cerebrovascular disease including migraine

G. Abnormal movement disorders not due to epilepsy (dystonia, tremors, tics, hyperexplexia, hemifacial spasms)

H. Other nonepileptic sensory disorders—paroxysmal vertigo, trigeminal neuralgia, peduncular hallucinosis

I. Psychogenic (pseudo) seizures

J. Dyscontrol states

K. Dissociative states and psychoses

L. Daydreaming

M. Nonpsychotic psychiatric disorders—panic attacks

IV. Treatment

A. General Principles

1. Treatment of generalized and complex partial seizures should aim for complete control.

2. All simple or brief nonconvulsive generalized seizures that do not interfere with daily function need not be eliminated.

3. Occasional seizures may be preferable to complete control in some patients because of impaired cognitive function associated with drug regimens and side effects.

B. Treatment Considerations

1. Risk from medication—severe reactions to antiepileptic drug (AED) about 1/30,000

2. About 15% of all patients may have a biologic, cognitive, or behavioral reaction to the first AED that will require it to be discontinued.

3. Almost no children need to be treated after a first seizure—overall risk of occurrence within 2 y is 40–50% and greatest (80–95%) in patients with abnormal neurologic examinations, complex partial seizures, and epileptiform discharges in EEG.

4. Overall risk of recurrence after first seizure in adults ranges from 30–60%.

5. Risk of seizure recurrence after two seizures is about 80–90%—common to begin therapy after two or more seizures.

C. Pharmacologic Treatment

1. Monotherapy preferrable to polytherapy

2. Give medication in therapeutic doses—monitor through AED levels.

3. Know pharmacology and pharmacokinetics of drugs prescribed (Table 77-1).

4. Be aware of drug interactions that enhance/reduce effectiveness

5. Toxic side effects
   a. Dose dependent
   b. Hypersensitivity

6. AED monitoring for incomplete seizure control
   a. Evaluate compliance.
   b. If drug therapy imperfect, is dose/schedule inappropriate or does drug need to be changed?
   c. Ascertain if seizures recur after period of control or side effects due to change in blood levels of drug.
   d. Assess if cognitive changes represent toxic dose of drug.
   e. Define dosing change if more than one AED is needed.

Table 77–1. Drugs Used for Treatment of Epilepsy

Drug	Seizure Type	Adult Dose mg/kg/d	Therapeutic Dose range (μg/mL)	$t_{1/2}$ (h)	Common Side Effects
Carbamazepine	P, CP, GC	15–25	8–12	10–12	Ataxia, sedation
Phenobarbital	GC	2–4	15–40	100	Sedation
Phenytoin	P, CP, GC	3–8	10–20	24	Dysequilibrium
Primidone	P, CP, GC	10–20	8–12	2	Sedation, nausea
Divalproex sodium	P, CP, GC	15–60	50–100	14	Nausea

P, partial; CP, complex partial; GC, generalized convulsive

V. Patient Education and Counseling

A. Compliance and outcomes are better when patients and their families are active participants in the process.

B. Children need realistic limits and knowledge of safe activities.

C. Adolescents and adults need specific advice about driving, activities of daily living, participation in sports, and alcohol consumption.

D. Adults require advice about work and career goals, legal rights, medical insurance, marriage counseling, and having/raising children.

VI. Indications for Referral

A. Seizures that are not easily controlled within 3 mon

B. If appropriate therapy has not yielded satisfactory results in 1 y, consider referral to an epilepsy center.

C. Disabling partial or complex partial seizures that continue for more than 2 y should be considered for surgical therapy.

VII. Indications for Hospitalization

A. Status epilepticus (see Chapter 6)

B. Video/EEG monitoring to establish diagnosis, plan, or adjust therapy

C. Toxic reactions/overdose that may be life-threatening

D. Evaluation for "seizure surgery" or resection of the epileptic focus

VIII. Annotated Bibliography

Engel, Jr. Seizures and Epilepsy. New York: FA Davis; 1989. Good review of principles and practice of management of patients with seizures.

Wyllie E. The Treatment of Epilepsy: Principles and Practice. Philadelphia: Lea & Febiger; 1993. Comprehensive current review of all aspects of seizure disorders.

Chapter 78: Tinnitus

David Zwillenberg

I. Clinical Presentation

A. General Information

1. Patient presents complaining of a constant or intermittent noise that others do not hear.
2. Does not include voices heard by those with auditory hallucinations

B. Symptoms and Signs by Type

1. Conductive causes
   a. Serous otitis media
      1) Tinnitus is usually pulsatile.
      2) Tympanic membrane will be dull, retracted.
      3) Tympanogram will be flat and there will be conductive hearing loss of mild to moderate severity.
   b. Otosclerosis
      1) Bony fixation of the stapes in the oval window
      2) More common in women after pregnancy or on birth control pills
      3) Familial tendency
      4) Accompanied by hearing loss that may be conductive or mixed
   c. Oscicular discontinuity or tympanic membrane perforation
      1) Secondary to head trauma or surgery or chronic ear infection
      2) Tinnitus often pulsatile and generally accompanied by hearing loss of a conductive nature
      3) Tympanogram will be hypermobile for ossicular discontinuity. No seal will be obtained with a perforation. There will be no reflexes elicited.
   d. Cerumen impaction—readily apparent on examination
   e. Barotitis
      1) Acute onset during diving or flying
      2) Painful
      3) Tinnitus usually pulsatile
      4) Flat tympanogram and hypomobile tympanic membrane to pneumotoscopy
      5) Fluid or blood seen behind tympanic membrane

    f. Cholesteatoma
       1) Erosive lesion generally arising in patients with a history of chronic ear infections although they may be congenital
       2) White pearly lesion visible behind intact tympanic membrane or perforation with recurrent drainage
    g. Exostoses
       1) Bone growth in external auditory canals
       2) Tinnitus when canal occluded by exostoses and/or cerumen in canal narrowed by exostoses
       3) Usually seen in swimmers
2. Sensorineural and systemic causes
    a. Hypothyroidism
       1) Often unaccompanied by other signs
       2) Obtain thyrotropin (TSH)
    b. Neurosyphilis
       1) Usually accompanied by discrimination scores that are disproportionately worse than the pure tone audiogram would suggest
       2) Obtain fluorescein treponemal antibody absorption or test CSF
    c. Meniere's syndrome
       1) Accompanied by complaints of
          a) Aural fullness
          b) Vertigo—generally recurrent, with nausea
          c) Normal otologic examination
    d. Noise exposure
       1) Patient will often be able to attribute the tinnitus and possible hearing loss to a particular incident in acute cases; often spontaneously improves initially over a few days.
       2) When exposure has been chronic (ie, occupational or recreational) typically hearing loss is maximal at 4000 cps.
    e. Head trauma
       1) Frequent cause of tinnitus
       2) May or may not be accompanied by hearing loss or vertigo
       3) May or may not have suffered temporal bone fracture
    f. Ototoxicity
       1) May be secondary to medications. May be gradual or acute onset
       2) Usually accompanied by high tone loss on audiogram, which may then spread to affect all frequencies
       3) Tinnitus is the best early warning sign of ototoxicity. Do not ignore it.
    g. Presbycusis
       1) Older population by definition
       2) Bilaterally symmetrical hearing loss although tinnitus may or may not be bilateral
       3) Typically, sloping predominately high-tone loss on audiogram
    h. Acoustic neuroma
       1) Unilateral
       2) May be accompanied by asymmetic hearing loss and/or vertigo
    i. Herpes zoster oticus

1) Patients complain of ear pain, which starts before the onset of vesicular eruptions around the ear.
2) Tinnitus, hearing loss, and facial nerve paralysis may occur and may be permanent.

j. Bell's palsy
   1) Typically presents as an acute onset of facial paralysis; may be accompanied by tinnitus
k. Sudden sensorineural hearing loss
   1) Patient suddenly notices no hearing in one ear.
   2) Acoustic neuroma must be ruled out, although often is idiopathic.
   3) Usually accompanied by tinnitus
l. Illness and neuropathies
   1) Mumps
      a) *Accompanied by total unilateral hearing loss*
      b) *Meningitis*
         i. Sudden onset, near total bilateral hearing loss and tinnitus
      c) *Diabetes*
      d) *Mononucleosis*
      e) *Multiple sclerosis*
         i. Hearing loss and/or tinnitus may fluctuate with other symptoms.
         ii. May be unilateral or bilateral
m. Idiopathic

II. Diagnostic Approach

A. History

1. Noise exposure
   a. Avocation
   b. Vocation

2. Gradual versus acute onset

3. Infectious diseases

4. Systemic diseases

5. Medications particularly diuretics, erythromycin, aminoglycosides

B. All patients should have an audiogram.

1. If no air–bone gap, sensorineural loss or normal hearing

2. If air–bone gap—conductive loss

C. For patients with sensorineural hearing loss that is bilaterally symmetrical

1. Consider
   a. Presbycusis

b. Hypothyroidism
   c. Rheumatoid disease
   d. Ototoxicity
   e. Noise exposure
   f. Mumps
   g. Meningitis
   h. Syphilis
   i. Diabetes
2. Obtain
   a. Serologic tests for syphilis
   b. Antinuclear antibody, erythrocyte sedimentation rate
   c. TSH
   d. Fasting glucose

D. **For patients with sensorineural hearing loss that is asymmetric**

1. Consider
   a. Unilateral noise exposure
   b. Multiple sclerosis
   c. Acoustic neuroma
   d. Meniere's syndrome
2. Obtain
   a. Electronystagmography (ENG) if patient has vertigo
   b. Brain stem evoked response (BSER) audiometry if the difference between the ears is < 20 db
   c. MRI of the brain and auditory canals with gadilinium if BSER or ENG suggests central pathology or if asymmetry is > 20db

III. Treatment

A. **Conductive Causes**

1. Serous otitis media—An initial trial of antibiotics (such as trimethoprim/sulfamethoxisole) should be attempted for a 3-4 wk course.
   a. If unsuccessful, myringotomy with tube insertion may be appropriate.
   b. Nasopharyngoscopy may be necessary in adults.
2. Otosclerosis—Stapedectomy may alleviate the tinnitus and almost always corrects the hearing loss.
3. Ossicular discontinuity or tympanic membrane perforation—Surgical correction should be performed if the symptoms are troublesome.
4. Cerumen impaction—Debride the ear.
5. Barotitis—Manage conservatively with decongestants, antiobiotics, and the modified Valsalva maneuver. If intensely painful or if another pressure change is imminent (ie, another airplane flight), a myringotomy may be needed.

6. Exostoses—Debride any cerumen present. May need operative excision if the problem recurs frequently
7. Cholesteatoma—Surgical excision via mastoidectomy is indicated.

B. Sensorineural and Systemic Causes

1. Metabolic causes—Detection and correction of the hypothyroidism and hyperglycemia will halt and may somewhat reverse the progression of the hearing loss and tinnitus.
2. Ototoxicify—Serial audiograms should be obtained with patient on ototoxic drugs. Patients should be asked about tinnitus, vertigo, and hearing changes. Peak and trough levels should be obtained as appropriate. Drugs should be stopped as soon as possible.
3. Otosyphilis—Should be treated as neurosyphilis. High-dose oral steroids should be started and slowly tapered as guided by the audiogram and discrimination scores.
4. Noise exposure—Avoid noise; use ear protection during exposure.
5. Acoustic neuroma—This slow-growing benign tumor shoud be removed if the patient's overall condition warrants it.
6. Herpes zoster oticus—High-dose steroids (prednisone 60 mg/d, tapered slowly) are indicated to prevent permanent changes, particularly in the facial nerve.
7. Bell's palsy—An oral steroid taper of prednisone 60 mg to 0 over several days is suggested. A more protracted course may be necessary, depending on response.
8. Sudden sensorineural hearing loss—Many very complicated protocols exist for treating this entity. A course of steroids and a period of rest probably are indicted. All other treatment is presently a matter of disagreement.
9. Meniere's syndrome—Low-salt diet, decreased caffeine intake, and elimination of alchohol intake are suggested. Agents to suppress the vertigo, eg, Antivert 25 mg t.i.d. (12.5 mg t.i.d. in the elderly) or diazepam 5 mg t.i.d. should be tried first. A diuretic (eg, hydrochlorthiazide 50 mg 3 times a week) may be useful. In highly disabling causes surgery may be needed.
10. Posthead trauma, postmeningitis, idiopathic, presbycusis, etc.—No treatment has eradicated tinnitus successfully. The following are helpful.
    a. Masking—a hearing aid or background noise generator (eg, TV, radio)
    b. Biofeedback, psychotherapy, or support groups are available and may help some individuals deal with the anxiety or depression that tinnitus may engender.
    c. Antidepressants

IV. Indications for Referral

A. All patients with tinnitus should be referred to an otolaryngologist if the primary physician is unfamiliar with the otoscopic examination (rarely) or unfamiliar with the work-up of tinnitus.

B. All patients with an audiogram showing

1. An air–bone gap should be referred

2. Asymmetric sensorineural hearing loss should be referred

3. Symmetric sensorineural hearing loss should have a medical work-up as mentioned above

C. Patients who are severely depressed or anxious should have appropriate psychiatric care.

V. Indications for Hospitalization

A. Tinnitus is not an indication for hospitalization unless accompanied by

1. Overtly suicidal ideation

2. Severe vertigo with vomiting

3. A need for surgical correction of the underlying problem

VI. Annotated Bibliography

Meyerhoff W, Cooper J. Tinnitus. In: Paparella MM, Schumrock DA, Gluckman JL, Meyhoff WL, eds. Otolaryngology-Otology and Neuro-Otology, 3rd ed. Vol II. Philadelphia: WB Saunders; 1991:1169–1179.

Sataloff RT, Sataloff J. Tinnitus and vertigo. In: Sataloff RT, Sataloff J, eds. Occupational Hearing Loss. New York: Dekker; 1987:397–407. The best general source on this problem I've seen.

Tyler R, Babin R. Tinnitus. In: Cummings CW, Fredrickson JM, Harker LA, Krause CT, Schuller DE, eds. Otolaryngology-Head and Neck Surgery. St. Louis: CV Mosby; 1986:3201–3217.

Chapter 79: Tremor

Karen G. Kelly

I. Clinical Presentation

A. General Information

1. Tremor is defined as involuntary rhythmc oscillation of antagonistic muscles.
2. Tremors are classified on the basis of when the tremor occurs.

   a. Resting tremor is maximal at rest.
   b. Postural or static—Tremor is maximal with sustained postures, such as with hands outstretched.
   c. Kinetic or intentional—Tremor is maximal with intentional movement such as moving finger to nose.

B. History

1. When tremor occurs (eg, at rest, with motion) with particular action
2. What part of body affected
3. Age of onset
4. Family history of tremor or Wilson's disease
5. Associated neurologic symptoms—particularly

   a. Bradykinesia or stiffness suggestive of Parkinson's disease.
   b. Signs or symptoms of multiple sclerosis such as episodes of optic neuritis or paralysis
   c. Symptoms of cerebellar disease such as ataxia

6. Medications
7. Medical problems (particularly strokes)
8. Alcohol use and its effect on the tremor
9. Effect of tremor on activities of daily living
10. Effect of tremor on social functioning

C. Physical Examination

1. Observe the tremor with patient

a. At rest
b. Arms outstreched
c. During motion (eg, finger to nose)

2. Observe when it is present and when it is maximal

3. Perform a thorough neurologic examination with particular attention to

   a. Signs of parkinsonism, cogwheel rigidity, bradykinesia, postural instability
   b. Signs of cerebellar dysfunction, ataxia, nystagmus, dysmetria
   c. Signs of peripheral neuropathy in the affected ares.

II. Diagnostic Approach

A. History and physical examination are most important in distinguishing types of tremors.

B. Further work-up based on type of tremor (see below)

C. Neuroimaging may be part of work-up in patients with suspected cerebellar tremor or with symptoms of parkinsonism.

D. Thyroid function tests and thyrotropin should be done in patients with apparent essential tremors.

III. Differential Diagnosis

A. Other Movement Disorders

1. Rarely will be mistaken for tremor

2. Chorea—arrhythmic movements of a forcible, rapid, jerky, restless type

3. Athetosis—continuous slow purposeless movements, usually slower than chorea, but may be similar

4. Tics or myoclonus—brief, involuntary random muscle contractions

5. Asterixis—quick arrhythmic movements that interrupt muscular contractions

6. Hemiballismus—violent flinging motions of arm

B. Postural Tremors—Maximal with Sustained Posture

1. Physiologic tremors—small amplitude, high frequency usually asymptomatic

2. Exaggerated physiologic tremor

   a. Anxiety, fatigue
   b. Thyrotoxicosis
   c. Pheochromocytomia
   d. Hypoglycemia
   e. Drugs—theophylline, caffeine, adrenergic antagonists, tricyclics, lithium, phenothiazines, alcohol withdrawal

3. Essential—onset may be at young age or middle or old age, so called "senile" tremor
   a. Familial in 50–60% of cases with autosomal dominant inheritance
   b. No associated neurologic symptoms
   c. Temporarily suppressible by alcohol
   d. Worsens with alcohol withdrawal
   e. May affect head, neck, jaw, voice, or upper limbs; less commonly lower extremities
   f. Occasionally this type of tremor may be initial sign of Parkinson's disease.
4. Tremor with peripheral neuropathy—in distribution of peripheral neuropathy

C. Resting Tremor

1. Parkinson's disease—idiopathic or secondary to drugs

2. Can be asymmetrical or unilateral

3. Classic tremor is pill-rolling but may involve legs or jaw; but not whole head tremor

4. 20% of patients with Parkinson's disease never have tremor

5. Parkinson's disease can also cause a postural tremor.

D. Kinetic Tremor

1. Cerebellar dysfunction—cerebellar degeneration, multiple sclerosis, posterior circulation stroke, drug toxicity (eg, Dilantin, alcohol)

2. Cerebellar dysfunction can also lead to a postural tremor and kinetic tremor with dysmetria, the so-called rubral tremor; caused by lesions in the cerebellar outflow tract.

E. Task-Specific Tremors

1. Tremors associated only with particular tasks

2. Primary writing tremor

3. Vocal tremor

4. Orthostatic tremor: tremor of the legs that occurs only when standing and disappears with walking or voluntary motion of the legs

IV. Treatment

A. Goals of Therapy

1. Amelioration of tremor if possible

2. Education of the patient that abolition of the tremor may not be possible

3. Assisting the patient in returning to social activities if embarrassment about tremors has limited these

4. Monitoring of patient's ability to perform activities of daily living

B. Essential Tremor
   1. Limit stress, caffeine, and other exacerbating factors
   2. Propranolol or other β blockers—Start with low dose (80 mg qd) and increase to 320 mg qd if necessary.
   3. Alternative is primidone
      a. Start with very small dose 25 mg hs and increase as necessary to maximum dose of 250 mg t.i.d.
      b. Average dose required is 250 mg.
      c. About 10% of patients suffer first-dose phenomenon of dizziness, confusion, and nausea, which generally resolve with continued use.
   4. Patients who do not respond to β blockers may respond to primidone and vice-versa.
   5. Tremor may improve, but not go away entirely.
   6. Clonazepam has been useful in orthostatic tremor.

C. Parkinson's Tremor
   1. Variable response to either dopaminergic therapy *OR*
   2. Anticholinergic therapy (eg, trihexyphenidyl 4–10 mg qd)

D. Cerebellar Tremor
   1. No effective therapy for cerebellar tremor
   2. Rubral tremor in multiple sclerosis occasionally responds to 600–1200 mg isoniazid with pyridoxine.

V. Indications for Referral to a Neurologist

A. Unclear diagnosis

B. Lack of response to therapy

VI. Annotated Bibliography

Findley LJ, Keller WC. Essential tremor: a review. Neurology 1987;37:1194–1197.
Hallett M. Classification and treatment of tremor. JAMA 1991;266:1115–1117. A complete review with recommendations for therapy.
Koller WC. Evaluation of tremor disorders. Hosp Prac 1990;May:23–31. A briefer review.

Chapter 80: Vertigo

David Zwillenberg

I. Clinical Presentation

A. General Information

Definition—sensation of movement of the person relative to the immediate environment or of the environment

B. Symptoms and Signs

1. May be accompanied by sweating, nausea, vomiting, and nystagmus
2. Faintness, weakness, or lightheadedness are not suggestive of a vestibular system disorder.
3. Patient may present
   a. Acutely—sudden onset of vertigo, possibly with nausea, vomiting, falling, nystagmus, etc.
   b. Chronically—A history of mild vertigo, usually with minimal somatic signs or
   c. With an acute exacerbation of a chronic condition, as in Meniere's syndrome

C. Physical Examination

1. Otoscopic examination
   a. Otitis media—acute
      1) Tympanic membrane will be red and bulging.
      2) There will be a conductive loss.
      3) If labyrinthitis supervenes there will be a sensorineural conponent.
   b. Chronic otitis media with cholesteatoma
      1) Chronically or recurrently draining ear
      2) White mass or desquamating debris seen when ear is debrided
      3) If cholesteatoma is the cause of the vertigo, suctioning on it will produce vertigo.
   c. Fistula—A pneumotoscopy will often reproduce the vertigo (positive fistula sign).
   d. With the exception of the above, the otoscopic examination will be normal.

2. Positional testing—best administered with Frenzel glasses so patient can't use ocular fixation to reduce nystagmus
3. Romberg testing
4. General neurologic examination

II. Diagnostic Approach

A. Multiple sclerosis, diabetes, otosyphilis, hyperlipoproteinemia, meningitis, encephalitis, and herpes oticus should be treated as described elsewhere.

B. Vestibular Neuronitis (Labyrinthitis)

1. Typically acute onset of rotatory vertigo with or without tinnitus or hearing loss
2. Self-limited—generally days to 2–3 wk
3. Audiogram may show unilateral sensorineural loss. Repeat after resolution should show resolution of the hearing loss.
4. Electronystagmography (ENG) will show peripheral pathology with statistically significant functional decrease in the affected ear.

C. Meniere's Syndrome

1. Acute recurrent episodes of vertigo, tinnitus, hearing loss and aural pressure
2. Audiogram during the episode will show a sensorineural hearing loss, which will improve toward baseline after the attack. Over time the hearing will gradually worsen.
3. ENG will show definite unilateral progressive dysfunction.

D. Serous or Suppurative Labyrinthitis

1. Otitis media accompanied by sensorineural hearing loss on the audiogram
2. Myringotomy for culture

E. Cervical Vertigo

1. Normal calorics on ENG, normal hearing, abnormal positional testing
2. Usually history of neck pain or trauma

F. Postconcussive and after Cerebrovascular Accident

1. The capacity for ambulation must be carefully assessed before allowing the patient to do so unassisted.
2. Quad cane or walker may be helpful.

G. Posterior Fossa and Cerebello Pontine Angle Lesions

1. Some authors contend that all patients with even one episode of vertigo should undergo MRI or CT scanning. This is defensible. Others would argue that if the ENG is abnormal and the audiogram is normal or asymmetrical by < 20 db brain stem evoked response audiometry should be obtained. If normal, no MRI need be obtained. If abnormal, proceed to MRI.

H. Ototoxicity

1. Vestibulotoxic drugs will generally not change the audiogram initially but will eventually if the drug is not discontinued.
2. ENG will be symmetrical but relatively flat.
3. Stop the drug.

IV. Treatment

A. Vestibular Neuronitis (Labyrinthitis)

1. Treatment is supportive.
    a. Meclizine 12.5 mg up to t.i.d. in the elderly, up to 25 mg t.i.d. in most adults *OR*
    b. Benadryl 25–50 mg up to t.i.d. *OR*
    c. Valium 2–5 mg PO t.i.d.
    d. Bed rest

B. Meniere's syndrome

1. Treatment of acute episodes is supportive (see IV-A-1).
2. Avoidance of caffeine, alchohol, salt, and tobacco has been advocated.
3. Long-term diuretic treatment is often helpful.
4. Surgery—Endolymphatic shunt or vestibular nerve section have a place in refractory cases.

C. Cholesteatoma with Vertigo

1. Mastoidectomy is indicated.

D. Otitis media with vertigo

1. Myringotomy for drainage and culture is indicated.
2. IV antiobiotics depending on Gram stain

E. Serous or Suppurative Labyrinthitis

1. Drainage via the oval or round window may also be necessary.

F. Cervical Vertigo

1. Treatment may consist of

    a. Evaluation of the cervical spine radiographically
    b. Neurologic or physiatric evaluation and treatment with physical therapy
    c. Cervical collar
    d. Surgery may be necessary, eg, spinal fusion

G. Postconcussive and after Cerebrovascular Accident

1. Treatment with suppressive drugs (see IV-A-1) may be helpful.

H. Fistula

1. Suppressive treatment

2. Bed rest

V. Patient Education

A. People with vertigo should not drive or operate heavy machinery when vertiginous or on suppressive medicine.

B. In some states patient may have driver's license revoked for vertigo.

VI. Indications for Referral

A. Unfamiliarity on the part of the primary doctor with otoscopy (rare)

B. Unfamiliarity with the interpretation of audiograms and ENG data

C. Need for myringotomy or other intervention

D. To aid in decision-making regarding the need for further testing

VII. Indications for Hospitalization

A. Acute otitis media with severe vertigo

B. Cholesteatoma with vertigo

C. Vertigo resulting in dehydration

D. Severe vertigo in those living alone, particularly the elderly

E. In cases requiring surgical treatment

VIII. Annotated Bibliography

Black F. Peripheral vestibular disorders. In: Cummings CW, Fredrickson JM Harker LA, Krause CJ Schulle DE, eds. Otolaryngology-Head and Neck Surgery. St. Louis: CV Mosby, 1986.

Harker L, Baloh R. Central vestibular system. In: Cummings CW, Fredrickson JM Harker LA, Krause CJ Schulle DE, eds. Otolaryngology-Head and Neck Surgery. St. Louis: CV Mosby, 1986.

Sataloff R, Sataloff J. Tinnitus and vertigo. In: Occupational Hearing Loss. New York: Dekker; 1987:397–407. Contains very fine review of otologic problems with an explanation of the various tests. Only very basic information on treatment.

Schapiro R. Clinical neurology for the otolaryngologist. In: Paparella MM, Schumrock DA, Gluckman JL, Meyerhoff WL, eds. Otolaryngology-Plastic and Reconstructive Surgery and Related Disciplines, vol IV. Philadelphia: WB Saunders; 1991:2971–2982.

Part XVI: Psychiatry/Behavioral Medicine

Chapter 81: Anxiety

Susan E. West

I. Clinical Presentation

A. Anxiety Disorders

1. Generalized anxiety disorder, including panic disorder
2. Phobias
3. Obsessive/compulsive disorder
4. Posttraumatic stress disorder

B. This chapter will review only generalized anxiety disorders and panic disorder. The treatment of phobias, obsessive/compulsive disorder, and posttraumatic stress disorder usually requires referral to a mental health professional.

II. Generalized Anxiety Disorder

A. Definition

B. Prevalence

1. 5% of general population
2. 15–30% of general medical practice

C. Symptoms—generalized, severe anxiety of at least 1 mo duration

1. Motor tension
   a. Muscle spasms and aches
   b. Headache
   c. Jitteriness
   d. Fatigability
   e. Inability to relax
   f. Insomnia

2. Autonomic hyperactivity
   a. Heart pounding

- b. Sweating
- c. Cold, clammy hands
- d. Dizziness
- e. Upset stomach, "butterflies"
- f. Frequent urination
- g. Diarrhea
- h. Sensation of lump in throat
- i. Flushing, hot flashes
- j. Dry mouth
- k. Shortness of breath or smothering sensation

3. Apprehensive expectation

    a. Worry, fear, anxiety
    b. Rumination
    c. Anticipation of misfortune

4. Vigilance and scanning

    a. Inability to concentrate
    b. Heightened startle reaction
    c. Insomnia

5. Idiosyncratic symptoms at odds with anatomy, physiology, or physical examination

D. Signs

1. Shaking or trembling

2. Tachycardia

3. Tachypnea

4. Cool, clammy extremities; diaphoresis

5. Muscle tension; inability to elicit reflexes because of inability to relax

6. Fidgeting, restlessness

7. Easy startle

8. Deep, sighing respirations

9. Flushing

E. Differential Diagnosis

1. "Normal" anxiety, which is milder, of shorter duration, and precipitated by an event that would make average person nervous.

2. Hyperthyroidism

3. Hypoglycemia

4. Pheochromocytoma

5. Cushing's syndrome

6. Cardiac arrhythmias
7. Hyperventilation
8. Excess caffeine or other stimulants
9. Medication side effect
10. Withdrawal reaction to alcohol or benzodiazepines
11. Often coexists with substance abuse, alcoholism and/or depression

F. Treatment

1. Behavioral therapy
   a. Meditation
   b. Guided muscle relaxation
   c. Self-hypnosis
   d. Breathing exercises

2. Reassurance; may require frequent visits at first

3. Pharmacotherapy
   a. If symptoms interfere with functioning
   b. If symptoms cannot be managed by behavioral modification
   c. Benzodiazepines
      1) Are effective but sedating with strong risk of addiction
      2) Interact with alcohol and other sedating drugs
      3) Avoid in unstable patients or patients with substance or alcohol abuse; use with caution in elderly or persons with liver disease.
      4) Specific agents—with usual starting doses
         a) *Diazepam 2–5 mg b.i.d.–t.i.d.*
         b) *Alprazolam 0.25–0.5 mg t.i.d.*
         c) *Lorazepam 0.5–1.0 mg b.i.d. or t.i.d.*
         d) *Oxazepam 10–15 mg t.i.d. or q.i.d*
   d. Imipramine
      1) Lacks abuse or addiction potential
      2) Start with 75 mg qd; increase to 150–250 mg qd if necessary
   e. Buspirone
      1) Nonbenzodiazepine without sedative, withdrawal or addiction potential
      2) Delayed onset of action; may take 2–4 wk
      3) Initial dose 5 mg b.i.d, titrated up to 10 mg t.i.d.
   f. β Blockers—may be used to control the catecholamine-induced symptoms

G. Indications for Referral to Psychiatrist

1. Severe impairment in functioning

2. Poor response to, or intolerance of, drug therapy

3. Patient at high risk for benzodiazepine dependence

4. Biofeedback training
5. Concomitant phobia, obsessive compulsive disorder, or posttraumatic stress disorder

III. Panic Disorder

A. Epidemiology

1. 1.6–2.9% of women; 0.4–1.7% of men
2. 13% of a general medical practice
3. Mean age of onset is 26 y but may occur at any age.
4. Strong familial component; two thirds have affected family member

B. Diagnosis

1. Discrete periods of sudden onset of intense fear or discomfort, which are unexpected and not predictable
2. Defined as four such attacks within a 4-wk period or one or more attacks followed by a month of persistent fear of another attack. Latter often leads to agoraphobia.
3. Symptoms—At least four of the following should be present for the diagnosis
   a. Shortness of breath or smothering sensation
   b. Dizziness, lightheadedness, or unsteadiness
   c. Palpitations or racing heart
   d. Trembling or shaking
   e. Sweating
   f. Choking, sensation of throat closing off
   g. Nausea or abdominal distress
   h. Depersonalization or derealization
   i. Paresthesias
   j. Hot flushes or chills
   k. Chest pain or tightness
   l. Fear of dying or "impending doom"
   m. Fear of going crazy or doing something uncontrolled.

C. Differential Diagnosis

1. Hyperthyroidism
2. Coronary artery disease, arrhythmias
3. Asthma, hyperventilation
4. Transient ischemic attacks, migraine, complex partial seizures
5. Pheochromocytoma
6. Hypoglycemia

7. Withdrawal from barbiturates, alcohol, or benzodiazepines
8. Cocaine, LSD, amphetamine, PCP use
9. Phobias, depression, schizophrenia

D. Treatment

1. Educate patient and offer reassurance.
2. There is a strong association with suicidal ideation. It is essential to ask about this.
3. Pharmacologic—Ask if patient or a family member has responded to a drug for panic attacks in the past; if so, start with that one.
   a. Benozodiazepines
      1) Alprazolam
         a) *Only drug currently approved by Food and Drug Administration for panic disorder*
         b) *Rapid onset of action*
         c) *Start at 0.5 mg t.i.d.; increase by 0.5 mg q 2–3 d, up to 4–6 mg/d*
         d) *Avoid in patients with substance or alcohol abuse.*
      2) Clonazepam
         a) *Less severe withdrawal reaction than alprazolam*
         b) *Start with 0.25 mg b.i.d.; increase by 0.5 mg/wk up to 2–4 mg/d*
   b. Tricyclic antidepressants—take 4–6 wk for effect
      1) Imipramine
         a) *Start with 10–25 mg qhs*
         b) *Increase q 4–6 d to 150–300 mg/d*
      2) Desipramine
         a) *Start with 10–25 mg qhs*
         b) *Increase q 4–6 d to 150–300 mg/d*
      3) Nortriptyline
         a) *Start with 10–25 mg/d*
         b) *Increase q 4–6 d to 75–125 mg/d*
   c. Selective serotonin reuptake inhibitors—take 4–6 wk for effect
      1) Sertraline causes fewer jittery or agitated side effects than fluoxetine.
      2) Start sertraline with 50 mg/d, increasing every 3–7 d up to 200 mg/d
   d. Monoamine oxidase inhibitors
      1) Only if above medications fail
      2) Suggest referral to psychiatrist

E. Indications for Referral

1. Suicidal ideation—Suicidal intent is grounds for immediate hospitalization.
2. Physician discomfort in prescribing pharmacologic therapy
3. Failure to respond to pharmacologic therapy
4. Agoraphobia or other disabling fear of attack recurrence

IV. Annotated Bibliography

American Psychiatric Association. Diagnostic and Statistical Manual of Mental Disorders, 4th ed. Washington, DC: American Psychiatric Press; 1994. The definitive manual for the American Psychiatric Association. This book not only discusses diagnostic criteria, but also describes clinical presentation and differential diagnosis.

Appenheimer T, Noyes R. Generalized anxiety disorder. Patient Care 1987; 14:635-649. Clear, easily read descriptions with clinical, pragmatic approach.

Katon W, Sheehan DV, Whole JW, et al. Panic disorder: a treatable problem. Patient Care 1992;26:81-107. Thorough description of panic disorders from the point of view of a primary care provider. Gives suggested doses of individual drugs, as well as practical advice on nonpharmacologic treatment.

Shader RI, Greenblatt DJ. Use of benzodiazepines in anxiety disorders. N Engl J Med 1993;328,1398-1405. Good overview of uses of benzodiazepines as well as tolerance, abuse, and dependence.

Wesner R. Panic disorder and agoraphobia. Prim Care 1987;14:649-657. Clear description with pragmatic approach.

Chapter 82: Bipolar Affective Disorder

Susan E. West

I. Clinical Presentation

A. General Information

1. Bipolar disorder, or manic-depressive illness, has a lifetime prevalence of about 1%.
2. Unlike major depression, men and women are equally affected.
3. Unlike major depression, which can occur at any age, bipolar disorder usually presents before age 30 (mean age of onset: early 20s).
4. Bipolar disorder runs in families. First-degree relatives of bipolar patients have a 12% risk of major depression and 12% risk of bipolar disorder. 80–90% of bipolar patients have a relative with depression.

B. Symptoms

1. Bipolar disorder is diagnosed if a patient has ever had a manic episode (see below). 95% of bipolar patients will eventually have a depressive episode.
2. Depression symptoms are same as for major depression (see Chapter 83), lasting at least 2 wk.
3. Diagnosis of manic episode
   a. One or more distinct periods of a prominent expansive, elevated, or irritated mood.
   b. Duration of at least 1 wk of three of the following symptoms (four if mood is only irritable)
      1) Increase in activity (social, sexual or work related) or physical restlessness
      2) Much more talkative (pressured speech)
      3) Flight of ideas ("thoughts are racing")
      4) Inflated self-esteem/grandiosity
      5) Decreased need for sleep
      6) Marked distractibility
      7) Excessive involvement in pleasurable activities without concern for harmful consequences (spending sprees, foolish business ventures, risky sexual behavior, reckless driving)

II. Diagnostic Approach

A. Patients may be brought in by family members concerned about patient's change in mood or lack of sleep.

1. With patient's permission, interviewing family member can help make diagnosis.

2. Patients themselves may view their increased energy, heightened creative thinking, and increased productivity as desirable.

B. Ask about history of mania in all depressed patients.

C. Ask about depression and bipolar disorder when taking family history.

D. Further questions and physical examination should be geared toward ruling out other causes of manic episodes.

III. Differential Diagnosis

A. Drug reaction—steroids, L-dopa, cocaine, amphetamines

B. Endocrinopathies—hyperthyroidism, Cushing's disease

C. Head Trauma

D. Multiple sclerosis or other neurologic diseases

E. Metabolic abnormalities—hemodialysis, liver failure

IV. Treatment

A. Complications if Untreated

1. Incidence of suicide is 10–15%

2. Increased "accidental deaths"

3. Consequences of illicit drug use, promiscuity, and other reckless behavior

B. Acute Management

1. Assess risk of suicide.

2. Assess physical consequences of manic state such as blood pressure and nutritional and fluid status.

C. Long-term Management

1. Lithium carbonate—70% get reduction in manic episodes and 20% become free of symptoms

a. Should not be given to patients with significant renal or cardiac disease, or dehydration
b. Adverse side effects are frequent and related to lithium levels. Lithium levels may rise with dehydration, diuretic use, salt depletion, indomethacin (possibly other nonsteroidal anti-inflammatory drugs), metronidazole, and control of acute mania.
c. Side effects can occur at any dose. Unusually sensitive patients may develop signs of toxicity with serum level < 1.0 mEq/L. In general, desired therapeutic level is 0.6–1.2 mEq/L, and in most patients there is a progression of toxic signs (Table 82–1).

Table 82–1. Progression of Toxic Signs

Approximate Levels	Side Effects
< 1.5 mEq/L	Hand tremor, thirst, polyuria, nausea
1.5–2.0 mEq/L	Diarrhea, vomiting, muscle weakness, incoordination
> 2.0 mEq/L	Ataxia, tinnitus, nephrogenic diabetes, insipidus

d. Starting dose—300–600 mg t.i.d. Drug levels should be drawn immediately prior to next dose.
e. Patient education
   1) Must be aware that salt depletion, diarrhea, sweating, can raise lithium levels
   2) Must be warned of possible side effects and need for blood levels to be drawn
2. If lithium is ineffective, consider referral to psychiatrist for prescription of carbamazepine or valproic acid.
3. Psychotherapy is generally needed to deal with the illness' effect on self-esteem, family, and work.

V. Indications for Referral to a Psychiatrist

A. Suicidal (without plans)

B. Poor prognosis for symptom relief

1. Rapid cyclers
2. No symptom-free intervals between mania and depression

C. Poor response to trial of lithium

D. Some generalists refer all bipolar patients to psychiatrists.

VI. Indications for Hospitalization

A. Acutely suicidal

B. Acute risk of self-injury

VII. Annotated Bibliography

American Psychiatric Association. Diagnostic and Statistical Manual of Mental Disorders, 3rd rev. ed. Washington, DC: American Psychiatric Press; 1987. The standard reference for diagnosis of psychiatric disorders with helpful examples and details to flesh out diagnostic criteria.

Goodwin FK, Jamison KR. Manic Depressive Illness. New York: Oxford University Press; 1990. Comprehensive discussion of diagnosis, treatment, and complications.

United States Department of Health and Human Services. Clinical Practice Guideline No. 5: Depression in Primary Care, vols 1 and 2; 1993. Clear, detailed discussion of depression and its less common presentation, bipolar disorder, with algorithms for diagnosis and treatment.

Chapter 83: Depression

Susan E. West

I. Clinical Presentation

A. General Information

1. The lifetime risk of a major depressive disorder is 7–12% for men, and 20–25% for women.

2. Risk factors

   a. Female gender
   b. First-degree relatives with depression
   c. Prior episodes of major depression
   d. Lack of social support
   e. Current substance abuse

3. Diagnosis—pervasive depressed mood or loss of interest. Not all patients with depression are "sad."

B. Symptoms—at least 5 of the following symptoms should be present for 2 weeks.

1. Depressed mood or irritability most of the day, almost every day; often worse at same time of day

2. Decreased interest or pleasure most of the day, nearly every day

3. Weight loss or gain; decreased or increased appetite

4. Insomnia or hypersomnia, nearly every day

5. Psychomotor agitation or retardation

6. Fatigue, loss of energy, loss of libido

7. Feelings of worthlessness or excessive or inappropriate guilt

8. Decreased ability to think or concentrate, or indecisiveness

9. Sense of hopelessness or despair

10. Recurrent thoughts of death; suicidal thoughts

11. May present with somatic manifestations—headache, backache, fatigue, chronic abdominal or pelvic pain, "diffusely positive review of systems"

C. Physical Examination

1. Psychomotor retardation
2. Poor eye contact
3. Examine for evidence of thyroid abnormalities or neurologic deficits

II. Differential Diagnosis

A. Medical Illness

1. Endocrinopathies—hypothyroidism, hyperthyroidism in the elderly, Addison's, Cushing's, hypercalcemia
2. Cancer—especially pancreatic and lymphoma
3. Dementing neurologic diseases—Parkinson's or senile dementia

B. Other Psychiatric Illness

1. Bipolar disorder
2. Anxiety
3. Substance abuse—may coexist with anxiety or depression

C. Medications

1. Antihypertensives—α-methyldopa, reserpine, propranolol, clonidine, thiazides
2. Digitalis
3. H_2 blockers
4. Barbiturates, benzodiazepines
5. Anticonvulsants
6. Hormones—glucocorticoids, anabolic steroids, oral contraceptives
7. Nonsteroidal anti-inflammatory medications, especially indomethacin
8. L-dopa
9. Withdrawal from cocaine, amphetamines

III. Treatment

A. Nonpharmacologic

1. Educate patient
2. Active listening, concern

3. Behavioral changes to treat symptoms—decrease alcohol, increase exercise, increase social supports

B. Indications for Drug Therapy

1. Poor sleep, energy, or concentration preventing patient from participating in usual activities
2. Home/work/school difficulties because of cognitive dysfunction
3. Lack of response to nonpharmacologic treatment
4. History of prior major depressive episode

C. Selection of Medication (Table 83–1)

1. Prior experience—If patient responded well in past, try the same medication unless contraindicated.
2. Prior good experience of a family member.
3. Specific characteristics of patient
   a. Lethargic, slowed cognition—Avoid sedating medications such as amitriptyline, doxepin, imipramine, or trazodone.
   b. Insomnia—Consider use of sedating antidepressant at bedtime. Avoid selective serotonim reuptake inhibitors (SSRIs).
   c. Anxious, agitated—avoid SSRIs.
   d. Obsessive/compulsive tendencies or concomitant eating disorder—Consider SSRIs.
   e. "Atypical" depression (increased weight, increased sleep, rejection sensitivity)—Consider SSRIs.
   f. Concomitant panic attacks—Consider imipramine, desipramine.
   g. Dysrhythmias, heart block—avoid tricyclic antidepressants (TCAs).
   h. Orthostatic hypotension, urinary retention, benign prostatic hypertrophy—avoid TCAs with prominent anticholinergic profiles (eg, amitriptyline, imipramine)
   i. Anorexia—avoid SSRI.
4. Ask all patients about suicidal ideation and plans. SSRIs have greater safety profile in overdoses. If patient is suicidal, refer to an emergency psychiatric facility. If patient has history of suicide attempts or ideation but no current plans, give only 1 wk supply at a time.

D. Long-term Therapy

1. Unless maintenance therapy is planned, antidepressant medication should be discontinued after 4–9 mo (TCAs should be tapered over several weeks).
2. If depressions recurs, reinstitute the medication for another 4–9 mo.

Table 83-1. Medications for Depression

	Sedation	Insomnia Agitation	Anticholinergic Effects	Cardiac Conduction Effects	Initial Dose (mg/d)	Usual Adult Dosage (mg/d)
TCAs						
Amitriptyline	4+	0	4+	3+	50	150–200
Desipramine	1+	1+	1+	2+	50	100–200
Imipramine	3+	1+	3+	3+	50	75–200
Doxepin	4+	0	3+	2+	50	75–150
Nortriptyline	2+	0	1+	2+	25	75–100
SSRIs						
Fluoxetine	0	2+	0	0	20	20–80
Sertraline	0	1+	0	0	50	50–200
Paroxetine	0	1+	0	0	20	20–50
Other						
Bupropion	0	2+	0	1+	200	300
Trazodone	4+	0	0	1+	50	150–400
Maprotiline	3+	0	2+	2+	50	100–150

TCAs, tricyclic antidepressants; SSRIs, selective serotonin reuptake inhibitors

3. Patients who have had three or more episodes of major depression are potential candidates for long-term maintenance antidepressant medication. Use same type and dosage as that found to be effective for acute management.

4. Strongly consider maintenance therapy if patient has had two episodes of major depression and

   a. Family history of bipolar disorder
   b. Age of onset < 20
   c. Both prior episodes were severe, sudden, or life threatening or both occurred in the last 3 y.

IV. Indications for Referral

A. To a Psychiatrist

1. Lack of response to trial of one or two drugs
2. Symptoms are severe or persistent (eg, significant weight loss because of not eating)
3. Concomitant substance abuse
4. Age > 70
5. Medical problem complicating treatment
6. Psychotic features
7. Suicidal ideation
8. Perceived need for monoamine oxidase inhibitor or electroconvulsive therapy

B. To Other Mental Health Professional

1. Patient has significant psychosocial problems that require lengthy psychotherapy
2. A common practice involves medication prescription and monitoring by the primary care provider, with counseling from therapist.

V. Indications for Hospitalization

A. Suicidal ideation with specific plan

B. Severe malnutrition

C. No social supports

VI. Annotated Bibliography

American Psychiatric Association. Diagnostic and Statistical Manual of Mental Disorders, 4th ed. Washington, DC: American Psychiatric Press; 1994. The definitive source for information on diagnosing depression, including differential diagnoses.

Depression in Primary Care, vol 1 and 2. U.S. Department of Health and Human Services, AHCPR Publication No. 93-0551, April 1993. These practice guidelines, devised by the U.S. Department of Health and Human Services, are thorough, well indexed and outlined with clarity. A physician's quick reference guide and patient's guide are also available. All are highly recommended and available by writing to AHCPR Publications Clearing House, P.O. Box 8547, Silver Spring, MD, 20907, or by calling (800) 358-9295.

Potter WZ, Rudorfer MV, Menji H, et al. The pharmacologic treatment of depression. N Engl J Med 1991;325:633-642. Compares the uses and side effects of antidepressants, although little attention given to serotonin reuptake inhibitors in 1991.

Shearer SL, Kaplin Adams G. Nonpharmacologic aids in treatment of depression. Am Fam Phy 1993;47:435-441.

Part XVII:
Pulmonary

Chapter 84: Asthma

Marvin E. Gozum

I. Clinical Presentation: History and Physical

A. General Information

1. Asthma is defined as an increased responsiveness of the trachea and bronchi to various stimuli and manifested by widespread narrowing of the airways that change in severity either spontaneously or as a result of treatment.
2. Pathology reveals hypertrophy of bronchial smooth muscle, mucosal edema, thickening of epithelial basement membrane, hypertrophy of mucous glands, acute inflammation, and plugging of airways by thick viscid mucus.
3. Pathogenesis is multifactorial most likely resulting from effects of release of neuropeptides, vasoactive intestinal peptide, substance P, histamines, leukotrienes, prostaglandins, thromboxanes, bradykinins, chemotactic factors, platelet-activating factors, mast cells, and platelets.
4. The major classifications are
   a. Extrinsic asthma or allergic asthma—often allergen related; IgE mediated; clear trigger factors; family history of asthma; responds to allergic desensitization.
   b. Intrinsic asthma or complex asthma—everything *not* classified as extrinsic asthma; unclear trigger factors.
   c. Triad asthma—intrinsic asthma, aspirin sensitivity and nasal polyposis; due to the effects of aspirin or nonsteroidal anti-inflammatory drugs (NSAIDs), tartrazine dye, and related compounds on arachidonic acid metabolism.

B. Symptoms

1. Acute shortness of breath
2. Diffuse expiratory wheezing
3. Cough
4. Chest tightness

C. Physical signs, in order of severity

1. Coughing and tachypnea

2. Diffuse expiratory wheezing
3. Use of accessory muscles of respiration
4. Intercostal muscle retractions
5. Loss of breath sounds or wheezing
6. Cyanosis

II. Diagnostic Approach

A. History

1. Elicit a prior history of asthma
2. Elicit history of probable trigger factors such as allergens, chemicals, and upper respiratory infections.
3. Determine seasonal pattern
4. Determine any history of heart disease.

B. Pulmonary Function Testing (see Chapter 88)

1. Bronchial provocation testing with methacholine or histamine is helpful but not solely diagnostic of asthma.
2. Allergic skin testing

C. Laboratory Studies

1. Follow peak expiratory flow rates. Maintain rates at > 200 L/min.
2. New onset of asthma attacks: check sputum Gram stain and culture.
3. New onset of asthma attacks: check chest x-ray.
4. Baseline and periodic spirometry testing to follow disease progression.

III. Differential Diagnosis

A. Asthma is likely the etiology of wheezing if eosinophilia, "Curshmann's spirals," mucous airway casts, or Charcot-Leyden crystals in mucus are found in a sputum examination.

B. Cardiac asthma—Wheezing is due to an exacerbation of congestive heart failure causing bronchoconstriction. It is important to differentiate cardiac asthma from other causes of wheezing. For treatment of cardiac asthma, see Chapter 25. Treatment for asthma may aggravate "cardiac" asthma.

C. Asthmatic bronchitis—a bronchospastic episode rather then true asthma, often occurring in patients with chronic bronchitis or chronic obstructive pulmonary disease (COPD).

D. Gram stains suggestive of infectious bacterial bronchitis should be treated with antibiotics. Sputum culture yields are usually low so antibiotics may have to be started empirically.

IV. Treatment

A. Asthmatic Attack Management (see also Chapter 25).

B. Goals

1. Eliminate trigger factors.
2. Alleviate hypoxemia.
3. Treat bronchoconstriction.
4. Attain a peak expiratory flow rate of > 200 L/min.
5. Attain a wheeze-free state.
6. Add medications incrementally.
7. Prophylaxis against future asthma attacks

C. Chronic or Maintenance Asthma Therapy

1. Mild to moderate asthma—inhaled β-agonists and/or topical steroids.

    a. Albuterol inhaler: 2–4 puffs of metered-dose inhaler q 4–6 h
    b. Metaproterenol inhaler: 2–4 puffs metered-dose inhaler q 3–4 h
    c. Beclomethasone by metered-dose inhaler 2–4 puffs q 6–12 h. Triamcinolone inhaler 2–4 puffs q 6–8 h may cause less coughing. Flunisolide 2–4 puffs q 12 h offers longer duration of action.
    d. In extrinsic or exercised-induced asthma, cromolyn 2 puffs q.i.d. before exercise may prevent asthma.

2. Moderately severe asthma

    a. Increase use of inhaled steroids
    b. Oral aminophylline—Use long-acting theophyllire preparation to maintain serum levels at 5–12 µg/mL but not to exceed 20 m/mL. Consider starting dose at 0.5 mg/kg/h, based on lean body weight, in divided doses.

3. Severe asthma

    a. Oral steroids—Begin with Prednisone 60 mg every day and taper off 10 mg q 3 d. Actual maintenance dose depends on the minimal dose required to achieve a wheeze-free goal. Every-other-day dosing may prevent adrenal suppression and is recommended.

4. Other prophylactic measures

    a. Allergic trigger factors should be eliminated or patients desensitized to allergens.

b. Upper airway infections are often trigger factors; prevention of common infections through *Pneumococcal* vaccinations or yearly influenza vaccination is recommended.
c. Active infections can be treated with oral antibiotics such as amoxicillin 500 mg q 8 × 10 d, erythromycin 250 mg q 6 h × 10 d, or Bactrim DS b.i.d. × 10 d.

V. Indication for Referral

A. An asthmatic, in an acute attack, unrelieved by hand-held nebulizers should be referred to an emergency room for further treatment.

B. An asthmatic who revisits an emergency room twice in a month for emergent therapy, despite maximum outpatient therapy, should be referred to a pulmonologist for further evaluation.

VI. Annotated Bibliography

Spitzer W, Suissa S, Ernst P, et al. The use of beta-agonists and the risk of death and near death from asthma. N Engl J Med 1992;326;501–506. Emphasizes the critical nature of inhaled agonists, its complications, and when to consider the need for additional therapy.

Stauffer J. Pulmonary Disease. In: Tierney L, Schroeder S, Krupp MA, et al, eds. Current Medical Diagnosis and Therapy. Los Altos, CA: Lange, 1993. A very concise, well written, up to date text (revised annually) and geared toward clinicians. For many topics, this book may be all you need to read. Highly recommended.

Chapter 85: Chronic Cough

Sandra B. Weibel

I. Clinical Presentation

A. General Information

1. Cough is often a persistent symptom after an upper respiratory infection (URI), but it is only considered chronic if it lasts for > 8 wk after a URI.
2. Cough is the body's basic defense mechanism to clear airways of both secretions and inhaled particles.
3. Many stimuli initiate cough, either mechanical or chemical
4. Afferent receptors for cough are located on mucosal neural receptors in the nasopharynx, larynx, trachea, large airways, and in the auditory canal and stomach.
5. Most common cause of chronic cough is cigarette smoking.
6. In nonsmokers, postnasal drip, asthma, and gastroesophageal reflux are the most common etiologies.

B. History

1. Chronic cough is a common reason that medical advice is sought. Although it can be associated with other symptoms, the cough itself is usually the most disturbing symptom.
2. Usually is dry but can be productive
3. The associated symptoms are often helpful in distinguishing the cause.
4. Postnasal drip—most will complain of one or all of the following
   a. Postnasal drip
   b. Throat clearing
   c. Nasal discharge
5. Cough variant asthma (see Chapter 84).
   a. Can be associated with wheezing and shortness of breath
   b. Often dry cough is the only complaint.
   c. May have family history of asthma

6. Gastroesophageal reflux (see Chapter 50).
    a. May complain of heartburn or sour taste in mouth
    b. Cough may be worse after meals or at bedtime.
    c. Cough may be the only symptom.
7. Weight loss, hemoptysis, and other systemic symptoms suggest carcinoma.

C. Physical Examination

1. Respiratory rate
    a. Usually normal
    b. If abnormal, suggests a more serious underlying pulmonary disease
2. Cobblestoning of oropharynx or mucus in the nares can be seen with rhinitis.
3. Lung examination often normal but may reveal wheezing or crackles

II. Diagnostic Approach

A. The anatomic location where cough receptors are located along with suggestive findings in history and physical examination will guide the work-up.

B. History and physical examination will suggest the diagnosis in a majority of cases.

C. Chest x-ray should be performed. However, in most cases, it will be negative.

D. Pulmonary function studies with evaluation of a bronchodilator response should be done if asthma suspected (see Chapter 88).

E. Methacholine challenge—if asthma is still considered and pulmonary function studies are normal (see Chapters 25 and 84).

F. Upper GI to evaluate for gastroesophageal reflux. If the upper GI is negative, then can proceed to 24-h pH probe with recording of symptoms (see Chapter 50).

G. Sinus films are rarely helpful but should be performed if sinusitis suspected.

H. Bronchoscopy is indicated only in patients in whom lung cancer is considered or when the cause of cough is not identified by the above methods.

III. Differential Diagnosis

A. Postnasal drip

B. Asthma

C. Gastroesophageal reflux

D. Chronic bronchitis—mainly smokers with daily cough productive of sputum

E. Post infectious—following URI, cough can last for > 6 wk.

F. Angiotensin-converting enzyme (ACE) inhibitor induced.

G. Lung cancer and multiple other miscellaneous disorders that are much less common.

IV. Treatment

A. It is most important to diagnose the underlying etiology and then direct the treatment. Antitussives are rarely indicated.

B. Postnasal Drip

1. Intranasal steroid 2 puffs in each nostril b.i.d.
2. Antihistamine and decongestant preparation (eg, brompheniramine maleate plus psuedoephedrine hydrochloride) particularly with allergic rhinitis.
3. If sinusitis is present, treatment with antibiotics and decongestant nasal spray can be used for short-term therapy.

C. Asthma (see Chapter 84).

1. β-agonists up to 2 puffs q.i.d. as needed.
2. For more severe symptoms add inhaled steroids (eg, triamcianolone 4 puffs b.i.d.)
3. Oral steroids may occasionally be needed for short period of time.

D. Gastroesophageal Reflux (see Chapter 50).

1. Limit eating—none for 2–3 hours prior to bedtime.
2. Elevate the head of the bed (30°)
3. Drug therapy

    a. H_2 blocker (cimetidine 400 mg b.i.d.)
    b. Metoclopramide 10 mg t.i.d.

E. Chronic Bronchitis (see Chapter 86).

   a. Avoid irritant—in particular stop smoking

F. Discontinue ACE inhibitors.

G. Often cough can be multifactorial and will need treatment of all etiologies.

V. Patient Education

A. If patients smoke they must be encouraged to stop to relieve the cough.

B. To ensure that the cough resolves, patients must remain compliant with therapy.

C. Patients will need encouragement and reassurance because the work-up and the time from initiation of treatment to resolution of the cough may be prolonged.

VI. Long-term Management

A. Dependent on disease and degree of continued symptoms

B. Often the cough will resolve completely (particularly patients with chronic bronchitis). Follow-up is only needed for recurrences.

C. When cough worsens or does not improve, often further etiologies need to be examined.

VII. Indications for Referral to Pulmonologist

A. Cough not diagnosed by the initial history, physical, and diagnostic studies as outlined above.

B. Cough that has been diagnosed but does not respond to the specific therapy

C. Patients with abnormal chest x-rays

D. Patients in whom lung cancer is suspected for bronchoscopy

VIII. Indications for Hospitalization

A. Rarely is hospitalization needed.

B. Only if other symptoms and underlying disease necessitate.

IX. Annotated Bibliography

Irwin RS, Corrao WM, Pratter MR. Chronic persistent cough in adults: the spectrum and frequency of cases and successful outcome of specific therapy. Am Rev Respir Dis 1981;123:413–417. Initial article looking at etiology and treatment of cough in a large series.

Irwin RS, Curley FJ, French CL. Chronic cough—the spectrum and frequency of causes, key components of the diagnostic evaluation, and outcome of specific therapy. Am Rev Respir Dis 1990;141:640–647. Recent review of etiologies of cough.

Kamei RK. Chronic cough in children. Pediatr Clin North Am 1991;38(3):593–605. Good review of pathophysiology, etiologies, and treatment of cough.

Poe RH, Harder RV, Israel RH, Kallay MC. Chronic persistent cough—experience in diagnosis and outcome using an anatomic diagnostic protocol. Chest 1989; 95:723–728. Thorough approach to the work-up of chronic cough.

Poe RH, Israel RH, Utell MJ, Hall WJ. Chronic cough: bronchoscopy or pulmonary function testing? Am Rev Respir Dis 1982;126:160–162. Brief review of these diagnostic tests in evaluation of cough.

Chapter 86: Chronic Obstructive Pulmonary Disease

Sandra B. Weibel

I. Clinical Presentation

A. General Information

1. Chronic obstructive pulmonary disease (COPD) is really not one disease process but is a term that refers to patients with emphysema, chronic bronchitis, and sometimes long-standing asthma.

2. COPD is characterized by airflow limitation and obstruction. This can be the result of loss of elastic recoil or obstruction of the conducting airways.

3. Pathophysiology—two basic groups but there is much overlap

    a. Chronic bronchitis
      1) Bronchial mucous gland hypertrophy and hyperplasia
      2) Smooth muscle hyperplasia
      3) Plugging the bronchioles with mucus
    b. Emphysema
      1) Abnormal enlargement of air spaces
      2) Can be further described based on where the acinar are involved; centrilobular emphysema most common usually related to cigarette smoking
      3) Larger areas of air space enlargement are bullae.

4. COPD is the leading cause of pulmonary disability

    a. Estimated in 1987 that there are 11.1 million patients in the United States with chronic bronchitis and 2 million with emphysema
    b. In 1985, these disorders accounted for 5% of office visits and 13% of hospitalizations.

5. Chronic bronchitis is defined as a clinical syndrome with cough and sputum production that occurs on most days for at least a 3-mo period for 2 consecutive years.

6. Emphysema is defined in anatomic terms when permanent abnormal dilation and destruction of the alveolar ducts and terminal bronchioles has occurred.

7. Associated risk factors for the development of COPD

    a. Cigarette smoking is the most significant factor—increases the rate of decline of forced expiratory volume in 1 sec (FEV_1).

b. Gender—men greater than women.
   c. Age—increasing age and declining pulmonary function seen with aging
   d. Occupational exposures—Inorganic dusts increase the risk. Higher and longer levels of exposure are associated with greatest risk.
   e. Hereditary
      1) α-1-antitrypsin deficiency
      2) Appears to be familial predisposition for development of COPD
   f. Socioeconomic status—inversely related

B. History

1. Gradual onset and steady progression of symptoms

2. Dyspnea is the usual presenting symptom with emphysema. The dyspnea may progress so gradually that the patient describes the dyspnea as occurring over a short time period, but family members may have noted changes for many years.

3. Cough with productive sputum occurs in patients with chronic bronchitis in particular. Patients with emphysema may also complain of cough but it is often nonproductive. Purulent sputum production can occur with exacerbations.

4. Hemoptysis can occur with chronic bronchitis, but not usually with emphysema. Should always consider lung cancer in these patients.

5. Wheezing may be noted in some patients, especially during acute exacerbations.

6. Weight loss can be the initial presenting complaint. Look for evidence of occult malignancy particular lung cancer, but if other etiologies are excluded, can be secondary to severe end stage disease.

7. Cor pulmonale—Lower extremity edema is noted.

C. Physical Examination

1. Historically patients were divided into pink puffers (emphysema) and the blue bloaters (chronic bronchitis). Now there is thought to be significant overlap between the two groups.

2. Vital signs
   a. Respiratory rate can often be increased especially with acute exacerbation.
   b. Use of accessory muscles of respiration (sternocleidomastoids)
   c. Tachycardia with exacerbations and severe disease (multifocal atrial tachycardia can be seen)

3. Lung examination
   a. Increase in anteroposterior diameter of the chest.
   b. Percussion—increased resonance
   c. Breath sounds—may be diminished, exhibit a prolonged expiratory phase, or reveal wheezing or rhonchi

d. Cardiac examination—often distant heart sounds
   e. Extremities—Clubbing and/or cyanosis can be seen.
   f. Cor pulmonale: if present, can have peripheral edema, jugular venous distention, and loud P_2.

II. Diagnostic Approach

A. Chest x-ray—posteroanterior and lateral films. Changes may include

1. Hyperinflation with increased anterior posterior diameter
2. Flattened diaphragms
3. Decreased or sometimes increased lung markings
4. Bullous changes particularly at the apices
5. Small vertical heart

B. Pulmonary Function Tests (see Chapter 88)

1. Spirometry
   a. FEV_1/forced vital capacity (FVC) < 75%
   b. FEV_1 < 80% of predicted
   c. May or may not have response to bronchodilators
   d. Rate of fall of FEV_1/y is significantly greater in smokers than in nonsmokers.

2. Lung volumes
   a. Residual volume (RV) is increased.
   b. Increased RV/total lung capacity (TLC) suggests air trapping.
   c. TLC may be increased if hyperinflation present.
   d. Lung volumes can be underestimated by helium dilution technique if bullae are present.

3. Diffusing capacity
   a. Often reduced in emphysema
   b. Can help distinguish from asthma as the diffusing capacity is normal in asthma

4. Pulmonary function and disease course
   a. Decline in FEV_1 does follow progressive lung destruction.
   b. Severity of COPD by FEV_1 does not always correlate with degree of dyspnea. However, most patients will be very symptomatic with FEV_1 < 1 L.

C. Arterial Blood Gases

1. Hypercapnia—more common in bronchitis but if present, suggests an FEV_1 < 1 L
2. Hypoxemia—often present with more severe disease
3. pH—usually close to normal except during episodes of respiratory decompensation when a respiratory acidosis can develop

D. Laboratory

1. Hemoglobin—may be elevated if there is chronic hypoxemia

2. Elevated bicarbonate with a chronic respiratory acidosis

3. Sputum—cultures are indicated when there is change in amount or color of sputum. Usual organisms are streptococci, *Haemophilus influenzae*, or *Moraxhella*.

E. Special Studies

1. CT scan of the chest—helpful in better defining bullous disease or evaluating for lung cancer

2. Echocardiogram—indicated to assess right and left ventricular function if cor pulmonale felt to be present.

3. α-1-Antitrypsin level if patient is young and there is a significant family history of emphysema. If low, can proceed to check phenotype.

III. Differential Diagnosis

A. Asthma—if the obstructive lung disease is actually reversible with treatment

B. α-1-Antitrypsin deficiency

C. Cystic fibrosis in younger patients

D. Bronchiectasis: usually more productive sputum and will have ectatic airways noted on either chest x-ray, CT scan, or bronchoscopy.

IV. Treatment

A. Goals

1. Improve symptoms and decrease disability.

2. Aggressively treat acute exacerbations.

3. Remove irritants that may be worsening disease.

B. Prevention

1. Patient must stop smoking.

   a. Rate of decline of FEV_1 can return to non-smoking rate.

2. Avoidance of inorganic dusts especially if high exposure in the workplace

3. Pharmacologic therapy

   a. β-agonists; ie, albuterol 2 puffs q.i.d.
      1) Can improve dyspnea even if no bronchodilator response by pulmonary function tests

2) Oral preparations rarely indicated because they often have more adverse than therapeutic effects
    b. Theophylline—controversial what effect it has; bronchodilation and possibly increased diaphragmatic strength
        1) Would use if no serious contraindications such as tachyarrhythmias or significant side effects
        2) Dose to keep blood level between 8–12 mg/mL
    c. Anticholinergic agents
        1) Can be more potent than β-agonists in COPD
        2) Would start initially iprotropium bromide 2 puffs q.i.d. Can then increase to 4 puffs q.i.d.
    d. Corticosteroids
        1) Oral useful for acute exacerbations or as 2 wk tapering trial to evaluate for change in FEV_1
        2) Not usually indicated for long-term treatment
        3) Inhaled steroids—A portion of patients who respond to oral steroids will benefit from inhaled steroids.
    e. Mucolytic agents
        1) Iodide or guaifenisin useful only in a small number of patients with significant sputum production.
    f. Antibiotics
        1) Helpful in acute exacerbations especially with changes in sputum production or color
        2) Any agent to cover *Streptococcus*, *H. influenzae* and *Moraxhella* such as:
            a) Amoxicillin-clavulonic acid 250–500 mg t.i.d.
            b) Trimethoprim-sulfa one double-strength, b.i.d.
4. Other therapy
    a. Oxygen
        1) If PaO_2 < 55 mm Hg at rest or oxygen saturation decreases to 85% with exercise
        2) If there is evidence of cor pulmonale or polycythemia
        3) Has been shown to improve survival
        4) Must be used for 12 h or more a day.
        5) O_2 flow rate to keep PaO_2 > 60 mm Hg.
    b. Pulmonary rehabilitation
        1) Has not been shown to change pulmonary function tests but can improve symptoms by reconditioning a sedentary patient
        2) Relaxation and pursed-lip breathing also can be taught.
    c. Nutrition
        1) Should try to keep nutritional status optimal but there is no evidence that increasing the caloric intake to promote weight gain actually changes survival.

V. Patient Education

A. Smoking cessation is the most important aspect.

B. If there is significant work exposure to inorganic dusts, the patients need to change jobs or use protective masks.

C. Patients need to learn how to use their inhalers correctly and if there is difficulty, then a spacer should be prescribed such as the InspirEase or AeroChamber to help with coordination.

D. Patients should be advised to have influenza vaccine yearly and Pneumovax.

E. Patients must be aware of changes in symptoms and seek physician's advice early, particularly for upper respiratory infections.

VI. Long-term Management

A. No further smoking

B. Compliance with medication needs to be monitored.

C. Spirometry at least yearly to evaluate progression of disease

D. Follow-up examination 1–2 times a year and as needed for acute exacerbations

VII. Indications for Referral to Pulmonologist

A. α-1 Antitrypsin deficiency

B. Disease that is poorly responsive to routine management

VIII. Indications for Hospitalization

A. Acute exacerbations—increasing shortness of breath unresponsive to outpatient therapy or with hypercapnia or hypoxemia

B. Patients who develop pneumonia

IX. Annotated Bibliography

Bleecker ER, Smith PL. Obstructive airways disease. In: Barker LR, Burton JR, Zieve PD eds. Principles of Ambulatory Medicine. Baltimore: Williams and Wilkins; 1986:637–669. Basic review of the disease with some good tables.
Hodkin JE, ed. Chronic obstructive pulmonary disease. Clin Chest Med 1990:11(3). Numerous articles on the various aspects of COPD from pathophysiology to treatment. Good discussion of the current controversies.
Snider GL. Chronic bronchitis and emphysema. In: Nadel JA, Murray JF, eds. Textbook of Respiratory Medicine. Philadelphia: WB Saunders; 1988:1069–1106. Excellent but very detailed review of the disease.

Chapter 87: Hemoptysis

Sandra B. Weibel

I. Clinical Presentation

A. General Information

1. Common symptom that may account for 8–15% of a pulmonary referral population
2. Can range from blood-streaked sputum to massive hemoptysis
3. Massive is defined as > 600 mL of blood in 24 h.
4. Usually arises from the high-pressure bronchial circulation
5. Life-threatening hemoptysis is a rare event. It occurs in 5% of those with hemoptysis. However, the mortality can be as high as 85%.
6. Hemoptysis can be caused by a wide variety of tracheobronchial, cardiovascular, and hematologic disorders.
7. Historical information such as recent travel, smoking history, age, recent infection, previous pulmonary history, and any other significant systemic disease will help in diagnosing the etiology of the hemoptysis.

B. History

1. Hemoptysis—blood in sputum. Initially need to make sure that it is not blood from the upper respiratory tract or GI tract.
2. Amount of hemoptysis and time course is also important in deciding on the etiology (eg, repeated hemoptysis over several years may suggest bronchiectasis).
3. Cough—may have productive sputum with blood. Often associated with upper respiratory infection (URI).
4. Systemic complaints can include fevers, chills, chest pain, weight loss, or shortness of breath.
5. Paroxysmal nocturnal dyspnea and orthopnea may be present and suggest a cardiac etiology such as mitral stenosis or congestive heart failure.

C. Physical Examination
1. Vital signs
   a. Fever may be present especially with infectious etiology.
   b. Respiratory rate will be increased with significant underlying pulmonary disease or if significant aspiration of blood has occurred.
2. Skin and mucous membranes
   a. Telangiectasia in hereditary diseases such as Osler Weber Rendu
   b. Ecchymoses and petechiae if there is an underlying hematologic disorder
3. Upper airway—A careful examination of the nose, mouth, and oropharynx must be performed to distinguish hemoptysis from bleeding at an upper airway site such as the nose.
4. Lung
   a. Isolated wheeze suggests that there is an endobronchial lesion.
   b. Crackles may be present but are nonspecific.
   c. Often is normal
5. Cardiac
   a. Diastolic murmur if mitral stenosis is cause of hemoptysis
   b. S_3 is often heard if there is congestive heart failure.
   c. Loud P_2 suggests pulmonary hypertension.

II. Diagnostic Approach

A. Most important initial step is to distinguish other sources of bleeding such as upper airway or GI from true hemoptysis.
1. Upper airway bleeding can be diagnosed by a good history and physical examination.
2. GI bleeding—hematemesis
   a. Usually darker
   b. Can see partially digested food particles, whereas hemoptysis contains pulmonary macrophages.
   c. pH is acidic; hemoptysis is alkaline

B. Chest X-ray
1. Normal suggests airway source of bleeding
2. Abnormal—may often be able to diagnose by the particular x-ray abnormality
   a. Infiltrate
      1) May be actual source of bleeding or can be aspirated blood
      2) Upper lobe infiltrate: suspect tuberculosis

b. Mass
   1) Tumor or arteriovenous malformation
   2) Aspergilloma in cavity
c. Cardiac—Signs of left atrial enlargement can suggest mitral stenosis

C. Laboratory

1. Complete blood count

   a. Elevated white cell count suggests infection.
   b. Anemia can be related to an underlying disease or to significant bleeding.
   c. Thrombocytopenia can be the etiology for the bleeding.

2. Coagulation studies—Abnormalities in prothrombin time or partial thromboplastin time can lead to hemoptysis or suggest an underlying hematologic disorder.

3. Sputum evaluation for Gram stain, culture, acid-fast bacilli and cytology.

D. Bronchoscopy—Massive Hemoptysis

1. Can only be done in acutely bleeding patients if the airway and respiratory status are adequate

2. Performed as soon as the patient is stable to localize the site of bleeding

3. Often large amounts of blood make visualization difficult.

4. Flexible bronchoscopy is usually preferred except for foreign body removal or for better ventilation of patient.

E. CT Scan of Chest

1. Additional information about the lung parenchyma

2. Is more sensitive than routine chest x-rays for localizing the source

3. High-resolution CT scan can diagnose bronchiectasis.

F. Special Studies

1. Ventilation perfusion scan—if history is suggestive of pulmonary embolus or infarct

2. Echocardiography—to evaluate potential cardiac etiologies and to assess pulmonary arteries if pulmonary hypertension is suspected.

3. Miscellaneous laboratory studies for systemic diseases (urinalysis, liver function studies, antineutrophil cytoplasmic antibodies, antinuclear antibodies, etc.)

III. Differential Diagnosis

A. Pseudohemoptysis

1. Upper respiratory tract

2. Hematemesis
3. Pneumonia with *Serratia marcescens*
4. Malingering

B. **Massive Hemoptysis**

1. Tuberculosis (TB)
2. Bronchiectasis
3. Lung carcinoma
4. Aspergilloma
5. Lung abscess

C. **Hemoptysis (Not Massive)**

1. Bronchitis most common
2. Extensive differential diagnosis.
   a. Tracheobronchial disorders (eg, endobronchial tumor)
   b. Cardiovascular disorders (eg, mitral stenosis)
   c. Hematologic disorders (eg, coagulopathy)
   d. Localized parenchymal disease (eg, TB)
   e. Diffuse parenchymal disease (eg, pulmonary hemorrhage)

IV. Treatment

A. **Massive Hemoptysis**

1. All these patients should be hospitalized.
2. Treatment is aimed first at stabilization of airway and hemodynamics and then can proceed with work-up.

B. **Submassive Hemoptysis (< 600 mL in 24 h)**

1. If the amount of bleeding is small and there is no significant underlying disease such as severe coagulopathy or significant pulmonary disease, then not all patients need to be hospitalized. However, each patient has to be evaluated on an individual basis.
2. If antecedent history of URI and normal chest x-ray, can empirically treat for bronchitis. All patients with a smoking history and age > 40 will need further evaluation.
3. A definitive diagnosis needs to be made in most cases before treatment.
4. Surgical resection of abnormal lung is sometimes indicated for recurrent hemoptysis or for a localized etiology (ie, bronchiectasis).

5. Cough suppressants are indicated only acutely with significant hemoptysis.
6. Bronchial artery embolization can be performed in some cases where a source is found and there is continued bleeding.

V. Long-term Management

A. Cryptogenic hemoptysis (no source found)

1. Follow-up examination and chest x-rays at least q 6 mo initially.
2. Prognosis is usually good and often no recurrence.

B. Largely dependent on the etiology of the hemoptysis

VI. Patient Education

A. Patient needs to report promptly any worsening or recurrence of the hemoptysis especially if managed as an outpatient.

B. It is important that patient be able to quantitate the amount of hemoptysis.

C. If the patient smokes, should be encouraged to quit.

VII. Indications for Referral to a Pulmonologist

A. All cases of massive hemoptysis should be immediately referred. There should also be a surgical evaluation.

B. All smokers who develop hemoptysis

C. Most cases of hemoptysis will need referral for bronchoscopy.

D. Some cases may not need referral such as a young person with no other medical problems, a recent history of URI, and self-limited hemoptysis.

VIII. Indications for Hospitalization

A. Massive hemoptysis—All cases should be hospitalized and monitored carefully.

B. Submassive

1. All patients with chest x-ray abnormalities that are undiagnosed
2. Patients with previous history of massive hemoptysis or if suspected etiology may have tendency for massive hemoptysis (ie, aspergilloma)

IX. Annotated Bibliography

Adelman M, Haponk EF, Bleecker ER, Britt EJ. Cryptogenic hemoptysis: clinical features, bronchoscopic findings, and natural history in 67 patients. Ann Intern Med 1985:102:829–834. Review of patients with hemoptysis and normal chest x-rays, their diagnoses, and outcome.

Irwin RS, Hubmayr RD. Hemoptysis. In: Rippe JM, Irwin RS, Alpert JS, et al. eds. Intensive Care Medicine. Boston: Little Brown; 1985:413–422. Concise well written chapter in textbook of critical care medicine.

Thompson AB, Teschler H, Rennard SI. Pathogenesis, evaluation, and therapy for massive hemoptysis. Clin Chest Med 1992;13:69. Good review of hemoptysis with emphasis on massive.

Chapter 88: Pulmonary Function Tests

Daniel Holleran

I. General Information

A. Specific Measurements

1. TLC = total lung capacity
2. RV = residual volume left after maximal exhalation
3. FVC = forced vital capacity on maximal exhalation
    a. FVC = TLC − RV.
    b. Analysis of FVC is the basis of formal pulmonary function testing.
4. FEV_1 = volume of exhalation expelled in first second.
5. Peak flow
    a. Maximum expiratory flow rate—usually obtained early in expiration
    b. Fastest and easiest single breath pulmonary function test available
6. Diffusion capacity
    a. Reflects the amount of functional alveolar–capillary surface area available for gas exchange
    b. Dependent on alveolar–capillary wall thickness and the time that blood spends in the alveolar capillary

B. Methods

1. Pulmonary function testing requires motivated patient with reproducible effort.
2. Spirometry equipment ranges from simple time-volume curves to flow-volume loops with computer-calculated indices (Figure 88–1A)
3. Peak flow determination requires an inexpensive hand-held flowmeter.
    a. Flow rate is simply read from the dial.
    b. Complete expiration not necessary so procedure well tolerated
4. Diffusion capacity determination requires expensive instrumentation in a pulmonary function laboratory.

II. Clinical Correlation

A. Obstructive Disease (Figure 88-1B)

1. Key points

   a. Definition of obstructive lung disease is $FEV_1/FVC < 70\%$
   b. FVC is generally preserved.

2. Etiology not distinguished by pulmonary function tests

   a. Bronchospasm (asthma)
   b. Airway inflammation (chronic bronchitis)
   c. Loss of elastic support (emphysema)

3. Patients are usually asymptomatic until FEV_1 is < 2L.

4. 800-1000 cc FEV_1 is usually necessary to survive weaning off mechanical ventilation.

5. Peak flow rates have a wide variation.

   a. 400-700 L/min is normal.
   b. Flow rates > 150 are acceptable for patients with obstructive pulmonary disease.

B. Restrictive Lung Disease (Figure 88-1C)

1. Key points

   a. Definition of restrictive lung disease is a general decrease in lung volume.
   b. FEV_1/FVC ratio is preserved unless there is superimposed obstructive plus restrictive disease.

2. Etiology

   a. Interstitial parenchymal disease—the five "i's"
      1) Inhalation—hypersensitivity (organic agent) or pneumoconiosis (inorganic agent)
      2) Infection
      3) Immunologic—eg, systemic lupus erythematosis
      4) Iatrogenic—drugs and radiation therapy
      5) "Idema" (edema)—congestive heart failure
      6) Idiopathic
   b. Mechanical factors
      1) Kyphoscoliosis
      2) Ankylosing spondylitis
      3) Obesity
      4) Neuromuscular disease—eg, myasthenia gravis, Guillain-Barré syndrome.

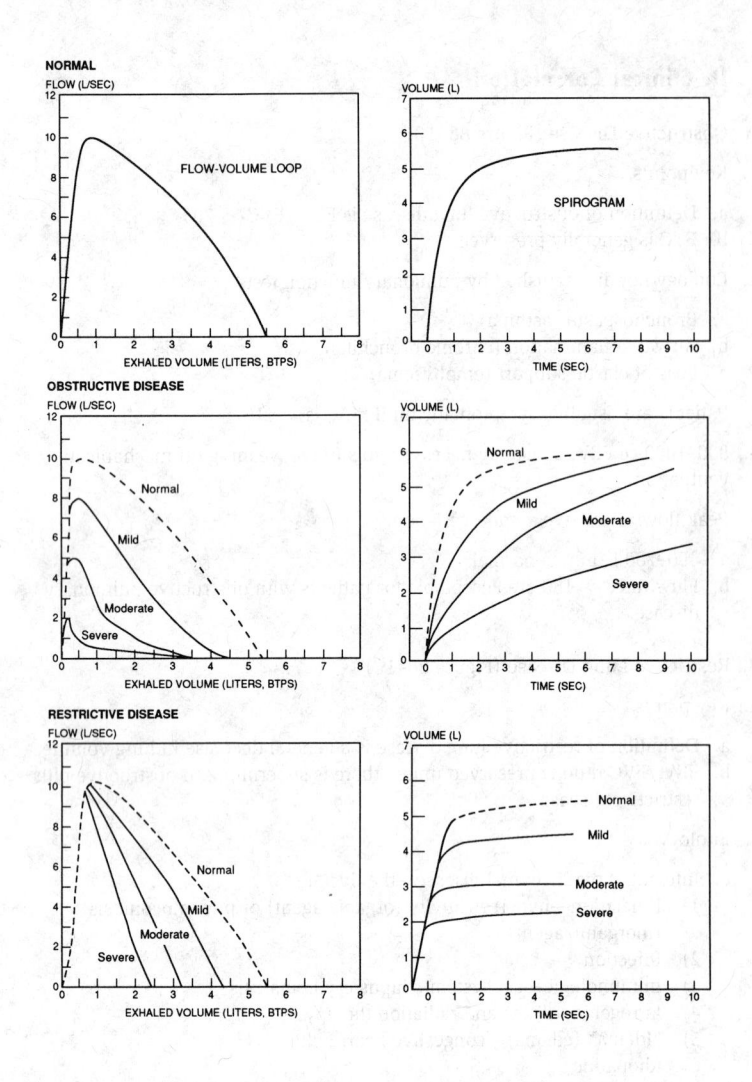

Figure 88-1. Pulmonary function testing.

III. Indications for Pulmonary Function Tests

A. Evaluation of unexplained dyspnea

B. Evaluation of bronchial hyperreactivity

C. Evaluation of chronic cough

D. Evaluation of response to pulmonary therapy

E. Evaluation of occupational exposures

F. Part of preoperative risk assessment

IV. Preoperative Assessment

A. Thoracic Surgery with Pneumonectomy

1. Assume pulmonary parenchymal surgery will require total pneumonectomy.
2. If FEV_1 preoperatively is < 2 L, then quantitive assessment of individual lung function must be obtained.
   a. Technique requires split function ventilation perfusion scans.
   b. Determines percentage of FEV_1 from each lung.

B. Thoracic Surgery without Pneumonectomy

1. Minimal impact on lung function
2. Pulmonary function testing may be helpful in patients with moderate to severe pulmonary disease.

C. Nonthoracic Surgery

1. Upper abdominal surgery has the greatest impact on pulmonary function and can cause up to a temporary 50% loss in FEV_1 (microatelectasis).
2. Preoperative pulmonary function tests helpful if patient has underlying pulmonary disease.

V. Indications for Referral

A. Symptomatic disease despite aggressive therapy

B. Progressive disease because evaluation may require bronchoscopy

VI. Indications for Hospitalization

A. No specific pulmonary function value automatically indicates admission.

VII. Annotated Bibliography

Chusid EL. The Selective and Comprehensive Testing of Adult Pulmonary Function. Mt. Kisco, NY: Futura Publishing, 1983. Chapters 1, 2, 11, 13 relevant for primary care; other chapters aimed at pulmonologists and respiratory technicians.

Weinberger SE, Drazen JM. Disturbances of respiratory function. In: Wilson JD, Braunwald E, Isselbacher KJ, et al, eds. Harrison's Principles of Internal Medicine, 12th ed. New York: McGraw-Hill, 1991. Excellent source for various causes of obstructive and restrictive disease.

Wright W, Hodgkin JE. Pulmonary functions tests. In: Burton GG, Hodgkin JE, Ward JJ. Respiratory Care—A Guide to Clinical Practice, 3rd ed. Philadelphia: JB Lippincott,1991:157–164. Easy to read guide for understanding pulmonary function test graphs.

Chapter 89: Pulmonary Nodule

Sandra B. Weibel

I. Clinical Presentation

A. General Information

1. Solitary pulmonary nodules are defined as opacities completely surrounded by lung and are < 4 cm. Lesions > 4 cm are called masses and are usually malignant.

2. Because bronchogenic carcinoma is the most common fatal malignant lesion, it is important to evaluate pulmonary nodules in a systematic and timely manner.

3. Most patients are asymptomatic at the time of discovery of the nodule. The chest x-rays are often done for other reasons and the nodule is found incidentally.

4. Increasing age and a smoking history increase the odds that a lesion is malignant.

B. History

1. Patients are often asymptomatic but previous history is important.

    a. History of prior malignancy
    b. Recent travel to an area where certain diseases are endemic such as southwest United States or Ohio River area (ie, coccidiomycosis or histoplasmosis)
    c. Previous smoking history
    d. Previous pulmonary history

2. Systemic symptoms such as fever and weight loss are sometimes present and suggest malignancy or systemic disease such as Wegener's granulomatosis.

3. Either pleuritic or nonspecific pain can occur in some cases (ie, trauma, pulmonary infarct) but is not common.

C. Physical Examination

1. Usually unremarkable

2. Certain findings will suggest the diagnosis.

    a. Hypertrophic pulmonary osteoarthropathy (bronchogenic carcinoma).

b. Nasal lesions such as nasal ulcers in Wegener's granulomatosis.
  c. Telangiectasias (pulmonary arteriovenous malformations)

II. Diagnostic Approach

A. Pseudonodules

1. If the lesion is visible in only one projection of the x-ray may not actually be a parenchymal nodule
2. Skin lesions or opacities on the chest wall
3. Nipple shadows—if you suspect this, can mark with radiopaque marker.
4. Loculated pleural effusions may also simulate a nodule.

B. Characteristics of Benign Nodules

1. Slow growth; no change in size by chest x-ray over 2 y.
2. Calcifications. Certain types increase the likelihood that the lesion is benign (central, laminated, diffuse, and popcorn).
3. Size of the nodule—usually < 3 cm but occasionally are larger
4. Shape not as specific but may be suggestive (ie, angular with smooth margins suggest nodule is benign)
5. Location and presence of cavitation are not helpful.

C. Malignant Nodule Characteristics

1. Rapid growth and larger nodules
2. Irregular, shaggy borders, the corona radiata, is usually indicative of malignancy.
3. Older age (> 40 y) and smoking history make malignancy more likely.

D. Radiologic Evaluation

1. Chest x-ray—good posteroanterior and lateral
   a. Will aid in eliminating possibility of pseudonodule
   b. Obtain old films preferably including x-rays 2 y ago or greater
   c. If stable over a 2 y period, can follow with serial chest x-rays initially at 4–6 mo intervals
   d. Evaluate for calcifications.
2. Conventional tomography
   a. Useful to delineate actual size, shape, and presence of calcifications
   b. Largely superseded by CT scans
3. CT
   a. Large lesions that are presumed malignant can be further staged.

b. Small lesions can be better defined.
   c. Densitometric studies (phantom studies) with high resolution are more sensitive for detecting calcification and may suggest the lesion is benign.
   d. Some morphologic characteristics can allow a diagnosis to be made (ie, fat density in hamartoma, pleural plaques, or arteriovenous fistula).
   e. Occasionally multiple nodules are visualized by CT, which were not apparent by plain films.
4. MRI has little to offer over CT scan.
5. Biopsy if lesion is indeterminate or higher probability of malignancy
   a. Bronchoscopy
      1) Small, peripheral lesions low yield
      2) High yield if lesion seen endobronchially
      3) Low-risk procedure
   b. Transthoracic needle aspiration
      1) Used with fluoroscopy or CT to localize the lesion
      2) High yield for malignant lesions and has positive predictive value of 99%.
      3) Biopsy often indeterminate for benign lesions
      4) Risk of pneumothorax 33% but is usually not life-threatening
   c. Surgical
      1) In past most lesions were excised.
      2) Thoracoscopy has been used increasingly.
      3) Can diagnose and resect at the same time.
      4) Approximately one third of resected pulmonary nodules are benign.
      5) If nodule is indeterminate by radiologic evaluation and patient is in high-risk group for cancer, may wish to proceed directly with resection.
      6) Morbidity and mortality are higher than with the other biopsy techniques.
      7) Prior to surgery, pulmonary function studies need to be obtained to determine resectability (forced expiratory volume in 1 sec [FEV_1] > 2.0 for pneumonectomy and FEV_1 > 1.2 L for lobectomy).
      8) If lung function is borderline, can obtain split function perfusion scan and quantitate function of each lung. It is preferable to leave patient with FEV_1 of 1 L or greater after surgery.

III. Differential Diagnosis

A. Pseudonodules—pleura, nipple shadows or external objects.

B. Benign

1. Granulomatous disease (TB, sarcoidosis, or histoplasmosis)

2. Arteriovenous malformations

3. Hamartomas and other benign tumors

4. Infectious lesions (abscess, parasitic, *Nocardia*, and *Aspergillus*)

5. Rheumatoid nodules or Wegener's granulomatosis

C. **Malignant**
1. Metastatic disease—often multiple nodules (colon, breast, kidney, and melanoma are common primaries)
2. Bronchogenic carcinoma
3. Lymphoma

IV. Treatment

A. **Diagnosis**
1. Initially must decide whether it is more likely to be malignant or benign
2. If not clearly benign, then will often have to pursue a biopsy
3. Once diagnosis made, can treat the etiology appropriately

B. **Benign**
1. Often no treatment needed as with old granulomas and hamartomas
2. Arteriovenous malformations will need no treatment unless a significant shunt exists. They will then need to be resected or embolized.
3. Infectious etiologies such as *Nocardia*, *Aspergillus*, etc. will need treatment with the appropriate antibiotic.

C. **Malignant**
1. Metastatic
   a. If it is the only metastatic site it can sometimes be resected (some sarcomas and colon carcinoma with otherwise controlled primary site).
   b. Chemotherapy depending on the primary site
2. Bronchogenic carcinoma
   a. Metastasic work-up needs to be completed first with CT scan to the level of the adrenals; bone scan, pulmonary function studies, and CT head as indicated.
   b. If non-small cell and stage IIIa or less then resection is indicated
   c. Small cell carcinomas, although rarely present as solitary pulmonary nodule, have been resected with some success.
   d. If not a surgical candidate then radiation therapy and/or chemotherapy

V. Patient Education

A. Need to discuss with patient all the risks and benefits of watching and waiting versus biopsy; also the advantages and risks of one biopsy procedure over another

B. If bronchogenic carcinoma is diagnosed, need to strongly advise to stop smoking. Even if they are resected, they are at increased risk for second primary lesion.

VI. Long-term Management

A. Largely dependent on the diagnosis

B. If felt to be benign or indeterminate and in low-risk group for carcinoma, then they need follow-up chest x-rays q 4–6 mo until it is documented to be stable over 2 y.

C. If a nodule is being observed and increases in size, it should be resected.

D. Bronchogenic carcinoma, even if resected, needs to have chest x-ray q 6 mo initially and then yearly.

VII. Indications for Referral to a Pulmonologist

A. Anyone with a lesion > 3 cm.

B. If the lesion is indeterminate or the patient is in a group at increased risk for carcinoma (ie, smoking history or age > 40)

C. Most pulmonary nodules will need to be seen by a pulmonologist unless they can be assumed to be benign by the criteria listed above with a high degree of confidence.

VIII. Indications for Hospitalization

A. Immunocompromised patients in whom infection is suspected

B. Otherwise only if other significant symptoms are present such as dyspnea or hemoptysis.

IX. Annotated Bibliography

Gurney JW. Determining the likelihood of malignancy in solitary pulmonary nodules with Bayesian analysis. Radiology 1993;186:405–421. A somewhat tedious analysis of odds of nodule being benign versus malignant but then can aid in diagnostic work-up.

Lillington GA. Management of solitary pulmonary nodules. DM 1991;274–318. Extensive review of differential diagnosis and work-up of pulmonary nodules.

Swenson SJ, Jett JR, Payne WS, Viggiano RW. An integrated approach to evaluation of the solitary pulmonary nodule. Mayo Clin Proc 1990;65:173–186. A concise and well organized approach to the management of solitary pulmonary nodules.

Part XVIII:
Renal/Urologic Diseases

Chapter 90: Evaluation of Renal Dysfunction

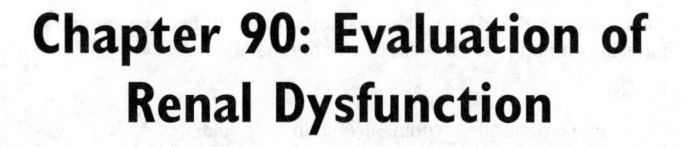

Herman J. Michael, Jr.

I. Clinical Presentation

A. Patients with renal dysfunction can present in many ways.

1. Signs and symptoms can be directly referable to the urinary tract.

   a. Flank pain
   b. Gross hematuria

2. Patients can have systemic manifestations of renal disease.

   a. Edema
   b. Hypertension
   c. Signs and symptoms of uremia such as nausea, vomiting, anorexia, and asterixis.

3. Patients can be asymptomatic and are incidentally found to have

   a. An elevated plasma creatinine concentration
   b. Abnormal findings on urinalysis

II. Diagnostic Approach

A. A critical issue is whether the azotemia is chronic, ie, stable and long-standing, or is acute, ie, recent with increasing azotemia.

B. Acute and chronic renal failure are classified separately.

1. Acute renal failure can be grouped according to the following functional classifications.

   a. Prerenal disease in which reduced perfusion is the primary abnormality
   b. Postrenal disease in which obstruction at a site in the urinary tract impedes the flow of urine
   c. Intrinsic renal disease, which can be caused by glomerular, vascular, tubular, or interstitial damage

2. Chronic renal failure almost always includes a component of intrinsic renal disease.

C. Examination of the urine is the most important noninvasive method for distinguishing among the different causes of renal disease.

1. Urinalysis
   a. Should be performed within 30–60 min after voiding.
   b. In the male, a midstream specimen is adequate but in the female, the external genitalia should first be cleaned to avoid contamination of the specimen with vaginal secretions.
   c. The urinalysis is diagnostically useful because different patterns of urinary findings are associated with different renal diseases.
      1) Hematuria and red cell casts point toward glomerulonephritis or vasculitis.
      2) Proteinuria and lipiduria point toward glomerular disease.
      3) Renal tubular epithelial cells and granular casts in a patient with acute renal failure point toward acute tubular necrosis.
      4) Pyuria with white cells and granular casts and mild or no proteinuria point toward tubular or interstitial disease or obstruction.
      5) Hematuria alone and pyuria with no casts may be seen in glomerular disease, vasculitis, obstruction, renal infarction, or acute interstitial nephritis.
      6) Hematuria alone is suggestive of vasculitis or obstruction in acute renal failure but also may be found in patients with mild glomerular disease, polycystic kidney disease, or extrarenal problems such as prostatic disease, calculi, or trauma.
      7) Pyuria alone is usually indicative of urinary tract infection but can occur in noninfectious tubulointerstitial diseases such as analgesic nephropathy.
      8) Normal or near normal urinalyses
         a) In acute disease may be found in prerenal disease, obstruction, hypercalcemia, intratubular obstruction, and acute tubular necrosis
         b) In chronic disease may be seen in prerenal disease, obstruction, tubular or interstitial disorders, or nephrosclerosis

2. Urine volume—is diagnostically quite important
   a. Oliguria refers to a urine volume insufficient to sustain life (usually < 400 mL/d), and commonly occurs in prerenal azotemia and acute tubular necrosis.
   b. Anuria, which is absence of urinary flow, may be caused by
      1) Urinary obstruction, which must be excluded in the initial evaluation
      2) Renal arterial or venous occlusion
      3) Shock, which is accompanied by intense renal vasoconstriction and usually hypotension
      4) Less commonly by rapidly progressive glomerulonephritis, hemolytic uremic syndrome, or renal cortical necrosis
   c. Wide fluctuations in daily urine output suggest intermittent obstructive uropathy.
   d. Polyuria (> 3 L/d) can be a hallmark of partial urinary tract obstruction in a patient with renal insufficiency.

D. Chemical analysis of urine composition is helpful in differentiating acute tubular necrosis from prerenal azotemia in the oliguric patient.
1. In patients with prerenal azotemia and with oliguria
   a. Reduced renal perfusion leads to appropriate sodium and water retention.
      1) The urine sodium concentration is usually low (< 20 mmol/L).
      2) The fractional excretion of filtered sodium (FENa) is usually low (< 1%).

$$\text{FENa} = \frac{(\text{Urine Na/Serum Na})}{(\text{Urine creatinine/Serum creatinine})} \times 100$$

      3) The urine osmolality may exceed 500 mosmol/kg.
   b. Urine/plasma creatinine ratio is usually > 40.
2. Patients with tubular necrosis, impairment of tubular function, and oliguria have
   a. An increased rate of sodium excretion
      1) Urine Na > 40 mmol/L
      2) FENa > 1%.
   b. A urine osmolality similar to that of plasma (< 350 mosmol/kg)
   c. Urine/plasma creatinine ratio usually < 20

E. Assessment of Glomerular Filtration Rate (GFR)

1. Measurement of urea and creatinine concentration are useful because they both vary inversely with the GFR.
2. Urea nitrogen is less useful because it may change independently of the GFR due to variations in the rates of urea production and reabsorption.
   a. Urea nitrogen production can be increased with
      1) High-protein diet
      2) Hemolysis and gastrointestinal bleeding
      3) Trauma
      4) Corticosteroids
   b. Approximately 40–50% of the filtered urea is passively reabsorbed.
      1) In volume dehydration, the enhanced sodium and water absorption is paralleled by an increase in urea reabsorption. Therefore, the urea nitrogen measurement will rise out of proportion to any change in the GFR or plasma creatinine concentration.
      2) An elevation in the ratio of the plasma urea nitrogen to creatinine therefore is useful in assessing prerenal disease.
3. Plasma creatinine concentration is more useful in monitoring renal disease.
   a. Creatinine production tends to be rather consistent.
   b. Creatinine is a more reliable index of GFR than urea because creatinine does not back diffuse from tubular lumen to peritubular blood.
4. Therefore, the creatinine clearance provides a reasonably accurate evaluation of the true GFR.

a. The creatinine clearance is given by the formula

$$\text{Creatinine Clearance} = \frac{(\text{Urine creatinine concentration}) \times (\text{Urine flow rate})}{(\text{Plasma creatinine concentration})}$$

b. It is measured with a 24-h urine collection and a venous blood sample.
c. There are two major sources of error.
   1) The 24-h urine collection is often incomplete because of patient error in collecting specimens.
   2) Approximately 15% of urinary creatinine is normally derived from secretion in the proximal tubule. This can result in an overestimation of the GFR, which becomes more important as the true GFR begins to decline.

F. Renal Ultrasonography

1. Used to assess kidney size, cortical thickness, echogenicity, and hydronephrosis caused by urinary tract obstruction

2. Probably should be performed in every patient with acute renal failure

G. Renal biopsy—usually performed when less invasive procedures cannot establish the diagnosis

III. Differential Diagnosis

A. One should differentiate between acute and chronic renal failure.

1. Chronic renal failure is suggested by the presence of uremic osteodystrophy, uremic neuropathy, bilateral small kidneys on ultrasound, or unexplained anemia.

2. Acute renal failure is suggested by a rapid rise in serum creatinine, little uremic osteodystrophy, or normal-sized kidneys on ultrasound.

B. Causes of Renal Failure

1. Prerenal azotemia causes 40–80% of cases of acute renal failure. Etiologies include:
   a. Volume depletion
   b. Heart failure
   c. Hepatic cirrhosis
   d. Peripheral vasodilation
   e. Drugs
      1) Nonsteroidal anti-inflammatory drugs (NSAIDs)—primarily in patients with an increase in endogenous renal vasoconstrictors and increased renal adrenergic neural tone
      2) Angiotensin-converting enzyme inhibitors, particularly in patients with bilateral renal artery stenosis, unilateral renal artery stenosis without a contralateral kidney, or other high-renin disorders

2. Postrenal failure or obstructive nephropathy accounts for 10% or less of all cases of acute renal failure.
   a. Can result from prostatic disease, pelvic or retroperitoneal cancer, calculi, or congenital abnormalities.
   b. Intrarenal obstruction is usually due to intratubular precipitation of poorly soluble material such as uric acid, oxalic acid, acyclovir, sulfonamides, and myeloma proteins.
3. Renal causes of azotemia
   a. Glomerular disease
      1) Glomerulonephritis
      2) Nephrotic syndrome
   b. Vascular disease
      1) Disorders of the large renal arteries such as thrombosis, emboli, and dissection
      2) Disorders of the smaller renal arterial vessels including vasculitis, malignant hypertension, hemolytic uremic syndrome, thrombotic thrombocytopenic purpura, disseminated intravascular coagulation, and scleroderma
   c. Tubular Disease = Acute Tubular Necrosis
      1) 60% of cases are related to surgery or trauma
      2) 40% occur in a medical setting
      3) The most common cause of acute tubular necrosis is renal ischemia.
      4) Nephrotoxic agents can cause acute tubular necrosis—aminoglycoside antibiotics and radiographic contrast agents are the leading nephrotoxic agents responsible for acute renal failure.
      5) Another common cause of acute tubular necrosis is the release of large amounts of myoglobin into the circulation.
   d. Interstitial disease
      1) usually drug induced
      2) Common agents include furosemide, penicillin, phenytoin, sulfonamides, rifampin, NSAIDs, trimethoprim, cimetidine, and captopril.

IV. Treatment

A. Exclude causes of renal failure that are potentially reversible such as prerenal state, obstruction, glomerulonephritis, renal vascular and interstitial disease and intrarenal crystal precipitation.

B. Once the diagnosis of acute tubular necrosis is made, little specific therapy is needed.

1. In the oliguric patient in whom prerenal factors have been corrected, a loop diuretic can be administered to enhance urine output.
2. Low-dose infusion of dopamine (1–3 µg/kg/min) may increase renal blood flow and allow a response to diuretics.

3. Conservative therapy
   a. Fluid restriction if patient oliguric and prerenal factors corrected
   b. Provide adequate nutrition—decrease intake of nitrogen, water, sodium, and potassium to match excretion.
   c. Only treat acidosis if serum bicarbonate < 10 mmol/L. If rapid correction of acidemia occurs with alkali administration, ionized calcium concentration can decrease and precipitate tetany.
   d. Hypocalcemia usually is asymptomatic and rarely requires therapy.
   e. Hyperphosphatemia should be controlled with phosphate binders.
   f. The secondary hyperuricemia of acute renal failure usually does not require treatment because the decreased glomerular filtration rate limits the filtered load and intratubular deposition of uric acid.
   g. Alter medication therapy if drugs are excreted by the kidneys.
4. Hyperkalemia
   a. If serum potassium is < 6 mmol/L would treat with elimination of any sources of potassium.
   b. Serum potassium > 6.5 mmol/L with ECG changes
      1) Emergent therapy
         a) IV calcium—10 mL of 10% solution of calcium gluconate given IV over 2–5 min and repeated at 10–15 min intervals will temporarily antagonize the cardiac and neuromuscular effects of hyperkalemia.
         b) 1 ampule of 7.5% Na HCO_3 (44.6 mEq HCO_3) can be given IV over 5 min and repeated at 10–15 min intervals to shift potassium from the extracellular space to the intracellular space.
         c) Glucose and insulin infusions act to shift potassium from extracellular space into cells. 10 units of regular insulin can be given IV at the same time as 1 ampule of 50% glucose (25 g) is given IV over 5 min. The combination of nebulized albuterol with insulin and glucose has been shown to be effective in dialysis patients.
      2) Nonemergent therapy
         a) Use cation-exchange resins to bind potassium in exchange for another cation in the intestinal tract.
         b) Oral therapy consists of 15–30 g sodium polystyrene sulfonate (Kayexalate) mixed in 50–100 mL of 20% sorbitol.
         c) Rectal therapy consists of a retention enema given as a mixture of 50–100 g sodium polystyrene sulfonate in 200 mL of 20% sorbitol or 20% dextrose in water.
5. Indications for dialysis
   a. Symptomatic uremia
   b. Resistent hyperkalemia
   c. Severe acidemia not responsive to medical therapy
   d. Severe fluid overload not responsive to medical therapy.

V. Indications for Referral

A. Urology consult to evaluate or rule out obstruction

B. Nephrology consult for renal dysfunction not responsive to elimination of prerenal causes

VI. Indications for Hospitalization

Severe renal dysfunction especially with rapidly rising creatinine and with oliguria or anuria

VII. Annotated Bibliography

Anderson RJ, Schrier RW. Acute renal failure. In: Wilson JD, Braunwald E, Isselbacher KJ, et al., eds. Harrison's Principles of Internal Medicine, 12th ed. New York: McGraw-Hill; 1991:1144–1156. A good basic overview of acute renal failure.

Coe FL. Alterations in urinary function. In: Wilson JD ed., Harrison's Principles of Internal Medicine, 12th ed. New York: McGraw-Hill; 1991:271–278. A basic overview of how to approach disturbances in urinary function.

O'Shea MH. Fluid and electrolyte management: potassium. In: Woodly M, Whelon A. Manual of Medical Therapeutics, 27th ed. Boston: Little, Brown; 1992:50–54. As always, this source presents a clear concise management scheme.

Rose BD. Approach to the patient with renal disease. In: Rubenstein E, ed. Scientific American Medicine 10, Nephrology III, 1992:1–10. A very concise detailed summary of the approach to renal disease.

Chapter 91: Hematuria

Herman J. Michael, Jr.

I. Clinical Presentation

A. General Information

1. Gross or microscopic hematuria may be due to serious urologic disease including malignancy or renal parenchymal disease.
2. Up to 18% of normal persons excrete red blood cells (RBCs) into the urine, averaging approximately 2 million RBCs in 24 h or 2 RBCs/high power field (hpf).
3. Detection
   a. Cellulose strips impregnated with peroxidase, orthotolidine, and buffers detect the peroxidase activity of heme in urinary RBCs, hemoglobin, or myoglobin with a sensitivity of 91–100% and a specificity of 65–99%.
   b. Therefore, a negative dipstick rules out significant hematuria but the lower specificity of a positive result requires the microscopic examination of the urinary sediment.
4. Pigmenturia
   a. Must be ruled out before the diagnosis of hematuria can be made
   b. Causes of pigmenturia
      1) Hemoglobin/myoglobin—Dipstick is positive but microscopic examination of urine reveals few to no RBCs.
      2) Foods—Examples include beets, berries, fava beans, and food coloring.
      3) Drugs—Examples include phenytoin, primaquine, rifampin, phenothiazines, and nitrofurantoin.
5. At least one of the following three criteria should be met before working up hematuria.
   a. > 3 RBCs/hpf in two of three properly collected clean-catch specimens.
      1) Patients should abstain from exercise and not have urethral instrumentation for 48 h before examination.
      2) Urinalysis should not be performed on women during menses.
   b. One episode of gross hematuria
   c. One episode of high-grade microhematuria (> 100 RBCs/hpf)

B. History

1. Intensity

    a. Gross hematuria suggests a urologic cause.
    b. Microscopic hematuria suggests a medical/glomerular cause.

2. Color

    a. Renal parenchymal bleeding is smoky, hazy or brownish red.
    b. Urologic hematuria is often bright red with clots.

3. Timing

    a. Initial hematuria (blood at the start of voiding) is usually from an anterior urethral site.
    b. Terminal hematuria is associated with bladder neck or prostate bleeding.
    c. Total hematuria results from bleeding at or above the level of the bladder.

4. Associated symptoms

    a. Bleeding may be associated with exercise or menses.
    b. Frequency, urgency or dysuria may indicate urinary tract infection or carcinoma.
    c. Renal colic may indicate a calculus.
    d. A recent sore throat or impetigo may indicate poststreptococcal glomerulonephritis.

5. Review of medications

    a. Drugs that affect coagulation (coumadin, heparin) may predispose to hematuria. It is important to look for underlying genitourinary lesions as the etiology of the hematuria.
    b. Many drugs can induce hematuria by causing glomerulonephritis, vasculitis, thrombotic microangiopathy, or intersititial nephritis.

6. Social history—A history of tobacco use and occupational exposure to a carcinogen may be associated with bladder tumors.

7. Family history

    a. Alport's syndrome
    b. Hereditary nephritis
    c. Sickle cell disease

8. Sex and age

    a. Men have a greater chance of having hematuria due to a life-threatening lesion (urologic malignancy).
    b. For both sexes the risk for significant lesion increases after the age of 40 and rises sharply after the age of 50.

C. Physical Examination

1. A medical cause of hematuria may be associated with

    a. Hypertension
    b. Edema

c. Rash/petechiae/angiomas
   d. Heart murmurs
   e. Hearing loss
2. Abdominal mass may point to a renal tumor, cystic renal disease, or hydronephrosis from obstruction.
3. Genitourinary examination—Inspect for lesions of the prostate, external genitalia, and urethral opening.

II. Diagnostic Approach

A. Urinalysis—three factors important

1. RBC morphology via light or phase contrast microscopy

   a. Glomerular RBCs (medical cause of hematuria) are distorted with crenated membranes and an uneven hemoglobin distribution.
   b. Nonglomerular RBCs (urologic cause) are typically disc shaped with an even hemoglobin distribution.

2. Character of the sediment

   a. RBC casts are pathognomonic of glomerulonephritis.
   b. Leukocyte casts may be found in pyelonephritis.

3. Presence or absence of significant proteinuria

   a. Urologic hematuria usually has a reading of less than 2+ protein on dipstick.
   b. Medical hematuria usually has a reading of ≥ 2+ on dipstick. A 24-h urine collection for total protein is performed to confirm a result of ≥ 2+ on dipstick. In the nephritic syndrome, gross or microscopic hematuria, RBC casts, and proteinuria are seen.

B. Urine culture to rule out urinary tract infection

C. Serum blood urea nitrogen (BUN) and creatinine levels to evaluate renal function

1. Impaired renal function is seen more commonly with medical etiologies.
2. 24-h urine collection for creatinine clearance is useful to further evaluate renal function.

D. Complete blood count can indicate the severity of blood loss or the presence of infection.

E. Coagulation studies to screen for a coagulopathy

F. Skin tests for TB depending on the patient's history and geographical location

G. A sickle cell preparation should be performed in all African American patients with hematuria.

H. Immunologic Studies

1. The third and fourth components of complement should be measured in patients with nephritic syndrome.

2. In hypocomplementemia, the presence of

   a. Antistreptococcal antibodies increases the likelihood of poststreptococcal glomerulonephritis
   b. Antinuclear antibodies increase the likelihood of lupus nephritis
   c. C3 nephritic factor increases the likelihood of membranoproliferative glomerulonephritis
   d. Mixed cryoglobulins increases the likelihood of cryoglobulonemic glomerulonephritis

3. In normocomplementemia, the presence of

   a. IgA fibronectin aggregates increases the likelihood of IgA nephropathy but its diagnostic utility has not been definitively determined
   b. Antineutrophil cytoplasmic antibodies increases the likelihood of idiopathic crescentic glomerulonephritis
   c. Antiglomerular basement membrane antibodies increases the likelihood of antiglomerular basement membrane glomerulonephritis

I. Serum and urine electrophoresis should be performed in patients with nephrotic syndrome, nephritic syndrome, and patients for whom there is clinical suspicion for myeloma.

J. Urine cytology can increase the index of suspicion for malignancy prior to intravenous pyelogram (IVP) or cystourethroscopy especially in patients who are at risk.

K. Ultrasound of kidneys should be performed in all patients with hematuria to

1. Evaluate kidney size
2. Rule out hydronephrosis
3. Determine if cystic disease is present
4. Detect large renal masses

L. IVP

1. Classically, the mainstay in the evaluation of the upper urinary tract for lesions
2. Renal ultrasound could replace IVP with a minimal decrease in diagnostic yield and is preferable in the patient at high risk for contrast nephropathy

M. CT scan could be used when other imaging studies are equivocal.

1. More sensitive than an IVP or a renal ultrasound in detecting renal lesions < 3 cm or those lesions not impinging directly on the urinary collecting system.

N. The role of MRI remains to be defined.

O. Cystoscopy is indicated in patients with hematuria especially those at increased risk for urinary malignancies.

1. Cystoscopy with washing for cytology may reveal the cause of bleeding.
2. Abnormalities can be defined by biopsy.

P. Retrograde pyelography should be performed in those patients in whom the IVP only partially visualizes the lower urinary tract.

Q. Renal biopsy is indicated if renal function is decreasing or proteinuria is > 1 g/d.

III. Differential Diagnosis

A. Urologic Causes

1. Urologic cancer
   a. Bladder
   b. Renal
   c. Prostate
   d. Ureteral

2. Nephrolithiasis

3. Urinary tract infection/tuberculosis

4. Papillary necrosis

5. Prostatic hyperplasia

B. Medical Causes

1. Menstruation

2. Viral illness

3. Physical exercise

4. Mild trauma

5. Food or pollen allergies

6. Cryoglobulinemia

7. Lupus nephritis

8. Alport's syndrome/thin basement membrane disease

9. Glomerulonephritis
   a. Rapidly progressive glomerulonephritis
      1) Antibasement membrane antibody disease (Goodpasture's disease)
      2) Idiopathic crescentic glomerulonephritis or pauci-immune glomerulonephritis (Wegener's granulomatosis)

b. Mesangial proliferative glomerulonephritis (IgA nephropathy)
c. Diffuse proliferative glomerulonephritis

10. Renal vein thrombosis

IV. Treatment

Treatment is specific for the etiology of the hematuria determined from the above evaluation.

V. Indications for Referral

A. Urology consult for cystoscopy and possible retrograde pyelography for nonglomerular hematuria

B. Nephrology consult for glomerular hematuria (especially if RBC casts) and evidence of renal dysfunction

VI. Indications for Hospitalization

A. Severe, uncontrollable bleeding

B. Infection resulting in fever, chills, and "toxic" state

C. Obstruction resulting in severe renal dysfunction

D. Renal dysfunction (especially if creatinine is rising rapidly associated with RBC casts)

VII. Annotated Bibliography

Jennette JC, Falk RJ. Serologic diagnostic techniques in renal disease. In: Narins RG, ed. Contemporary Issues in Nephrology Volume 25: Diagnostic Techniques in Renal Disease. Series editor, JH Stein. New York: Churchill Livingstone; 1992. Very detailed nephrologist-oriented review of serologic tests.

Mariani AJ. The evaluation of adult hematuria. AUA Update Series, vol. 8, lesson 23. Bellaire, TX: American Urological Association; 1989. Urologically slanted review of the subject on which most other reviews are based.

Paola AS. Hematuria: essentials of diagnosis. Hosp Pract 1990;25(11):144–152. Clear basic overview of hematuria.

Sutton JM. Evaluation of hematuria in adults. JAMA 1990;263(18):2475–2480. More detailed review of hematuria with comprehensive tables reviewing all aspects of evaluation.

Chapter 92: Urinary Incontinence

Karen G. Kelly

I. Clinical Presentation

A. General Information

1. Definition

    a. Involuntary loss of urine
    b. Incontinence is a symptom not a disease and should prompt a work-up.
    c. Although common, incontinence is not normal at any age.

2. Epidemiology

    a. Prevalence increases with age
    b. Prevalence in females > males
    c. Estimates of 15–30% in free living elderly, 50% or more of nursing home residents.
    d. Age, gender, and parity are established risk factors; other risk factors are unknown.

3. Classification

    a. Transient versus chronic
    b. Classification of chronic based on pathophysiology
        1) Urge incontinence—secondary to detrusor overactivity
        2) Stress incontinence—secondary to outlet incompetence
        3) Overflow incontinence—secondary to detrusor inactivity or outlet obstruction
        4) Functional—inability to get to toilet because of limitation in mentation or mobility
        5) Mixed—more than one mechanism

B. History

1. Screening

    a. All elderly patients should be asked directly about incontinence because patients may not raise it out of embarrassment or a feeling that it is an inevitable result of aging.
    b. If incontinence exists, the physician must take a thorough medical history with particular attention to neurologic problems, previous surgery, functional problems, and medications.

c. A voiding diary should be kept in which all episodes of voiding and incontinence, along with precipitants of incontinence, are recorded by patient or caregiver. If the quantity voided can be recorded as well, this can be useful.

2. Acute or transient (Table 92-1)—Ask about

   a. Symptoms of infections (dysuria, new urgency)
   b. Acute change in mental state
   c. Depressive symptoms
   d. Possibility of fecal impaction
   e. Excessive urine output
   f. Acute restrictions in mobility
   g. Medications (see Table 92-1)

3. Chronic

   a. Urge incontinence, detrusor overactivity
      1) Most common cause of incontinence in elderly
      2) Frequent, precipitous incontinence
      3) Moderate to large in volume
      4) Nocturnal incontinence common
      5) Sometimes associated with inpaired bladder contractability as well
   b. Stress incontinence, outflow incompetence
      1) Occurs with increased abdominal pressure (eg, coughing, laughing)
      2) Small or moderate amounts of daytime loss
      3) Rare at night
      4) Rare in men unless they have had surgery or are on medications that compromise sphincter function
   c. Overflow incontinence—detrusor inactivity or outlet obstruction
      1) Leakage of small amounts frequently
      2) Day and night
      3) Patient may note hesitancy, diminished and interrupted flow, a need to strain, and a sense of incomplete emptying.
   d. Functional
      1) Patient knows he or she has to void, but cannot get to toilet in time because of functional restrictions.
      2) May contribute to urge incontinence

C. Physical Examination

1. Pay particular attention to mental status and neurologic examination.

   a. Delirium, dementia
   b. Evidence of spinal cord compression

2. Percuss for bladder distention
3. Rectal examination for tone and impaction
4. Functional impairments
5. Edema or congestive heart failure which may contribute to polyuria

Table 92–1. Common Causes of Transient Incontinence

Mental Status Changes—delirium or depression
Urinary Tract Infection
Medications—Sedatives or hypnotics
  Diuretics
  Drugs with anticholinergic side-effects
    eg, antipsychotic agents
    tricyclic antidepressants
    antiparkinsonian agents
    opiates
    anti-diarrheals
  α-adrenergic agonists and antagonists
Polyuria—eg, secondary to hypercalcemia or hyperglycemia
Decreased mobility—eg, enforced bed rest

6. Pelvic examination in women
   a. Cystocele/rectocele or uterine prolapse
   b. Atrophic vaginitis

II. Diagnostic Approach

A. History and physical examination along with voiding record will often provide significant clues as to etiology and type of incontinence.

B. A postvoid residual (PVR) should be checked in all patients. A PVR > 50–100 mL suggests outlet obstruction or impaired bladder contractility.

C. Diagnostic Tests

1. Urinalysis
2. Creatinine
3. Culture and sensitivity if there are symptoms or abnormal urinalysis
4. Glucose and calcium if polyuria

D. Full Urodynamics

1. If cause not determined by clinical evaluation
2. When empirical therapy has failed
3. When surgery is planned
4. To exclude correctable obstruction in patient with overflow incontinence

III. Differential Diagnosis

A. Urge/Detrusor Overactivity

1. Can occur with or without bladder contractility problems
2. Seen with damage to CNS inhibitory centers, eg, stroke, Alzheimer's disease, Parkinson's disease
3. Seen with local irritation to urinary tract such as radiation or interstitial cystitis, bladder tumor, or stone
4. Often idiopathic

B. Stress/Outlet Incompetence

1. Usually in women secondary to pelvic floor laxity
2. In men only postsurgery
3. Occasionally secondary to intrinsically weak sphincter
   a. Surgery
   b. Diabetes
   c. Occasionally idiopathic

d. May leak while sitting quietly if bladder filled
   e. Atrophic urethritis may contribute

C. **Overflow—Outlet Obstruction/Bladder Contractility Problems**

1. Prostatic enlargement
2. Urethral stricture
3. Spinal cord lesions
4. Detrusor underactivity
5. Injury to nerves supplying bladder either from spinal cord or autonomic neuropathy

D. **Functional**

1. May contribute to urge incontinence.
2. Can be caused by any process that affects
   a. Mobility
   b. Cognition
   c. Motivation
   d. Manual dexterity

IV. Therapy

Important to treat urinary incontinence because it often limits activities and is associated with depressive symptoms. Therapy is often effective in at least improving symptoms.

A. **Acute—identification and treatment of acute precipitants**

1. Discontinue medications responsible for delirium.
2. Treat symptomatic urinary tract infections.
3. Eliminate medications that can cause incontinence.

B. **Chronic—Therapy is based on results of clinical evaluation as outlined above.**

1. Exacerbating factors listed under causes of transient incontinence should be sought and corrected.
2. Detrusor overactivity
   a. Behavioral
      1) Frequent scheduled voiding in demented individuals
      2) Bladder training if not demented (Table 92-2)
   b. Medications (combined with behavioral recommendations)
      1) Oxybutynin, usual dose is 2.5-5 mg up to t.i.d., has anticholinergic and smooth muscle relaxant properties
      2) Anticholinergics

Table 92-2. Bladder Training

Tell the patient to schedule urination q 30–60 min, depending on how long it is possible to wait comfortably without voiding. The bladder should be emptied as completely as possible at each scheduled time, regardless of the desire to void. If urgency occurs before the scheduled voiding time, the patient should suppress the urge as long as possible. Patients should try not to void off schedule, but if they must they should void the next scheduled time and resume the process. Patients who are experiencing fewer incontinent episodes and who are able to keep to their schedules comfortably should extend the intervals between voiding by 30 min each week until a voiding interval of 2.5–3 h is reached.

---

      3) Smooth muscle relaxants, eg, Flavoxate 100–200 mg t.i.d.
      4) Calcium cannel blockers (usual doses may be tried)
      5) Imipramine, lowest effective dose, with usual tricyclic precautions
      6) Doxepin, lowest effective dose
   c. Choice of agent will depend on comorbidity and side effects expected.
      1) Anticholinergics and drugs with anticholinergic side effects, such as tricyclic antidepressants, are poorly tolerated in demented or very elderly patients.
      2) Watch for urinary retention in patients with impaired bladder contractility

3. Stress incontinence

   a. Behavioral
      1) Pelvic floor muscle exercises (Kegel)
      2) Bladder training may help here as well.
      3) Frequent voiding in demented patients
      4) Weight loss if obese
   b. Medications
      1) Estrogen if atrophic urethritis (topical or oral) (see Chapter 55)
      2) α-Adrenergic agonists (watch for increased blood pressure)
      3) Imipramine (if patient is not demented) especially if urge and stress (check orthostatic pulse)

4. Overflow secondary to obstruction—usually requires referral to urologist or gynecologist

5. Overflow secondary to underactive detrusor

   a. Decompress bladder for 7–14 d
   b. Exclude obstruction
   c. Voiding trial after decompression
   d. $α_2$ Blockers, eg, terazosin (up 10 mg if blood pressure can tolerate it) to decrease outlet resistance

6. Indwelling catheters should be used infrequently

   a. Nonhealing sacral ulcers
   b. Terminal illness

V. Indications for Referral to Specialist in Incontinence

A. Obstruction

B. Significant PVR (> 100 mL)

C. Previous surgery that may have damaged sphincter

D. Lack of response to therapy

VI. Indications for Hospitalization

A. Acute obstruction

B. Coexisting illnesses that require hospitalization

VII. Annotated Bibliography

Fantl JA, Wyman JF, McClish DK, et al. Efficacy of bladder training in older women with urinary incontinence. JAMA 1991;265:609–613. A trial of bladder training that was successful in reducing incontinent episodes by 57% regardless of whether the cause was detrusor instability or outlet incompetence.

NIH Consensus Development Conference. Urinary incontinence in adults. J Am Geriatr Soc 1990;38:265–272. A consensus statement. In this same issue are a whole series of articles on incontinence.

Resnick NM. Initial evaluation of the incontinent patient. J Am Geriatr Soc 1990;38:311–316. Recommendations from an expert in the field.

Chapter 93: Impotence

Daniel Holleran

I. Clinical Presentation

A. General Information

1. Definition: inability to achieve or maintain an erection to complete a sexual act.
2. Organic and psychological causes of impotence must be considered.

B. Symptoms

1. Manifestations of occlusive aortoiliac disease such as bilateral leg claudication
2. Evidence of spinal cord trauma causing leg pain or weakness
3. Androgen failure leading to loss of libido
4. Pituitary tumor causing headache or vision problems

C. Signs

1. Evidence of aortoiliac disease—abdominal or femoral bruits or decreased distal pulses
2. Evidence of spinal cord neuropathy
   a. Diminished or exaggerated deep tendon reflexes
   b. Loss of leg strength
   c. Loss of anal sphincter tone after compression of glans penis (loss of bulbo cavernosus reflex)
3. Evidence of parkinsonism
   a. Resting tremor
   b. Cog wheel rigidity
   c. Masked facies
4. Androgen failure
   a. Small testes
   b. Loss of facial and pubic hair
5. Previous prostatic surgery

II. Differential Diagnosis

A. Psychological
1. Anxiety
2. Depression

B. Organic
1. Medication effect
    a. Antihypertensives are most commonly implicated.
        1) Thiazides
        2) β Blockers
        3) Centrally acting agents, eg, clonidine
    b. Tricyclic antidepressants
    c. Antihistamines
    d. Phenothiazines
    e. Cimetidine
2. Endocrinopathy
    a. Androgen failure
    b. Prolactinoma
3. Neurologic syndromes
    a. Lumbosacral plexus lesion
    b. Parkinsonism
    c. Multiple sclerosis
    d. Local damage to nerves following transurethral or suprapubic prostatic resection
4. Occlusive aortoiliac disease

III. Treatment

A. Acute
1. Eliminate any potential offending medications.
2. Reassurance pending results of tests

B. Long-term
1. Dependent on etiology
2. Treatment of potentially reversible primary medical disorder
3. Psychotherapy with or without medication for psychological disorder

C. Patient Education
1. Encourage patient to stop smoking, which will aggravate aortoiliac disease
2. Reassurance

IV. Indications for Referral to Urologist

A. High suspicion of occlusive arterial disease after medical evaluation

B. Inability to determine etiology

C. Failure of medical psychotherapy

D. Intracavernous pharmacotherapy

E. Penile implant

V. Annotated Bibliography

Rajfer J. Common Problems in Infertility and Impotence. Chicago: Yearbook Medical Publishers; 1990:235–376. Thorough readable coverage stressing diagnostic evaluation.

Wagner G, Green R. Impotence—Physiological, Psychological, Surgical Diagnosis and Treatment. New York: Plenum Press; 1981:24–131. Covers all the topics but not as readable as the Rajfer text.

Zerghiotti AW, Lizza EF. Diagnosis and Management of Impotence. Philadelphia: BC Decker; 1991:13–34. Concise evaluation of impotence stressing atherosclerotic disease and therapy.

Chapter 94: Prostatic Hyperplasia

Daniel Holleran

I. Clinical Presentation

A. General Information

1. Symptoms of prostatic hyperplasia (prostatism) occur to some degree in 75% of men over age 50.

2. Prostatic hyperplasia is an insidious process starting around age 30–49.

B. Symptoms

1. Often aggravated by medications including OTC antihistamines

2. Obstructive

    a. Hesitancy
    b. Intermittent stream
    c. Decreased force of urinary stream

C. Physical Examination

1. Examination by digital rectal examination may reveal the prostate to be:

    a. Smooth and nontender—not necessarily "large," likely benign prostatic hyperplasia (BPH)

    b. Large, boggy and tender—acute prostatitis

    c. Irregular or nodular—must exclude neoplasia

2. Evaluation of the abdomen may demonstrate a palpable or percussible bladder if obstruction of the bladder is present.

II. Diagnostic Approach

A. Eliminate drugs with anticholinergic activity.

1. Antihistamines

2. Tricyclic antidepressants

3. Diisopyramide

B. Evaluate for infection with urinalysis and urine culture.

C. Assess renal function.

1. Obstruction can lead to renal failure, which is potentially reversible after restoring urine flow.
2. Measure serum creatinine.

D. Evaluate for presence of obstruction.

1. Physical examination is most important.
2. Ultrasound can confirm bladder obstruction.

E. Exclude cancer.

1. Obtain prostatic specific antigen on all men over age 50.
2. See Chapter 9 for details of recommendations on screening for prostatic cancer.

III. Differential Diagnosis

A. BPH

B. Anticholinergic effect of medication

C. Acute prostatitis

1. Presents with low inguinal pain and fever
2. Physical examination reveals a tender swollen prostate

D. Cystitis—may lead to bladder spasm

E. Urethral stricture

F. Prostate carcinoma

IV. Treatment

A. Acute

1. Stop medications that may exacerbate obstruction.
2. Insert Foley catheter if acutely obstructed or with renal decompensation.
    a. Avoid too rapid collapse of distended bladder to avoid hematuria.
    b. Clamp Foley after 200 mL urine drains.
    c. After 10 min can let remaining urine drain in 200 mL increments.
3. Antibiotic therapy for prostatitis or cystitis
    a. Gram-negative—*Escherichia coli* and *Klebsiella*

b. Gonorrhea is less common.
c. Route of delivery (IV or PO) depends on systemic assessment of patient.
d. Specific agents
   1) Trimethoprim-sulfa 1 double-strength tablet b.i.d. for 10 d.
   2) Norfloxacin: 400 mg 1 b.i.d. for 10 d

B. Long-term

1. Finasteride

   a. 5-α reductase inhibitor, which blocks conversion of testosterone to dehydrotestosterone
   b. Leads to a 23% increase in maximal urine flow rate and a 18% decrease in prostatic volume
   c. Also causes a 3–6% incidence of impotence and decreased libido
   d. Dosage—5 mg qd

2. α Blockers

   a. Relieve blockage by relaxing the prostatic urethra—approximately 70% effective
   b. Specific agents
      1) Terazosin 1–20 mg qd
      2) Dixazosin 1–16 mg qd
   c. Major side effect is orthostasis (up to 23% of patients).
   d. Indications
      1) Hypertensive patient with BPH
      2) Problems with impotence or decreased libido on finasteride

3. Surgical options exist for patients who prefer surgery or who have failed medical therapy.

   a. Transurethral resection—85% successful in relieving prostatism; frequently causes retrograde ejaculation resulting in sterility but rarely causes impotence
   b. Balloon dilation—safe, only requires local anesthesia but long-term relief disappointing
   c. Stent—inserted after balloon dilation, only requires local anesthesia but long-term efficacy unknown
   d. Laser—ultrasound-guided resection using special catheter; no long-term data but may cause temporary worsening of symptoms

V. Indications for Referral to Urologist

A. Acute obstruction

B. Palpable nodule-biopsy may be performed by urologist or ultrasonographer.

C. Progressive prostatism if patient considering surgery

VI. Indications for Hospitalization

A. Obstruction requiring Foley catheter

B. Renal decompensation

C. Acute prostatitis with systemic toxicity

VII. Annotated Bibliography

Bruskewitz RC. Benign prostatic hyperplasia: Intervene or wait. Hosp Pract 1992; 27:99–115. Thorough article written by a urologist to be used by primary care practitioners.

Gormley GJ, Stoner E, Bruskewitz RC, et al. The effect of finasteride in men with benign prostatic hyperplasia. N Engl J Med 1992;327:1185–1191. Well written and informative.

Sobel JD, Kaye D. Urinary tract infections. In: Mandell CL, Douglas RG Jr, Bennett JE, eds. Principles and Practice of Infectious Diseases, 3rd ed. New York: Churchill Livingstone; 1990:600–601. Good review of infectious problems of the prostate.

Chapter 95: Proteinuria

Herman J. Michael, Jr.

I. Clinical Presentation

A. General Information
1. Proteinuria is a marker for renal disease.
2. Normal urinary protein excretion
   a. The glomerulus acts as a molecular sieve, allowing easy passage of water and small molecules such as glucose and urea, while hindering the filtration of larger plasma proteins into the ultrafiltrate.
   b. Passage of molecules across the glomerular barrier is a function of
      1) Molecular size—Proteins with a relative molecular mass > 40,000 daltons are almost completely prevented from entering the glomerular ultrafiltrate.
      2) Charge—There is decreased filtration of anionic substances such as albumin because the glomerular basement membrane contains negatively charged components.
      3) Configuration
   c. The following three proteins originate in the kidneys.
      1) Tamm-Horsfall protein—a mucoprotein synthesized by epithelial cells in the distal tubule that possesses antiviral activity and is involved in cast formation
      2) Urokinase-thrombolytic enzyme that is secreted by tubular cells
      3) Secretory IgA—Synthesized by renal tubular epithelial cells
   d. Healthy adults excrete < 150 mg of total protein in 24 h. Approximately one third is albumin and two thirds is globulins.
3. Proteinuria may be isolated or associated with hematuria. The presence of hematuria with proteinuria localizes the cause of the proteinuria to some type of glomerular process.
4. Proteinuria may be intermittent or persistent.
   a. Intermittent proteinuria—see differential diagnosis in III below
   b. Persistent proteinuria defined by positive tests for protein in repeated specimens

5. Proteinuria may be classified by the site of the lesion.
   a. Prerenal or overflow proteinuria
      1) Caused by a nonrenal disorder where excess low-molecular mass proteins are filtered by the glomerulus and exceed the reabsorptive capacity of the tubules
      2) Types of prerenal proteinuria include
         a) *Hemoglobinuria*
         b) *Myoglobinuria*
         c) *Lysozymuria associated with myelomonocytic leukemia immunoglobulin*
         d) *Immunoglobulin light chain proteinuria associated with multiple myeloma; the commonest example of overload proteinuria*
   b. Renal proteinuria—may be glomerular or tubular
      1) Glomerular disease can disrupt any of the glomerular filtration barriers.
         a) *Injury limited to the polyanion glycoproteins of the glomerular basement membrane tends to produce selective losses of anionic proteins such as albumin.*
         b) *Extensive injury that involves the entire basement membrane may cause losses of very large proteins as well as albumin.*
      2) Glomerular proteinuria may be mild or nephrotic range.
         a) *Nephrotic range proteinuria is defined as > 3 g/1.73m^2 body surface/d.*
         b) *The nephrotic syndrome is characterized by*
            i.) Nephrotic range proteinuria
            ii.) Hypoalbuminemia
            iii.) Edema
            iv.) Hyperlipidemia and lipiduria
      3) Tubular
         a) *If proximal tubular reabsorption is impaired, normally filtered serum proteins appear in the urine in increased amounts.*
         b) *These proteins include $β_2$-microglobulin, retinol binding protein, lysozyme.*
   c. Postrenal—can be caused by inflammatory or degenerative lesions of the renal pelvis, ureter, bladder, prostate, urethra, or external genitalia

B. **History**

1. History of renal disease
2. Urinary symptoms suggestive of infection
3. Family history of hereditary nephritis or other genetic renal diseases
4. Medications
   a. Minimal change disease may be secondary to probenecid or nonsteroidal anti-inflammatory drugs (NSAIDs)
   b. Membranous glomerulonephritis may be due to gold, penicillamine, captopril, or trimethadione.

C. Physical Examination

1. Signs related to renal disease

   a. Hypertension
   b. Costovertebral angle tenderness
   c. Edema

2. Signs related to systemic disease

   a. Diabetic retinopathy
   b. Joint involvement

II. Diagnostic Approach

A. The dipstick method detects urinary proteins using a buffered indicator that changes color in the presence of protein.

1. It is most sensitive to albumin.

2. Initially patients with a positive test should have the test repeated because a large proportion of patients will show disappearance of the proteinuria within several days.

3. False positive tests

   a. Dehydration
   b. Gross hematuria
   c. Highly alkaline urine

4. False negative results

   a. Dilute urine
   b. The presence of large amounts of nonalbumin protein in the urine such as immunoglobulin light chains in multiple myeloma

B. Protein precipitation methods such as sulfosalicylic acid detect proteins other than albumin. A finding of more protein by precipitation than by dipstick methods may indicate the presence of multiple myeloma.

C. If the patient has two or more repeatedly positive qualitative tests, a 24-h urine collection for protein and creatinine levels should be done.

1. Urinary creatinine excretion is measured to ascertain the adequacy of the urine collection (normal range in men is 15–25 mg/dL/d and in women 10–22 mg/dL/d).

2. Untimed urine samples have been used to estimate total 24-h protein excretion. A ratio of the concentration of total protein (mg/dL) to creatinine (mg/dL) > 3.5 is suggestive of nephrotic range proteinuria, whereas a ratio of < 0.2 is suggestive of normal protein excretion.

D. If persistent fixed proteinuria is found, the following work-up should be done.

1. A complete urinalysis

2. Urine culture
3. Assay of serum creatinine
4. Renal ultrasound
5. Serum albumin
6. Total serum protein and serum protein electrophoresis
7. Total cholesterol
8. C_3 and C_4 complement levels
9. Streptococcal studies such as antistreptolysin levels especially in patients with impetigo or a recent sore throat
10. Cryoglobulins
11. Urine protein electrophoresis
12. Hepatitis studies when clinically indicated
13. Blood glucose—Diabetic nephropathy is presumed if the patient has diabetes for 15–20 y, diabetic retinopathy, and proteinuria.
14. Antinuclear antibody test

E. If the patient has heavy proteinuria, hematuria with proteinuria, persistent hypocomplementemia, decreased renal function, or hypertension, there is probably a significant glomerular abnormality, and the patient should undergo a renal biopsy.

III. Differential Diagnoses

A. Intermittent proteinuria is characterized by an occasional urine specimen that has an abnormal quantity of protein. Classified as

1. Benign transient proteinuria
   a. Describes the isolated finding of urine containing abnormal amounts of protein that remits within a few days
   b. Most often seen in children or young adults

2. Functional proteinuria
   a. Excessive proteinuria in the absence of renal disease
   b. May be seen with
      1) Fever
      2) Strenuous exercise
      3) Cold or emotional stress
      4) Congestive heart failure
      5) Seizures
      6) Abdominal surgery
      7) Therapy with sympathomimetic drugs

3. Postural or orthostatic proteinuria
   a. Occurs only in the upright position
   b. 15-20% of young men with proteinuria on routine urinalysis have this pattern of proteinuria as do some patients with resolving acute pyelonephritis or glomerulonephritis.
   c. First morning voided specimen is invariably normal in protein content in these individuals.
   d. Is considered to be benign. Recheck periodically, because a few patients with an orthostatic pattern develop constant proteinuria in both the upright and recumbent position.

B. **Glomerular Proteinuria**

1. Primary glomerular diseases

   a. Minimal change disease/lipoid nephrosis can be idiopathic as well as associated with Hodgkin's disease.
   b. Focal glomerular sclerosis can be idiopathic as well as associated with HIV disease, heroin use, massive obesity.
   c. Membranous glomerulonephritis can be idiopathic as well as associated with hepatitis B, carcinoma, lymphoma.
   d. Mesangiocapillary glomerulonephritis/membranoproliferative glomerulonephritis may be idiopathic as well as associated with hepatitis (both B and C), cryoglobulinemia, and malignancy.

2. Secondary causes of proteinuria

   a. Hypertension
   b. Diabetes
   c. Drug side effect (ie, gold, captopril, NSAIDs, and penicillamine)
   d. Systemic lupus erythematous
   e. Amyloidosis
   f. Multiple myeloma
   g. Polyarteritis nodosa
   h. Subacute bacterial endocarditis

C. **Tubular proteinuria**

1. Chronic pyelonephritis

2. Fanconi syndrome

IV. Indications for Referral

A. **Refer to nephrologist for possible renal biopsy for**

1. Nephrotic range proteinuria

2. Hematuria and proteinuria

3. Declining renal function

B. Refer to hematologist for bone marrow biopsy if monoclonal immunoglobulin spike found on evaluation of proteinuria

V. Indication for Hospitalization

A. Intractable edema

B. Rapidly declining renal function

VI. Annotated Bibliography

Abuelo JG. Proteinuria: diagnostic principles and procedures. Ann Intern Med 1983;98:186–191. Good concise review of how to approach proteinuria.

Coe FL. Alterations in urinary function. In: Wilson JD, Braunwald E, Isselbacher KJ, et al. eds. Harrison's Principles of Internal Medicine, 12th ed. New York: McGraw-Hill; 1991:271–278. A basic overview of how to approach disturbances in urinary function.

Glassock RJ, Adler SG, Ward HJ, Cohn AH. Primary glomerular diseases. In: Brenner BM, ed. The Kidney, 4th ed. Philadelphia: WB Saunders; 1991: 1182–1279. Comprehensive, nephrologist-oriented review of primary glomerular disease.

Levey AS, Madaio MP, Perrone RD. Laboratory assessment of renal disease: clearance, urinalysis and renal biopsy. In: Brenner BM, ed. The Kidney, 4th ed. Philadelphia: WB Saunders; 1991:919–968. Comprehensive, nephrologist-oriented review of the diagnostic tools used to assess renal disease.

Waller KV, Ward KM, Mahan JD, Wismaltt DK. Current concepts in proteinuria. Clin Chem 1989;35:755–765. A good, more detailed review with clear definitions, detailed tables and a review of analytical methods.

Chapter 96: Kidney Stones

Karen G. Kelly

I. Clinical Presentation

A. General Information

1. Epidemiology

   a. Common—The lifetime risk may be as high as 20% for white men. Less common in African American patients and women.
   b. 80% of kidney stone patients are men.
   c. Peak age of onset is 20–30.
   d. Recurrence rate is as high as 50% within 5 y.
   e. Frequently familial

2. Stone composition

   a. 70–80% are calcium oxalate. Some of these contain a small amount of hydroxyapatite and some contain uric acid.
   b. 10–20% are struvite (magnesium ammonium phosphate).
   c. 5% are pure uric acid.
   d. 5% are calcium monohydrogen phosphate (brushite) or hydroxyapatite.
   e. < 1% are cystine and are caused by cystinuria, a rare hereditary disease.

3. Stones can only form when urine is supersaturated by crystals. This may be caused by hyperexcretion of ions, abnormal levels of inhibitory ions (eg, citrate), abnormal pH, or infections. Stone formation is not yet completely understood.

B. History

1. Renal colic—sudden onset of severe pain that may be steady or spasmodic. It typically occurs in the flank and may then progress downward to the groin area.

2. Large stones may present with painless obstruction or back pain.

3. Hematuria is common and may be the only symptom.

4. Urgency and frequency may occur as the stone reaches the uterovesicular junction.

5. Stones in the kidney may be entirely asymptomatic.

6. The clinician should inquire about
   a. Previous stones, their frequency, and whether their composition is known
   b. Family history of stones
   c. History of gout
   d. History of inflammatory bowel disease or intestinal bypass
   e. Urinary tract infections
   f. All medications, including vitamins, particularly C and D.
   g. Diet, climate, and fluid intake will also influence the formation of stones.

C. Physical Examination

1. Is typically negative or shows only slight flank tenderness
2. Peritoneal signs are usually absent.
3. Patients are often restless, pacing, and in severe pain.

II. Diagnostic Approach

A. Goals

1. Identify the number, size, and location of stones
2. Analyze a stone's composition
3. Identify metabolic abnormalities or diseases that have led to the stone's formation. Not all patients will require complete metabolic work-up, but stone identification and a basic work-up should be done in all cases.

B. Identifying Stones

1. Radioopaque stones (calcium stones, struvite, and cystine) can be seen on abdominal flat plate or intravenous pyelogram (IVP).
2. CT scans can distinguish nonopaque stones (uric acid) from kidney tissue or blood clots.

C. Stone Analysis

Patients should be instructed to strain all urine until a stone fragment is obtained for analysis.

D. Metabolic Work-up

1. All patients should have a basic work-up consisting of
   a. Urinalysis and culture, if infection is suspected
   b. Blood tests for calcium, phosphate, uric acid, electrolytes, and creatinine
   c. Urinalysis for qualitative cystine should be done if the composition of the stone is unknown.
   d. Further work-up is required if any of the above tests are abnormal.

2. Patients who have recurrent or growing stones within a 1 y follow-up should have further evaluation including 24-h urine collection for volume, pH, calcium, phosphorus, sodium, uric acid, oxalate, citrate, and creatinine. More than one sample may be useful because of variability. Treatment will be based on the results of this evaluation.

III. Differential Diagnosis

A. Will depend on the kind of stone formed

B. Calcium Oxalate Stones

1. Primary hyperparathyroidism results in hypercalcemia and hypercalciuria. Hypercalcemia is usually mild and the serum phosphorus is usually low. Occasionally other causes of hypercalcemia result in kidney stones. (See Chapter 40 for a full discussion of work-up and management.)
2. Idiopathic hypercalciuria—> 250 mg of calcium in 24 h of urine in women or > 300 mg in men, in the absence of hypercalcemia, represents hypercalciuria. More than half of all patients with calcium oxalate stones have hypercalciuria. It may be familial and affects both sexes equally.
3. Low urine citrate—may be seen in people with bowel disease and renal tubular acidosis as well as others with calcium oxalate stones. Citrate lowers calcium oxalate supersaturation.
4. Hyperoxaluria—> 45 mg/d is considered excessive and may be due to dietary excess (spinach, pecans, peanuts, and chocolate among other foods), ileal disease, vitamin C excess, or inherited forms of hyperoxaluria
5. Hyperuricosuria—> 750 mg/d in women and 800 mg/d in men.
6. No identifiable abnormalities will be found in some patients.
7. More than one mechanism may be at play in some patients.

C. Calcium Phosphate Stones

1. The majority of patients with calcium phosphate stones have renal tubular acidosis.

D. Uric Acid Stones

1. Low urine pH
2. Hyperuricosuria

E. Struvite

1. Infection with bacterial organisms that express urease. Struvite stones tend to be large and cause bleeding or obstruction.

F. Cystine Stones

1. Hereditary cystinuria

IV. Treatment

A. Treatment includes both management of the existing stones and therapy designed to prevent further stones. Successful therapy to prevent further stones will depend on the correct diagnosis.

B. Management of stones involves

1. Pain control, often with parenteral narcotics and hydration
2. Urologic consultation will be required for further management if the stone does not pass spontaneously.
3. Current methods of stone management include ureteroscopy to remove the stone, percutaneous nephrolithomy, and percutaneous or in situ extracorporeal shock wave lithotripsy. Open surgery may be required in complicated cases.
4. Stone management should be accompanied by medical management to prevent recurrences.

C. Medical Management

1. Conservative therapy is reasonable for all stone formers and as the only therapy for those in whom a limited work-up has failed to reveal a treatable cause.
2. It consists of increasing fluid intake to cause a urine output of > 2 L/d.
3. Diet should be limited in sodium and oxalate. Animal proteins may be limited in those with high protein intakes and in those with hyperuricosuria.

D. Calcium Oxalate Stones

1. Hypercalcemia—Hyperparathyroidism should be corrected surgically. Other causes should be treated appropriately.
2. Hypercalcuria—Drug treatment with thiazides reduces calcium excretion and reduces stone formation. Potassium should be replaced with potassium citrate (30–60 mEq in divided doses). Low-calcium diets are controversial.
3. Low urinary citrate—potassium citrate supplementation
4. Hyperoxaluria—dietary restriction of oxalate. In the presence of ileal disease, oral calcium supplements (1–4 g calcium carbonate in divided doses), cholestyramine (4–16 g in divided doses with meals) and oral citrate have been recommended.
5. Hyperuricosuria—dietary restriction of purines. Alkalinization of the urine to a pH of 6.5 with bicarbonate or citrate. Allopurinol should be considered, especially if uric acid excretion is > 1200 mg/d.

E. Calcium phosphate stones—can be treated with potassium alkali (bicarbonate or citrate) and thiazides

F. Uric acid stones—alkalinization of urine with potassium salts to pH 6–6.5; allopurinol if necessary

G. Struvite—Stones must be removed. After removal of the stones, long-term antibiotics may be helpful.

H. Cystine—High fluid intake; alkalinization and use of penacillamine (1–2 g/d) or other agents

V. Indications for Referral

A. A urologist will often need to be involved in the acute management of the stone.

B. Referral to an expert in stone management should be made in cases where failure of initial management occurs or where diagnosis is uncertain.

C. Patients with hyperparathyroidism should be referred for surgery.

VI. Indications for Hospitalization

A. For pain management

B. For stone removal

VII. Annotated Bibliography

Coe FL, Parks JH, Asplin JR. The pathogenesis and treatment of kidney stones. N Engl J Med 1992;327:1141–1152. A review with an extensive bibliography.

Consensus Conference. Prevention and treatment of kidney stones. JAMA 1988;260:977–981. A consensus statement.

Preminger GM. Renal calculi: pathogenesis, diagnosis, and medical therapy. Semin Nephrol 1992;12:200–216. A review with a more detailed discussion of pathogenesis and treatment of hypercalcuria.

Part XIX:
Rheumatology/Orthopedics

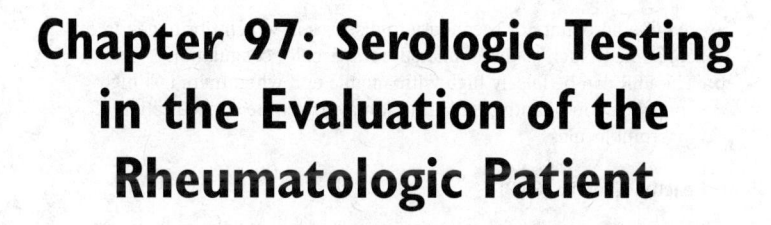

Chapter 97: Serologic Testing in the Evaluation of the Rheumatologic Patient

John M. Spandorfer

I. Acute Phase Reactant

A. Erythrocyte Sedimentation Rate (ESR)

1. Definition

   a. The ESR measures the rate of fall of red blood cells (RBCs) in a standard tube and is used as a nonspecific measure of inflammation.
   b. RBCs in inflammatory disorders may form stacks, resulting from an increase in plasma proteins such as fibrinogen or macroglobulins, thus causing a quicker sediment.
   c. The normal ESR for males is 0–15 mm/h and for females is 0–20 mm/h.
   d. The ESR is affected by age. It increases by 0.85 mm/h for each 5-y interval increase in age.

2. Association with diseases

   a. A normal ESR may help exclude active inflammatory diseases.
   b. Malignancy, infection, and connective tissue disease may cause mild to moderate (30–50 mm/h) elevations of ESR.
   c. ESR of > 100 mm/h is associated with various systemic vasculitides, polymyalgia rheumatica, very active rheumatoid arthritis, infection (such as endocarditis, abscesses, osteomyelitis, and TB), chronic renal failure, and states with an absolute increase in globulins such as multiple myeloma, lymphoma, and cryoglobulinemia.

3. Clinical use

   a. An aid to help diagnose or rule out an inflammatory condition
   b. Can also be used to follow the activity or response to therapy of an inflammatory disease

4. Limitations

   a. Falsely low ESR is found in conditions in which RBCs do not undergo rouleaux formation as in anisocytosis, spherocytosis, polycythemia, and sickle cell anemia and other hemoglobinopathies. An ESR of 20 mm/h in a patient with sickle cell anemia may equate to a value of 100 mm/h in a normal patient. It may also be falsely low in hypofibrinogenemia, which

may be hereditary or secondary to diseases in which fibrinogen is consumed (such as disseminated intravascular coagulation).
   b. The ESR can be falsely high with anemia and when there is a high concentration of anticoagulant that may lower the concentration of macromolecules.

B. C-Reactive Protein (CRP)

1. CRP is an acute reacting protein that may increase rapidly with an inflammatory stimulus.
2. Similar to ESR, it is nonspecific and can supplement or complement the ESR.
3. CRP, in contrast to ESR, more closely approximates the degree of ongoing tissue damage. In systemic lupus erythematosus (SLE) and scleroderma, CRP levels are inappropriately low unless infection or other tissue damage is present. Also in contrast to ESR, CRP can be used on freeze-stored serum.

II. Autoimmune Serologies (Table 97–1)

Table 97–1. Prevalence of Autoantibodies in Specific Diseases

Antibody	Associated Diseases (% prevalence)
Rheumatoid factor	Rheumatoid arthritis (80–90%)
	SLE (20–40%)
	Scleroderma (30%)
	Dermatomyositis (10–15%)
Antinuclear	Mixed connective tissue disease (100%)
	Drug-induced lupus (100%)
	SLE (95–100%)
	Sjögren's syndrome (90%)
	Scleroderma (60–95%)
	Rheumatoid arthritis (30–50%)
	Dermatomyositis and polymyositis (25–50%)
Anti-DNA	SLE (60–70%)
Anti-Sm	SLE (5–30%)
Anti-Ro	Sjögren's syndrome (75%)
	SLE (25–30%)
Anti-La	Sjögren's syndrome (40–60%)
	SLE (5–10%)
Antihistone	Drug-induced lupus (95%)
	SLE (70%)
Anti-RNP	Mixed connective tissue disease (100%)
	SLE (25–30%)
Anti-Jo1	Dermatomyositis and polymyositis (25–30%)
Anti-Scl-70	Scleroderma (20%)

A. Rheumatoid factor (RF)

1. Definition
   a. RF is a group of autoantibodies that are reactive with the Fc portion of IgG.
   b. They were first described in its association with rheumatoid arthritis (RA) but are not specific for RA.
   c. All classes of immunoglobulins are included in the RF but classically RF is IgM directed against IgG.

2. Association with disease
   a. 80% of patients with RA will have titers of at least 1:160. See Table 97-1 for RF's association with other diseases.
   b. Low titers, which are 1:20 to 1:80, are seen with chronic active hepatitis, TB, subacute bacterial endocarditis, syphilis, pulmonary fibrosis, sarcoidosis, and viral and parasitic infection. These low titers may be the result of RF responding to stimulation with altered IgG.
   c. 30% of patients over age 65 may be RF positive without any associated rheumatologic disease; 5–10% of these patients may have a high titer.

3. Clinical use
   a. RF can be of prognostic significance because patients with high titers tend to have more aggressive disease and have extra-articular manifestations.
   b. Presence of RF does not establish disease because fewer than one third of unselected patients with positive RF will be found to have RA.
   c. RF is not useful as a screening procedure but can help confirm or exclude a diagnosis in patients with suspected RA.

B. Antinuclear Antibody (ANA)

1. Definition—ANAs are a wide array of antibodies directed against nuclear and cytoplasmic cellular antigens. They are found in many rheumatic diseases and assayed through immunofluorescence, radioimmunoassay, and immunodiffusion.

2. Association with disease (see Table 97-1)

3. Clinical use
   a. ANA should be requested when an autoimmune disease is suspected.
   b. The presence or absence of ANA is helpful in confirming or negating the clinical impression.
   c. ANA may be a good screening test because it includes a wide variety of antibodies to nuclear antigens.
   d. A significant amount of variability exists between laboratories; thus, the level for a significant titer may vary. In general, a titer of < 1:80 is not considered significant.
   e. When a positive ANA is obtained one should interpret the result in context with the clinical picture. The pretest suspicion of autoimmune disease, the age of the patient, the use of ANA-inducing drugs, and the titer all should be considered to help exclude false positives.

4. Pattern of immunofluorescence—There are four patterns associated with different diseases.
   a. Homogenous and peripheral correlate with SLE and RA.
   b. Speckled is seen with mixed connective tissue diseases and, less commonly, SLE, RA, and scleroderma.
   c. Nucleolar is associated with scleroderma and Sjögren's.
5. False positives are seen with many medications such as hydralazine, procainamide, isoniazid, methyldopa, and phenytoin. A low titer is seen in 18% of people over age 65 and 4% below age 30.

C. Specific Antinuclear Antibodies

The ANA is able to determine if the patient's serum contains ANA, but it is not immunologically specific. After a positive ANA is obtained, the following antoantibodies can be requested, depending on what specific disease is clinically suspected.

1. Anti-DNA antibody (anti-dsDNA)
   a. Anti-dsDNA is relatively specific for SLE and may help in its diagnosis. After a long period of observation, 70% of patients with SLE are positive for this antibody. The level of anti-dsDNA may correlate with activity of SLE.
   b. Positive results occur less commonly in RA, systemic sclerosis, chronic hepatitis, and chronic infections.
2. Antibodies to Sm—Anti-Sm are named after a patient, Smith, in whom this antibody was first described. They are seen in 5–30% of patients with SLE and are uncommon in any other connective tissue disease.
3. Anti-Ro antibody (also known as SS-A antibody)
   a. This is a relatively common antibody found in 75% of patients with primary Sjögren's and 30% of those with SLE. Those patients with primary Sjögren's and a positive anti-Ro are at increased risk for vasculitis and nervous system complications.
   b. Anti-Ro antibodies occur with increased frequency in certain SLE patients—those with thrombocytopenia, cutaneous lupus and ANA-negative SLE.
4. Anti-La antibody (or SS-B)—Often associated with anti-Ro antibody, anti-La appears in 40% of patients with primary Sjögren's and 10% of patients with SLE.
5. Antibodies to histones—These antibodies are present in 95% of patients with drug-induced lupus and 70% of SLE.
6. Antibodies to RNP—RNP antibodies in low titers are present in 25% of patients with SLE and less often in those with systemic sclerosis, polymyositis,

and Sjögren's. A high titer anti-RNP of > 1:10,000 is a hallmark of mixed connective tissue disease.

7. Antibodies to Jo-1—Present in 25% of patients with dermatomyositis and polymyositis, antibodies to Jo-1 are specific for these disorders.

8. Antibodies to Sc1-70—Although these antibodies are only present in 20% of patients with scleroderma, they are specific for the disease because they are rarely found in other conditions.

D. Other Autoantibodies

1. Antineutrophil cytoplasmic antibodies (ANCA)—Two types have been described.

   a. ANCA with a cytoplasmic staining pattern (cANCA) is highly specific (> 98%) and sensitive (80%) for extended Wegener's granulomatosis. The test is less useful for limited Wegener's granulomatosis and other vasculitides.

   b. ANCA with a perinuclear staining pattern (pANCA) are not common in Wegener's granulomatosis but are highly specific (> 94%) for Churg-Strauss, polyarteritis nodosa and vasculitic overlap syndromes.

2. Antiphospholipid antibodies—Those with very high titer are predisposed to thrombotic complications such as deep venous thrombosis, pulmonary emboli, myocardial infarction, cerebrovascular accidents, and placental insufficiency. Elevated levels are seen with 40% of patients with SLE.

E. HLA

The clinical usefulness of HLA typing for diagnosis is limited to examining HLA B27 in patients suspected of having ankylosing spondylitis. The sensitivity and specificity for this association is 90%.

F. Recommendation for Initial Autoantibody Testing When Specific Conditions Are Suspected

1. RA—RF is recommended and serves as a criteria for the diagnosis.

2. SLE—ANA and anti-DNA can both help to establish the diagnosis of SLE. If the ANA and anti-DNA are both positive, the anti-Sm, although specific for SLE, is not necessary.

3. Drug-induced SLE—ANA and antihistone should be ordered. The anti-DNA can also be helpful because it is rarely present and will therefore help to distinguish drug-induced SLE from idiopathic SLE.

4. Dermatomyositis and polymyositis—No autoantibody testing is needed. An elevated creatinine phosphokinase level and a characteristic electromyogram and muscle biopsy are diagnostic.

5. Scleroderma—Although no test is specific, an ANA, RF, and anti-Sc1-70 may be helpful.
6. Sjögren's—No autoantibodies are needed to help with the diagnosis. The classic triad of keratoconjunctivitis sicca, xerostomia, and a mononuclear cell infiltration of the salivary gland is diagnostic.
7. Wegener's—An ANCA is recommended.

III. Complement

A. The complement system consists of a network of interacting proteins that aid in the humoral immune system.

B. Serum complements are often decreased with active SLE. The specific complements, C3 and C4, as well as the total hemolytic complement, CH50, can be low (the CH50 is a functional assay that measures the ability of test serum to lyse 50% of sheep erythrocytes coated with antibody). C3, C4 and CH50 can be used as markers of disease activity.

C. Serum complements are also decreased in 25% of patients with Sjögren's syndrome. Other connective tissue diseases typically have normal complement levels.

D. A decreased serum complement level may be helpful to distinguish SLE and Sjögren's from other connective tissue diseases.

IV. Annotated Bibliography

Bedell SA, Bush BT. Erythrocyte sedimentation rate. Am J Med 1985;78:1001–1009. In-depth review of the historical background, physics, and clinical utility of the ESR.

Harmon C. Antinuclear antibodies in autoimmune diseases. Med Clin North Am 1985;69:547–563. An excellent and well referenced review of the clinical significance of antinuclear antibodies.

Kollenberg CG, et al. Antineutrophil cytoplasmic antibodies: a still-growing class of autoantibodies in inflammatory disorders. Am J Med 1992;93:675–681. ANCA's association with various rheumatologic diseases is explored with emphasis on its sensitivity and specificity.

Shmerling RH, Delbanco TL. How useful is the rheumatoid factor. Arch Intern Med 1992;152:2417–2420. Original investigation elucidating the sensitivity, specificity, and predictive value of the RF.

Chapter 98: Degenerative Joint Disease

John M. Spandorfer

I. Clinical Presentation

A. General Information

1. Degenerative joint disease (DJD), or osteoarthritis, is characterized by a progressive degeneration of articular cartilage and reactive changes resulting in new bone formation at the base of the cartilage lesion and joint margins.
2. It is the most common rheumatologic disease and most common cause of disability in the elderly. Approximately 50% of adults show degenerative changes on radiographs but only 20% are symptomatic. 90% of people over 65 have radiographic evidence of DJD.
3. DJD may be classified as primary and secondary.
   a. Primary DJD is when there are no known predisposing factors. It may be the result of the normal aging process of the joint and chronic mechanical factors.
   b. Secondary DJD may result from prior joint disease resulting from trauma, inflammation, metabolic diseases, bone disease, or steroid injections into the joint.

B. History

1. Complaints
   a. Patient complains of an insidious onset of a deep aching pain in usually one or a few joints.
   b. Pain is aggravated by joint use and can be relieved by rest. Later in the course of the disease, pain can occur at rest and may awaken the patient from sleep.
   c. There may be stiffness on awakening that typically is of short duration.
2. Distribution—DJD most commonly involves the distal interphalangeal (DIP) joint, first carpometacarpal joint, first metatarsal phalangeal (MTP) joint, lumbar and cervical spine, hips, and the knees. Except in secondary DJD there is rare involvement of the metacarpophalangeal (MCP), wrist, elbow, or shoulder joints.

3. Past medical history—The patient can be questioned about history, which may differentiate primary from secondary DJD.
   a. Obesity and repetitive stress may be involved in the development of primary DJD, but this remains controversial.
   b. Prior inflammatory joint disease as in infectious arthritis, rheumatoid arthritis (RA), systemic lupus erythematosus (SLE), gout, and pseudogout may cause secondary DJD. Neuropathic joint disease from any cause, repetitive cases of hemarthroses, and the repeated use of intra-articular steroids can also result in secondary disease.

C. Physical Examination
1. Appearance—As the disease progresses there may be enlargement of the joint from synovitis or proliferative changes in the cartilage resulting in osteophytes. Osteophyte of the DIP joint is referred to as Heberden's node and of the proximal interphalangeal (PIP) joint as Brouchard's node.
2. Palpation
   a. Joints may be locally tender and warm.
   b. There may be crepitus and pain on passive motion.
   c. Osteophytes may be palpated at the joint margin.
   d. Progression of disease may result in severe deformities and subluxation of the joint.

D. Specific Joints
1. Hand
   a. Heberden's nodes of the DIP joint may be single but are usually multiple. They often develop slowly over years after age 45 and may be genetically acquired. Women are affected 10 times as frequently as men.
   b. Small gelatinous cysts often appear on the dorsal aspect of the finger joints and precede the development of nodes.
   c. Degenerative changes at the base of the thumb are frequent and result in difficulty with grip and thumb apposition.
2. Spine
   a. Osteoarthritis of the spinal joints is common. It often results from degenerative changes of the intervertebral discs and apophyseal joints.
   b. Patients commonly complain of pain and stiffness at the site.
   c. Osteophytes can impinge on the nerve root. This may initially result in radicular pain and paresthesias and later in reflex and motor loss in the distribution of the affected nerve.
3. Knees
   a. When DJD involves the knee it often leads to pain that is worsened with weight-bearing.
   b. There may be few objective changes on examination except for crepitus, mild tenderness, and joint effusion.
   c. Muscle atrophy and joint enlargement can also be present.

4. Hip
   a. Osteoarthritis involving the hip may be significantly disabling.
   b. Patients may complain of pain with walking, resulting in a characteristic limp (antalgic gait).
   c. The pain may be referred to the buttocks, sciatic region, or distal thigh.
   d. The examination may reveal decreased range of motion and pain on motion.
   e. The inability to internally rotate the leg during flexion may be one of the earliest signs.
5. Feet
   a. One of the most common sites of DJD is the first MTP joint.
   b. It may be aggravated by wearing tight fitting shoes.
   c. Bony enlargement and a valgus deformity may result.

II. Diagnostic Approach

A. History—Osteoarthritis is likely when a patient over the age of 40 complains of joint pain (as described above) and lacks systemic complaints.

B. Physical—Tenderness, restricted range of motion, and mild swelling and warmth may all be consistent with DJD.

C. Laboratory Findings

1. No specific laboratory abnormality exists in osteoarthritis.
2. Laboratory studies may be helpful in excluding other joint diseases. The erythrocyte sedimentation rate (ESR), complete blood count, and chemistries are all typically normal. Synovial fluid reveals a normal viscosity and a mildly elevated cell count, findings consistent with a noninflammatory arthritis. An arthrocentesis, however, is not needed if presentation is suggestive of DJD.

D. Radiographic Findings

1. If the changes are mild the radiograph may appear normal.
2. With progressive disease there are characteristic findings—joint-space narrowing (results from degeneration and destruction of the articular cartilage), subchondral bony sclerosis, and cysts in the periarticular bone.
3. These findings are common in elderly patients and therefore may not exclude the presence of other causes of arthritic pain.

III. Differential Diagnosis

Osteoarthritis may be difficult to differentiate from other causes of joint pain because many rheumatologic diseases lead to joint pain, stiffness, swelling, and warmth. These diseases may coexist with DJD.

A. RA—is more inflammatory that DJD and has a characteristic distribution. RA is generally polyarticular. When it involves the hand, the MCP, PIP, and wrist are involved. In osteoarthritis the DIP and PIP are commonly affected. RA has less knee involvement and more hand involvement than DJD. Morning stiffness lasts longer than 30 min. The synovial fluid is inflammatory, the ESR is elevated, and the rheumatoid factor is often positive. Osteophyte development with RA is rare.

B. Seronegative spondylarthropathy—When these diseases involve the hand they may be confused with DJD. The associated clinical findings of psoriasis, inflammatory bowel disease, ankylosing spondylitis, and Reiter's syndrome aid in the differentiation.

C. Crystal-induced arthritis—Gout typically involves the joints of the lower extremity and pseudogout involves the ankle, knee, wrist, and shoulder. Both lead to a more inflammatory process than DJD. The diagnosis is confirmed by observance of crystals in synovial fluid.

D. Infectious arthritis—Inflammatory and monoarticular infectious arthritis may need to be ruled out by examining and culturing the synovial fluid.

IV. Treatment

A. Rest

1. Resting or reducing the load on a joint may be helpful. Rest periods for 30–60 min in the morning and afternoon may be adequate. Prolonged rest can be deleterious as it may interfere with cartilage metabolism, worsen the stiffness, and cause muscle atrophy.

2. Weight-bearing joints can be unloaded by the use of a cane or walker.

B. Physical Therapy

1. Exercising and strengthening the surrounding muscles will help to improve the range of motion, maintain joint alignment, prevent muscle atrophy and avoid a sensation of gelling of the joint.

2. To minimize the stress to the joint, isometric exercises are preferable to isotonic exercises.

C. Heat

1. Heat may provide symptomatic relief of muscle spasm.

2. A warm bath, electric blanket, paraffin baths, ultrasonography, and diathermy are available modalities.

3. No one method has been proven to be more effective than another.

D. Drug Therapy
1. Nonsteroidal anti-inflammatory drugs (NSAIDs)
   a. Although NSAIDs are the most common drug used for relief of pain, recent studies have questioned their advantage over analgesics such as acetaminophen. It is unclear how much synovial inflammation leads to pain and therefore an anti-inflammatory agent may not be required. Their efficacy may, however, be independent of their anti-inflammatory activity.
   b. No single agent has been proven more effective than others.
   c. Side effects such as renal insufficiency, gastropathy, and hypertension are frequent. These complications most commonly occur in the elderly.
2. Analgesics
   a. A recent large randomized double-blind trial demonstrated acetaminophen at 1000 mg q 6 h was as effective as ibuprofen 1200–2400 mg/d during a 4-wk period, in relieving symptoms from osteoarthritis of the knee.
   b. To avoid NSAID-induced side effects, it may be reasonable to use acetaminophen initially. NSAIDs can be reserved when acetaminophen is not effective.
3. Intra-articular corticosteroids
   a. Many controlled studies have demonstrated only short-term benefits.
   b. Injections should not be given more than q 4–6 mo. More frequent injections can cause direct cartilage injury and possibly depress collagen and proteoglycan biosynthesis.
   c. The patient should be cautioned to minimize joint loading after an injection.
4. Topical agents
   a. The use of topical agents has occurred for centuries but only recently have scientific studies supported their role.
   b. Capsaicin results in the depletion of substance P, a cytokine that mediates pain. Recent studies have shown the effectiveness of capsaicin when applied to the affected area 3–4 times daily.

E. Surgery
1. Orthopedic surgical procedures may be offered to the patient who has pain or disability refractory to conservative therapy.
2. In most series, more than 90% of patients receiving joint replacement have good to excellent results in long-term follow-up.
3. Potential benefits of surgery should be weighed against known risks including infection, nerve injury, thromboembolic disease, and joint failure.
4. For knee and hip replacement the patient must be able to undergo proper deep vein thrombosis prophylaxis.

5. The patient should be instructed preoperatively about the importance of physical therapy after the operation.

F. **Patient Education**

1. The patient should be instructed that DJD is not reversible, but that pain and function of the joint can be improved.
2. Risks and benefits of each type of treatment modality should be discussed.
3. Exercise and weight loss in some cases may be helpful.

V. Indications for Referral

A. Referral to an orthopedic surgeon is indicated when medical management has failed and surgery is considered.

B. Physical and occupational therapists can be helpful in recommending types of exercise and methods to more easily perform the activities of daily living.

VI. Annotated Bibliography

Bradley JD, Brandt KD, Katz BP, Kalasinski LA, Ryan SI. Comparison of an antiinflammatory dose of ibuprofen, an analgesic dose of ibuprofen, and acetaminophen in the treatment of patients with osteoarthritis of the knee. N Engl J Med 1991;325:87–91. A randomized double-blind study showing acetaminophen's efficacy is equal to ibuprofen in the short-term treatment of DJD of the knee.

Brandt KD. Should nonsteroidal anti-inflammatory drugs be used to treat osteoarthritis? Rheum Dis Clin North Am 1993;19:29–44. A review of the role of NSAIDs in the treatment of DJD and whether analgesics should be preferentially used.

Deal CL, et al. Treatment of arthritis with topical capsaicin: a double blind trial. Clin Therap 1991;13:383–395. Trial demonstrates capsaicin utility in treating osteoarthritis.

Felson DT. Osteoarthritis. Rheum Dis Clin North Am 1990;16:499–512. General review of osteoarthritis that emphasizes epidemiology.

Moskowitz RW. Clinical and laboratory findings in osteoarthritis. In: McCarty DJ, ed. Arthritis and Allied Conditions, 11th ed. Philadelphia: Lea & Febiger;1989:1605–1630. A thorough review of osteoarthritis with many illustrations and radiographs.

Chapter 99: Evaluation of the Hot, Tender Joint

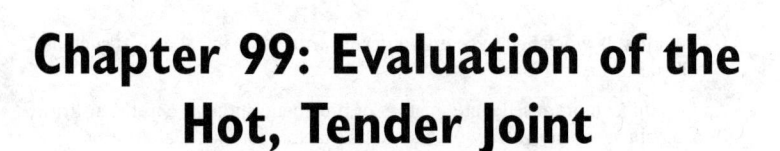

John M. Spandorfer

I. Clinical Presentation

A. General Information

1. History and physical examination vary depending on the etiology of the monoarticular arthritis.
2. Any form of polyarthritis may initially present with monoarthritis.

B. History

1. Onset of pain
   a. Extremely rapid (minutes)—suggests fracture, trauma, or loose body
   b. Hours to weeks—bacterial or crystal induced
   c. Weeks-months-years—osteoarthritis, tumor, tuberculosis, or fungal arthritis
   d. Recurrent—gout, pseudogout, and disease secondary to autoimmune cause such as rheumatoid arthritis.

2. Location—may be variable but some diseases have classic locations.
   a. Gout is common in the distal joint of lower extremity.
   b. Pseudogout is common in the knee.
   c. Bacterial arthritis often affects the large joints.
   d. Osteoarthritis frequently involves the knees and hips.

3. Age
   a. Osteoarthritis and pseudogout are more common in the elderly.
   b. Gonococcal arthritis usually occurs in the healthy and young.

4. Associated symptoms
   a. Fever can occur with any inflammatory condition but is most dramatic with bacterial arthritis.
   b. Associated back pain and stiffness is suggestive of spondylarthropathy.
   c. Recent conjunctivitis or urethritis is suggestive of Reiter's.
   d. Skin lesion of psoriasis or erythema chronicum migrans may be associated with arthritis secondary to psoriasis or Lyme disease.
   e. Morning stiffness or waxing and waning course unrelated to use of joint suggests an inflammatory cause.

f. Pain that is worsened by exertion occurs with mechanical causes such as osteoarthritis.
5. An immunocompromised state, history of prosthetic surgery, chronic arthritis, IV drug abuse, or puncture wounds are risk factors for bacterial arthritis.

C. Physical Examination
1. Check body temperature.
2. Examine the joint to differentiate between true articular swelling secondary to synovial effusion and that of a synovial proliferation or periarticular involvement. On palpation, synovial proliferation is harder than a synovial effusion. Periarticular involvement should extend beyond the normal boundaries of the joint.
3. Note crepitus, which is associated with degenerative disorders.
4. Look for joint deformity and muscular atrophy, both of which suggest chronic disease.
5. Search for skin lesions associated with infections or psoriasis. Note track marks suggestive of recent IV drug use. Look for rheumatoid nodules or tophi.
6. Examine for any source of infection that may lead to septic arthritis, such as evidence of gonococcal infection or cellulitis.

II. Diagnostic Approach

A. The examination of synovial fluid is the most helpful study. The fluid can be classified according to appearance, viscosity, cell count, presence of crystals, glucose level, and microbiologic studies. Identification of crystals is highly sensitive and 100% specific.

1. Noninflammatory synovial fluid is clear or amber colored, viscous, has a cell count < 2000, and a glucose level similar to the serum glucose level.
2. Inflammatory fluid is turbid, less viscous, glucose is normal to low, and the cell count is > 3000 with a predominance of neutrophils. The following diseases also have additional findings:
   a. Gout—Monosodium urate crystals are seen under polarized light and are needle shaped and strongly birefringent. The birefringence disappears when their long axis is parallel to polarized light.
   b. Pseudogout—Calcium pyrophosphate dihydrate crystals under polarized light are rod or rhomboid shaped and birefringent. Their birefringence extinguishes when their long axis is oblique to the axis of polarized light.
   c. Infectious arthritis—most important condition to rule out because permanent joint damage can be prevented by appropriate antibiotics
      1) Nongonococcal bacterial arthritis—Cell count is usually > 50,000. Gram stain of the synovial fluid is positive in approximately 75% of patients with staphylococcus infection and 50% with gram-negative infections. The culture will be positive in almost all patients.

2) Gonococcal arthritis—organism is usually recovered from synovial fluid if cell count is > 80,000, rarely if count is < 20,000. Overall the Gram stain of the synovial fluid is positive in 25% of patients and the culture is positive in < 50%.
3) Tuberculosis—cell count usually 5–50,000. Acid-fast bacilli are often not seen on smear of fluid but culture of fluid or synovial tissue positive in 80–90% of cases.

B. Radiographs—generally no change with acute arthritis but may serve as baseline. May show some distinguishing features such as subchondral sclerosis and spur formation (seen with osteoarthritis), chondrocalcinosis (seen with pseudogout) and fracture or neoplasm.

C. Synovial biopsy—may help in diagnosis of chronic unexplained monoarticular arthritis. TB and fungal arthritis may be diagnosed by biopsy.

D. If a systemic connective tissue disease is suspected, appropriate autoantibodies may help in the diagnosis (see Chapter 97).

III. Differential Diagnosis

Other conditions may be confused with monoarthritis.

A. Tendinitis or bursitis is usually localized to one side of the joint and worse with active range of motion. Often caused by overuse or trauma.

B. Bone pain that is secondary to fracture, primary or secondary malignancy, or sickle cell anemia. Radiographs are helpful with diagnosis.

C. Structural change of joint such as loose body, torn meniscus, or ligaments. Clicking or laxity may be noted on physical examination.

D. Soft tissue infection, such as cellulitis, myositis or abscesses, if located near a joint may be confused with arthritis. Radiographs and synovial fluid analysis are usually normal.

IV. Treatment

A. Infectious

1. Antibiotics
   a. If synovial fluid is purulent but bacteria are not seen on the smear antibiotics should be empirically started.
   b. A young, healthy, sexually active patient should be given ceftriaxone (1–2 g IV q 24 h) or cefotaxime (1–2 g IV q 8 h) for gonococcal arthritis.
   c. An elderly patient should be started on anti-staph and strep coverage as well as gram-negative coverage.

d. If Lyme arthritis is suspected ceftriaxone 2 g IV qd for 14 d, both amoxicillin and probenicid (500 mg each PO q.i.d. for 30 d) *OR* doxycycline (100 mg PO b.i.d. for 30 d) can be used.
e. The selection can be narrowed when culture results are available.

2. Drainage can be performed by closed-needle aspiration in all joints except hips. Open drainage is preferable for the infected hip or any joint that cannot be adequately drained by closed needle.

3. Over 95% of patients with gonococcal arthritis recover completely. < 50% of patients with non-gonococcal arthritis recover without significant residual joint damage.

B. Osteoarthritis (see Chapter 98)

C. Gout

1. Acute
    a. The anti-inflammatory agent colchicine is most effective if given shortly after symptoms begin. It can be given 0.5 mg PO q 2 h until one of the following occurs: the patient improves, nausea or diarrhea develop, or a maximum of 6 mg is taken without relief. If the patient is unable to take cochicine orally it may be given IV at a dose of 1 mg. which can be repeated only once in 24 h. Contraindications to IV use are a creatinine clearance of < 10 mL/min, liver disease, and bone marrow suppression.
    b. Alternatively, NSAIDs may be tried. Indomethacin, at a dose of 25–50 mg q 8 h, is the agent most commonly used.
    c. Systemic or intra-articular steroids may help if the patient is refractory to anti-inflammatory drugs.

2. Chronic—The use of a drug to lower serum urate is indicated for the patient with recurrent attacks, visible tophi, or radiographic evidence of urate deposits. Allopurinol is the drug of choice unless the patient is well managed with a uricosuric agent (probenicid, sulfinpyrazone, or salicylates in high doses). The usual dose of allopurinol is 300 mg/d.

3. Patient education—Weight loss, moderate alcohol consumption and avoidance of diet rich in purines may help.

D. Pseudogout—Anti-inflammatory drugs are the first choice. If the patient is unable to tolerate this then IV colchicine may be effective at controlling inflammation. Another method to reduce pain is to aspirate the joint and inject steroids intra-articularly.

V. Indication for Referral

A. To a rheumatologist if a monoarticular arthritis remains undiagnosed

B. To an orthopedic surgeon for open drainage when required

VI. Indication for Hospitalization

Septic arthritis requires parenteral antibiotics.

VII. Annotated Bibliography

Freed JF. Acute monoarticular arthritis: a diagnostic approach. JAMA 1980; 243:2314–2319. Reviews the prevalence of the types of monoarthritis and useful diagnostic tests.

Goldenberg DL, Reed JI. Bacterial arthritis. N Engl J Med 1985;312:764–771. Classic review of bacterial arthritis. Details pathophysiology, clinical and microbiological characteristics, diagnostic evaluation, and treatment.

McCune JW. Monoarticular arthritis. In: Kelley W, ed. Rheumatology, 3rd ed. Philadelphia: WB Saunders;1989:442–453. A thorough clinical review of monoarthritis.

Chapter 100: Joint Pain

Barry Ziring

I. General Considerations

A. General Information

1. Although usually secondary to musculoskeletal causes, joint pain can also be due to vascular or neurologic disease.
2. If pain occurs following a traumatic injury, neurovascular status distal to the injury should always be checked.
3. If more than one joint is involved, the patient may have a systemic disease.
4. Infection, neoplasm, or significant occult trauma should always be considered when there is localized bony tenderness.
5. Until a diagnosis can be made, most musculoskeletal injury can be treated with cold, compression, elevation, and immobilization.

B. History and Symptoms

1. The patient should be questioned about the duration of symptoms, precipitating, and relieving factors.
2. History of trauma or overuse
3. History of arthritis or gout
4. Does the joint lock or collapse?
5. Is the pain localized to the joint or does it appear to radiate?
6. Is the pain articular or periarticular?
   a. Articular pain usually gives pain on movement of the joint in all directions.
   b. Perarticular conditions result in pain on movement only in certain directions (Figure 100–1).
   c. If joint has pain-free range of motion and no significant tenderness, pain is usually referred from other structures.

C. Physical Examination

1. Warmth or redness implies an acute inflammatory process.

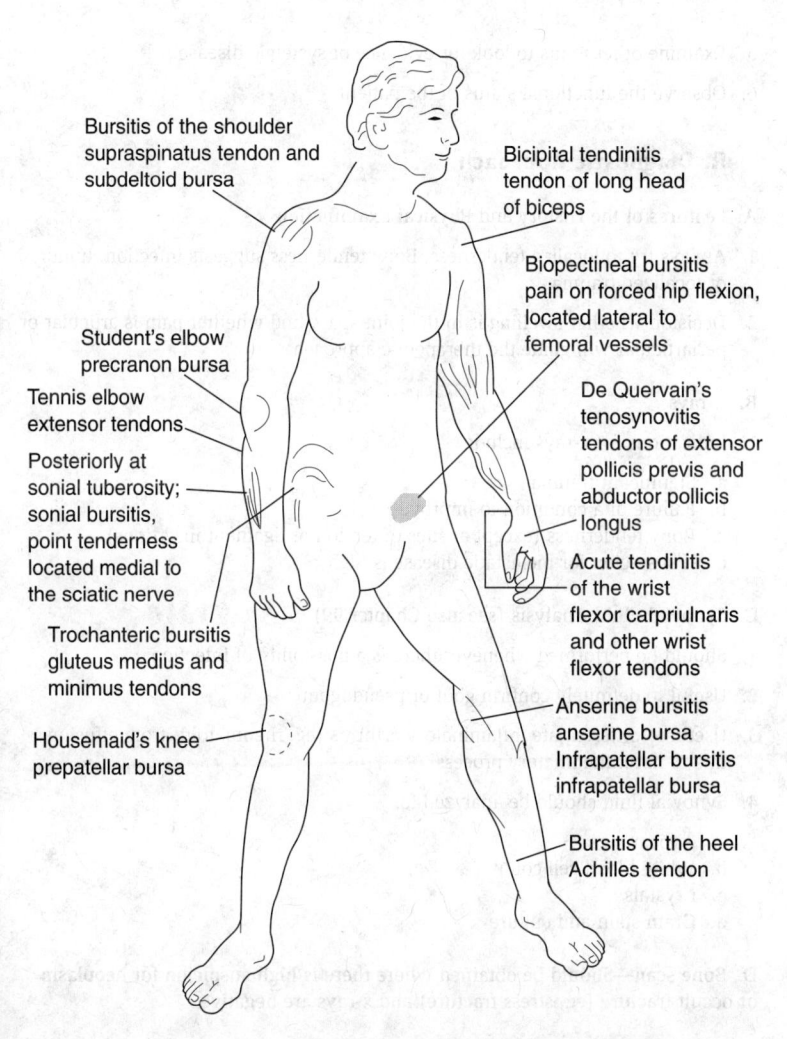

Figure 100–1. Common sites of periarticular pain. (Reproduced by permission from Branch W. Office Practice of Medicine. Philadelphia: WB Saunders; 1987.)

Labels on figure:
- Bursitis of the shoulder supraspinatus tendon and subdeltoid bursa
- Bicipital tendinitis tendon of long head of biceps
- Biopectineal bursitis pain on forced hip flexion, located lateral to femoral vessels
- Student's elbow precranon bursa
- Tennis elbow extensor tendons
- De Quervain's tenosynovitis tendons of extensor pollicis previs and abductor pollicis longus
- Posteriorly at sonial tuberosity; sonial bursitis, point tenderness located medial to the sciatic nerve
- Acute tendinitis of the wrist flexor carpriulnaris and other wrist flexor tendons
- Trochanteric bursitis gluteus medius and minimus tendons
- Anserine bursitis anserine bursa Infrapatellar bursitis infrapatellar bursa
- Housemaid's knee prepatellar bursa
- Bursitis of the heel Achilles tendon

2. Range of motion should be tested to distinguish articular from periarticular pain, as above.
3. Always check distal neurovascular examination after injury.
4. Try to differentiate swelling in joint space from soft tissue swelling.

5. Examine other joints to look for evidence of systemic disease.
6. Observe the functional status of the patient.

II. Diagnostic Approach

A. **Features of the History and Physical Examination**

1. Always try to localize tenderness. Bony tenderness suggests infection, tumor, or localized trauma.
2. Decision whether swelling is in the joint space and whether pain is articular or periarticular will guide the therapeutic approach.

B. **X-rays**

1. Indications for x-rays include
   a. Significant trauma
   b. Failure of a condition to improve
   c. Bony tenderness (except at sites of tendon or ligament insertions)
   d. If suspicion for metastatic disease is high

C. **Synovial Fluid Analysis (see also Chapter 99)**

1. Should be performed whenever there is a possibility of infection
2. Useful to definitely confirm gout or pseudogout
3. Useful to differentiate inflammatory arthritis (eg, rheumatoid) from effusion due to noninflammatory process
4. Synovial fluid should be analyzed for
   a. Appearance
   b. White blood cell count
   c. Crystals
   d. Gram stain and culture

D. **Bone scan**—Should be obtained where there is high suspicion for neoplasm or occult fracture (eg, stress fracture) and x-rays are negative.

E. **MRI**—becoming increasingly helpful for the noninvasive diagnosis of injuries to cartilage and ligaments

F. **Arthroscopy**

1. The most expensive and invasive technique for diagnosis
2. Allows definitive diagnosis and sometimes treatment

100A Ankle Pain (Figure 100A–1)

I. Traumatic Injuries

A. Sprains of Lateral, Medial, and Cruciate Ligaments

1. Soft tissue swelling is often present.
2. The joint should be tested for stability.

   a. Pull the foot forward. If the talis can move > 4 mm, rupture of the talofibular ligament is suspected.

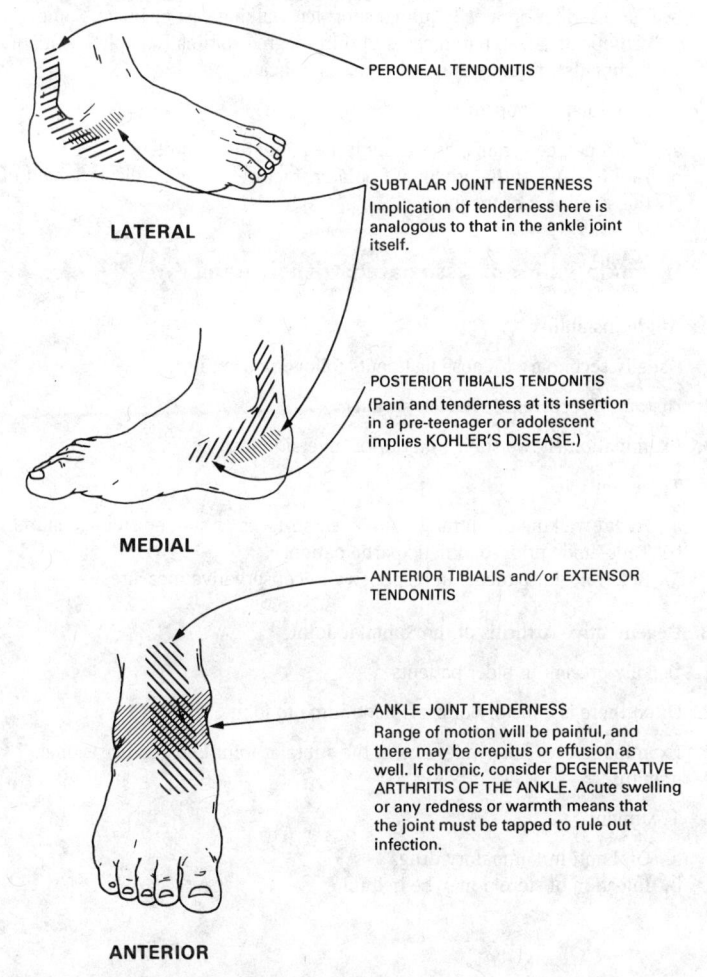

LATERAL
- PERONEAL TENDONITIS
- SUBTALAR JOINT TENDERNESS
  Implication of tenderness here is analogous to that in the ankle joint itself.

MEDIAL
- POSTERIOR TIBIALIS TENDONITIS
  (Pain and tenderness at its insertion in a pre-teenager or adolescent implies KOHLER'S DISEASE.)

ANTERIOR
- ANTERIOR TIBIALIS and/or EXTENSOR TENDONITIS
- ANKLE JOINT TENDERNESS
  Range of motion will be painful, and there may be crepitus or effusion as well. If chronic, consider DEGENERATIVE ARTHRITIS OF THE ANKLE. Acute swelling or any redness or warmth means that the joint must be tapped to rule out infection.

Figure 100A–1. Sites of tenderness: the ankle. (Reproduced by permission from Birnbaum JS. The Musculoskeletal Manual. New York: Academic Press, 1982:213.)

b. Invert the foot. The ability to tilt the foot more than 30° implies rupture of the anterior talofibular and calcaneofibular ligaments.
3. Check for tenderness over the medial aspect of the ankle (deltoid ligament).
4. Most traumatic injuries of the ankle that result in pain require x-ray to rule out an avulsion fracture (a fracture in which a small chip of bone is broken off at the insertion of a tendon or ligament). Sometimes avulsion fractures require surgical repair.
5. Treatment
   a. Minor sprains can be treated with ice, compression, and elevation. Weight-bearing should be limited with progression to walking as tolerated.
   b. More serious sprains require a short leg walking cast or brace. Some orthopedists feel that in cases of third-degree sprains (complete tears of ligaments), primary surgical repair is indicated.
6. Referral to an orthopedist
   a. Third-degree sprains, especially if the patient is an athlete
   b. Any fracture of the proximal fibula or fracture involving displacement of the structures of the joint

II. Ankle Pain not Associated with Trauma

A. Ankle Instability

1. Usually secondary to loose ligaments following a sprain
2. History of recurrent inversion sprains
3. Examination shows some anterior or inversion laxity
4. Treatment
   a. Avoid walking or running on uneven surfaces or sudden stops or starts.
   b. Tape ankle prior to athletic participation.
   5. Referral—for patients unresponsive to conservative measures.

B. Degenerative Arthritis of the Subtalar Joint

1. Usually present in older patients
2. Often there is a history of previous trauma to joint.
3. Examination reveals tenderness at the subtalar joint line and occasional crepitus.
4. Treatment
   a. Oral anti-inflammatory drugs
   b. Injection of steroid may be helpful.

C. Synovitis

1. Isolated ankle synovitis is uncommon.
2. When present, usually is secondary to degenerative arthritis, gout, sarcoid, gonococcal arthritis, or one of the spondyloarthropathes or collagen vascular diseases.
3. Signs include warmth and swelling.
4. Diagnosis is made by aspiration of the joint.

D. Uncommon causes of ankle pain and synovitis include chronic infectious arthritis (eg, TB) and tumor of the bone or joint.

E. Pain in the Achilles Tendon Area

1. Achilles tendinitis (see also Chapter 103)

    a. Pain located at the Achilles tendon insertion
    b. Due to excessive stretch from uphill walking or new shoe
    c. Treatment consists of stretching exercise, heel lift, cold compresses, and oral nonsteroidal medication.

2. Posterior calcaneal bursitis (rare)

    a. Pain over Achilles tendon
    b. Treatment is usually conservative.

100B Shoulder Pain
(Figures 100B-1 and 100B-2)

I. Traumatic or Acute Injuries

A. Dislocations (see also Chapter 103)

1. Patient usually in intense pain after

   a. Fall, injury, or seizure
   b. Holds the arm across the chest or abdomen
   c. Shoulder has squared off appearance
   d. Diagnosis is easily made for anterior dislocations on an anteroposterior film. Posterior dislocations are more difficult to diagnose.
   e. Treatment is manual reduction, which may require referral.

B. Acromioclavicular Joint Sprain

1. Usually caused by a fall

2. Tenderness over acromioclavicular joint

3. X-ray is diagnostic using a 5–10-lb weight in each hand

4. Treatment

   a. Treated with a sling until pain resolves
   b. Referral should be made for third-degree sprains involving significant displacement of the distal end of the clavicle.

C. Rotator Cuff Tear

1. Rarely occurs in patients under age 50

2. May be caused by acute trauma (throwing) or repetitive trauma and muscular and tendinous degeneration

3. Physical examination reveals complete passive range of motion, which sometimes must be done with anesthetization.

4. The patient is unable to actively abduct the arm. However, if the arm is raised to 90° the patient can continue abduction using the deltoid.

5. Treatment

   a. Partial tears are treated with rest, analgesics, and physical therapy.
   b. Complete tears often require surgical repair. Diagnosis of complete tears may require MRI or arthrography.

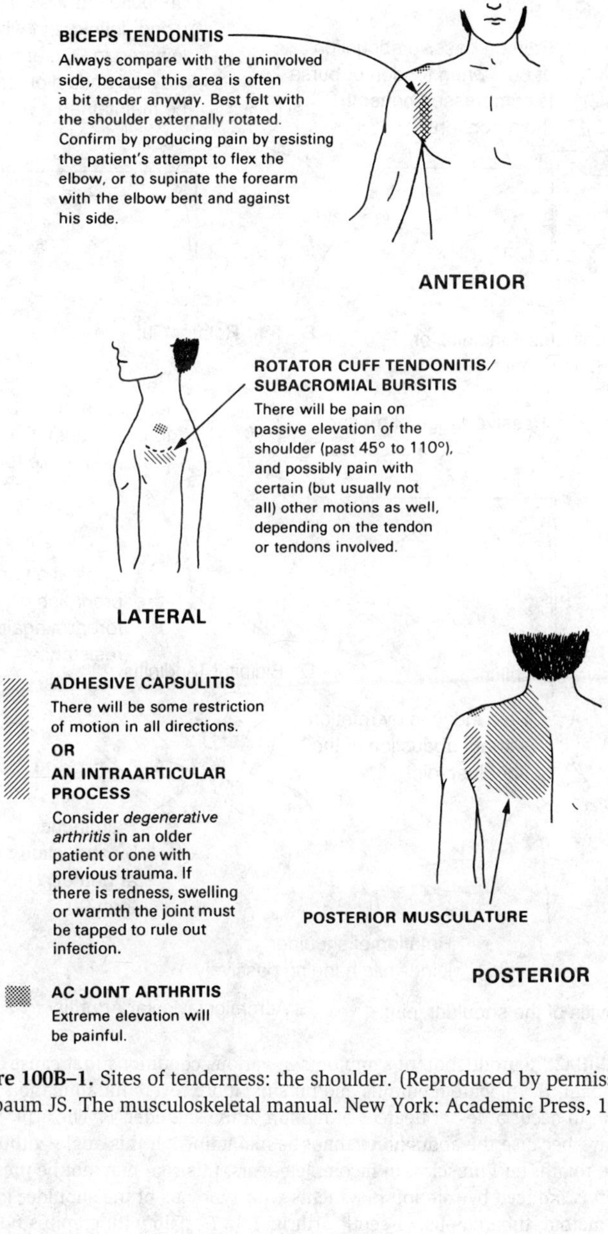

BICEPS TENDONITIS
Always compare with the uninvolved side, because this area is often a bit tender anyway. Best felt with the shoulder externally rotated. Confirm by producing pain by resisting the patient's attempt to flex the elbow, or to supinate the forearm with the elbow bent and against his side.

ANTERIOR

ROTATOR CUFF TENDONITIS/ SUBACROMIAL BURSITIS
There will be pain on passive elevation of the shoulder (past 45° to 110°), and possibly pain with certain (but usually not all) other motions as well, depending on the tendon or tendons involved.

LATERAL

ADHESIVE CAPSULITIS
There will be some restriction of motion in all directions.
OR
AN INTRAARTICULAR PROCESS
Consider *degenerative arthritis* in an older patient or one with previous trauma. If there is redness, swelling or warmth the joint must be tapped to rule out infection.

AC JOINT ARTHRITIS
Extreme elevation will be painful.

POSTERIOR MUSCULATURE

POSTERIOR

Figure 100B–1. Sites of tenderness: the shoulder. (Reproduced by permission from Birnbaum JS. The musculoskeletal manual. New York: Academic Press, 1982:72.)

A. Supraspinatus Tendinitis or Subdeltoid Bursitis — Pain on passive abduction at 60°, when tendon or bursa is compressed beneath the acromion

B. Torn Rotator Cuff — Patient can maintain abduction at > 90° by using deltoid, but when lowered to 90°, arm gives way, as abduction cannot be maintained

C. Adhesive Capsulitis — Passive range of motion is limited in all directions

D. Bicipital Tendinitis — Pain at site of biceps tendon, induced by forceful supination and pronation of the forearm. Supination and pronation of forearm against resistance

E. Synovitis of the shoulder joint. — Pain induced by rotation without abduction of the shoulder joint. Rotation of shoulder joint while hanging passively

F. Acromioclavicular Arthritis — Pain induced by abduction at greater than 90°

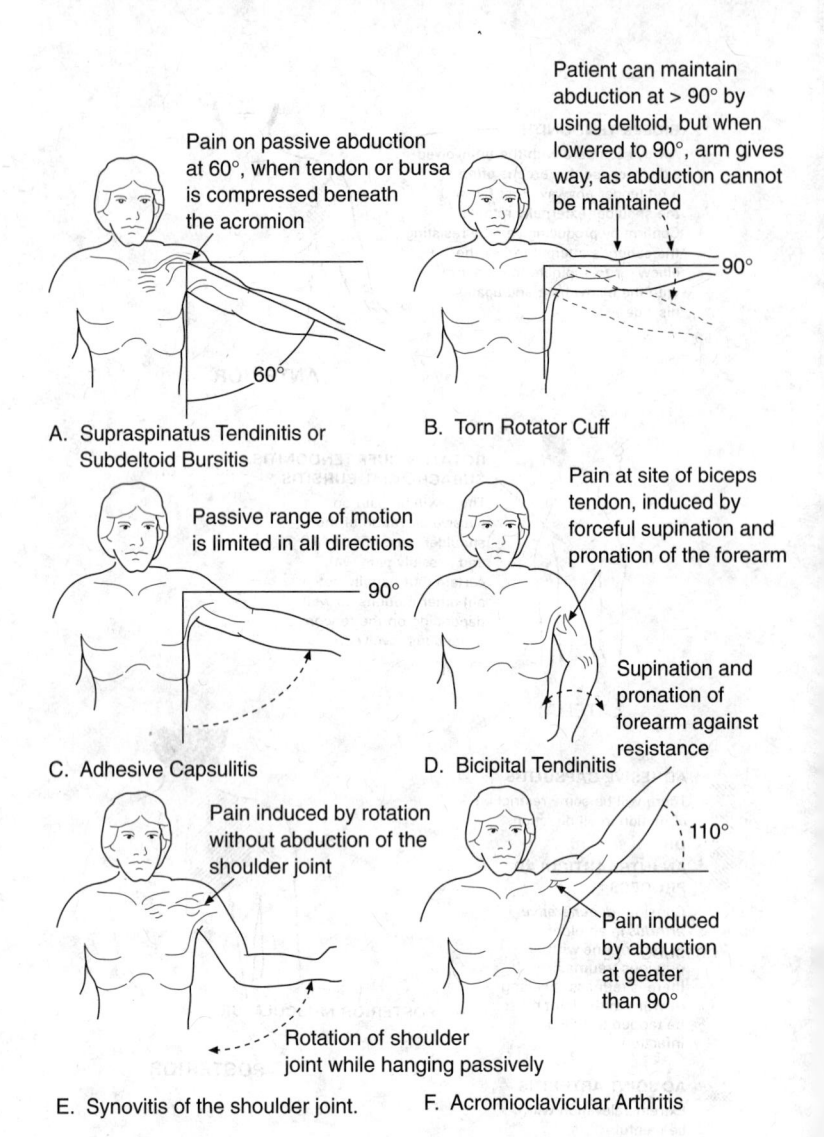

Figure 100B–2. Reproduction of symptoms in various conditions that cause shoulder pain. *A.* In acute tendinitis and bursitis, more severe inflammation can cause pain to occur at lesser degrees of motion of the shoulder. *B.* The arm "gives way" because the abduction cannot be maintained at this angle without use of the rotator cuff muscles. In incomplete tears, this sign may not be present. In *E.*, pain is induced by rotation in patients with synovitis of the shoulder joint (eg, rheumatoid, tuberculous, or septic arthritis). In *F.*, pain with crepitus noted at greater than 90° of abduction suggests the possibility of acromioclavicular arthritis. (Reproduced by permission from Branch W. Office Practice of Medicine. Philadelphia: WB Saunders; 1987.)

II. Periarticular Disorders

A. Degenerative tendonitis (pericapsulitis, subacromial bursitis, subdeltoid bursitis, supraspinatous tendonitis, bicipital tendonitis, or impingement syndrome) comprises 90% of painful disorders.

1. Pain localized along the anterior lateral aspect of the acromion
2. Secondary functional impairment
3. Pain increases with elevation of the shoulder (especially between 60° and 90°)
4. Diagnosis of bicipital tendonitis is made by demonstrating tenderness when rolling the biceps tendon beneath the fingers as it passes from within the joint down the biceps groove or when pressing at the insertion of the supraspinatous.
5. X-rays usually are normal in early stages.
6. Treatment
    a. Nonsteroidal anti-inflammatory drugs (NSAIDs)
    b. Physical therapy (Figure 100B-3)
    c. Local injection of steroids
    d. Avoid immobilization for more than 24 h.
    e. After initial immobilization, exercise should include bending at the waist, hanging the shoulder in forward flexion, and drawing circles with the hand. Also lying on the back, holding a stick in both hands, and lifting the stick overhead.

B. Adhesive Capsulitis (Frozen Shoulder)

1. Progressive limitation of motion associated with generalized pain in shoulder
2. Usually over age 50, women more frequently
3. Unclear whether limitation of motion is due to lack of motion secondary to a preexisting painful condition or whether there is idiopathic capsular inflammation
4. Treatment—usually NSAIDs, steroid injections, and long-term physical therapy. Occasionally, manipulation under anesthesia is required.

III. Intra-articular Disorders

A. Rheumatoid arthritis—most common inflammatory disease of shoulder

B. Systemic lupus erythematosus and gout can affect shoulder.

C. Osteoarthritis—rare unless there is preexisting damage or trauma.

D. Infections rare in shoulder

E. Osteonecrosis of the humeral head most commonly follows fracture, steroid treatment, alcohol use, or is secondary to hemoglobinopathy.

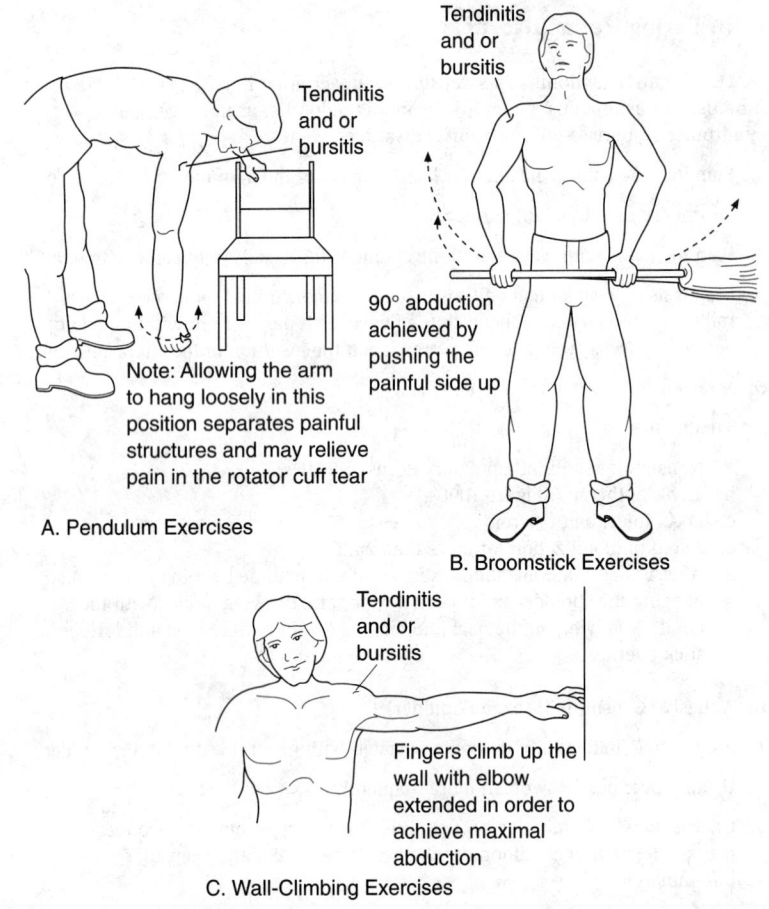

Figure 100B–3. Active range-of-motion exercises for patients with tendinitis or bursitis of the shoulder. *A.* Pendulum exercises. The patient relaxes by leaning and supporting his weight on a chair. This allows the affected arm to hang freely. If a tear of the rotator cuff is present, this may relieve discomfort. For performing exercises, with the arm hanging freely, a pendulum motion is initiated by moving the body and can be gradually increased to extend the range of motion, first for flexion-extension and later for abduction-adduction. This is the least painful exercise to perform when acute tendinitis is present. *B.* Broomstick exercises. The patient holds the broomstick in front of the body and initiates motion by pushing upward with the nonpainful arm. This motion can be repeated in a backward and forward manner. By pushing with the unaffected arm, one can achieve more abduction of the affected shoulder. *C.* Wall-climbing exercises. The patient stands next to the wall and "walks up the wall with his fingers." If the elbow is extended and the patient moves at the shoulder joint rather than by shrugging, significant abduction can be achieved. (Reproduced by permission from Branch W. Office Practice of Medicine. Philadelphia: WB Saunders; 1987.)

IV. Other Causes of Shoulder Pain

A. Neurologic

1. Cervical radiculopathy (usually neck and suprascapular area)
2. Brachial plexopathy
3. Nerve entrapment syndrome
4. Reflex sympathetic dystrophy

B. Referred visceral pain

1. Coronary ischemia
2. Pulmonary infarction
3. Pancoast tumor
4. Gallbladder disease (scapular pain)
5. Intraabdominal condition (often at trapezius)

100C Knee Pain

I. General History

A. Swelling that occurs immediately after injury. Is usually associated with ligament tear. Swelling that occurs hours later is usually due to an intra-articular lesion such as meniscus tear.

B. Is there warmth or redness?

C. Does the knee lock? Often secondary to meniscus tear

D. Does the knee collapse? Consider ligamentory instability, torn meniscus, loose body, or dislocating patella.

E. Is there a grinding or grating sensation? Common in degenerative arthritis

II. General Examination (Figure 100C–1)

A. Check for effusion (see below).

B. Check for warmth or redness.

C. Examine and document range of motion.

D. Check for sites of tenderness.

E. Check medial and lateral stability with knee flexed and straight.

F. Press patella down into femur and move it proximally and distally.

G. Pull lower leg forward and backward against thigh with knee flexed (anterior and posterior drawer test).

H. Have patient do a deep knee bend. Ability to do this without difficulty makes meniscal problems unlikely.

III. Knee Swelling (Figure 100C–2)

A. Knee Effusion

1. There is usually swelling of the *entire* joint.

2. Pain and stiffness on active or passive movement

3. Relatively large amounts of fluid may be detected by ballottement of the patella.

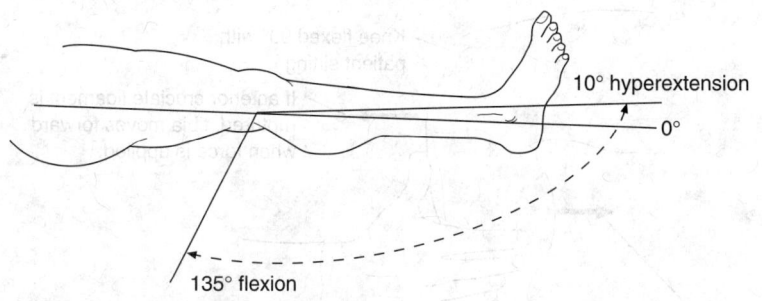

A. Normal range of motion of the knee joint

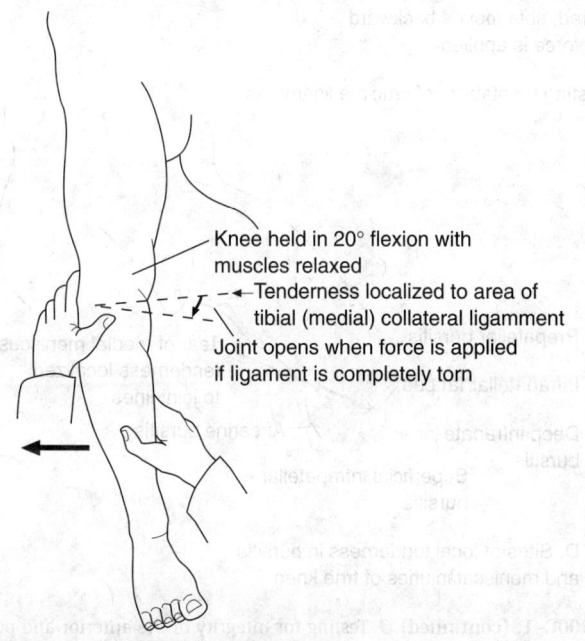

A. Normal range of motion of the knee joint

Figure 100C-1. Clinical examination of the knee joint. *A.* Following inspection, palpation of the suprapatellar pouch, and ballotement of the patella to detect joint effusion, the range of motion of the joint should be tested while one palpates for crepitus during motion. *B.* The stability of the tibial (medial) collateral and fibular (lateral) collateral ligaments should be tested with the knee held in 20 degrees of flexion. Force is applied, and if the ligaments are intact, even though sprained, pain but not instability results. Complete ligamentous tear results in instability of the joint as illustrated in the figure.

(continued)

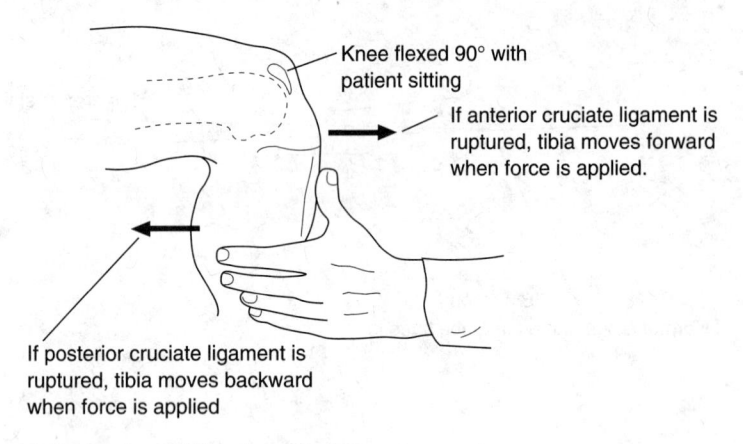

810 • Manual of Office Medicine

Knee flexed 90° with patient sitting

If anterior cruciate ligament is ruptured, tibia moves forward when force is applied.

If posterior cruciate ligament is ruptured, tibia moves backward when force is applied

C. Testing for stability of cruciate ligaments

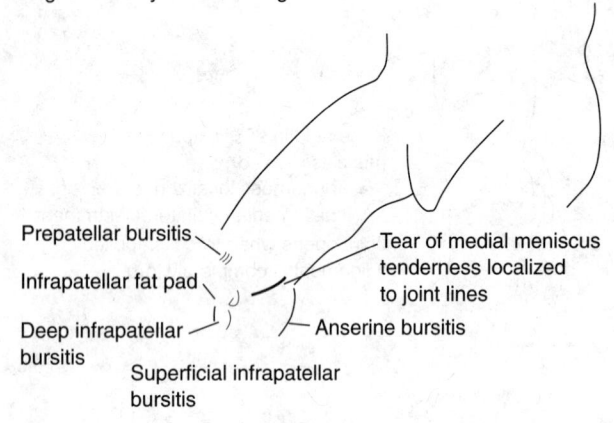

Prepatellar bursitis
Infrapatellar fat pad
Deep infrapatellar bursitis
Superficial infrapatellar bursitis
Tear of medial meniscus tenderness localized to joint lines
Anserine bursitis

D. Sites of local tenderness in bursitis and meniscal injuries of trhe knee

Figure 100C–1. (continued) *C.* Testing for integrity of the anterior and posterior cruciate ligaments is accomplished with the patient sitting and the knee flexed at 90 degrees. The examiner applies pressure in the posterior direction to detect abnormal movement of the joint, which is present in complete tear of the posterior cruciate ligament, and applies force in the anterior direction to detect abnormal movement of the joint and complete tear of the anterior cruciate ligament. *D.* Sites of local tenderness in bursitis and meniscal injuries of the knee. In bursitis, tenderness is localized (as shown) to the area of the prepatellar, superficial or deep infrapatellar, or anserine bursa. The infrapatellar fat pad may also be the site of tenderness following trauma. Tear of the medial meniscus results in tenderness localized to the tibial joint line. Likewise, tenderness is localized laterally in sprain or tear of the lateral meniscus, but this injury is less common than injury of the medial meniscus. (Reproduced by permission from Branch W. Office Practice of Medicine. Philadelphia: WB Saunders; 1987.)

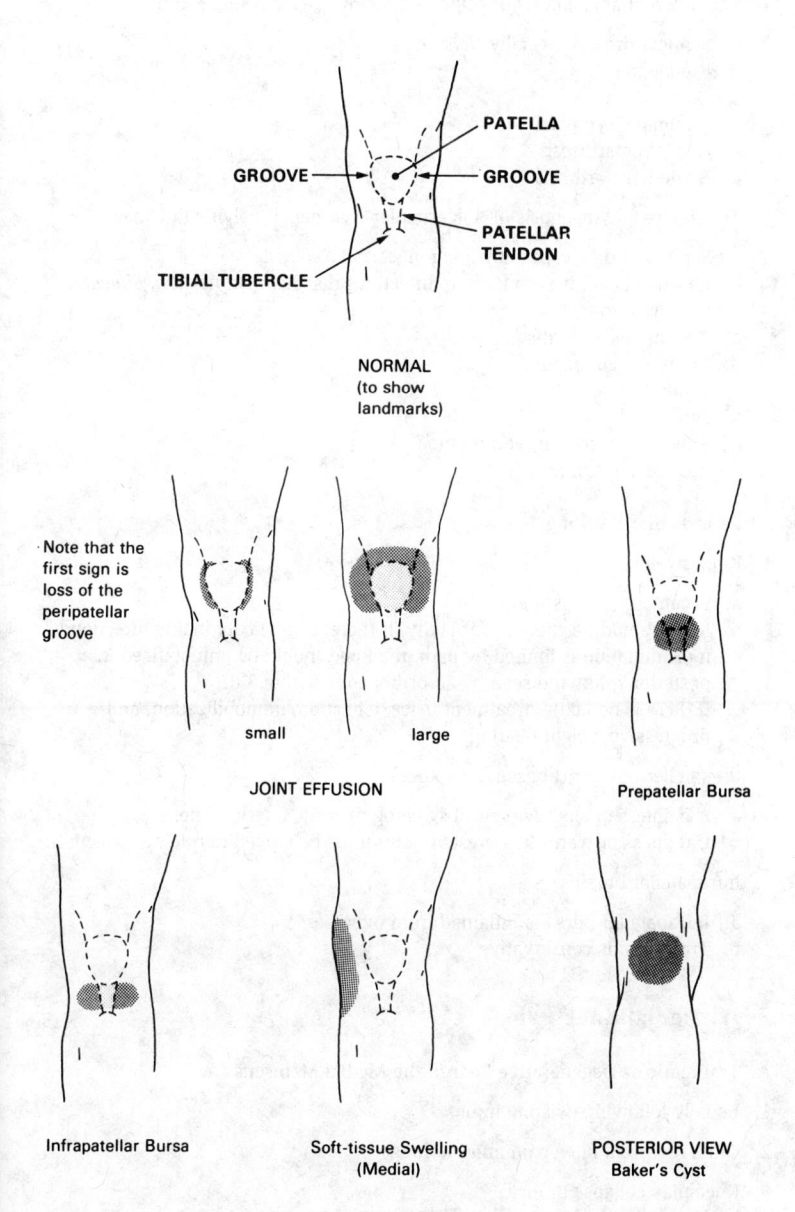

Figure 100C–2. Knee swelling. (Reproduced by permission from Birnbaum JS. The musculoskeletal manual. New York: Academic Press, 1982:180.)

4. The differential diagnosis of acute effusion involving a single joint

   a. Septic arthritis especially *Neisseria*
   b. Pseudogout
   c. Gout
   d. Traumatic synovitis
   e. Acute hemarthrosis
   f. Acute lyme arthritis

5. The differential diagnosis of polyarticular disorders involving the knee

   a. Septic arthritis, especially nongonococcal *Neisseria*.
   b. Reactive arthritis secondary to infectious diarrhea (*Salmonella, Shigella, Campylobacter*).
   c. Rheumatoid arthritis
   d. Gout or pseudogout
   e. Lyme disease
   f. Serum sickness
   g. Rubella, hepatitis B, and mumps
   h. Reiter's syndrome

B. Periarticular Swelling

1. Knee swelling

   a. Secondary to twisting injury
   b. Knee should be checked for laxity. If there is any laxity in any direction or if examination is limited by pain, the knee should be immobilized in a posterior splint and seen by an orthopedist within 3 d.
   c. If there is no laxity, treatment is ice, elevation, immobilization, and progressive weight-bearing.

2. Prepateller bursitis (housemaid's knee)

   a. A painless or slightly painful swelling over the inferior patella
   b. If redness or warmth is present, joint must be tapped to rule out infection.

3. Infrapatellar bursitis

   a. Infrapatellar bursa is inflamed from overuse.
   b. Treatment is conservative.

IV. Medial Knee Pain

A. Traumatic or Degenerative Tear of the Medial Meniscus

1. Usually following twisting injury

2. Often recurrent knee pain and swelling

3. Knee may collapse or lock.

4. Warmth, swelling, and tenderness sometimes localized to medial joint line

5. Diagnosis confirmed by MRI

6. Treatment may require arthroscopy.
7. Quadriceps strengthening exercises should be used to avoid atrophy.

B. Anserine tendonitis or bursitis—pain, local tenderness, and swelling over the anteromedial pattern of the upper tibia below the joint line.

C. Semimembranous Tendonitis

1. Aching pain over the posteromedial aspect of the knee provoked by walking, bending, lifting, climbing, or running.
2. More common in distance runners
3. Bone scan might demonstrate increased uptake at the site of insertion of the tendon on the tibia.

V. Lateral Knee Pain

A. Lateral Meniscus Tear

1. Secondary to twisting injury
2. Local tenderness over lateral joint line
3. MRI or arthroscopy may be diagnostic.

B. Lateral Collateral Ligament Tear

1. Usually secondary to fall in forward direction with lower leg internally rotated
2. Local tenderness over ligament
3. Flexion and internal rotation of knee can allow detection of tender ligament defect.

VI. Anterior Knee Pain

A. Chondromalacia Patellae

1. Common aching pain especially when going up or down stairs
2. Sometimes a grating sensation
3. Stiffness after immobility
4. Especially in young women
5. Developed due to irregularity or roughness of cartilage under patella
6. Pain and crepitus on pressing the patella and moving it proximally and distally
7. Treatment consists of conservative measures, quadriceps strengthening exercise, and occasionally surgery.

B. Patellar tendonitis ("jumper's knee")—anterior knee pain in athletes after jumping, climbing, or kicking

C. Quadriceps Tendon Rupture

1. Patient unable to extend the joint
2. Aching pain and soreness in region of proximal patella
3. X-ray may show avulsed bone.

VII. Posterior Knee Pain

A. Baker's Cyst

1. A painless or slightly painful swelling in popliteal space
2. Cystic
3. Cyst can rupture leading to swollen calf, which can resemble deep venous thrombosis.
4. Treatment consists of treatment of underlying knee problem.

B. Popliteal artery aneurysm—Rupture can occur causing posterior knee pain and popliteal hematoma.

I. Degenerative Arthritis

A. Uncommon limited to wrist

B. Common site of polyarticular disease

C. Degenerative arthritis of thumb is common.

D. Treatment consists of rest, NSAIDs.

E. Steroid injection of carpometacarpal joint is usually helpful.

II. De Quervain's Tenosynovitis

A. Tenderness proximal to anatomic "snuff box."

B. Pain can be reproduced by active abduction and hyperextension of thumb.

C. Pain also reproduced if the patient puts thumb inside curled fingers and the examiner pushes wrist to ulnar side.

D. Treatment consists of rest, wrist splint, and NSAIDs. Injection also helpful.

100D Wrist Pain (Figures 100D–1 and 100D–2)

THE "SNUFF BOX"
The patient may have an unsuspected *navicular fracture*. A negative X ray (including a navicular view) will rule out this possibility if the trauma was more than two weeks previous; but if more recent or not sure, referral is wise.

DE QUERVAIN'S TENDONITIS
There will be much pain if the patient puts his thumb inside his curled fingers and you move the wrist toward the ulnar side (Finkelstein's test).

DEGENERATIVE ARTHRITIS OF THE FIRST CARPAL-METACARPAL JOINT
Passive motion of this joint will give pain and/or crepitus.

EXTENSOR TENDONITIS

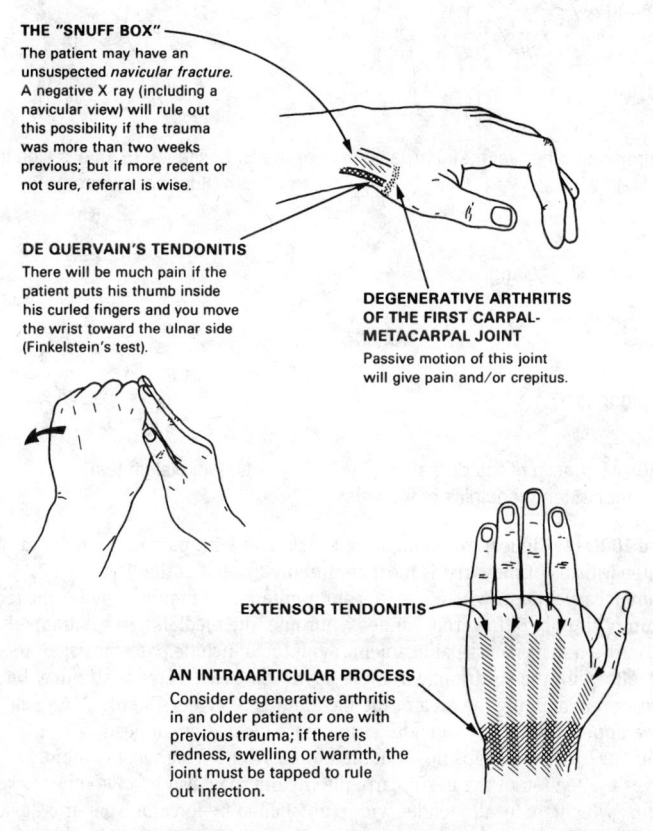

AN INTRAARTICULAR PROCESS
Consider degenerative arthritis in an older patient or one with previous trauma; if there is redness, swelling or warmth, the joint must be tapped to rule out infection.

Figure 100D–1. Sites of tenderness: the wrist. (Reproduced by permission from Birnbaum JS. The musculoskeletal manual. New York: Academic Press, 1982:94.)

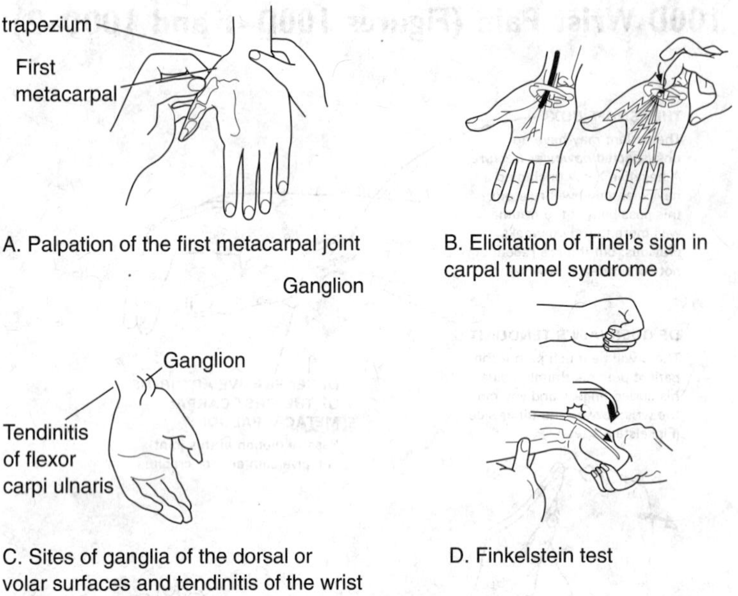

A. Palpation of the first metacarpal joint

B. Elicitation of Tinel's sign in carpal tunnel syndrome

C. Sites of ganglia of the dorsal or volar surfaces and tendinitis of the wrist

D. Finkelstein test

Figure 100D–2. Clinical examination of the patient with pain in the wrist or hand. *A.* Osteoarthritis of the wrist is most commonly located at the first carpometacarpal joint, where crepitus and limitation of motion may be elicited on rotation of thumb. *B.* In carpal tunnel syndrome, the median nerve is trapped beneath the transverse carpal ligament. Symptoms include paresthesias of the first four digits, with thenar atrophy in more advanced cases. Paresthesias may be reproduced by tapping the area of the median nerve (Tinel's sign). *C.* A ganglion may be appreciated as a nontender cystic mass located in connection with a tendon sheath or joint capsule. Acute tendinitis of the wrist most commonly involves the tendon of the flexor carpi ulnaris but may also involve other flexor tendons, which are locally tender with pain elicited by forceful isometric flexion of the wrist. *D.* De Quervain's tenosynovitis refers to inflammation of the extensor pollicis brevis and abductor pollicis longus near the first carpometacarpal joint; in tenosynovitis, pain is reproduced by palpating the tendon or with the Finkelstein test. *(Adapted from Hoppenfeld S, Physical Examiniation of the Spine and Extremities. East Norwalk, CT: Appleton-Century-Crofts, 1976.)*

III. Wrist Synovitis

A. May result from rheumatoid arthritis, gout, pseudogout, sepsis, tuberculosis.

B. Joint aspiration is diagnostic.

IV. Carpal Tunnel Syndrome (see Chapter 72)

A. Pain felt in first three fingers and radial side of hand

B. Paresthesias and numbness

C. Secondary to repetitive overuse

D. Decreased sensation in medial nerve distribution

E. Check for atrophy of thenar eminence.

F. More common with diabetes, rheumatoid arthritis, thyroid disease, and pregnancy

G. Tapping the middle of the underside of the wrist may produce distal paresthesias.

H. Nerve conduction studies are confirmatory.

I. Treatment (see Chapter 72)

V. Ganglion

A. Usually painless

B. Cystic structure connected to joint space or tendon

C. Usually no treatment necessary

VI. Annotated Bibliography

Bateman JE. The Shoulder and Neck, 2d ed. Philadelphia: WB Saunders; 1978. A complete text devoted to management of shoulder problems.

Birnbaum JS. The Musculoskeletal Manual. New York: Academic Press; 1982. A thorough text covering most common musculoskeletal complaints. The text is designed for primary care practitioners.

Branch WT. Pain in the shoulder, neck and arm. In: Branch WT ed. Office Practice of Medicine. Philadelphia: WB Saunders; 1987.

Liang MH, Hartley RM. Elbow, hand, knee, and foot pain. In: Branch WT, ed. Office Practice of Medicine. Philadelphia: WB Saunders; 1987. These two chapters are a good review of common orthopedic complaints.

Rothenberg MH, Graf BK. Evaluation of knee injuries. Postgrad Med 1993;93:75–86.

Swain RA, Holt WS. Ankle injuries. Postgrad Med 1993;93:91–100. Two recent articles for the primary care practitioner regarding knee and ankle injuries.

Chapter 101: Neck and Back Pain

Ellen M. O'Connor

101A Cervical Pain Syndromes

I. Clinical Presentation

A. General Information

1. Cervical disk injuries and degenerative changes usually happen at approximately the C-5–6, C-6–7 levels.
2. Ligament and nerve root damage are more likely to occur if neck is rotated at the time of injury.
3. Herniated cervical disks rarely cause nerve root compression.
4. There is minimal correlation between radiographic arthritic changes and degree of neck pain.
5. Persistent pressure on a nerve root > 3 mo duration may result in permanent damage even after surgical repair.

B. Symptoms

1. Pain
   a. Onset
      1) Gradual—typical in osteoarthritis
      2) Delayed—seen often in whiplash injury
      3) Acute—usually muscular caused by identifiable injury
   b. Location
      1) Posterior triangle of neck—seen with muscular injury
      2) Interscapular area—associated with poor posture
      3) Occipital region—may reflect stress
      4) Shoulder—may be referred from neck
   c. Radiation
      1) Lateral aspect of arm (C-8–T-1)
      2) Radial aspect of forearm (C-5–6, C-6–7)
      3) Thumb (C-6–7)
      4) Middle finger/anterior chest wall (C-7)
      5) Fifth finger (C-8, T-1)

d. Aggravating factors
   1) Cervical disk disease—sneezing, coughing
   2) Acute cervical myalgia—movements stretching affected muscles
2. Neurologic symptoms
   a. Decreased strength
      1) C-5—arm abduction, external arm rotation
      2) C-6—elbow flexion, forearm supination
      3) C-7—elbow extension, wrist and forearm pronation, extension of thumb distal phalanx
      4) C-8—abduction and adduction of fingers
   b. Paresthesias
      1) C-6—thumb
      2) C-7—middle finger
      3) C-8–T-1—fifth finger
3. Associated symptoms secondary to sympathetic chain and brain stem injury
   a. Tinnitus
   b. Vertigo
   c. Blurred vision
   d. Palpitations
   e. Near syncope

C. Physical Examination

1. Visualization
   a. Full inspection of neck, thorax, upper extremities
   b. Observation of posture
2. Palpation
   a. Determination of focal tenderness
   b. Check for shoulder joint tenderness
   c. Assess thyroid size, presence of tenderness
3. Active and passive range of motion
   a. Neck
      1) Flexion and extension
      2) Left and right rotation
      3) Left and right lateral flexion
   b. Shoulder
      1) Adduction and abduction
      2) Internal and external rotation
4. Strength testing
   a. Upper extremities
   b. Lower extremities
5. Neurologic testing
   a. Upper and lower extremity reflexes
   b. Upper and lower extremity sensory testing

6. Miscellaneous
   a. Adson test—reproduction of symptoms and obliteration of the radial pulse when patient turns head to side of affected extremity, abducts the arm then takes and holds a deep breath
   b. Babinski sign—dorsiflexion of the big toe possibly associated with dorsiflexion and fanning of other toes and dorsiflexion of the foot when noxious stimulus applied to the plantar surface of the foot

II. Diagnostic Approach

A. Most episodes of neck pain are self-limited or resolve after short course of conservative therapy. Radiographic and laboratory tests are not indicated unless conservative therapy has failed or if clinical suspicions point to more serious diagnosis.

B. Radiographic Test

1. Cervical films
   a. Views
      1) Anteroposterior
      2) Oblique
      3) Open mouth (in trauma)
      4) Flexion–extension lateral (in trauma)
   b. Indications
      1) Severe cervical sprain
      2) Severity/presence of trauma
      3) Neurologic deficit
      4) Unresolved pain after 4 wk conservative therapy
   c. Disadvantages
      1) Variance in interpretation
      2) Least useful in disk pathology

2. CT scan
   a. Advantages
      1) Excellent for bone pathology
      2) Good for disk abnormalities
   b. Disadvantages—localization of level should be determined before testing

3. MRI
   a. Advantages
      1) Excellent at demonstrating presence/severity of disk disease and spinal stenosis
      2) Good for bone pathology
      3) Demonstrates entire cervical spine
   b. Disadvantages—Findings must be related strictly to clinical setting due to frequency of asymptomatic pathology

4. Myelogram

    a. Indications—not indicated in neck pain due to many disadvantages
    b. Disadvantages
        1) Many asymptomatic protrusions found
        2) Neck position alters findings.
        3) Level of dye does not always reach level to be assessed.
        4) Invasive procedure

5. Bone scan

    a. Indications—extremely useful in evaluation of tumors, infection, or trauma

C. Laboratory Tests

1. Complete blood count—sensitive in detecting infection or occult malignancy in appropriate clinical setting

2. Erythrocyte sedimentation rate—helpful in collagen vascular disorder, tumors, rheumatoid arthritis, polymyalgia rheumatica

3. Creatinine phosphokinase—assists in setting where polymyalgia rheumatica, collagen vascular disorder, dermatomyositis, polymyositis are considered

D. Neurologic Testing

1. Electromyography

    a. Can localize nerve root damage
    b. Differentiates between nerve root and brachial plexus injury
    c. May be normal for up to 3 wk after acute injury
    d. Indicated for presurgical evaluation of nerve impingement

2. Somatosensory evoked potential

    a. Helpful in diagnosis of radiculopathy
    b. May show abnormal conduction earlier than nerve conduction velocity

III. Differential Diagnosis

A. Mechanical Problems

1. Traumatic

    a. Vertebral fracture
    b. Muscular strain—stretch injury to muscles alone
    c. Musculoligamentous sprain—stretch injury to muscles, deep fascia, and ligamentum nuchae
    d. Disk injury

2. Atraumatic

    a. Acute cervical myalgia
    b. Disk pathology—herniation, bulge, annular cyst

c. Degenerative changes—spondylosis with osteophytosis
   d. Space-occupying lesions
   e. Spinal stenosis

B. **Systemic Disease**

1. Osteomyelitis
2. Metastatic cancer
3. Multiple myeloma
4. Inflammatory spondyloarthropethies
5. Osteoporosis with compression fracture

C. **Locally Referred Pain**

1. Compression syndromes
   a. Scalene anticus syndrome—clumsy movement of arm/hand with dull/deep ache, positive Adson test
   b. Claviculocostal syndrome—clumsy movement of arm/hand with dull/deep ache, negative Adson test
   c. Pectoralis minor syndrome—clumsy movement of arm/hand with dull/deep ache, negative Adson test
2. Scapulocostal syndrome—interscapular pain secondary to round back posture
3. Pericapsulitis shoulder pain—supraspinatus tendonitis causing painful arm abduction or rotator cuff tear causing inability to abduct arm

D. **Miscellaneous Causes**

1. Angina pectoris
2. Meningitis
3. Thyroiditis
4. Lymphadenopathy
5. Apical carcinoma of the lung

IV. Treatment

A. **Acute Management**

1. Minor muscular or ligamentous strain is usually self-limited.
2. Pain control
   a. Antiinflammatory drugs beneficial
   b. Muscle relaxants helpful through general sedation
   c. Narcotics discouraged unless severe pain

3. Local care

    a. Ice 15 min q.i.d.
    b. Gentle massage
    c. Heat after 48 h

4. Immobilization

    a. Soft collar
       1) Helpful in severe sprain, disk injury
       2) Not to be worn > 4 wk
    b. Hard collar—indicated for instability pending further evaluation

5. Traction

    a. Indications
       1) Cervical spondylosis with severe pain
       2) Disk herniation with radiculitis
       3) Neck pain unresponsive to 6 wk conservative therapy

6. Exercises

    a. Indications
       1) Mild strain after 3 days
       2) Severe sprain after 1 week immobilization
       3) Unstable injury if done with collar in place
    b. Types
       1) Neck strengthening
          a) *Patient pushes with hand against forehead resisting movement with neck muscles while keeping head level.*
          b) *Patient pushes with hand against temple resisting movement with neck muscles while keeping head level and chin in. Repeat on opposite side.*
       2) Posture improvement
          a) *Half squats against wall with head back, chin in, low back against wall, heels flat*
          b) *Shoulder rotation moving both shoulders up, back, down, and front slowly*
          c) *Holding 2–5-lb weight on top of head for 5 min with head level*
       3) Flexibility—patient moves head in all directions of range of motion and holds to stretch.

V. Patient Education

A. Advise patient most episodes of neck pain are not medically serious.

B. Regular exercise routine improves flexibility.

C. Rest includes avoidance of excessive driving, stressful situations, and prolonged computer work.

VI. Indications for Referral to Orthopedist, Neurosurgeon, or Neurologist

A. Persistent radicular symptoms in disk disease

B. Long tract signs

C. Unstable fracture or subluxation as seen on plain films

VII. Annotated Bibliography

Cailliet R. Neck and Arm Pain, 2nd ed. Philadelphia: FA Davis; 1981. A concise book of anatomy and pathophysiology related to the clinical setting.

Dvorak J, Janssen B, Grob D. The neurologic workup in patients with cervical spine disorders. Spine 1990; 15(10):1017–1022.

LaBan M. "Whiplash": its evaluation and treatment. In: Physical Medicine and Rehabilitation: State of the Art Reviews. 1990; 4(2):293–307. A thorough review on the subject.

MacNab I. Degenerative disorders. In: The Cervical Spine Research Society Editorial Committee. The Cervical Spine 2nd ed. Philadelphia: JB Lippincott; 1989:599–616. Short summary of the differential diagnosis of neck pain including useful algorithms.

Naylor J, Mulley G. Surgical collars: a survey of their prescription and use. Br J Rheum 1991;30:282–284.

Ramamurti CP. The wry neck. In: Tinker RV, ed. Orthopedics in Primary Care. Baltimore: Williams & Wilkins;1982:1–13. Excellent chapter on "The Wry Neck" for the nonorthopedist.

101B Low Back Pain

I. Clinical Presentation

A. General Information

1. 80% of Americans will experience back pain in their lifetimes.
2. L-4–5 is the most susceptible disk space.

B. Symptoms

1. Pain
    a. Location
        1) Lumbar area—most common
        2) Hip—may reflect sciatica
        3) Leg—Dermatomal pattern points to nerve root involved.
    b. Quality
        1) Dull ache suggests inflammation of ligaments, muscle, or joint capsule.
        2) Sharp, burning pain indicates radiculopathy.
    c. Radiation patterns
        1) Anterior thigh to lower leg (L-3–4)
        2) Down posterior leg (L-5–S-1)
        3) Into buttocks (L-3–4, L-4–5, L-5–S-1)
    d. Aggravating factors
        1) Standing (degenerative disease)
        2) Supine position (space-occupying lesions)
        3) Walking (spinal stenosis)
        4) Sitting (disk disease)
2. Neurologic deficits
    a. Decreased strength
        1) L-3–4—knee extensors
        2) L-4–5—ankle dorsiflexors, great toe extensors
        3) L-5–S-1—ankle plantar flexor
    b. Numbness or tingling
    c. Incontinence or urinary retention suggests sacral root compression.

C. Physical Examination

1. Observation
    a. Gait
    b. Posture
    c. Spinal malalignment
    d. Atrophy of lower extremity muscles

2. Palpation
    a. Focal tenderness
    b. Flank tenderness
3. Range of motion
    a. Back
    b. Hip
4. Nerve root compression testing
    a. Straight leg lift
        1) With patient in recumbent position and knee fully extended, each leg is raised to 90°, if possible.
        2) Degree at which pain is reproduced or worsened is noted. Positive test is pain between 30°–60°, which indicates a problem in lower lumbar spine.
    b. Femoral nerve stretch test
        1) With patient in prone position, leg is bent at knee to 90°. Leg is lifted by ankle.
        2) Pain increase or reproduction means nerve root compression at upper lumbar spine.
5. Strength testing
6. Neurologic testing
    a. Pin prick
    b. Light touch
    c. Babinski

II. Diagnostic Approach

A. Lumbosacral plain films not recommended prior to 4 wk of conservative therapy unless:

Patient's age > 50
Significant trauma
Neuromotor deficits
Systemic symptoms
Drug/alcohol abuse history
Cancer history
Chronic steroid use
Possibility of hereditary condition

1. Interpretation—variations common
2. Problems
    a. Large dose of radiation to pelvic area
    b. Many radiographic abnormalities present in asymptomatic people

B. Laboratory Tests

1. Erythrocyte sedimentation rate—sensitive in detecting cancer or infection in appropriate clinical setting

2. Complete blood count—helpful in detecting occult malignancy or infection

C. CT Scan
1. Indicated for degenerative joint disease
2. Good for disk pathology

D. MRI Scan
1. Excellent at demonstrating disk disease and spinal stenosis
2. Most costly
3. Gadolinium enhancement indicated for "failed back syndrome" only
4. Asymptomatic pathology frequently seen

E. Myelogram
1. 95% accurate for disk disease
2. Invasive procedure usually reserved for surgical candidates

F. Bone Scan—helpful to rule out inflammatory, neoplastic or traumatic problems

G. Electromyography
1. Diagnostic of radiculopathy
2. Positive results may be permanent even after recovery

III. Differential Diagnosis

A. Mechanical Problems
1. Disk pathology
2. Degenerative changes
3. Spinal stenosis
4. Spondylolisthesis

B. Systemic Disease
1. Metastatic disease
2. Multiple myeloma
3. Osteomyelitis
4. Inflammatory spondyloarthropathies
5. Osteoporosis

C. Miscellaneous Visceral Problems
1. Dissecting aortic aneurysm

2. Prostatitis
3. Nephrolithiasis
4. Pancreatitis
5. Perforated ulcer

IV. Treatment

A. Pain Control

1. Bed rest to reduce intradiscal pressure for 2–3 d
   a. Longer periods of up to 1 wk beneficial in presence of neurologic symptoms
   b. Prolonged bed rest results in deconditioning.
2. Analgesics
   a. Short-term narcotics helpful in severe, acute pain
   b. Anti-inflammatory medications indicated
   c. Muscle relaxants beneficial through general sedation
3. Antidepressants—useful in chronic pain

B. Exercises

1. Limited program of stretches initially with gradual increase to strengthening routine
   a. Abdominal tuck—Patient lies on back and grabs one bent knee pulling it to chest for 10 sec. Repeats with opposite leg. Patient then grabs both flexed knees and rolls backward and forward stretching back muscles.
   b. Cat back—Patient gets on hands and knees. Patient arches his back up while inhaling and then pushes back down toward the floor while exhaling. Five repetitions.
   c. Arm/leg stretch—While on hands and knees, patient stretches out one arm and opposite leg holding stretch for 5 sec. Repeats with opposite arm/leg for 5 sec. Five repetitions.
2. Abdominal muscle strengthening indicated as well

V. Patient Education

A. Weight reduction reduces stress of the spine.

B. High heels increase hyperlordosis and worsen symptoms.

C. Use of an armrest when rising decreases intradiscal pressure by 30%.

D. Standing in one place for long periods of time may tighten back muscles and increase pain. Frequent changes of position are recommended.

E. Bending at the waist should be avoided. Bending at the knees with a straight back is the preferred position.

F. Proper lifting technique of bending at the knees and contracting abdominal muscles while lifting should be stressed.

G. Overall physical conditioning, particularly abdominal muscle strengthening, is an important part of back injury prophylaxis.

VI. Long-term Management

A. Physician awareness of somatization and secondary gain

B. Realistic explanation to patient of medical and surgical therapy with possible recurrence of pain

VII. Indications for Referral to Surgeon

A. Persistent radiculopathy for > 1 mo

B. Immediate referral for cauda equina syndrome—bowel/bladder dysfunction with sacral or peroneal pain and sensory loss

VIII. Annotated Bibliography

Allan D, Waddell G. An historical prospective on low back pain and disability. Acta Orthop Scand 1989 (suppl 234):60.

Deyo R. The early diagnostic evaluation of low back pain. J Gen Intern Med 1986;1:335. Helpful chart.

Deyo R. Lumbar spine films in primary care: current use and the effects of selective ordering criteria. J Gen Intern Med 1986;1:20–25. Useful criteria for ordering plain films.

Deyo R, Rainville J, Kent D. What can the history and physical exam tell us about low back pain. JAMA 1992;268(6):760–765. Necessary reading for any physician treating low back pain.

Sack B. Acute and chronic low back pain: how to pinpoint its cause and make the diagnosis. Mod Med 1993;60:58–83. Excellent summary with informative diagrams.

Sack B. Acute and chronic low back pain: how to treat and when to refer. Mod Med 1993;60:84–92. Very informative with practical recommendations.

Sontag M. Functional assessment of the spinal pain patient. Phys Med Rehab 1990;4(2):271–283.

Waddell G. A new clinical model for the treatment of low back pain. 1987; Spine 12(7):632–644.

Chapter 102: Myalgias

John M. Spandorfer

102A Fibrositis

I. Clinical Presentation

A. General Information

Fibrositis (also called fibromyalgia) is a generalized musculoskeletal pain syndrome associated with local tenderness. The prevalence in the general population may be as high as 5%. 80–90% of the cases occur in women.

B. History

1. Pain—There may be several patterns of muscle pain. The pain is usually diffuse and deep, commonly affecting the back, shoulder, pelvic girdle, arms, and hands. Patients may complain of joint pain and diffuse headaches. The pain may be worsened by damp weather, overexertion, and increased stress.
2. Stiffness—This is a common complaint. It is usually worse on awakening and improved with movement.
3. Fatigue and sleep disturbances may be the predominant symptom.
4. Past medical history may reveal the presence of migraines, irritable bowel syndrome, or dysmenorrhea.
5. Patient may have a history of anxiety or abnormalities on psychiatric testing.

C. Physical Examination

1. The only abnormal finding on the physical examination is the presence of numerous tender points, which are predictable in location and usually symmetrical.
2. The American College of Rheumatology (ACR) in 1990 defined 18 bilateral sites of involvement (Figure 102A–1).
   a. Occiput—at the suboccipital muscle insertion
   b. Low cervical—at the anterior aspect of the intertransverse spaces at C-5–C-7
   c. Trapezius—at the midpoint of the upper border
   d. Supraspinatus—above the scapula spine near the medial border

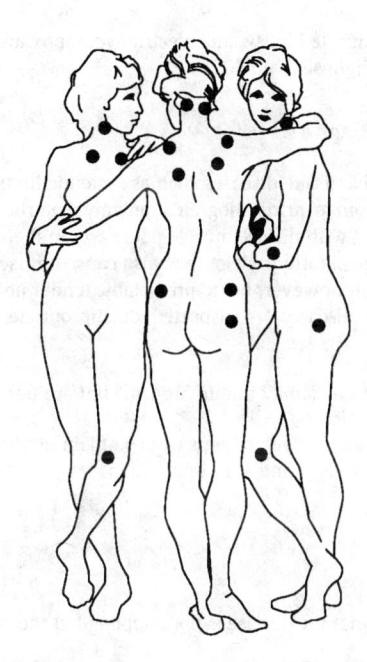

Figure 102A-1. Eighteen tender points required by the 1990 American College of Rheumatology criteria for the classification of fibromyalgia (Reproduced by permission from Wolfe F, Smythe HA, Yunus MB, et al. The American College of Rheumatology 1990 criteria for the classification of fibromyalgia: Report of the Multicenter Criteria Committee. Arthritis Rheum 1990, 33:160–172.)

    e. Second rib—at the second costochondral junction, just lateral to the junction on the upper surface
    f. Lateral epicondyle—2 cm distal to the epicondyle
    g. Gluteal—in upper outer quadrants of buttocks in anterior fold of muscle
    h. Greater trochanter—posterior to the trochanteric prominence
    i. Knee—at the medial fat pad proximal to the joint line

3. The patients are usually not aware of the tender point discreteness.

II. Diagnostic Approach

A. In 1990 the ACR defined criteria for the classification of fibrositis (both a specific history and physical examination must be obtained).

1. A history of widespread pain including each of the following—pain on the left and right side, above and below the waist and axial skeleton pain (cervical, thoracic, lumbar, sacral or anterior chest wall pain).
2. Pain in 11 of 18 of the above-mentioned tender point sites. Digital palpation with approximately 4 kg of force should elicit pain.

B. Laboratory studies, muscle biopsy, and electromyography are not considered helpful in obtaining a diagnosis.

III. Differential Diagnosis

A. Many of the connective tissue diseases such as systemic lupus erythematosus, rheumatoid arthritis, Sjögren's, polymyalgia rheumatica, and polymyositis may present with diffuse muscle pain early in their course. Hypothyroidism and hypoparathyroidism may also cause diffuse muscle complaints. There should, however, be no predictable tender points found on the examination. If these diseases are suspected, do appropriate work-up (see specific chapters).

B. Myofascial pain syndromes may mimic fibrositis but are frequently regional.

C. Psychosomatic and malingering patients can complain of diffuse muscle aches but will lack the tender points on examination.

IV. Treatment

A. Education

1. Reassure the patient that the disease is not crippling but the symptoms are real.
2. Try to decrease stress and improve sleep habits.
3. Stress that the patient should continue with former activities. Exercise can be increased even if it worsens symptoms.
4. Recommend that the lower neck should be supported during sleep. A firm mattress should be used.
5. Suggest heat or massage.

B. Medication

1. Pain, stiffness, and fatigue are typically not relieved by aspirin, nonsteroidal anti-inflammatory drugs, or systemic steroids. There is no role for narcotics.
2. Amitriptyline 10–75 mg qhs may improve sleep.

V. Annotated Bibliography

Henriksson KG, Bengtsson A. Fibromyalgia—a clinical entity? Can J Physiol Pharmacol 1991;69:672–677. A thorough review that emphasizes pathophysiology.

Smythe H. Fibrositis syndrome: a historical perspective. J Rheumatol 1989; (suppl)19:2–6. A good historical review of fibrositis.

Wolfe F, Smythe HA, Yunus MB, et al. The American College of Rheumatology 1990 Criteria for the Classification of Fibromyalgia. Arthritis Rheum 1990;33:160–172. A report from an ACR multicenter committee on a new classification of fibrositis.

102B Polymyalgia Rheumatica

I. Clinical Presentation

A. General Information

1. Polymyalgia rheumatica (PMR) is characterized by pain and stiffness in the neck, shoulders and pelvic girdle.

2. It occurs almost exclusively in patients over 50 y of age. The mean age of involvement is 70.

3. It often occurs in association with temporal arteritis, leading some authorities to suggest that both may represent the same disorder.

B. History

1. Abrupt onset of severe pain in the neck, back, shoulders, and pelvic girdle. One area may predominate or all may be affected.

2. Morning stiffness is common and may be severe enough to prevent the patient from arising from bed.

3. Weakness is unusual.

4. Nonspecific symptoms such as fever, weight loss, and depression may occur.

5. PMR is rare in patients < 50 y and in nonwhites. Women predominate in a ratio of 2:1.

C. Physical Examination

1. Physical examination is essentially normal except for mild tenderness and occasional joint swelling of the involved area.

2. Strength is usually normal.

II. Diagnostic Approach

A. Patients will likely have PMR if the following criteria are met:

1. Age ≥ 50

2. Pain and morning stiffness in at least two of the following muscle groups—neck, shoulder, and pelvic girdle

3. Persistence of symptoms for at least 1 mo

4. The erythrocyte sedimentation rate (ESR) is > 40 mm/h (may be > 100 mm/h).

5. Symptoms are not attributable to another cause.

B. In addition to the ESR, acute phase reactants are elevated.

C. Rheumatoid factor and antinuclear antibodies are usually negative.

III. Differential Diagnosis

A. Fibrositis has a normal ESR and has multiple tender sites.

B. Osteoarthritis has a normal ESR.

C. Viral myalgia does not persist > 1 mo.

D. Polymyositis is associated with muscle weakness, elevated creatine phosphokinase, abnormal muscle biopsy, and abnormal electromyography.

E. Rheumatoid arthritis is associated with synovitis in affected joints and frequently a positive rheumatoid factor.

IV. Treatment

A. Acute—The response of PMR to corticosteroids is dramatic. A dose of 10–15 mg/d of prednisone (or its equivalent) should be started. Nonsteroidal anti-inflammatory drugs are less effective.

B. Chronic—After several weeks of prednisone the dose should be tapered to a low dose, such as 2.5–7.5 mg/d. Most patients require these low doses for up to 2 y, some may need up to 5 y of therapy. Monitoring for relapse should continue 1 y after the cessation of steroids. If the patient is unable to tolerate corticosteroids a referral to a rheumatologist may be necessary for antimalarial or cytotoxic therapy.

C. Patient Education

1. Reassurance that the condition, despite possibly persisting for years, is self-limited
2. Normal activities can be continued
3. Education regarding chronic steroid therapy

V. Indications for Referral

A. May consider referral to a rheumatologist if the patient is unable to wean from steroids after 2 y

B. A rheumatologist may also be helpful if cytotoxic or antimalarial drugs are considered.

VI. Annotated Bibliography

Chuang TY, Hunder GG, Ilstrap DM, Karland, CT. Polymyalgia rheumatica: a 10 year epidemiologic and clinical study. Ann Intern Med 1982;97:672–680. Ten year clinical course of 96 patients diagnosed with PMR.

Cohen MD, Ginsburg WW. Polymyalgia rheumatica. Rheum Dis Clin North Am 1990;16:325–339. Thorough review of clinical manifestations and treatment of PMR.

Healey LA. Polymyalgia rheumatica and giant cell arteritis. In: McCarty DJ, ed. Arthritis and Allied Conditions, 11 ed. Philadelphia: Lea & Febiger; 1989:1234–1238. An overview of both disorders.

Chapter 103: Common Sports Injuries

Ellen M. O'Connor

I. Introduction

A. The goals of treatment for all sports injuries are pain relief, avoidance of complications, and rapid return to activity.

B. Most injuries respond to the RICEMS protocol.

1. Rest
2. Ice
3. Compression
4. Elevation
5. Medication
6. Stabilization

II. Common Fractures

A. Stress Fractures
1. General information
   a. Four types
      1) Oblique—most common
      2) Compression
      3) Transverse—most dangerous
      4) Longitudinal
   b. Commonly involved bones
      1) Tibia
      2) Fibula
      3) 2–4th metatarsal shafts
      4) Calcaneus
      5) Femur
      6) Rib
      7) Pars interarticularis of lumbar vertebrae

2. Symptoms
   a. Bone pain
      1) Worse at night
      2) Relief with rest
3. Physical Examination
   1) Focal tenderness on percussion
   2) Swelling over fracture
4. Diagnostic approach
   a. X-rays—may be negative for 2–8 wk after injury
   b. Bone scan
      1) Helpful when x-ray is negative, but pain persists
      2) Positive within few days of injury
5. Treatment
   a. RICEMS—heat rather than ice after initial swelling resolved
   b. Return to sports activity variable
6. Patient education—Overzealous return to sport may result in recurrence.

B. Clavicular Fracture

1. General information
   a. Usually occurs at middle third of clavicle
   b. Common with fall on outstretched arm or on point of shoulder
2. Symptoms—pain localized to site of fracture
3. Physical examination
   a. Visible deformity at site of fracture
   b. Tenderness at site
   c. Ecchymosis at site
4. Diagnostic approach
   a. X-ray—diagnostic and may rule out other fractures
5. Treatment
   a. Ice immediately
   b. Figure eight support

C. Metacarpal Fracture

1. General information—Fractures may be transverse, oblique or spiral.
2. Symptoms—pain and swelling over the hand after the injury
3. Physical examination
   a. Tenderness over fracture
   b. Crepitus over unstable fracture

c. Pain on firm percussion of fully extended fingertip
d. Nail malalignment when hand flexed at metaphalangeal and proximal interphalangeal (PIP) joints

4. Diagnostic approach

   a. X-rays—establish diagnosis

5. Treatment

   a. Ice
   b. Compression
   c. Elevation of the limb
   d. Referral to orthopedist after x-ray diagnosis for immobilization or open reduction as needed

III. Common Dislocations

A. Elbow Dislocation

1. General information

   a. Usually secondary to hyperextension force
   b. Emergency secondary to possibility of neurovascular compromise
   c. Usually associated with coronoid fracture

2. Symptoms

   a. Intense pain at elbow
   b. Patient usually aware of dislocation

3. Physical examination

   a. Rapid swelling over joint
   b. Apparent shortened forearm
   c. Inability to extend elbow
   d. Prominent olecranon

4. Diagnostic approach

   a. Usually confirmed on physical examination
   b. X-ray of joint to rule out fractures

5. Treatment

   a. Ice
   b. Immobilization
   c. Immediate referral to orthopedic care

B. Shoulder Dislocation

1. General information

   a. Anterior dislocation is most common
   b. Ideal time for reduction is immediately after injury.

c. Complications include damage to axillary, musculocutaneous or ulnar nerve, rotator cuff tears, fracture of humerus or glenoid.

2. Symptoms

   a. Intense pain at initial dislocation
   b. Possible numbness or tingling down arm

3. Physical Examination

   a. Prominent acromion
   b. Inability to rotate internally and adduct
   c. Normal neurovascular examination of arm

4. Diagnostic approach

   a. Usually diagnosed on physical exam.
   b. X-ray—anteroposterior view usually diagnostic in anterior dislocation; other views may be necessary to rule out associated fractures.

5. Treatment

   a. Immediate reduction or referral to orthopedist for reduction
   b. 3–4 wk immobilization
   c. Physical therapy for return to preinjury status
   d. Orthopedic referral for associated rotator cuff tears or glenoid or humeral fractures

6. Patient education

   a. Younger athletes have increased risk for recurrent dislocations.
   b. Older patients have higher risk of developing frozen shoulder.

IV. Common Sprains

A. Collateral Ligament Sprain of Proximal Interphalanged Joint

1. General information

   a. Most common athletic injury
   b. Inadequate treatment may lead to permanent disability.

2. Symptoms

   a. Rapid swelling
   b. Pain along lateral finger

3. Physical examination

   a. Tenderness over collateral ligament
   b. Joint swelling
   c. Instability of joint in third-degree sprain due to avulsion fracture

4. Diagnostic Approach—X-ray usually done to exclude fracture or avulsion fracture

5. Treatment

   a. Ice
   b. Compression
   c. Immobilize by dorsal splint with PIP at 20°–30° flexion for 1–3 wk
   d. Orthopedic referral for joint instability or associated fracture

B. Ulnar Collateral Ligament Sprain (Gamekeeper's Thumb)

1. General information

   a. Abduction or hyperextension forces are usual mechanism of injury.
   b. Ligament most frequently torn at distal end

2. Symptoms

   a. Pain at web space at base of thumb
   b. Difficulty grasping

3. Physical examination

   a. Tenderness at base of thumb
   b. Pain with thumb abduction
   c. Inability to hold thumb to index finger

4. Diagnosis

   a. X-ray—usually diagnostic of second-degree sprains
   b. Arthrography by orthopedist—helpful in difficult cases

5. Treatment

   a. Ice
   b. Compression
   c. Elevation
   d. Referral to orthopedic care for joint laxity or persistent pain without diagnosis

C. Ankle Sprain

1. General information

   a. More than 80% of ankle injuries are with inversion.
   b. Associated fractures are relatively uncommon.
   c. Talofibular ligament is most commonly injured with inversion injuries.
   d. Evaluation should include anatomic diagnosis, severity of injury, and joint stability.

2. Symptoms

   a. Pain—localized over injured ligament
   b. Swelling may be immediate or delayed
   c. Ecchymoses
   d. Inability to bear weight

3. Physical examination

   a. Determine whether swelling, ecchymoses present
   b. Palpate for point tenderness
   c. Evaluate stability
      1) Eversion stress to check deltoid ligament
      2) Talus side-to-side movement for tibiofibular ligament stretch
      3) Anterior drawer test for anterior talofibular ligament rupture
      4) Inversion stress to check calcaneofibular ligament

4. Differential diagnosis

   a. Osteochondral fracture of dome of talus
   b. Subluxing peroneal tendons
   c. Os trigonum injury
   d. Achilles tendon sprain
   e. Bifurcated ligament sprain
   f. Avulsion fracture of fifth metatarsal

5. Diagnostic approach

   a. Physical examination and history will support diagnosis
   b. X-ray to rule out fracture—may be negative for 1 wk after injury

6. Treatment

   a. Rest without weight-bearing for 5–7 d
   b. Ice for 15 min q 4 h for 48 h
   c. Compression with an ACE wrap
   d. Elevation·
   e. Anti-inflammatory drugs indicated if hemarthrosis not present
   f. Stretching exercises may start within 24 h in stable sprain

7. Patient education

   a. Daily Achilles tendon stretching can reduce recurrent sprains.
   b. Ankle taping with high-top shoes may reduce the incidence of ankle sprains in athletes.
   c. Swimming is good ankle exercise.

8. Referral to orthopedic care

   a. Associated fracture
   b. Ankle instability

D. Knee Sprain (see also Chapter 100C)

1. General information

   a. Complete history aids greatly in diagnosis.
   b. Early orthopedic referral recommended in all but trivial injuries.

2. Symptoms

   a. Rapid swelling within 12 h

1) Anterior cruciate ligament tear
2) Subluxed patella
3) Osteochondral fracture
 b. Swelling > 12 h after injury
1) Synovial irritation
2) Meniscal tear
 c. "Pop" sound with injury
1) Anterior cruciate ligament injury
2) Subluxed patella
 d. Joint locking
1) Meniscal tears
2) Hamstring spasm
 e. Joint giving way without rotation—meniscal injury
 f. Pain on ascending or descending stairs—retropatellar irritation
 g. Pain under patella after jumping—patellar tendonitis
3. Physical Examination
 a. Observation
1) Gait
2) Swelling
3) Leg alignment
 b. Palpation
1) Patellar ballottement
2) Ligament tenderness check
 c. Ligament testing
1) anterior drawer—anterior cruciate ligament (ACL)
2) Posterior drawer—posterior cruciate ligament (PCL)
3) Hyperextension test—ACL/PCL
4) Varus and valgus stress at 30° flexion—medial collateral ligament (MCL)/lateral collateral ligament (LCL)
5) Varus and valgus stress at 0° flexion—MCL/LCL and ACL/PCL
6) Lachman test—ACL
   a) With the knee flexed at 10° and the thigh supported with one hand, the tibia is brought forward on the femur.
   b) Excessive movement suggests a torn ACL.
 d. Meniscal testing
1) McMurray test—While patient is supine, knee is flexed toward buttock. Examiner steadies knee with one hand and holds the heel with the opposite hand. Lateral meniscus is tested by internally rotating leg with slight varus stress then slowly extending the leg. Medial meniscus is tested by externally rotating leg with slight valgus stress then extending the leg. A painful click can be felt as the meniscus moves in/out of its normal position.
2) Apley grinding test—While patient is prone, the knee is flexed 90° and rotated as a compression force is applied. Pain indicates torn meniscus.

4. Diagnostic approach

   a. X-ray
      1) Helpful to rule out associated fractures only
      2) May demonstrate old meniscal tear and degenerative changes
   b. Arthroscopy by orthopedist—usually necessary to confirm diagnosis of ACL/PCL tear

5. Treatment

   a. Medial/lateral ligament injury
      1) First-degree sprain (intact ligament)—RICEMS protocol
      2) Second-degree sprain (partial tear of ligament)—RICEMS and referral to orthopedic care for immobilization
      3) Third-degree sprain (complete rupture of ligament)—RICEMS with immediate referral to orthopedics for possible surgical repair
   b. Cruciate ligament injuries—referral to orthopedist for confirmation of diagnosis
   c. Meniscal tears—referral to orthopedist for surgical repair

6. Patient education

   a. Increasing leg musculature strength can decrease incidence of knee injuries.
   b. Athletic shoes with a large number of low, wide cleats are safest for contact sports.

V. Common Tendonitis Syndromes

A. Lateral Epicondylitis (tennis elbow)

1. Characteristics—usually seen due to overuse of forearm with poor technique

2. Symptoms—pain at elbow with movement, especially pronation of forearm

3. Physical examination

   a. Focal tenderness over lateral epicondyle
   b. Weakness of extensor muscles on lateral side
   c. Decrease in wrist flexibility

4. Diagnostic approach

   a. History and physical examination usually diagnostic
   b. X-ray—to rule out calcium deposits on the lateral epicondyle of humerus if no improvement

5. Treatment

   a. Acute case
      1) Ice packs for 15 min q.i.d. for 48–72 h
      2) Arm sling to rest arm for 1 wk
      3) No activity for at least 1 wk
      4) Anti-inflammatory medication until pain resolves

5) Injection at the point of tenderness with 3 mL 2% Xylocaine and 1 mL glucocorticoid if unimproved after anti-inflammatory medication
  b. Chronic case
    1) Heat or ice to area 1 h before playing
    2) Passive stretching of extensor carpi radialis muscle before playing
    3) Gentle warm up before playing racquet sport
    4) Muscle strengthening of the upper arm, forearm, and shoulder
6. Patient education
  a. Backhand technique should be improved
  b. Racquets with lighter weight, larger "sweet spot," less tension, and smaller grip are best.

B. Achilles Tendonitis

1. Characteristics
  a. Inflammation of the heel tendon
  b. Usually seen by repetitive tendon stretching in the deconditioned athlete
  c. Predisposing conditions
    1) Tibia vara (bowlegged deformity)
    2) Tight hamstring and calf muscles
    3) High arch of foot
2. Symptoms—burning sensation in heel at start of running and again at completion of run
3. Physical examination
  a. Local tenderness of Achilles tendon
  b. In chronic patients, nodule, crepitus, and swelling in tendon
4. Diagnostic approach—history and physical examination are diagnostic
5. Treatment
  a. Ice pack for 15 min q.i.d. for 1 wk
  b. Aspirin or acetaminophen 650 mg q.i.d. for 1 wk
  c. Rest for 1 wk
  d. Return to running with reduced mileage and no hills for 1 wk
  e. Gentle stretching exercises of the Achilles tendon b.i.d.
6. Patient education
  a. Regular stretching necessary to prevent further injury
  b. Running shoes with flexible sole recommended
7. Referral to orthopedist—may be necessary in refractory cases for casting and possible surgery

C. Shoulder Tendonitis

1. Characteristics
  a. Usually self-limited for up to 2 wk

b. Subdeltoid bursa may become inflamed secondarily.

2. Symptoms

   a. Rapid onset of severe pain over anterior or lateral aspect of shoulder
   b. Radiation as far as elbow only

3. Physical examination

   a. Pain on arm abduction
   b. Localized tenderness over one of the rotator cuff tendons or biceps tendon

4. Diagnostic approach

   a. History and physical exam sufficient
   b. X-ray—may show calcium within rotator cuff tendons or biceps tendon

5. Treatment

   a. Arm sling for 3–4 d
   b. Anti-inflammatory medication until pain resolves
   c. Moist/dry heat to area 20 min t.i.d. for 1 wk
   d. Gentle range of motion exercises recommended as pain subsides for 10 min b.i.d.
      1) "Walking" the fingers up the wall while facing a wall with the arm flexed at the elbow
      2) Swinging the arm in a circle while bending forward 90° at the waist and dangling the arm down toward the floor

6. Referral to orthopedist/physical therapy

   a. Incomplete range of motion after 2–4 wk warrants physical therapy consultation
   b. Significant calcium deposit in the tendon as seen on x-ray may require aspiration by an orthopedist.

VI. Bursitis

A. Ischial Bursitis

1. Characteristics—most commonly caused by trauma as in bicycling

2. Symptoms

   a. Abrupt onset of pain
   b. Pain increased on sitting or lying
   c. Pain may radiate into the leg

3. Physical examination

   a. Sharp pain with pressure over the ischial tuberosity
   b. Induration near ischial tuberosity on rectal exam

4. Diagnostic approach—history and physical examination diagnostic

5. Treatment

   a. Heat to area 20–30 min q.i.d.
   b. Anti-inflammatory medications for 10 d

B. **Semimembranous—Gastrocnemius Bursitis (Baker's Cyst)**

1. Characteristics—commonly seen in patients with preexisting knee problems, rheumatoid arthritis, osteoarthritis

2. Symptoms—pain with repetitive squatting or knee movement

3. Physical Examination

   a. Tenderness in popliteal fossa
   b. Fullness in popliteal fossa
   c. Possibly secondary calf swelling/tenderness

4. Diagnostic approach

   a. History and physical examination diagnostic
   b. Must consider deep venous thrombosis in proper clinical setting and use appropriate testing

5. Treatment

   a. Unruptured cyst—decreased ambulation until symptoms resolved
   b. Ruptured cyst
      1) Elevation
      2) Bed rest for 5–7 d
      3) Heat to area
      4) Anti-inflammatories until pain resolves

6. Referral to orthopedist

   a. For arthroscopy to rule out meniscal tear if indicated
   b. For injection of joint if pain unresponsive to conservative measures

VII. Annotated Bibliography

Birrer R. Sports Medicine for the Primary Care Physician. Norwalk, CT: Appleton-Century-Crofts; 1984. Extensive description of sports medicine.

Howe W. Common Sports Injuries. In: Rakel RE, ed. Conn's Current Therapy. Philadelphia: WB Saunders; 1992:936–939. Brief chapter with general information for sports injuries.

Hutson MA. Sports Injuries, Recognition and Management. Oxford, England: Oxford University Press; 1990. Detailed text for sports injuries.

Roy S, Irvin R. Sports Medicine, Prevention, Evaluation, Management and Rehabilitation. Englewood Cliffs, NJ: Prentice-Hall; 1983:170–189, 200–209, 235–244, 305–33, 379–391. Good explanation of relevant history, physical examination, and practical rehabilitation with excellent illustrations.

Part XX:
Vascular Disease

Chapter 104: Peripheral Vascular Disease

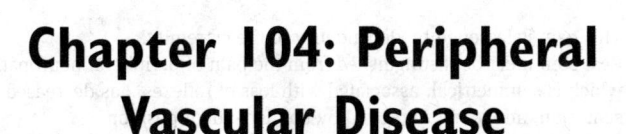

Geno J. Merli

I. Clinical Presentation

A. General Information

1. It has been documented that 1.5% of men under the age of 49 and 5% of men over 50 develop intermittent claudication during their lifetime. Women have the same incidence but it occurs 10 y later and has a more benign course.
2. In patients with claudication, the prognosis with respect to limb loss is most closely related to the severity of disease assessed by the ankle-brachial index or other noninvasive methods.
3. The need for amputation or revascularization to prevent amputation occurs annually in 4–8% of claudicants.
4. Diabetes mellitus increases the 5-y risk of amputation for claudicants as much as sevenfold.
5. Patients with claudication who continue to smoke will require amputation in 11% of cases.

B. Symptoms

1. Claudication
   a. This is an exercise-induced pain or cramping sensation in the muscle group distal to the site of arterial occlusion. This could include either the buttock, thigh, or calf.
   b. This pain or cramping in the muscle group can be relieved by rest.
   c. The degree of arterial insufficiency can be estimated by the amount of exercise or walking that the patients can do before pain begins.
   d. Claudication can easily be confused with pseudoclaudication, which is secondary either to lumbar spinal stenosis, herniated disk, or hypertrophic ridging. These symptoms may occur while lying in bed or with activities and are frequently described as a sensation of tingling, weakness, or incoordination, which requires 5–10 min to be relieved.
2. Rest pain
   a. This pain is characterized as a burning or constantly aching discomfort in the lower extremity, which is exacerbated by elevation and worse at night.

b. This pain is lessened by dependency of the extremity.
   c. Rest pain must be distinguished from the pain of peripheral neuropathy, which is symmetrical, associated with loss of reflexes, has decreased sensation, and is not improved by the dependent position.

C. Physical Examination

1. Pulses

   a. The femoral, popliteal, dorsalis pedis, and the posterior tibial pulse should be palpated and graded on a scale of 0 to +3.
   b. The abdominal aorta should be palpated for any enlargement and subsequently auscultated for bruits. The femoral pulses can be assessed at the same time.

2. Color/temperature

   a. The involved extremity frequently has pallor and is cooler than the opposite side.
   b. Rubor is reddening of the foot in the dependent position and is the result of reactive hyperemia secondary to large vessel disease.

3. Elevation/dependency test

   a. This consists of elevation of both extremities to 30° for 30 sec and then returning the legs to the horizontal position.
   b. The extremity should have capillary filling and pinkness within 10 sec

II. Diagnostic Approach

A. Ankle-Brachial Index (ABI)

1. The ABI is the simplest test for evaluating the lower extremity circulation. The ABI is obtained by dividing the ankle systolic blood pressure by the arm systolic blood pressure. The normal range for the index is 0.9–1.3.

2. Patients with a history of intermittent claudication will often have an ABI of 0.9–0.35. Ulceration or impending gangrene has been correlated with ABIs < 0.25. This index can also be used in patients with normal pulses but claudication history. These patients may manifest a drop in their ABI following exercise.

3. This noninvasive test can be easily performed in the office or at the patient's bedside and provides an accurate assessment of the presence of peripheral vascular disease.

4. Calcified vessels may result in falsely normal ABI results.

B. Segmental Limb Pressure (SLP)

1. SLPs can provide a simple assessment of pressures at four levels of the studied extremity.

2. This test is completed by placing cuffs on the most proximal thigh, just above and below the knee, and proximal to the malleoli at the ankle. The arterial signal is assessed by a Doppler probe as each segmental cuff is deflated. A gradient of > 20 mm Hg between high thigh and above knee pressure and below the knee pressure indicates superficial femoral or popliteal artery disease. A gradient of > 20 mm Hg between the below knee and ankle pressure is indicative of tibial or peroneal arterial disease. Using these criteria segmental pressures accurately predicted the site of occlusive arterial lesions in 83% of limbs studied arteriographically.

C. Pulse Volume Recordings (PVR)

1. This method of evaluating the lower extremity arterial circulation is based on the principle of assessing volume changes.

2. Pneumatic segmental cuffs with pressure transducers detect momentary volume changes in a limb and these are displayed as segmental pressure pulse contours. This type of study better localizes arterial disease than the segmental limb pressure technique and its results are more qualitatively reproducible.

3. This test has a 95% accuracy for defining occlusive disease when compared to arteriography. Combining the SLP and PVR provides a more accurate assessment of lower extremity arterial disease than either test alone.

D. Transcutaneous Oxygen Tension ($TCpO_2$) Determination

1. $TCpO_2$ determination is a method of assessing the amount of oxygen that is delivered to the area of the extremity being evaluated, in excess of local metabolic consumption.

2. The measured value of $TCpO_2$ depends on both the volume of blood flowing to the region and the degree to which it is oxygenated (% saturation of hemoglobin) when it arrives. This measure reflects the metabolic state of the tissue being examined, whereas the previous tests assess for hemodynamic and anatomic disease.

3. The greatest utility of $TCpO_2$ appears to be in assessing the diabetic patient with incompressible vessels and in predicting the healing potential of ischemic lesions and amputation incisions.

E. Duplex Scanning

1. The duplex scan system combines a B-mode ultrasound image of the vessel being studied with a pulsed Doppler flow detector to obtain velocity information from specific locations along the artery. This study can provide hemodynamic and anatomic information whereas the SLP and PVR only detect hemodynamically significant lesions.

2. The anatomic information provided by duplex is able to categorize the degree of stenosis and its location along the vessel. When coupled with flow velocity,

the hemodynamic significance of the lesion can be documented. This study can be used to evaluate graft patency and the status of the proximal and distal anastomosis in patients who have undergone revascularization of the lower extremity.

F. Arteriography

1. The major purpose of arteriography in patients with peripheral vascular disease is to provide a precise, high-resolution definition of anatomy for nonsurgical interventional therapy or surgical revascularization. This study should only be done when definitive treatment is planned. It is not a diagnostic study for peripheral vascular disease.

2. The incidence of idiosyncratic contrast reactions is approximately < 4%.

3. Patients with low renal blood flow states, preexisting renal insufficiency, diabetes mellitus, proteinuria, and dehydration are at increased risk for contrast induced renal failure. These patients should be well hydrated before and after arterial studies.

4. Local complications of arteriography occur in 0.5% of procedures. These include hemorrhage, thrombosis, pseudoaneurysm, and arteriovenous fistula.

III. Differential Diagnosis

A. Lumbar spinal stenosis

B. Lumbar disk disease

C. Degenerative joint disease of the hip and back

D. Popliteal artery entrapment syndrome

E. Thromboangitis obliterans (Buerger's disease)

IV. Treatment

A. Goal of Treatment

The goal of therapy is to maintain the viability of the lower extremity tissues by medical modalities, nonsurgical interventional therapy, or surgical revascularization.

B. Noninvasive Modalities

1. A walking exercise program that emphasizes cardiovascular conditioning improves lower extremity resting blood flow, reduces the onset of claudication, and increases maximal walking time.

2. Smoking cessation can be accomplished by physician counseling, professional program, or the use of transdermal nicotine patches. The latter must be used with caution in patients with peripheral vascular disease.

3. Good diabetic control

4. Skin care to prevent drying or cracking of the tissues can be provided by such agents as Nivea, Eucerin, Alpha Keri, Carmol, Lachydrin, or products that moisturize the skin

5. Appropriate footwear that provides comfort and prevents tissue injury

6. When these measures fail to provide symptomatic relief or when the patient develops acute ischemia or gangrene or rest pain the patient needs to proceed to invasive modalities of therapy.

7. Pentoxifylline (400 mg, PO t.i.d.) has been used in chronic intermittent claudication to improve exercise tolerance. Approximately 20% of patients taking this medication will subjectively note improvement. The major side effect is GI intolerance, which can be minimized if the medication is taken with meals. If no improvement occurs after 8 wk of therapy, the medication should be discontinued.

C. Invasive Modalities

1. Percutaneous transluminal angioplasty is the ideal procedure for single, short, stenotic segmental lesions in medium to large size vessels. This modality of therapy will be decided on at the time of the arteriogram.

2. Revascularization procedures such as aortoiliac-femoral, perfunda femoris, femoropopliteal, or femorotibial reconstruction are indicated depending on the extent of disease diagnosed by arteriography.

3. In very high-risk patients with aortoiliac disease, an axillofemoral or femoral-femoral bypass is an alternative form of revascularization.

4. Amputation of an extremity is indicated in the following circumstances

    a. Extensive tissue necrosis such that salvage of the extremity is not possible
    b. Ischemia accompanied by extensive soft tissue infection with signs of sepsis

V. Indications for Referral to a Vascular Surgeon

A. Claudication that impairs the patient's function

B. Rest pain

C. Rest pain with gangrene

VI. Indications for Hospitalization

Patients presenting with rest pain and gangrenous changes in the lower extremities must be admitted for diagnostic evaluation and surgical revascularization.

VII. Annotated Bibliography

DeWeese J, Leather R, Porter J. Practice guidelines: lower extremity revascularization. J Vasc Surg 1993;18:280–294. This paper is a very good overview of management strategies for nonsurgical physicians caring for patients with peripheral vascular disease.

Imparato A, Kim G. Intermittent claudication: its natural course. Surgery 1975;78:795–799. This is the classic clinical paper on the natural course of peripheral vascular disease presenting with claudication.

Loscalzo J, Creager M, Dzau V, eds. Vascular Medicine: A Textbook of Vascular Biology and Diseases. Boston: Little, Brown; 1992. An excellent text for physicians involved in the care of patients with vascular diseases. This book is heavily weighted toward medical management.

Rutherford R, Flanigan O, Gupta S, et al. Ad Hoc Committee on Reporting Standards of the SVS and ISCVS: Suggested standards for reports dealing with lower extremity ischemia. J Vasc Surg 1986;4:80–94. The purpose of this article is to review the noninvasive studies recommended for assessing lower extremity peripheral vascular disease.

Young J, Graor R, Olin J, Bartholomew J. eds. Peripheral Vascular Diseases. St. Louis: Mosby-Year Book; 1991. A classic textbook devoted strictly to peripheral vascular disease. The authors bring a wealth of experience from the Cleveland Clinic vascular programs.

Chapter 105: Peripheral Venous Disease

Geno J. Merli

105A Deep Vein Thrombosis

I. Clinical Presentation

A. General Information

1. Venous thrombosis remains a major cause of disability and death in all patient populations. In hospitalized patients autopsy studies have demonstrated that massive pulmonary embolism is the cause of death in 5–10% of all hospital deaths and have suggested that two thirds of all clinically important venous thromboemboli are never recognized during life.

2. It has also been estimated by population studies that 170,000 patients are treated for clinically recognized initial episodes of venous thromboembolism in U.S. hospitals each year and that 90,000 will be treated for recurrent disease.

3. Whenever a patient presents with a painful extremity and has a risk factor such as obesity, malignancy, recent surgery, using oral contraceptives, has varicose veins, or has had a previous deep vein thrombosis (DVT), the presence of thrombosis should be suspected.

B. Symptoms

1. Patients will frequently complain of pain in the extremity, which gradually increases in intensity and is exacerbated by weight-bearing. This pain is described as squeezing, knotlike, or tightness deep in the extremity.

2. Swelling often occurs beginning in the ankle and progressing proximally. This swelling characteristically increases with prolonged standing or sitting and is not decreased by elevation.

3. A sensation of warmth has also been reported in some cases.

4. Often the patient will recall an event or situation that preceded the above symptoms such as a prolonged car or airplane trip, traumatic injury, recent surgery, or medications that are thrombogenic.

C. Physical Examination

1. The lower extremities should be inspected for signs of trauma, color, and superficial venous distention.
2. The circumference of the lower extremities may be measured 15 cm above and below the medial tibial plateau. A leg girth discrepancy between extremities of > 1 cm may be considered significant depending on other clinical findings.
3. Next swelling in the extremity should be described as pitting or nonpitting (the former seen with thrombosis), the extent of involvement, and the degree of induration. Induration can be determined by palpating the involved and noninvolved extremity simultaneously and sensing the degree of doughiness of the tissues.
4. Induration is a result of increased venous pressure secondary to impaired venous outflow from thrombosis. This results in leaking at the capillary level with excess interstitial fluid in the tissues. This causes firmness in the extremity.
5. The temperature of the extremity should be checked by placing the back of the hand on the skin surface. Increased temperature may be present in cellulitis, gout, or arthritis as well as DVT.
6. Frequently the extremity will appear mottled or dusky blue in color. In cases of severely impaired venous drainage the extremity could become cyanotic with acute tissue necrosis.
7. The pulses of the lower extremity are always examined to assess for concomitant arterial disease.

II. Diagnostic Approach

A. Venography

1. Venography is the gold standard for the diagnosis of DVT.
2. Radiopaque contrast medium is injected into veins on the dorsum of the foot to outline the lower extremity venous system. This study will visualize the calf, popliteal, femoral, external iliac, and common iliac veins.
3. The most reliable criterion for the diagnosis of acute DVT is the presence of an intraluminal filling defect that is constant in all films and seen in a number of projections. Nonfilling of vessels could mean complete occlusion or an inadequate study. Clinical correlation is most important in these circumstances.
4. The literature has reported a 1–2% incidence of superficial phlebitis and acute DVT in patients with negative venograms poststudy.
5. The usual contrast allergies, impaired renal function, diabetes mellitus, multiple myeloma, and dehydration should be all taken into consideration when ordering this test for diagnosis.

B. Impedance Plethysmography (IPG)

1. IPG is based on the principle that changes in the blood volume of the calf (produced by inflation and deflation of a pneumatic thigh cuff) result in changes in electrical resistance (impedance), which is detected by skin electrodes placed circumferentially around the calf.

2. IPG is sensitive (95%) and specific (96%) for the detection of occluding thrombi in the proximal venous system. It is not sensitive and specific for calf vein or partially occluding thrombi. In addition IPG will not distinguish between thrombotic and nonthrombotic obstruction to venous outflow.

3. Two studies have concluded the following about IPG for suspected DVT.
   a. A positive result by IPG in a patient with clinically suspect DVT is highly predictive of acute proximal vein thrombosis.
   b. It is safe to withhold anticoagulant therapy in patients with clinically suspected DVT who have had negative serial IPG studies over a 10–14-day period. Studies have shown that the incidence of embolic disease in this group is low.

C. Venous Duplex Imaging

1. This test is a combination of Doppler and B-mode ultrasound.

2. It is useful in assessing the deep venous system from the ankle to the external iliac vein.

3. Thrombi are visualized and confirmed by demonstrating noncompressibility by probe assessment.

4. Advantages of venous duplex imaging include that extrinsic compression can be differentiated from intrinsic obstruction, and small, nonocclusive, and free-floating thrombi are distinguishable from occluding and adherent thrombi.

5. In screening symptomatic patients the sensitivity and specificity approach 95% in proximal DVT.

6. The sensitivity of this test in screening asymptomatic patients is 54%.

7. The study best identifies thrombosis developing from the popliteal upward with less sensitivity for calf vein thrombosis.

III. Differential Diagnosis

A. Trauma to the extremity

B. Cellulitis

C. Ruptured Baker's cyst

D. Lymphedema

E. Arthritis of knee or ankle

F. Tumor

G. Congestive heart failure

H. Gout

IV. Treatment

A. Goals

The goals of treatment are to prevent propagation of clot, pulmonary embolism during the acute phase of treatment, and recurrence of DVT/pulmonary embolism.

B. Acute Management
1. There are four approaches to managing heparin for acute DVT (Table 105A–1).
   a. Standard heparin therapy
      1) Bolus 5000 units followed by 1000 units/h (25,000 units/250 D5W)
      2) Infusion adjusted at 6-h intervals to achieve a partial thromboplastin time (PTT) of 1.5–2.5 times the patient's baseline.
      3) Once achieved a PTT is checked daily and appropriate dosing adjustment made to maintain the target PTT
      4) Check platelets every other day while on heparin therapy and observe for 30% decrease from baseline as suspicious for the development of heparin-induced thrombocytopenia.
   b. Weight-based nomogram
      1) Bolus 80 units/kg followed by 18 units/kg/h
      2) Infusion adjustment at 6-h interval by nomogram
      3) Once the desired range is achieved PTT is checked daily and appropriate dosing is by the nomogram.
      4) Platelets should be checked as above.
   c. Hull method
      1) Bolus 5000 units followed by 1600 units/h for patients at low risk of bleeding
      2) Bolus 5000 units followed by 1200 or 1300 units/h for patients at high risk of bleeding
      3) Initial infusion adjustments are made at 6-h intervals to achieve PTT of 55–75 sec.
      4) Once achieved PTT is checked daily and the infusion rate is adjusted to maintain the desired 55–75 sec.
      5) Platelets should be checked as above.
   d. Adjusted high-dose subcutaneous heparin
      1) 250 units/kg SQ q 12 h

Table 105A–1. Heparin Dosing Regimens

Standard	Weight-based	Hull Method
1. Bolus 5000 units IV	1. Bolus 80 units/kg, IV	1. Bolus 5000 units IV
2. Infusion 1000 units/h	2. Infusion 18 units/kg/h	2. Infusion 1200–1300 units/h
3. Target PTT 1.5–2.5 pt's baseline	3. Target PTTs a. PTT < 35 sec 80 units/kg bolus then increase infusion by 4 units/kg/h b. PTT 35–45 sec 40 units/kg bolus then increase infusion by 2 units/kg/h c. PTT 46–70 sec no change d. PTT 71–90 sec decrease infusion 2 units/kg/h e. PTT > 90 sec Hold infusion 1 h then decrease to 3 units/kg/h recheck in 6 h	3. Target PTT 55–75 sec
4. PTT in range continue infusion		4. PTT in range continue infusion
5. If PTT is low a. 5000 unit-bolus then b. Increase drip by 200 units/h c. PTT q 6 h until desired PTT obtained		5. PTT is low a. 5000-unit bolus b. Increase drip by 200 units/h c. PTT q 6 h until desired PTT obtained
6. PTT > 99 sec a. Decrease by 200 units/h recheck in 6 h b. Stop drip 1 h then decrease drip by 200 units/h recheck in 6 h and continue until desired range obtained		6. PTT > 99 sec a. Decrease by 200 units/h then recheck in 6 h b. Stop drip 1 h then decrease drip by 200 units/h recheck in 6 h and continue until desired range obtained

  2) Check PTT 5 h following the morning dose of day 2 and adjust the heparin dose to achieve PTT of 1.5–2.5 times the patient's baseline level.
  3) Platelets should be checked as above.

C. Long-term Management

1. Warfarin (standard therapy)

   a. The traditional method is to begin warfarin on the evening of the third night of therapy. The target INR is 2–3.
   b. Newer approach is to begin warfarin in the first 24 h following the initiation of heparin therapy. The INR sought is 2–3.
   c. Therapy is maintained 3–6 mo.

2. Subcutaneous adjusted dose heparin

   a. 10,000 units SQ SC, q 12 h for the first 24 h
   b. On day 2 an activated PTT (aPTT) is obtained 6 h following the morning dose.
   c. The desired aPTT is 1.5 times the patient's baseline.
   d. Therapy is maintained 3–6 mo.

D. Patient Education

1. The major focus of education is compliance with the use of anticoagulation therapy as an outpatient. This includes regular dosing, appropriate outpatient laboratory testing of the prothrombin time to adjust medications, and reporting of symptoms or signs of bleeding. Patients should be cautioned about using OTC medications that contain aspirin or nonsteroidal anti-inflammatory drugs and the avoidance of alcohol.
2. If the patient has other concomitant medical problems that may affect the metabolism of warfarin or heparin, appropriate precautions such as frequent assessment of anticoagulation and dosage adjustment must be taken to ensure safety during oral anticoagulation therapy.
3. Premenopausal women should be made aware of increased menstrual flow and vaginal bleeding following sexual intercourse. Male patients have reported blood in their ejaculate while on anticoagulant therapy.
4. My rule of thumb for when to reassess outpatients with recurrent leg symptoms at any point in time after DVT is to place them at bed rest with leg elevation for 24 h. If the symptoms persist, evaluation for recurrence of thrombosis must be completed.

V. Indications for Referral

Patients with a cyanotic, edematous, painful extremity may require a thrombectomy for management. A vascular surgery consultation in this case would be indicated.

VI. Indications for Hospitalization

Patients with a symptomatic lower extremity and a very strong history for the development of DVT should be referred for evaluation of the extremity. If thrombosis is discovered, the patient is admitted and treated with one of the previously described regimens of therapy.

VII. Annotated Bibliography

Anderson F, Wheeler H, Goldberg R, et al. A population based perspective of the hospital incidence and case fatality rate of deep vein thrombosis and pulmonary embolism: the Worcester DVT study. Arch Intern Med 1991;151:933–938. This is one of the best reviews on thromboembolic disease as it relates to hospitalization and fatality rates from a multihospital system.

Cruickshank M, Levine M, Hirsh J, et al. A standard heparin nomogram for the management of heparin therapy. Arch Intern Med 1991;151:333–337. The author achieved a more rapid therapeutic PTT using a dosing nomogram compared to the standard dosing regimen.

Glazier R, Crowell E. Randomized prospective trial of continuous vs intermittent heparin therapy. JAMA 1976;236:1365–1367. This is the classic article that converted heparin to continuous infusion therapy.

Hommes C, Bura A, Mazzolai L, et al. Subcutaneous heparin compared with continuous intravenous heparin administration in the initial treatment of deep venous thrombosis: a metaanalysis. Ann Intern Med 1992;116:279–284. This is an excellent meta-analysis of all the papers evaluating the treatment of DVT by subcutaneous heparin.

Hull R, Delmore T, Carter C, et al. Adjusted subcutaneous heparin versus warfarin sodium in the long-term treatment of venous thrombosis. N Engl J Med 1982;306:189–194. This is the classic paper on the use of adjusted dose, subcutaneous heparin compared to warfarin for the prevention of DVT. Adjusted dose heparin was as effective and safer than warfarin therapy.

Hull R, Hirsh J, Jay R, et al. Different intensities of oral anticoagulation therapy in the treatment of proximal vein thrombosis. N Engl J Med 1982;307:1676–1681. This paper evaluated the different intensities of warfarin for prevention of recurrence of DVT. Essentially this is the paper in which the current INR of 2–3 is derived.

Hull R, Raskob G, Rosenbloom D, et al. Heparin for 5 days as compared with 10 days in the initial treatment of proximal venous thrombosis. N Engl J Med 1990;322:1260–1264. In this paper the authors demonstrated that a heparin dosing schedule based on risk of bleeding by the patient achieved a therapeutic aPTT more rapidly and warfarin was safely begun within the first 24 h of initiation of therapy.

Kramer F, Teitelbaum G, Merli G. Panvenography and pulmonary angiography in the diagnosis of deep venous thrombosis and pulmonary embolism. Radiol Clin North Am 1986;243:397–418. This article reviews all the studies, both pulmonary and low extremity, for the assessment of thromboembolic disease. There are numerous tables and decision tree for assessing thromboembolic events.

105B Chronic Venous Insufficiency

I. Clinical Presentation

A. General Information

1. Over 1.6 million Americans have some form of chronic venous insufficiency that accounts for 30,000 hospitalizations, 50,000 surgical procedures, and 10,000 days absent from work.
2. The first step in understanding chronic venous insufficiency is the classification of this disease and recognizing that valvular incompetence is the major pathophysiologic abnormality of this disease.

B. Symptoms

1. The most frequently used terms by patients to describe their lower extremities are heaviness, tightness, tiredness, fatigue, aching, or painful.
2. The symptoms begin on arising and assuming the upright posture and gradually increase as the day progresses. The only position that provides relief is elevation of the lower extremities.

C. Physical Examination

1. Inspection of the lower extremities for varicosities, pigmentation, ulceration, and leg size is important. Varicose veins, either familial or secondary, may be present bilaterally. Their distribution could be from the greater saphenous and/or lesser saphenous venous system. These varices may be large grapelike clusters or multiple small superficial venules over the foot and ankle area.
2. The pigmentary changes are secondary to hemosiderin deposition in the subcutaneous tissue. This is a result of increased venous pressure and the extrusion of red cells in the interstitial space. The red cells are reabsorbed leaving behind hemosiderin pigmentation. The distribution of the hemosiderin is predominantly in the distal medial aspect of the ankle, called the gaiter area.
3. Ulcers are commonly located over the distal medial aspect of the extremity over the medial malleolus. The ulcer may occur spontaneously or secondary to trauma. The base of the ulcer has extensive granulation tissue with serosanguinous drainage present. These ulcers may or may not be painful. Sometimes stasis dermatitis will accompany venous ulceration. This is located around the periphery of the ulcer and frequently can resemble macerated tissue.

II. Diagnostic Approach

A. Photoplethysmography

1. The density of the skin and its ability to reflect light partly depends on the volume of blood in the capillaries within the skin. Photoplethysmography is

an indirect measure of blood volume and correlates with superficial venous pressure but does not provide information about the communicating or deep venous system.

2. The probe, which contains both an infrared light source and a photoelectric cell to measure the reflectivity of the skin, is placed 4–5 inches (10–12.5 cm) above the medial malleolus. The patient is asked to sit with the feet resting on the floor and then to perform regular heel raises.

3. Alternatively, the patient may stand with all the weight on one leg while performing the heel raising with the non–weight-bearing leg. This posture will provide greater hydrostatic pressure and maximize venous filling.

4. Venous refilling after exercise is provided by the arterial circulation. Therefore if the superficial and deep venous systems are incompetent, the increase in refluxed blood will be picked up by the superficial probe. The usefulness of this test is primarily for assessing the severity of venous reflux and excluding venous disease.

B. Air Plethysmography (APG)

1. APG is a more comprehensive modality for evaluating lower extremity venous function. This test operates on the principle of volume change in the lower extremity both with and without exercise. The information provided by these changes in volume reflects the ambulatory venous pressure, venous reflux, and calf muscle pump function.

2. The venous filling index indicates the degree of valvular insufficiency.

3. The ejection fraction is more of a measure of calf muscle pump function.

4. The residual volume fraction (RVF) indicates the overall performance of the venous system.

5. Patients with venous ulcers have a higher venous filling index, a lower ejection fraction, and a higher RVF compared to asymptomatic volunteers. A shortcoming of APG is the need for the patient to be able to stand as well as perform tip-toe exercises.

C. Venography—This study is rarely used as the diagnostic test for venous insufficiency because it is invasive and has potential risk of complications.

D. Recommendations—At the present time APG is recommended as the best test to document chronic venous insufficiency in conjunction with the history and physical examination.

III. Differential Diagnosis

A. Cellulitis

B. Superficial phlebitis

C. Acute deep vein thrombosis (see Chapter 105A)

IV. Treatment

A. Goals

1. Control swelling
2. Provide good skin care
3. Provide aggressive ulcer therapy
4. Prevent venous thrombosis

B. Acute and Chronic Management

1. The control of swelling is an ongoing process. The primary mode of management is the use of gradient elastic stockings.
   a. These come in a variety of compression pressures and lengths. 30 mm Hg compression is used for most patients. Higher or lower pressures have been used depending on the patient's symptoms.
   b. Stocking length—Use calf length for calf-only swelling and full leg for proximal extremity involvement. The latter could be a half panty hose style or full bilateral leg garment.
   c. Gradient stockings can be purchased from many manufacturers including Jobst, Sigvarus, Medi, or Juzzo.
2. Frequently swelling cannot be controlled with gradient stockings alone. In this case external pneumatic compression sleeves can be used at the end of the day to reduce swelling before the patient retires.
   a. Combined with overnight leg elevation, this approach results in decreased swelling in the patient's lower extremities on arising.
   b. The external pneumatic compression stockings are worn for 1 h each evening and set initially at 30 mm Hg pressure. This can be increased based on the patient's improvement and tolerability.
   c. Pneumatic compression sleeves can be rented through third-party payers for a 3-mo period to allow time to monitor their effect on reducing lower extremity swelling. In severe cases of chronic venous insufficiency, the patient may require use of these devices indefinitely.
3. The primary focus of skin care is moisturization of the skin. The lower extremities of patients with chronic venous insufficiency are usually dry. This can result in cracking of the skin, allowing portals of entry for bacteria and increased risk for cellulitis. Twice per day moisturization is recommended with a topical cream such as Nivea, Eucerin, Carmol, and Lachydrin.
4. Ulcer care must be aggressive. At the first sign of breakdown the patient should be evaluated to identify any concomitant problems such as cellulitis, phlebitis, foreign body, trauma, etc. Lower extremity dependency should be reduced and compression provided, with medical care of the ulcer. This can be accomplished with an unna paste boot.

V. Indications for Referral

A. Recurrent episodes of superficial phlebitis in the same distribution of veins can be treated by selective surgical removal of these vessels.

B. Rarely a venous stasis ulcer will not heal due to a significant perforating vein. This can be remedied by surgical removal.

VI. Indications for Hospitalization

A. Acute deep vein thrombosis

B. Superficial phlebitis that extends above the knee into the deep femoral venous system

C. Extensive cellulitis

VIII. Annotated Bibliography

Angel M, Ramasastry S, Swartz W, et al. The causes of skin ulcerations associated with venous insufficiency: a unifying hypothesis. Plast Reconstruct Surg 1987;79:289. In this article the authors review all the theories put forth as the etiology for ulcer formation in patients with chronic venous insufficiency.

Browse N, Burnand K, Thomas M, eds. Diseases of the Veins: Pathology, Diagnosis, and Treatment. London: Edward Arnold Co; 1988. This is the most comprehensive textbook on this subject.

Browse N, Clemenson G, Thomas L. Is the postphlebitic leg always postphlebitic? Relationship between phlebographic appearance of DVT and late sequelae. Br Med J 1980;281:1167. This article is the classic review of postphlebitic syndrome with respect to the extent of clot and the disease outcome.

Lindner D, Edwards J, Phinney E, et al. Long-term hemodynamic and clinical sequelae of lower extremity DVT. J Vasc Surg 1986;4:436. This paper reviews the hemodynamic studies in conjunction with the clinical manifestation of DVT.

Strandness D, Langlois Y, Cramer M, et al. Long-term sequelae of acute venous thrombosis. JAMA 1983;280:1289. The author reviews the long-term experience in managing patients with acute thrombosis.

Train J, Schanzer H, Peirce C, et al. Radiological evaluation of the chronic venous stasis syndrome. JAMA 1987;258:941. In this paper the authors focus on venographic studies to document valvular incompetence as the etiology for chronic venous insufficiency.

Appendix A

Adult Immunizations

Kenneth R. Epstein

A. Recommendations for Healthy Adults (see section H below for dosing)

1. Adolescents and young adults
   a. Tetanus-diphtheria (Td) toxoid—initial series, then booster q 10 y
   b. Measles-mumps-rubella (MMR)—give combined vaccine for below indications
      1) Measles—if no evidence of live-virus immunization after first birthday, physician-documented infection, or laboratory proven immunity
      2) Rubella (women only)—if not pregnant and no evidence of prior immunization or laboratory-documented immunity. Avoid pregnancy for 3 months after immunization.
   c. Hepatitis B—if sexually active or otherwise high risk.

2. Age 25–64 y
   a. Td toxoid—document prior primary series, then booster q 10 y
   b. MMR—give combined vaccine for below indications
      1) Measles—if born after 1956 and no evidence of live-virus immunization after first birthday, physician-documented infection, or laboratory proven immunity
      2) Rubella (women only)—if not pregnant and no evidence of prior immunization or laboratory-documented immunity. Avoid pregnancy for 3 months after immunization.
   c. Influenza—can offer to healthy young adults

3. Age > 65 y
   a. Td toxoid—document prior primary series, then booster q 10 y
   b. Influenza—vaccinate annually
   c. Pneumococcal polysacharride—everyone should be immunized initially, then consider repeating after 6 y

4. Pregnant women
   a. MMR contraindicated
   b. Test for rubella antibody and hepatitis B surface antigen (HBSAg)
      1) If HBSAg negative and high risk, then immunize
      2) If rubella antibody negative, and rubella is contracted in the first 16 weeks of pregnancy, then there is a 15–20% risk of fetal or neonatal death, and a 20–50% risk of congenital rubella syndrome if the infant survives.

B. Recommendations for Specific Occupational Groups
1. College students
   a. Routine immunizations as listed above
   b. MMR—indicated almost universally, with exclusions as noted above
   c. Hepatitis B vaccine—consider for all students if:
      1) Homosexual or bisexual male
      2) Heterosexual with multiple partners
      3) Students with intimate or sexual contact with foreign students from endemic areas
      4) Students planning extended overseas travel to developing countries
2. Health care workers
   a. Hepatitis B—all health care workers should be immunized. It may not be cost effective to test prior serologic status.
   b. Influenza—vaccinate annually
   c. Rubella—all workers, male or female, should have documented immunity. Vaccinate with MMR.
3. Persons providing essential community services
   a. Influenza—vaccinate annually
   b. Hepatitis B—for emergency medical personnel
4. Day care center personnel
   a. MMR
   b. Poliomyelitis
   c. Influenza—vaccinate annually
5. Laboratory personnel
   a. Hepatitis B—if handle clinical specimens
   b. Consider specific risks based on type of laboratory
6. Veterinarians, animal handlers, rural workers, and other field personnel
   a. Rabies vaccine—recommended preexposure. Does not eliminate need for additional therapy postexposure.
   b. In southwestern United States or other high-risk area, consider plague vaccine.
   c. Anthrax vaccine—if exposed frequently to imported animal products

C. Recommendations for Specific Environmental Situations
1. Nursing home residents
   a. Influenza—vaccinate annually
   b. Pneumococcal Vaccine
   c. Td—booster dose (or primary series)
   d. Tuberculin skin testing

2. Institutionalized mentally retarded
   a. Hepatitis B vaccine
3. Prison inmates
   a. Hepatitis B vaccine
4. Homeless persons
   a. Review history of all vaccinations, especially dT
   b. Consider the need for influenza, pneumococcal, and hepatitis B vaccines.

D. Recommendations for Specific Life styles

1. Homosexual and bisexual men
   a. Hepatitis—serologic testing may be cost effective prior to immunization
2. Intravenous drug users
   a. Hepatitis B—serologic testing may be cost effective prior to immunization
   b. Td toxoid—important to maintain immunity
3. Prostitutes, persons with multiple sexual partners or sexually transmitted diseases
   a. Hepatitis B—serologic testing may be cost effective prior to immunization

E. Recommendations for Immunocompromised Adults

1. HIV infection and AIDS (see Part XIII)
   a. Pneumococcal vaccine—recommended
   b. *Haemophilus influenzae* type B vaccine—consider use
   c. Influenza—vaccinate annually
   d. Varicella zoster immune globulin—indicated postexposure regardless of prior serologic status
   e. Hepatitis B—if at high risk of exposure
2. Splenic disorders
   a. Pneumococcal vaccine—if possible, vaccinate at least 2 wk prior to an elective splenectomy
   b. Consider *H. influenzae* type B and meningococcal vaccine
3. Diabetes mellitus
   a. Pneumococcal Vaccine
   b. Influenza—vaccinate annually
4. Renal failure and dialysis
   a. Pneumococcal vaccine—especially for nephrotic syndrome
   b. Influenza—vaccinate annually
   c. Hepatitis B—Vaccine is indicated for patients with renal failure if dialysis or transplantation are possibilities in future.

5. Alcoholism and hepatic cirrhosis
   a. Pneumococcal vaccine
   b. Influenza annually
6. Organ transplantation and immunosuppressive therapy
   a. Pneumococcal vaccine
   b. Influenza annually
7. Malignant diseases
   a. Consider individually based on type of tumor and risk of infection
   b. Most patients should receive pneumococcal and annual influenza vaccine.

F. Recommendations for International Travel

   See Chapter 12

G. Tetanus Prophylaxis in Wound Management

Table 1. Summary Guide to Tetanus Prophylaxis* in Routine Wound Management, United States

	Clean, minor wounds		All other wounds[†]	
	Td[§]	TIG[¶]	Td[§]	TIG
Uncertain or < 3	Yes	No	Yes	Yes
≥ 3**	No[††]	No	No[§§]	No

* Refer also to text on specific vaccines or toxoids for contraindications, precautions, dosages, side effects, adverse reactions, and special considerations. Important details are in the text and in the ACIP recommendations on diphtheria, tetanus, and pertussis (DTP) (MMWR 1991: 40[RR-10]).

† Such as, but not limited to: wounds contaminated with dirt, feces, and saliva; puncture wounds; avulsions; and wounds resulting from missiles, crushing, burns, and frostbite.

§ Td, Tetanus and diphtheria toxoids, adsorbed (for adults use). For children < 7 y old, DTP (DT, if pertussis vaccine is contraindicated) is preferred to tetanus toxoid alone. For persons ≥ 7 y old, Td is preferred to tetanus toxoid alone.

¶ TIG, tetanus immune globulin.

** If only three doses of fluid toxoid have been received, a fourth dose of toxoid, preferably an adsorbed toxoid, should be given.

†† Yes, > 10 y since last dose.

§§ Yes, > 5 y since last dose. (More frequent boosters are not needed and can accentuate side effects.)

Reprinted with permission from Centers for Disease Control. Update on adult immunization: recommendations of the Immunization Practices Advisory Committee (ACIP). MMWR 1991;40 (RR-12): Table 8.

H. Dosage Schedule for Selected Immunizations

Table 2.

Name	Primary Schedule	Booster
Toxoids		
Tetanus-diphtheria toxoid (Td)	Two doses IM 4 wk apart, third dose 6–12 mo later	q 10 yr
Live Virus Vaccines		
Measles	MMR*: One dose SQ	No boosters if has had previous live vaccine. May want to re-vaccinate if previous vaccine was killed vaccine.
Mumps	MMR*: One dose SQ	No booster
Rubella	MMR*: One dose SQ	No booster
Live-Virus and Inactivated Virus Vaccines		
Enhanced-potency inactivated poliovirus (E-IPV); live oral polio (OPV)	E-IPV preferred vaccine for primary immunization in adults: 2 doses SQ 4–8 wk apart, third dose 6–12 mo later.	If booster indicated, can use either OPV or E-IPV
Inactivated Virus Vaccines		
Hepatitis B	2 doses IM 4 wk apart third dose 5 mo later.	No booster necessary for at least 7 y
Influenza	Vaccinate annually	
Rabies	Preexposure prophylaxis: 2 doses IM or ID 1 wk apart third dose 3 wk later	q 2 y
Inactivated Bacteria		
Haemophilus influenzae type B	One dose IM	
Pneumoccal polysaccharide (23 valent)	One dose IM	Consider after 6 y if high risk

*MMR recommended if person being vaccinated for measles, mumps, or rubella is likely to be susceptible to the other two.

Annotated Bibliography

American College of Physicians Task Force on Adult Immunization and Infectious Disease Society of America. Guide for Adult Immunization, 3rd ed. Philadelphia: American College of Physicians; 1994. An excellent, short book that summarizes current recommendations on adult immunization.

Centers for Disease Control and Prevention. Update on adult immunization: recommendations of the Immunization Practices Advisory Committee (ACIP). MMWR 1991;40 (RR-12). A summary of CDC's recommendations regarding adult immunizations.

Appendix B

Subacute Bacterial Endocarditis Prophylaxis

Kenneth R. Epstein

Table 1. Selected Cardiac Conditions for Which Endocarditis Prophylaxis Is Recommended

Prosthetic cardiac valves
Previous bacterial endocarditis
Most congenital cardiac malformations
Rheumatic and other acquired valvular dysfunction, even after valvular surgery
Hypertrophic cardiomyopathy
Mitral valve prolapse with valvular regurgitation

SOURCE: Adapted with permission from Dajani AS, Bisno AL, Chung KY, et al. Prevention of Bacterial Endocarditis. Recommendations by the American Heart Association. JAMA 1990;264:2919–2922.

Table 2. Selected Cardiac Conditions for Which Endocarditis Prophylaxis Is Not Recommended

Isolated secundum atrial septal defect
Surgical repair without residua beyond 6 mo of secundum atrial septal defect, ventricular septal defect, or patent ductus arteriosus
Previous coronary artery bypass graft surgery
Mitral valve prolapse without valvular regurgitation
Physiologic, functional, or innocent heart murmurs
Previous Kawasaki disease without valvular dysfunction
Previous rheumatic fever without valvular dysfunction
Cardiac pacemakers and implanted defibrillators

SOURCE: Adapted with permission from Dajani AS, Bisno AL, Chung KY, et al. Prevention of Bacterial Endocarditis. Recommendations by the American Heart Association. JAMA 1990;264:2919–2922.

Table 3. Selected Dental or Surgical Procedures

Endocarditis Prophylaxis Recommended

- Dental procedures known to induce gingival or mucosal bleeding, including professional cleaning
- Tonsillectomy and/or adenoidectomy
- Surgical operations that involve intestinal or respiratory mucosa
- Bronchoscopy with a rigid bronchoscope
- Sclerotherapy for esophageal varices
- Esophageal dilatation
- Gallbladder surgery
- Cystoscopy
- Urethral dilatation
- Urethral catheterization if urinary tract infection is present*
- Urinary tract surgery if urinary tract infection is present*
- Prostatic surgery
- Incision and drainage of infected tissue*
- Vaginal hysterectomy
- Vaginal delivery in the presence of infection*

Endocarditis Prophylaxis Not Recommended[†]

- Dental procedures not likely to induce gingival bleeding, such as simple adjustment of orthodontic appliances or fillings above the gum line
- Injection of local intraoral anesthetic (except intraligamentary injections)
- Shedding of primary teeth
- Tympanostomy tube insertion
- Endotracheal intubation
- Bronchoscopy with a flexible bronchoscope, with or without biopsy
- Cardiac catheterization
- Endoscopy with or without GI biopsy
- Cesarean section
- In the absence of infection for urethral catheterization, dilatation and curettage, uncomplicated vaginal delivery, therapeutic abortion, sterilization procedures, or insertion or removal of intrauterine devices

*In addition to prophylactic regimen for genitourinary procedures, antibiotic therapy should be directed against the most likely bacterial pathogen.

[†] In patients who have prosthetic heart valves, a previous history of endocarditis, or surgically constructed system-pulmonary shunts or conduits, physicians may choose to administer prophylactic antibiotics even for low-risk procedures that involve the lower respiratory, genitourinary, or GI tracts.

SOURCE: Adapted with permission from Dajani AS, Bisno AL, Chung KY, et al. Prevention of Bacterial Endocarditis. Recommendations by the American Heart Association. JAMA 1990;264:2919-2922.

Appendix B: Subacute Bacterial Endocarditis Prophylaxis

Table 4. Recommended Standard Prophylactic Regimen for Dental, Oral, or Upper Respiratory Tract Procedures in Patients Who Are at Risk.[*]

Drug	Dosing Regimen
Standard Regimen	
Amoxicillin	3.0 g PO 1 h before procedure, then 1.5 g 6 h after initial dose
Amoxicillin/Penicillin-Allergic Patients	
Erythromycin	Erythromycin ethylsuccinate, 800 mg or erythromycin stearate, 1.0 g PO 2 h before procedure, then half the dose 6 h after initial dose
Clindamycin	300 mg PO 1 h before procedure and 150 mg 6 h after initial dose

[*] Includes those with prosthetic heart valves and other high-risk patients. See Tables 1 and 2.
SOURCE: Adapted with permission from Dajani AS, Bisno AL, Chung KY, et al. Prevention of Bacterial Endocarditis. Recommendations by the American Heart Association. JAMA 1990;264:2919–2922.

Table 5. Alternate Prophylactic Regimens for Dental, Oral, or Upper Respiratory Tract Procedures in Patients Who Are at Risk

Drug	Dosing Regimen
Patients Unable to Take Oral Medications	
Ampicillin	IV or IM administration of ampicillin, 2.0 g 30 min before procedure, then IV or IM administration of ampicillin 1.0 g or oral administration of amoxicillin, 1.5 g 6 h after initial dose
Ampicillin/Amoxicillin/Penicillin—Allergic Patients Unable to Take Oral Medications	
Clindamycin	IV administration of 300 mg 30 min before procedure and IV or oral administration of 150 mg 6 h after initial dose
Patients Considered High Risk and Not Candidates for Standard Regimen[*]	
Ampicillin, gentamicin, and amoxicillin	IV or IM administration of ampicillin 2.0 g plus gentamicin, 1.5 mg/kg (not to exceed 80 mg), 30 min before procedure; followed by amoxicillin, 1.5 g orally 6 h after initial dose; alternatively, the parenteral regimen may be repeated 8 h after initial dose
Ampicillin/Amoxicillin/Penicillin—Allergic Patients Considered High Risk[*]	
Vancomycin	IV administration of 1.0 g over 1 h starting 1h before procedure; no repeated dose necessary

[*] If clinician desires a more stringent, parenteral regimen for patients with prosthetic valves, previous history of endocarditis, or surgically constructed systemic-pulmonary shunts or conduits.
SOURCE: Adapted with permission from Dajani AS, Bisno AL, Chung KY, et al. Prevention of Bacterial Endocarditis. Recommendations by the American Heart Association. JAMA 1990;264:2919–2922.

Table 6. Regimens for Genitourinary/GI Procedures

Drug	Dosage Regimen
Standard Regimen	
Ampicillin, gentamicin, and amoxicillin	IV or IM administration of ampicillin, 2.0 g plus gentamicin, 1.5 mg/kg (not to exceed 80 mg), 30 min before procedure; followed by amoxicillin, 1.5 g orally 6 h after initial dose; alternatively, the parenteral regimen may be repeated once 8 h after initial dose
Ampicillin/Amoxicillin/Penicillin—Allergic Patient Regimen	
Vancomycin and gentamycin	IV administration of vancomycin, 1.0 g over 1 h plus IV or IM administration of gentamicin, 1.5 mg/kg (not to exceed 80 mg), 1 h before procedure; may be repeated once 8 h after initial dose
Alternate Low-Risk Patient Regimen	
Amoxicillin	3.0 g PO 1 h before procedure; then 1.5 g 6 h after initial dose

SOURCE: Adapted with permission from Dajani AS, Bisno AL, Chung KY, et al. Prevention of Bacterial Endocarditis. Recommendations by the American Heart Association. JAMA 1990;264:2919–2922.

Appendix C

Topical Corticosteroid Potencies

Guy F. Webster

Table 1. Potency Ranking of Some Commonly Used Brand-Name Corticosteroids*

Group 1 (super-potent)
    Temovate cream 0.05%[a]
    Temovate ointment 0.05%[a]
    Diprolene cream† 0.05%[b]
    Diprolene ointment 0.05%[b]
    Psorcon ointment 0.05%[c]

Group 2 (potent)
    Cyclocort ointment 0.1%[d]
    Diprolene cream AF 0.05%[b]
    Diprosone ointment 0.05%[e]
    Elocon ointment 0.1%[f]
    Florone ointment 0.05%[g]
    Halog cream 0.1%[h]
    Lidex cream 0.05%[i]
    Lidex gel 0.05%[i]
    Lidex ointment 0.05%[i]
    Maxiflor ointment 0.05%[g]
    Topicort cream 0.25%[j]
    Topicort gel 0.05%[j]
    Topicort ointment 0.25%[j]

Group 3 (potent)
    Aristocort A ointment 0.1%[k]
    Cutivate ointment 0.005%[l]
    Cyclocort cream 0.1%[d]
    Cyclocort lotion 0.1%[d]
    Diprosone cream 0.05%[e]
    Florone cream 0.05%[g]
    Halog ointment 0.1%[h]
    Lidex E cream 0.05%[i]
    Maxiflor cream 0.05%[g]
    Valisone ointment 0.1%[m]

Group 4 (mid-strength)
    Cordran ointment 0.05%[n]
    Elocon cream 0.1%[f]
    Kenalog cream 0.1%[k]
    Synalar ointment 0.025%[o]
    Westcort ointment 0.2%[p]

(continued)

Table 1. Potency Ranking of Some Commonly Used Brand-Name Corticosteroids* (continued)

Group 5 (mid-strength)
    Cordran cream 0.05%[n]
    Cutivate cream 0.05%[l]
    Diprosone lotion 0.05%[e]
    Kenalog lotion 0.1%[k]
    Locoid cream 0.1%[q]
    Synalar cream 0.025%[o]
    Valisone cream 0.1%[m]
    Westcort cream 0.2%[p]

Group 6 (mild)
    Aclovate cream 0.05%[r]
    Aclovate ointment 0.05%[r]
    Aristocort cream 0.1%[k]
    Desowen cream 0.05%[s]
    Synalar solution 0.01%[o]
    Synalar cream 0.01%[o]
    Tridesilon cream 0.05%[s]
    Valisone lotion 0.1%[m]

Group 7 (mild)
    Topicals with hydrocortisone dexamethasone, flumethasone, prednisolone, and methyprednisolone

---

* Group 1 is the super-potent category; potency descends with each group. There is no significant difference between agents *within* groups 2 through 7; the compounds are simply arranged alphabetically. However, within group 1, Temovate cream or ointment is more potent than Diprolene cream or ointment and Psorcon ointment.

† Diprolene cream has been renamed Diprolene gel (whitener-free reformulation).

a Clobetasone propionate
b Betamethasone dipropionate (optimized vehicle)
c Diflorasone diacetate (optimized vehicle)
d Amcinonide
e Betamethasone dipropionate
f Mometasone furoate
g Diflorasone diacetate
h Halcinonide
i Fluocinonide
j Desoximetasone
k Triamcinolone acetonide
l Fluticasone propionate
m Betamethasone valerate
n Flurandrenolide
o Fluocinolone acetonide
p Hydrocortisone valerate
q Hydrocortisone butyrate
r Alclometasone dipropionate
s Desonide

Index

A

Accidents. *See* Injuries
Acne, 207–208
ACTH stimulation test, 254
Actinic keratosis, 224, 225
Activated partial thromboplastin time (aPTT), 471, 475–476
Activities of daily living, 421–424
Acute angle closure glaucoma, 644
Acute bronchitis, 576–578
Acute nausea and vomiting, 335–339
Acute otitis externa, 520–522
Acute otitis media, 525–526
Acute renal failure, 739, 742
Acute sinusitis, 568–570, 644
Acute urticaria, 103
Acute viral hepatitis, 401
Addison's disease, 251–257
Adrenal axis suppression, 259, 261
Adrenocortical hyperfunction, 231–249
Adrenocortical insufficiency, 200, 251–257
Age-related osteoporosis, 290
AIDS. *See also* HIV disease
  defining conditions of, 499t
  immunization recommendations, 873
  travel precautions, 59–60
Air plethysmography, 865
Alanine aminotransferase (ALT), 392
Albert's disease, 323
Alcohol use, 201, 429
Aldosterone levels, plasma, 240
Alkaline phosphatase, 392
Allergic asthma, 705
Allergic rhinitis, 85–91
Allergies
  contact dermatitis, 216
  insect stings/bites, 92–99
  plant dermatitis, 100–101
  skin testing for, 86
  urticaria, 103–105
Alopecia, 209–211
α_1-adrenergic blockers, 115t, 117
α_2 agonists, 117
Alzheimer's disease, 417t
Amantadine, 596, 597

Ambulatory cardiac arythmia monitor, 173
Anaphylaxis, 3–6, 92
Anemia, 479–485
  nonmegaloblastic, 483
  normochromic normocytic, 482–483
Angina pectoris, 122–137, 139
  Atypical angina, 122
Angiography, 164
Angiomas, 224, 225
  Acute chest pain, 11–13
Angiotensin-converting enzyme (ACE) inhibitors
  angina pectoris, 136
  congestive heart failure, 190
  hypertension, 115t, 116
Animal bites, 598–599
Ankle-brachial index (ABI), 852
Ankle pain, 799–801
Anoscopy, 343
Antacids, 373–374, 389
Antiarrhythmic agents, 176, 181, 190
Antibiotics, 352, 465
Anticoagulants, 190, 636–637, 860t, 861–862
Anticonvulsants, 31
Antihistamines, 88t, 89
Antineutrophil cytoplasmic antibodies (ANCA), 783
Antinuclear antibody (ANA), 781–783
Antiphospholipid antibodies, 783
Anuria, 740
Anxiety, 687–691
Aortic balloon valvuloplasty, 143, 144t
Aortic insufficiency (AI), 146–153, 147t
Aortic regurgitation (AR), 146–153, 149t
Aortic stenosis (AS), 138–145
Aphthous stomatitis, 517–519
Arrhythmias. *See* Cardiac arrhythmias
Arterial blood gases, 716–717
Arthroscopy, 798
Aspartate aminotransferase (AST), 392
Aspirin, 136, 428t
Asthma, 5–8, 705–708
Atopic dermatitis (eczema), 214–215
Atrial fibrillation (AF), 179–182

885

Atrial septal defect (ASD), 154–157
Atrophic urethritis, 542
Atrophic vaginitis, 433, 453, 455
Autoimmune serologies, 780t
Azotemia, 741, 743

B
Back pain, 818–829
Bacterial meningitis, 642
Bacterial vaginosis, 452–453, 454
Barium enema, 42–43, 382
Barium swallow, 371, 388
Basal cell carcinoma, 224, 225
Basedow's disease, 297–298
Bedbug bites, 97
Behavioral medicine. *See* Psychiatry/behavioral medicine
Bernstein test, 387
α-adrenergic blockers
　angina pectoris, 132t, 134–135
　arrhythmias, 176, 181
　congestive heart failure, 190
　hypertension, 115t, 116
Bile acids, dosages, 400
Biliary disease. *See* Hepatic and biliary disease Biphosphonates, 293
Bipolar affective disorder, 693–696
Bites
　animal, 598–599
　human, 599–600
　insect, 92–99
Bladder training, 757t
Bleeding disorders, 471–78
Blood pressure. *See* Hypertension
Bone mineral density (BMD) measurements, 291
Bone scan, 798, 821
Bone types, adult skeleton, 289
Bowel symptoms
　colonic diverticulosis and diverticulitis, 354–358
　constipation, 341–346
　diarrhea, 347–353
　irritable bowel syndrome, 359–363
　lactose intolerance, 365–368
Breast cancer, 35–39, 436
Breast masses
　nonpalpable, 39
　palpable, 38–39
Breast self-examination, 37
Bronchitis, 576–578
Bronchoscopy, 708, 710, 720, 722, 731
Bulking agents, 352–353

Bunion deformities, foot, 313–314
Bursitis, 322, 845–846

C
C-reactive protein (CRP), 780
Calcaneal spur, 323–324
Calcitonin, 293
Calcium, 284–287, 292
Calcium channel blockers
　angina pectoris, 133t, 135t, 135–136
　arrhythmias, 176, 181
　congestive heart failure, 190
Calluses, foot, 309–312
Cancer. *See also* Screening
　breast, 33
　cervical, 47
　colorectal, 38
　endometrial, 435
　as preoperative risk factor, 200
　prevention, in the elderly, 428
　prostate, 43
　skin, 224, 225, 226
Candidiasis, 220
Capsulitis, posterior foot, 322
Cardiac arrhythmias
　atrial fibrillation, 179–182
　drug therapy, 176, 181, 190
　palpitations, 172–174
　paroxysmal supraventricular tachycardia, 175–177
　ventricular, 183–184
Cardiac catheterization, 128–129, 142, 151
Cardiac emergencies, 11–13
Cardiac event recorders, 173–174
Cardiac risk factors, surgery, 195t, 196t
Cardiology. *See also* Coronary artery disease (CAD)
　angina pectoris, 122–137
　arrhythmias, 172–184
　congestive heart failure, 186–191
　heart murmurs, 138–167
　hypertension, 109–120
　prescribing safe exercise, 168–171
　SBE prophylaxis, 878–881
Carotid stenosis, as preoperative risk factor, 201
Carpal tunnel syndrome, 629–632, 816
Caterpillar rash, 97
CD4 cell counts, 508, 509t
Cellulitis, 601, 603–605
Centipede bites, 97
Cerebrovascular disease
　asymptomatic cervical bruits, 633

stroke, 634–637
  transient cerebral ischemic attacks, 634
  transient monocular blindness, 634
  vertebral-basilar insufficiency, 637–638
Cervical bruits, 633
Cervical cancer, 49–54, 51t
Cervical pain syndromes, 818–824
Cervicitis, 457–461
Cervicography, 52
Chancroid, 553, 555
Chemotherapy, as preoperative risk factor, 200
Chest pain, 11–13
Chigger bites, 98
Chlamydia trachomatis, 457, 459, 462, 542–543
Cholecystitis, 398
Cholelithiasis, 397–399
Cholera, 62
Cholesterol, 276–283
Cholesterol gallstones, 397
Cholestyramine, 281
Chronic fatigue syndrome (CFS), 69–74
Chronic obstructive pulmonary disease (COPD), 714–719
Cigarette smoking. *See* Smoking
Classic angina, 122
Claw toe, 315–316
Climacteric, 447
Clonidine suppression test, 246–247
Cluster headaches, 643, 647
Coagulation tests, 471–478
Colonic diverticulosis and diverticulitis, 354–358
Colonic transit studies, 343
Colonoscopy, 42, 382
Colorectal cancer screening, 40–43
Colposcopy, 52
Complement levels, 782
Congenital lactose intolerance, 365
Congestive heart failure (CHF), 186–191
Constipation, 341–346
Contact dermatitis, 216
Convulsions. *See* Seizures
Corneal abrasions, 20–22
Corns, foot, 309–312
Coronary artery disease (CAD). *See also* Angina pectoris
  hypercholesterolemia, 279f, 280f, 281f
  prevention, in the elderly, 428
  prevention with estrogen replacement therapy (ERT), 434–435
Cortical bone, 289

Corticosteroids, 89–90, 258–261, 883t–884t
Cough, 501–502, 709–712
  chronic, 709–712
Cranial (giant cell) arteritis, 644–645
Creatinine clearance, 741–742
Creatinine levels, plasma, 741–742
Cushing's syndrome, 231–237
Cystitis, 533–539

D

De Quervain's tenosynovitis, 814
Decongestants, 89, 89t
Deep vein thrombosis (DVT), 198–200, 857–862
Degenerative joint disease, 785–790
Dementia, 413–420
Dental care, 427, 879, 880
Depression, 697–701
Dermatitis
  atopic (eczema), 214–215
  plants, reactions to, 100–101
  seborrheic, 217
Dermatology
  acne, 207–208
  alopecia, 209–211
  atopic dermatitis (eczema), 214–215
  benign and malignant growths, 224–227
  contact dermatitis, 216
  fungal infections, 220–221
  pruritus, 212–213
  psoriasis, 222–223
  seborrheic dermatitis, 217
  xerosis (dry skin), 218–219
Dexamethasone suppression test, 233, 234–235
Diabetes mellitus
  clinical presentation, 262–264
  complications, 265–268, 273–275
  dermopathies, 268
  foot care, 324–329
  immunizations and, 871
  monitoring of therapy, 273–275
  neuropathies, 267, 660–661
  as preoperative risk factor, 201
  treatment, 269–272
Diabetic ketoacidosis (DKA), 16–19, 265
Dialysis, indications for, 744–745
Diarrhea, 60–61, 347–353
Didanosine (Videx, ddI), 509
Digital deformities, foot, 313–316
Digoxin, 181, 189
Diphtheria, 63
Dislocations, as sports injuries, 838–839

Disseminated gonococcal infection, 460
Diuretics, 115t, 116, 190
Diverticulosis and diverticulitis, 354–358
Doppler flow studies, 141, 150–151, 163
Drug use, 201, 427
Dry skin (xerosis), 218–219
Dual energy x-ray absorptiometry (DEXA), 292
Dual photon absorptiometry (DPA), 291
Dysmenorrhea, 444–445
    primary, 444
Dyspepsia, nonulcerative, 376–379
Dysphagia, 500–501
Dyspnea, 13–15, 139

E

Ear infections, 520–526
Echocardiography, 128, 141, 150–151, 163
Eczema, 214–215
Elderly. *See* Geriatrics
Electrocardiogram (ECG)
    angina pectoris, 125, 126–128
    aortic regurgitation, 150
    arrhythmias, 173
    mitral valve prolapse, 162–163
Electromyography (EMG), 659–660, 821
Endocrinology/metabolism
    adrenocortical hyperfunction, 231–249
    adrenocortical insufficiency, 251–257
    diabetes mellitus, 262–275
    glucocorticosteroids, management of, 258–261
    hypercalcemia, 284–287
    hypercholesterolemia, 276–283
    osteoporosis, 289–293
    thyroid disease, 295–306
Endometrial cancer, 435
Endoscopic retrograde cholangiopancreatography (ERCP), 399
Endoscopy, 371
Endourethral sampling, 541
Enzyme-linked immunosorbent assay (ELISA), 493, 498
Epididymitis, 545–548
Epigastric pain, 369–379
Epilepsy, 29–32, 667t
Ergotamine preparations, 646
Erysipelas, 601, 603–605
Erythrasma, 602
Erythrocyte sedimentation rate (ESR), 779–780
Erythropoietin, 484
Esophagogastroduodenoscopy (EGD), 388

Essential hypertension, 109–110
Estrogen replacement therapy (ERT), 433–438
Euthyroid sick syndrome, 300
Exercise
    contraindications, 170t
    HIV disease and, 512
    osteoporosis and, 292
    prescribing safe, 168–171
Exercise echocardiography, 128
Exercise tolerance testing
    angina pectoris, 126–127
    aortic insufficiency, 151
    aortic stenosis, 142
    mitral valve prolapse, 164
Exertional dyspnea, 139
Extracorporeal shock wave lithotripsy (ESWL), 400
Extrinsic asthma, 705

F

False Albert's disease, 323
Fatigue, 69
Fecal occult blood testing (FOBT), 41–42, 380–384
Fever, with HIV disease, 500
Fibrositis, 830–832
Flea bites, 97
Fluorides, 293
Fly bites, 99
Folate deficiency, 484
Folliculitis, 601
Foot problems
    hyperkeratotic lesions, 309–312
    pain, anterior foot, 317–319
    pain, digital deformities, 313–316
    pain, heel, 323–324
    pain, posterior foot, 320–322
    prevention, diabetic patient, 326–331
    rheumatologic diseases, 325
    subungual exostoses and spurs, 325
Foreign bodies, ophthalmologic, 23–25
Fractures, as sports injuries, 836–838
Fulminant hepatic failure, 408
Functional assessment, elderly patient, 421–424
Fungal otitis externa, 521
Fungal skin infections, 220–221
Furuncles, 602

G

Gait assessment, elderly, 423
α-glutamyl transpeptidase (GGTP), 392

Index • 889

Ganglion, 816
Gastroenterology
  bowel symptoms, 341–368
  epigastric pain, 369–379
  gastroesophageal reflux disease, 386–391
  heme-positive stool, 380–384
  hepatic and biliary disease, 392–410
  nausea and vomiting, acute, 335–339
Gastroesophageal reflux disease (GERD), 386–391
Gemfibrozil, 281
Generalized anxiety disorder, 687–690
Genital ulcers, 552–557
Genitourinary tract infections
  cervicitis, 457–461
  cystitis/pyelonephritis, 533–539
  epididymitis, 545–547
  genital ulcers, 552–557
  human papillomavirus infection, 467–468
  pelvic inflammatory disease, 462–466
  prostatitis, 549–551
  urethritis, 540–543
  vaginitis, 450–456
Geriatrics
  dementia, 413–420
  functional assessment of the elderly, 421–424
  immunization recommendations, 871, 872
  prevention in the elderly, 426–429
Gestational diabetes mellitus, 263
Glaucoma, 644
Glomerular filtration rate (GFR), 741
Glucocorticosteroids, 258–261
Glucose monitoring, 273
Goiters, 298–299, 301–302
Goldman Risk Assessment Scale, 196
Gonococcal infections
  pharyngitis, 564, 566
  treatment, 459–460
  urethritis, 540–543
Gout, 791, 792, 794
Granuloma inguinale, 554, 556
Graves's disease, 297–298
Gynecology
  estrogen replacement therapy, 433–438
  genital infections, 450–468
  menstrual abnormalities, 440–449

H

H_2 antagonists, 372, 389
Hallux limitus and hallux rigidus, 314–315

Hallux valgus, 313–314
Hammer toe, 315–316
Haugland's deformity, 323
Headache, 502–503, 640–649
  chronic relapsing, 642–643
  psychogenic, 643
Heart murmurs
  aortic insufficiency, 146–153
  aortic stenosis, 138–145
  atrial septal defect, 154–157
  mitral valve prolapse, 158–167
"Heartburn," 386
Heel pain, 323–324
Helicobacter pylori infection, 369, 371, 373
Hematology
  abnormal coagulation tests, 471–478
  anemia, 479–485
  lymphadenopathy, 486–489
Hematuria, 746–751
Heme-positive stool, 380–384
Hemoptysis, 720–724
Hemostasis, 471–478
Heparin, 860t, 861
Hepatic and biliary disease
  abnormal liver function tests, 392–395
  cholelithiasis, 397–400
  viral hepatitis, 402–410
Hepatitis, viral, 62–63, 402–410, 872
  chronic, 405, 408–409
Hepatobiliary scintigraphy (HIDA), 399
Herpes simplex, 554, 555, 607–610
Herpes zoster, 611–613
Hidradenitis suppritiva, 602
High-density lipoprotein (HDL), 277
Histamine headache, 643
HIV disease
  antiretroviral agents, 508–509
  CD4 count monitoring, 508, 509t
  early infection, management, 506–513
  immunization recommendations, 873
  pretest/posttest counseling, 493–497
  prophylaxis for opportunistic infections, 504–505
  symptomatic patient, management, 498–505
  syphilis and, 511–512, 624
  tuberculosis and, 511
HLA typing, 783–784
HMG coenzyme A (CoA) reductase inhibitors, 282
Hoarseness, 650–655
Holter monitor, 128, 173
Horton's headache, 643

Human bites, 599–600
Human papillomavirus (HPV), 50, 467–468
Hyperaldosteronism, 238–242
Hypercalcemia, 284–287
Hypercholesterolemia, 276–283
Hypercoagulable disorders, 476–477
Hyperkalemia, 744
Hyperkeratotic lesions, foot, 309–312
Hyperosmolar hyperglycemic nonketotic coma, 265
Hypertension
 classification, 109–110, 110t
 drug therapy, 115t, 116–118
 headaches and, 643–644
 as preoperative risk factor, 200
 secondary, 109–110
Hypertensive crisis, management of, 118–119
Hyperthyroidism, 296–299
Hypertrophic scars, 224, 226
Hypochromic microcytic anemia, 480
Hypoglycemia, 265
Hypothalamic-pituitary-adrenal axis suppression, 259
Hypothyroidism, 299–301

I
Immunizations
 adults, 871–875
 dosage schedule, 875
 early HIV disease and, 507–508
 elderly, 427
 hepatitis B, 872
 influenza vaccine, 596–597
 travel medicine, 62–64
Impedance plethysmography (IPG), 859
Impetigo, 601
Impotence, 759–761
Incontinence, urinary, 752–758
Infectious diseases
 aphthous stomatitis, 517–519
 ear infections, 520–526
 fungal skin, 220–221
 genitourinary tract, 450–468, 533–557
 Lyme disease, 527–531
 opportunistic, HIV disease, 504–505
 respiratory tract, 562–597
 skin, 598–617
 syphilis, 617–625
Inferior petrosal sinus (IPS) sampling, 235
Influenza, 594–597, 871
Inguinal lymphadenopathy, 552, 553

Injuries
 common sports, 836–846
 of the elderly, 427
 tetanus prophylaxis, 874
Insect allergies, 92–99
Insulin, 271–272
Insulin-dependent diabetes mellitus (IDDM), 262
Interferon, 409
Intracranial hemorrhage, 641–642
Intrinsic asthma, 705
Involuntary weight loss, 65–68
Iron deficiency anemia, 484
Irritable bowel syndrome, 359–363
Isolated systolic hypertension (ISH), 109, 118
Isoniazid, 560

J
Joints
 degenerative disease, 785–790
 hot, tender, 791–795
 pain, 796–801
 pain, knee, 808–813
 pain, shoulder, 802–807
 pain, wrist, 814–816

K
Keloids, 224, 226
Ketoacidosis, diabetic, 16–19, 265
Kidney stones, 772–776
Kissing bug bites, 97–98
Knee pain, 808–813

L
Labyrinthitis, 680
Lactose intolerance, 365–368
 secondary, 365
Lice infestation, 614–615
Liver biopsy, 406–407
Liver function tests, 392–395
Liver transplantation, 409
Low back pain, 825–829
Low-density lipoprotein (LDL), 277, 280t
Lutembacher's syndrome, 154
Lyme disease, 96, 527–531
Lymphadenopathy, 486–489
Lymphogranuloma venereum, 554, 556

M
Macrocytic anemia, 483
Malaria chemoprophylaxis, 61–62
Malignant otitis externa, 521, 523

Mallet toe, 315-316
Mammography, 38
Mantoux test, 511, 558
Measles-mumps-rubella (MMR immunization), 871, 872
Melanocytic nevi, 225, 226
Melanoma, 224, 226
Meniere's syndrome, 680, 681-682
Meningitis, 642
Menopause, 433-438, 447-449
Menstrual abnormalities, 440-449
Metabolism. *See* Endocrinology/metabolism
Metatarsalgia, 317-318
Metoclopramide, 389
Migraine headaches, 642-643, 646
Mini Mental Status examination, 416t
Mitral valve prolapse (MVP), 158-167
Myalgias, 830-835
Myelogram, 821

N
Nasal corticosteroids, 89-90, 90t
Nausea, 335-339
Neck and back pain, 818-829
Neisseria gonorrhoeae, 457, 462
Nephropathy, diabetic, 266-267
Nerve biopsy, 660
Nerve conduction studies (NCS), 659-660
Neuralgia, posterior foot, 321
Neuritis, posterior foot, 321
Neurology/ENT
  carpal tunnel syndrome, 629-631
  cerebrovascular disease, 633-638
  headache, 640-649
  hoarseness, 650-655
  peripheral neuropathy, 656-662
  seizures, 663-668
  tinnitus, 669-674
  tremor, 675-678
  vertigo, 679-682
Neuroma, posterior foot, 320
Neuropathy
  diabetic, 267, 660-661
  with HIV disease, 503-504
  peripheral, 656-662
Neurosyphilis, 623-624
Nevi, 225, 226
Nicotine dependence, 76-81
Nicotinic acid, 279
Nitrates
  angina pectoris, 131, 132t, 134
  congestive heart failure, 190

Nodules, pulmonary, 731-735
Non-insulin dependent diabetes mellitus (NIDDM), 262-263
Nongonococcal urethritis, 540
Nonmegaloblastic anemia, 483
Nonpalpable masses, breast, 39
Nonulcerative dyspepsia, 376-379
Normochromic normocytic anemia, 482-483
Nutrition, 426-427, 512

O
Old tuberculin (OT), 558
Oliguria, 740, 741
Omeprazole, 389
Onychomycosis, 220
Ophthalmologic emergencies, 20-28
Opportunistic infections, 504-505
Oral cholecystography, 399
Oral contraceptives, 50
Orthopedics. *See* Rheumatology/orthopedics
Osteoarthritis, 785-790
Osteoporosis, 289-293, 434, 448-449
  primary, 290
  secondary, 292-293
Ostium primum and ostium secundum ASD, 154
Otitis externa, 520-523
  chronic, 521, 522
  fungal, 521
Otitis media, 524-526
  chronic, 526

P
Pain
  acute chest, 11-13
  anterior foot, 317-319
  digital deformities, foot, 313-316
  epigastric, 369-379
  in the eye, 26-28
  heel, 323-324
  joints, 796-816
  neck and back, 818-829
  posterior foot, 320-322
Palpable masses, breast, 38-39
Palpitations, 172-174
Panic disorder, 690-691
Papanicolaou (Pap) smear, 51-52, 53-54
Parkinson's disease, 675-678
Paroxysmal atrial fibrillation (PAT), 181-182
Paroxysmal supraventricular tachycardia (PSVT), 175-177

Pediculosis, 614–615
Pelvic inflammatory disease (PID), 462–466
Peptic ulcer disease, 369–374
Peripheral neuropathy, 656–662
Peripheral vascular disease, 851–856
   chronic venous insufficiency, 864–967
   deep vein thrombosis, 857–862
Pes cavus and pes planus, 320
Pharyngitis, 562–567
Pheochromocytoma, 243–249
Photoplethysmography, 864–865
Physical examinations, yearly, 55–58
Pigment gallstones, 397
Plant dermatitis, 100–101
Plantar fasciitis, 323–324
Platelet function, 471, 475
   Antiplatelet drugs, 636–637
Plummers's disease, 298–299
Pneumocystis carinii pneumonia (PCP), 502t, 510–511, 585
Pneumonia, 579–593, 871
Poison ivy, poison oak, and poison sumac, 100
Polio immunizations, 63
Polymyalgia rheumatica, 644–645, 833–835
Polyneuropathies, 659t
Postmenopausal osteoporosis, 290
Postural tremors, 676–677
Pregnancy
   gestational diabetes, 263
   gonococcal infection during, 460
   immunizations and, 871
   Lyme disease in, 531
   syphilis and, 624–625
Premature ventricular contractions (PVCs), 183–184
Premenstrual syndrome (PMS), 445–446
Preoperative evaluation
   appropriate studies, obtaining, 201–202
   general considerations, 195
   pulmonary function, 729
   risk factor identification, 195t, 196–201
Pretest/posttest HIV counseling, 493–497
Prethrombic disorders, 476–477
Prevention
   in the elderly, 426–429
   opportunistic infections, HIV disease, 504–505
   subacute bacterial endocarditis, 878–881
Primary delayed onset lactose intolerance, 365
Primary dysmenorrhea, 444
Primary osteoporosis, 290
Primary prevention, in the elderly, 426
Primary syphilis, 618, 622
Prinzmetal's angina, 122
Prostate cancer, 45–48
Prostate specific antigen (PSA), 46–47
Prostatic hyperplasia, 762–765
Prostatitis, 549–551
Proteinuria, 766–771
Prothrombin time (PT), 471, 476
Proton pump inhibitors, 373
Pruritus, 212–213
Psoriasis, 222–223
Psychiatry/behavioral medicine
   anxiety, 687–691
   assessment, in the elderly, 422–423
   bipolar affective disorder, 693–696
   depression, 697–701
Psychogenic headaches, 643
Psychological support, HIV disease and, 512–513
Pulmonary disease. See also Respiratory tract infections
   asthma, 705–708
   chronic cough, 709–712
   chronic obstructive, 714–719
   hemoptysis, 720–724
   insufficiency, as preoperative risk, 201
   nodules, 731–735
Pulmonary function tests, 716, 726–729, 728f
Pulse volume recordings, 853
Purified protein derivative (PPD), 511, 558–560
Pyelonephritis, 533–539
Pyodermas, 601–602
Pyridoxine, 560

R

Rabies, 599
Radionuclide testing, 151
Rapid plasma reagent (RPR), 511–512, 620
Rectal examinations, 41, 46, 549
Red and painful eye, 26–28
Renal/urologic diseases. See also Genitourinary tract
   chronic renal failure, 739, 742
infections
   diabetic nephropathy, 266–267
   evaluation, renal dysfunction, 739–745
   hematuria, 746–750
   immunization recommendations, 873
   impotence, 759–761
   kidney stones, 772–776
   prostatic hyperplasia, 762–765

proteinuria, 766–771
urinary incontinence, 752–758
Renin activity, plasma, 240
Respiratory tract infections
  bronchitis, acute, 576–578
  influenza, 594–597
  pharyngitis, 562–567
  pneumonia, 579–593
  SBE prophylaxis, 880
  sinusitis, 568–575
Reticulocyte index (RI), 480, 481t
Retinopathy, diabetic, 266
Rheumatoid factor (RF), 781
Rheumatology/orthopedics
  degenerative joint disease, 785–790
  diseases of the foot, 325
  joint pain, 796–816
  joints, hot, tender, 791–795
  myalgias, 830–835
  neck and back pain, 818–829
  serologic testing, 777–784
  sports injuries, common, 836–846
Rhinitis, allergic, 85–91
Rifampin, 560
Rimantadine, 596, 597
Rocky Mountain spotted fever, 96

S
Scabies, 614, 616–617
Scorpion stings, 98–99
Screening, cancer
  breast, 35–39
  cervical, 49–54
  colorectal, 40–43
  prostate, 45–48
Seborrheic dermatitis, 217
Seborrheic keratosis, 225
Secondary dysmenorrhea, 444–445
Secondary hypertension, 109–110
Secondary lactose intolerance, 365
Secondary osteoporosis, 290–291
Secondary prevention, in the elderly, 426, 428–429
Secondary syphilis, 618, 622
Segmental limb pressure (SLP), 852–853
Seizures, 29–32, 663–668
Sensory assessment, elderly, 423
Serologic testing, rheumatology, 777–784
Serous otitis media, 524–525
Serum glutamic oxaloacetic transaminase, 392
Serum glutamic pyruvate transaminase, 392
Sesamoid disorders, 317

Sexually transmitted diseases. *See* Genitourinary tract infections; Gonococcal infections; HIV disease; Syphilis
Shingles, 611
Shoulder pain, 802–803
Sigmoidoscopy, 42, 343, 382
Simple nontoxic goiter, 301–302
Single photon absorptiometry (SPA), 291
Sinus venosus atrial septal defect (ASD), 154
Sinusitis, 568–575, 644
  chronic, 573–575
Sipple's syndrome, 243
Skin cancer, 224, 225, 226
Skin infections
  animal bites, 598–599
  cellulitis and erysipelas, 601, 603–605
  herpes simplex, 607–609
  herpes zoster, 611–613
  human bites, 599–600
  localized, 601–602
  pediculosis, 614–615
  pyodermas, 601–602
  scabies, 614, 616–617
Skin testing, allergen, 86
Smoking
  cervical cancer and, 50
  cessation of, 76–81
  in the elderly, 426
Social assessment, elderly, 423–424
Spider bites, 95–96
Sports injuries
  bursitis, 845–846
  dislocations, 838–839
  fractures, 836–838
  sprains, 839–843
  tendonitis syndromes, 843–845
Sprains, as sports injuries, 839–843
Squamous cell carcinoma, 225
Status asthmaticus, 7–9
Status epilepticus, 29–32
Stomatitis, aphthous, 517–519
Stool, heme-positive, 380–384
Streptococcal pharyngitis, 563, 566
Stress (exercise) testing, 126–128
Stress fractures, 836–837
Stroke, 634–637
  prethrombic/hypercoagulable disorders, 476–477
  prevention, 180, 190
Subacute bacterial endocarditis (SBE) prophylaxis, 878–881
Subarachnoid hemorrhage, 641–642
Subungual exostoses and spurs, foot, 325

Sucralfate, 373
Sudden death during exercise, 169
Sulfonylureas, 269–271
Surgery
   preoperative evaluation for, 196–202
   SBE prophylaxis, 878–881
Swimmer's ear, 521
Syncope, 139
Synovial fluid analysis, 798
Syphilis, 511–512, 618–625
   latent, 618, 622–623
   secondary, 618, 622

T

Tailor's bunion, 319
Temporomandibular joint (TMJ) dysfunction, 645
Tendonitis, 322, 843–845
Tenosynovitis, posterior foot, 322
Tension headaches, 643, 647
Tertiary syphilis, 618, 623
Tetanus-diphtheria (Td) toxoid, 871
Tetanus immunizations, 63, 874
Thalassemia, 481
Thallium 201
   perfusion scintigraphy, 127
Thrombocytopenia, 472–473
Thrombocytosis, 474–475
Thromboembolic stroke. *See* Stroke
Thyroid disease
   euthyroid sick syndrome, 302
   general information, 295–296
   hyperthyroidism, 296–299
   hypothyroidism, 299–301
   as preoperative risk factor, 200
   simple nontoxic goiter, 301–302
   thyroid nodules, 303–305
Thyroid function tests, 295–296
Thyroid nodules, 303–305
Thyroiditis, 299
Tic douloureux, 644
Tick bites, 96–97, 527
Tine test, 558
Tinea capitis, corporis, cruris, pedis, and versicolor, 220
Tinnitus, 669–674
Topical corticosteroids, 89, 90t, 883t–884t
Toxic nodular goiter, 298–299
Trabecular bone, 289
Transcutaneous oxygen tension (TCpO2) determination, 853
Transdermal estrogen, 437
Transient cerebral ischemic attacks (TIAs), 634
Transient incontinence, 754t
Transient monocular blindness, 634
Transrectal ultrasound (TRUS), 46
Travel medicine, 59–64
Tremor, 675–678
Treponemal tests, 620
Trichomoniasis, 453, 454
Trigeminal neuralgia, 644
Tuberculosis
   differential diagnosis, pneumonia, 585
   HIV disease and, 511
   management of positive PPD, 556
   prophylaxis, 560
   risk of developing active, 559
   travel medicine, 61
Typhoid immunizations, 63

U

Unstable angina, 122
Urethritis, 540–543
Urinalysis, 535–536, 740–741
Urinary incontinence, 752–758
Urinary tract. *See* Genitourinary tract
Urologic diseases. *See* Renal/urologic diseases
Urticaria, 103–105
   chronic, 103

V

Vaccines. *See* Immunizations
Vagal maneuvers, 176
Vaginal bleeding, abnormal, 440–444
Vaginitis, 450–456
Varicella-Zoster immune globulin (VZIG), 613
Vascular disease, peripheral, 849–867
Vascular surgery, as preoperative evaluation, 199f
Vasodilators, 117–118, 190
VDRL (Venereal Disease Research Laboratory) test, 620
Venography, 856, 863
Venous disease, peripheral, 857–865
Venous insufficiency, chronic, 862
Ventricular arrhythmias, 183–184
Vertebral-basilar insufficiency, 637–638
Vertigo, 679–682
Vibrio otitis externa, 522, 523
Viral hepatitis, 402–410
Vitamin B12 deficiency, 484

Vitamin D, osteoporosis and, 292
Voice, hoarseness of, 650–655
Vomiting, 335–339
von Recklinghausen's neurofibromatosis, 243
Vulvovaginal candidiasis, 453, 454–455
Vulvovaginitis, 450–456, 542

W
Warfarin, 859
Warts, 225, 227
Weight loss
  with HIV disease, 503
  involuntary, 65–68
  as preoperative risk factor, 201
Western blot test, 494, 498

Wolff-Parkinson-White syndrome (WPW), 175, 182
Wrist pain, 629–632, 814–816

X
Xerosis (dry skin), 218–219

Y
Yearly physical examinations, 55–58
Yellow fever immunizations, 64

Z
Zalcitabine (dideoxycitidine, ddC), 510
Zidovudine (AZT), 508–509
Zollinger-Ellison syndrome, 370, 371